Language Perspectives—
Acquisition,
Retardation,
and Intervention

Language Perspectives–
Acquisition,
Retardation,
and Intervention

Edited by
Richard L. Schiefelbusch, Ph.D.
Bureau of Child Research
University of Kansas

and

Lyle L. Lloyd, Ph.D.
Mental Retardation Program
National Institute of Child Health and Human Development

Technical Editor
Robert K. Hoyt
Bureau of Child Research
University of Kansas

University Park Press

Baltimore • London • Tokyo

University Park Press
International Publishers in Science and Medicine
Chamber of Commerce Building
Baltimore, Maryland 21202

Typeset in the United States of America by The Composing Room of Michigan
Printed in the United States of America by Universal Lithographers, Inc.
Published in the United Kingdom and Europe by The Macmillan Press Ltd.

Library of Congress Cataloging in Publication Data

Main entry under title:

Language perspectives—acquisition, retardation, and intervention.

Based on a conference held at Chula Vista Lodge, Wisconsin Dells, Wis., June 19-23, 1973, sponsored by the Mental Retardation Program of the National Institute of Child Health and Human Development.
   1. Speech disorders in children—Congresses.
2. Mentally handicapped children—Language—Congresses.
I. Schiefelbusch, Richard L., ed. II. Lloyd, Lyle L.,
ed. [DNLM: 1. Language development—Congresses.
2. Language disorders—In infancy and childhood—
Congresses. 3. Mental retardation—Congresses.
LB1139.L3 L289 1973]
RJ496.S7L354   618.9'28'55   74-11336
ISBN 0-8391-0687-4

Contents

To our wives Ruth and Myrna, with grateful acknowledgement of their encouragement, patience, and understanding through our professional involvements and occupational hazards, including the time we spend editing books.

Preface

The past decade saw major changes in linguistic theory and research. The increased activity in linguistics also had an impact on a number of new applied areas.

This book was prompted by a complex series of events that are only partially evident in the contents of these chapters. The book, in some respects, is the proceedings of the Chula Vista* conference on language intervention with the mentally retarded, sponsored by the Mental Retardation Branch of the National Institute of Child Health and Human Development (NICHD). Both the conference and this publication reflect recent developments in theory, research, and technology in normal *language acquisition* and development, *language retardation* and disability, *mental retardation*, and *language intervention* or remediation. This book undertakes to provide some *perspectives* on seven thematic areas designed to assist current research and stimulate new research and clinical activities.

For a number of years a few researchers scattered on campuses throughout the country, have attempted to teach language to retarded children. Identified with a number of different programs, their common aim was to develop valid procedures for clinical management, for language evaluation and planning, and for developmental programming. Each research effort also used an empirical model that included both a linguistic and a behavioral system. Many, but not all, language programs and procedures evolved from this research also reflect a strategy of early intervention for receptive and expressive functions and for operational processes. These aspects may be considered as a concern for language process features, including speech and communication features, and instructional features (the strategies used to teach language). The work, for the most part, was empirical and eclectic. It was data-oriented and was maintained by strategies derived from explicit events.

*Chula Vista Lodge, Wisconsin Dells, Wisconsin. June 19–23, 1973.

Many publications have resulted from work with retarded children. Much of the information has generalized to broader areas of language intervention and has influenced the field of clinical management. It has become apparent that many of the problems encountered in teaching language to retarded children are special ones in learning, in cognition, in auditory processing, in memory, in receptive and expressive functioning, in semantic mapping, and in early intervention.

There is literally nothing unique about the language problems of the retarded; however, what is learned by teaching of children with minimal language can inform the field of language in general. Similarly, progress in other areas of language and learning benefits our work with retarded speakers. The assumption is that exchanges across many areas of language activity serve a common purpose—the better understanding of language acquisition and intervention.

The Chula Vista Conference and book, *Language Perspectives—Acquisition, Retardation, and Intervention,* result from discussions among active language intervention researchers. The value of the results in certain critical respects was enhanced by a series of planning sessions that preceded the conference, wherein the planners undertook to isolate the critical areas in which knowledge should be sought and/or synthesized.

It was agreed that the fields of applied behavior analysis, audiology, child development, cognitive psychology, developmental linguistics, education of the hearing-impaired, special education, speech pathology, and psycholinguistics could be functionally synthesized for language intervention strategies. This decision was reached partly because important steps in combining these areas have already been taken in a number of language training programs. Likewise, the planners decided that the intricacies of infant research and early language acquisition might be productively examined; receptive and expressive processes related; acquisition and intervention processes compared; and nonspeech language acquisition systems examined for relevance to linguistic theory and intervention procedures. Thus evolved the seven thematic areas listed in the table of contents. The planners were emboldened to think that the conference might synthesize relevant information for a range of professional workers who study language events and attempt to change language behavior.

This book was developed in three phases. First, a format was designed, and conference participants were selected accordingly. From three to five participants were assigned to each thematic area, each of them capable of contributing to the discussions in several areas. Sixteen participants agreed to provide preconference papers which would form the nucleus of the book. Seven participants were selected to write postconference summaries, another participant to present concluding remarks. Other individuals involved in language programs in three Mental Retardation Research Centers were invited to participate in the conference discussions.

The second phase was the conference itself, which was designed to center not on the reading of the papers, prepared and reviewed in advance, but on a discussion of ideas generated by those papers. During the conference, brief preliminary discussion summaries of each of the seven thematic areas (each including two or more chapters) and concluding remarks were prepared.

The third phase was essentially an editing process. Authors revised their chapters. Discussion summaries and concluding remarks were refined with the aid of stenographic transcripts; the introduction was rewritten to reflect conference events, and an overall summary was prepared. Finally, the materials were edited by the technical editor and the conference co-chairmen.

A special note of recognition is due to the National Institute of Child Health and Human Development for the sponsorship (including staff effort and financial support) of the conference and manuscript preparation. The book is a testimony to the productive design of their Mental Retardation Research Centers and the continuing efforts of the Mental Retardation Branch to support research on the detection, diagnosis, prevention, and remediation of mental retardation. We also should recognize the role played by the University of Kansas, through its Bureau of Child Research, in providing support and behind-the-scenes manpower which contributed to both the conference and the publication.

The editors are especially grateful to Joseph Spradlin, David Yoder, Kenneth Ruder, and Melissa Bowerman for their contributions to the design of the conference plan. They are also indebted to Robert Hoyt for his editorial expertise and dedicated efforts. Finally, they wish to acknowledge the role played by David Yoder and colleagues at the University of Wisconsin and their doctoral students (Truman Coggins, Robin Dixon, Sharon James, Vickie Larson, Nathaniel Owings, and Larry Rider) for assisting with local arrangements and otherwise facilitating the development of this book.

L.L.L.
R.L.S.

Contributors

CONFERENCE CO-CHAIRMEN
AND EDITORS

Richard L. Schiefelbusch
Bureau of Child Research
University of Kansas
Lawrence, Kansas 66044

Lyle L. Lloyd
Mental Retardation Program
National Institute of Child Health
  and Human Development
Bethesda, Maryland 20014

NICHD CONFERENCE
SECRETARY

Mary P. Johnson
Mental Retardation Program
National Institute of Child Health
  and Human Development
Bethesda, Maryland 20014

TECHNICAL EDITOR

Robert Hoyt
Bureau of Child Research
University of Kansas
Lawrence, Kansas 66044

CONFERENCE PARTICIPANTS

Donald M. Baer
Department of Human Development
University of Kansas
Lawrence, Kansas 66044

Barbara Bateman
Department of Special Education
University of Oregon
Eugene, Oregon 97401

Lois Bloom
Department of Speech Pathology
  and Audiology
Columbia University
New York, New York 10027

Melissa F. Bowerman
Bureau of Child Research
University of Kansas
Lawrence, Kansas 66044

Diane Bricker
Toddler Research and Intervention
  Program
George Peabody College
Nashville, Tennessee 37203

William A. Bricker
John F. Kennedy Center for Research
  on Education and Human
  Development
George Peabody College
Nashville, Tennessee 37203

Earl C. Butterfield
Department of Psychology
University of Kansas
Lawrence, Kansas 66044

George F. Cairns
Smith Mental Retardation Unit
Kansas Center for Research in
  Mental Retardation
University of Kansas Medical Center
Kansas City, Kansas 66103

Robin S. Chapman
Department of Communicative
  Disorders
University of Wisconsin
Madison, Wisconsin 53706

Eve V. Clark
Committee on Linguistics
Building 100
Stanford University
Stanford, California 94305

Truman Coggins
Department of Communicative
  Disorders
University of Wisconsin
Madison, Wisconsin 53706

Richard F. Cromer
Developmental Psychology Unit
Medical Research Council
Drayton House, Gordon Street
London, WCIH OAN, England

Philip S. Dale
Department of Psychology
University of Washington
Seattle, Washington 98195

Richard Dever
Department of Special Education
Indiana University
Bloomington, Indiana 47401

Robin Dixon
Department of Communicative
  Disorders
University of Wisconsin
Madison, Wisconsin 53706

Enid Eilenberg
Child Development and
  Mental Retardation Center
University of Washington
Seattle, Washington 98195

Peter D. Eimas
Department of Psychology
Brown University
Providence, Rhode Island 02912

Doug Guess
Research Department
Kansas Neurological Institute
Topeka, Kansas 66614

Elsie D. Helsel
Washington Representative
United Cerebral Palsy Associations
Bellview Hotel
Washington, D.C. 20001

Kathryn B. Horton
Child Language Development Programs
Bill Wilkerson Hearing
  and Speech Center
Nashville, Tennessee 37212

David Ingram
Department of Linguistics
University of British Columbia
Vancouver 8, British Columbia
Canada

Sharon James
Department of Communicative
  Disorders
University of Wisconsin
Madison, Wisconsin 53706

D. D. Kluppel
Department of Communicative
  Disorders
University of Wisconsin
Madison, Wisconsin 53706

Vickie Larson
Department of Communicative
  Disorders
University of Wisconsin
Madison, Wisconsin 53706

Paula Menyuk
School of Education
Boston University
Boston, Massachusetts 02215

Jon F. Miller
Department of Communicative
  Disorders
University of Wisconsin
Madison, Wisconsin 53706

Fred D. Minifie
Department of Speech
University of Washington
Seattle, Washington 98195

Donald F. Moores
Research Development and Demonstration
  Center in Education of
  Handicapped Children
University of Minnesota
Minneapolis, Minnesota 55455

Ann Morehead
City College
San Francisco, California 93106

Donald M. Morehead
Department of Child Development
California State University
Hayward, California 94542

Philip A. Morse
Department of Psychology
University of Wisconsin
Madison, Wisconsin 53705

D. Kimbrough Oller
Child Development and
    Mental Retardation Center
University of Washington
Seattle, Washington 98195

Nathaniel Owings
Department of Communicative
    Disorders
University of Wisconsin
Madison, Wisconsin 53706

Ann James Premack
Department of Psychology
University of California
Santa Barbara, California 93106

David Premack
Department of Psychology
University of California
Santa Barbara, California 93106

Larry Rider
Department of Communicative
    Disorders
University of Wisconsin
Madison, Wisconsin 53706

Kenneth F. Ruder
Bureau of Child Research
University of Kansas
Lawrence, Kansas 66044

Wayne Sailor
Bureau of Child Research
University of Kansas
Lawrence, Kansas 66044

Izchak M. Schlesinger
Israel Institute of Applied
    Social Research
P.O. Box 7150
19 Washington Street
Jerusalem, Israel

Sue Seitz
Department of Communicative
    Disorders
University of Wisconsin
Madison, Wisconsin 53706

Michael D. Smith
Department of Linguistics
University of Kansas
Lawrence, Kansas 66044

Joseph E. Spradlin
Bureau of Child Research
University of Kansas
Lawrence, Kansas 66044

Arthur W. Staats
Department of Psychology
University of Hawaii
Honolulu, Hawaii 96822

Kathleen Stremel
Bureau of Child Research
University of Kansas
Lawrence, Kansas 66044

Lawrence J. Turton
Institute for the Study of Mental
    Retardation and Related Disabilities
University of Michigan
Ann Arbor, Michigan 48104

Carol Waryas
Bureau of Child Research
Parsons State Hospital
    and Training Center
Parsons, Kansas 67357

David E. Yoder
Department of Communicative
    Disorders
University of Wisconsin
Madison, Wisconsin 53706

INTRODUCTION

Richard L. Schiefelbusch and Lyle L. Lloyd

Bureau of Child Research, University of Kansas, Lawrence, Kansas 66045, and Mental Retardation Program, National Institute of Child Health and Human Development, Bethesda, Maryland 20014

This book was written to share as much recent information as possible on several intersecting language research themes which bear upon teaching language to language-delayed persons. The major areas of concern include early language acquisition, language retardation, and intervention strategies. The book is designed to stimulate others interested in language to undertake language training activities. The book may add substance to several productive controversies. These controversies cover a range of issues endemic to psycholinguistics, education, psychology, speech pathology, and audiology.

A number of critical issues are advanced which bear upon early developmental processes of language and which aid the language interventionist in planning for and designing a language teaching program. The content is slanted toward the teaching of language-retarded children, very young as well as older, largely nonverbal children. Considerable emphasis is devoted to the preschool deaf child and to older deaf persons who may be asked to learn both an oral and a gestural language system.

The book includes seven themes: I, infant reception; II, early development of concepts; III, development of receptive language; IV, the developmental relationship between expressive and receptive language; V, nonspeech communication; VI, early language intervention; and VII, language intervention for the mentally retarded. While there is considerable overlap, readers interested primarily in language acquisition should note that Sections I, II, III, and IV discuss critical features of the developmental process. Sections V, VI, and VII pertain more to the functions and the operations involved in language intervention.

AN OVERVIEW

Section I covers the receptive processes of infants and provides an intriguing basis for further research into the early responses of the infant and his environment. An especially provocative issue is raised by Eimas in suggesting that the infant may have a feature detector mechanism which allows selective processing of human speech in early infancy. The implication is that the infant comes equipped with a special capacity for processing speech and readily learns the segmental features as a consequence of limited social experience. In this view, the infant's early experiences are assumed to trigger speech mechanisms which result in language acquisition. This point of view contrasts with the developmental learning model which holds that the infant-child learns over time through feedback and with numerous successive approximations.

The data are inconclusive for either view. Butterfield and Cairns note that the conferees[1] agreed that a number of discriminations can be made by infants. For instance, by 2 months of age infants seem to discriminate between vowels, between fundamental frequency contours, and between different sequences of vowels and consonants. This tentative information is especially interesting when viewed against the obvious failure of infant research experiments to demonstrate infant discrimination of nonspeech auditory stimuli. Studies are practically unanimous in their failure to show that young infants discriminate among these auditory stimuli. Butterfield and Cairns recommend a position of caution, however, in making strong interpretations from the findings on speech discrimination of infants since the work is based primarily on findings of the high amplitude suck procedures which currently leave a large number of methodological issues unresolved. The conferees concurred that no clear cut interpretation can be made at this time.

Butterfield and Cairns also interpret the findings on infant speech perception as having significance for those who would like to improve the language development of abnormal infants. They point out that before we shall be able to speak about effective interventions we must determine if there are significant individual differences in speech perception. Do high risk infants, for instance, lack these discriminative capacities which are indicated for many of the infants studied by Eimas, by Morse, and by Butterfield and Cairns? A further question is whether infants who have discrimination limitations early in life develop these skills later on. The only current research which bears upon this issue has been reported by Trehub (1973). She reported that infants who are reared in orphanages from birth do not show the shift effects which she has demonstrated so repeatedly with infants reared at home. However, Butterfield and Cairns point out that this research does not rule out the effects of a number of confounding variables which might exist in the environment where the research was carried out. They also point out that this research calls for further investigations on the issue of individual differences. They suggest that, if individual differences can be found and if they are associated with abnormal language development or risk thereof, language

[1] The participants at the Chula Vista Conference.

interventionists might justifiably try to train speech discrimination in such infants. The question, then, would be, how does one train such discriminations? The needed research, therefore, is rather clear. First we must determine if there are major differences in discrimination abilities among children with normal and high risk characteristics to determine if there are discriminative deficits. Secondly, we need to develop a procedure for stimulating discrimination abilities so that children who may have deficits in early infancy may later on relate more normally to environmental stimuli. It may be possible to determine the degree of impact of naturally occurring environmental stimuli upon the perception of children. Early intervention procedures in years to come may utilize a discrimination training program that serves to develop certain precursors to the eventual receptive speech acquisition of children.

The infant research reported in the infant reception section also raises several issues regarding the content of other chapters. For instance, can responding be clearly demonstrated to vary with different stimuli (*i.e.*, human voice, music, singing, etc.)? The material prepared by Eimas, Morse, and Butterfield and Cairns represents first attempts to examine research on infant receptive processes and to combine the work with an extensive compendium of work on language acquisition and intervention.

Section II, "Development of Concepts Underlying Language," might be subtitled "The Concepts Preceding Language." The section is a complex discussion of concepts associated with early language acquisition. A natural assumption might be that Section VI, "Early Language Intervention," should be read in conjunction with Section II so that the issues of acquisition and intervention might be associated. The issues of motor and vocal imitation, language "precursors," and prelinguistic "entry behaviors" might be best considered with the discussions in Section II.

Each chapter in Section II, including Bowerman's summary chapter, makes a contribution to early intervention strategies. The theme of the section is introduced early in Clark's chapter and attributed to Slobin (1973), "... As the child develops cognitively, he will gradually learn to use more complex linguistic formulations." This statement agrees with Piaget's prelanguage formulations as presented in the chapter by Morehead and Morehead in a section dealing with Piagetian analysis of precursors to thought and language. Most of this discussion focuses upon the six substages of the sensorimotor period and covers development from birth to the end of the 2nd year. Thus it encompasses the "toddler stage" that Bricker and Bricker are describing. Even more specifically, the substages IV (a period for developing new forms or action schemes), V (a period of experimentation and refined imitations), and VI (a period of representation—the ability to evoke action schemes in the absence of immediate perception) are developed parts of the early intervention activity. Functions of the sensorimotor period are examined by Morehead and Morehead in regard to the concrete functions of agent-action-object relations described by Bloom and discussed by Schlesinger as *semantic relational concepts* for early language acquisition. Whereas Schlesinger is more intent upon relating early semantic relational concepts to the emerging syntactic system, the Piagetian system is more useful in linking emerging language functions to a larger symbolic system that includes "adultomorphic" forms and physico-logical-mathematical knowledge (both forms of reference) which herald the beginning of relational syntax.

Clark's emphasis is upon the relationship between cognitive-perceptual factors and the acquisition of word meanings. She points out that there is convincing evidence that conceptual factors play a crucial role in the acquisition of language. In addition, Clark emphasizes the importance of communicative intent. Schlesinger also proposes that the child's communicative intention in producing an utterance is crucial to its interpretation and syntactic analysis by the adult.

Bowerman, in the summary chapter for Section II, attempts to integrate the papers developed by Clark, Schlesinger, and Morehead and Morehead. In her analysis she extends and integrates the discussion under four major themes:

1. Language is only one manifestation of a very general ability to represent or symbolize experiences. (This is essentially the Piagetian formulation described by Morehead and Morehead in this volume.)
2. There are formal similarities between cognitive and linguistic structures and processes. (The work of Sinclair, 1971; Greenfield *et al.,* 1972; and Schlesinger, this volume, are examined to show an isomorphism between cognitive foundations and linguistic structures.)
3. Strategies for language acquisition are derived from the child's cognitive structuring of the world. (This refers primarily to the perception formulations of Clark and the *action* formulations of Sinclair and Greenfield.)
4. How should children's knowledge of linguistic structure be formalized? (A careful discussion of the positions of Chomsky 1969, Schlesinger, and Bowerman, this volume, is presented.)

Bowerman's analysis, together with the other papers in Section II and related papers not included in the conference, represents an interesting and productive analysis of the bases of cognitive and linguistic precursors of language. The work is further elucidated in Sections III and IV. Each section, although devoted to different topics, continues the theme of cognitive and linguistic relationships and also the analysis of complex structures and functions.

Section III, "Development of Receptive Language," includes papers by Menyuk and Cromer and a summary by Spradlin. It is clear that their interests and experimental preoccupations differ. It is also clear that they complement one another's formulations. Together they provide a comprehensive discussion of the early development of receptive language.

Menyuk presents her information in a framework that moves from the infant babbling period to the development of formal language. In certain respects she extends the discussion provided in Section I. Her interests, however, are not intently upon the experimental means for infant research but rather upon how the literature, including her own research, presents the child's perception of the structural properties of language and his comprehension of the communicative uses of these properties. Menyuk assumes that changes in perception over time are a product of the child's physiological maturation, his changing communicative needs, and his ability to relate these needs to particular aspects in the language. The last is due to his perceptual development.

Menyuk acknowledges that there are gaps in the data and that important controversies have arisen because of the methods used in obtaining and analyzing data:

> That is, in some instances, conclusions are based on reexaminations of previously collected data (old diaries), and in other instances, on the data of studies being carried out by the experimenters themselves. In some instances the data were obtained by audiorecording, either by written transcription or by tape recorder, and in other instances by audiovisual recording. . . . At each stage of development both the context of language generation and the structure of the utterances produced (both child and other) need to be more carefully analyzed and methods of data collection standardized.

Spradlin also points out the obvious need to achieve a more scientific rigor in pursuing research on the processes of early childhood. His stated interests in this regard cover a number of experimental functions. Primarily, however, he is concerned with the range of different experimental standards exhibited in the literature and the consequent difficulty in interpreting the validity and the reliability of results. He is concerned that in the academic analysis and interpretation of results and in the planning for further developments, in contexts similar to the conference at Chula Vista, there is no one set of operational or functional terms that discussants use to assure conceptual accuracy in discourse. This condition may reflect the fact that discussants come from diverse backgrounds, and it may reflect the lack of appropriate traditions of scientific rigor in the design and implementation of language research.

Cromer's strategy in discussing receptive language is to focus upon the mentally retarded. However, he finds few studies in which comprehension is the *raison d'être*. Instead he is able to report a number of studies in which comprehension is one aspect of the research or in which there is an important implication concerning receptive functions. He also advances a strategy: What is important in language acquisition is not so much *what* is comprehended by an individual or a group of individuals, but *how* they come to comprehend it, that is to say, the processes involved in language comprehension.

This strategy is especially valuable in the consideration of Cromer's own research, which comprises the last section of his paper. He devised a language game to test the validity of language universals in early sentence interpretation. This work may be significant as an example of experimental procedures in linguistic research and, more specifically, as an experiment for posing interesting questions about the theoretical bases of linguistic universals. This excitement is reflected in Cromer's analysis and in Spradlin's interpretation of the research information.

Section IV, "Developmental Relationships between Expressive and Receptive Language," includes papers by Ingram and Bloom. In summarizing Section IV Chapman emphasizes the clarity with which Ingram and Bloom approached comprehension and production as a relationship issue. Ingram analyzes the traditional meaning of the term, "comprehension precedes production." He concludes that, functionally, comprehension must precede production but that the two are much "closer than expected." This determination is based in part upon research findings of phonological acquisition. He further concludes that the real issue is the gap between comprehension and production apparent in children with language disorders. He assumes that productive research on this issue will emphasize the variable features of acquisition.

Bloom agrees that some kind of processing (comprehension) of a behavior has to take place before a child can use or produce that behavior. However, a review of the research indicates that children behave differently when they talk and when they are presented with sentences that presumably test their comprehension. Unfortunately, there are few studies that have investigated both speaking and understanding with the same young children.

Bloom concludes that there is not enough information at the present time to explain the relationship between speaking and understanding in language development. However, it is important to emphasize that "the relationship is probably never a static one but rather shifts and varies according to the experience of the individual child and his developing linguistic and cognitive capacities."

Chapman's summary highlights the issues, the gaps in information, and the probable lines of future research. For instance, she predicts that we probably will turn from models of *what* the child knows to models of *how* the child knows. Chapman is able to integrate both the formal papers and the conference discussion in a systematic discussion of comprehension and production issues. She adds further to the analysis and leaves the reader with a logical set of assumptions for further study and for research development. One concludes that a new set of events are likely to follow the careful designs that Bloom, Ingram, and Chapman have imposed upon this area of language study.

Section V, "Nonspeech Communication," concerns two primary areas of language intervention: early phases of language training (Premack and

Premack) and manual language of the deaf (Moores). In reality, however, each provides information that should be a significant contribution to strategies in the general field of language intervention. Although there are controversies related to each language system, there seems little doubt about current and future utility with retarded children. For instance, Carrier (1973) has adapted the Premacks' system extensively and successfully with severely retarded children, and Berger (1972) and Bricker (1972) have shown the utility of visual language with hearing-impaired retarded and severely retarded children, respectively.

The application possibilities, however, are only part of the excitement of each system. Dever's summary discussion delineates several issues that relate to the general possibilities of each system. He summarizes the Premacks' system as an

> enterprise . . . to arrive at some of the dispositions that are critical to language development, and to devise tests to discover if these dispositions are present or not present in a specific organism. Behind this statement was his contention that an animal cannot be expected to develop a linguistic representation for a concept if it does not have a prior conceptual representation of that concept. Therefore, a way must be found to discover whether or not the concept is present before any attempt at language training can be made. Then, if the concepts are found to be testable, effective training based upon the results of that testing can proceed.

Dever describes Moores' review and research on visual language as an important movement to get the oral-manual controversy out of the realm of prejudice and guesswork. The value of Moores' work can be inferred from its generalizable nature with the deaf, the deaf-retarded, the young retarded, and the profoundly retarded. Moores also points out the durability of manual language systems even against the hostility of many detractors. The value of sign language systems has recently become more generally apparent, and there is the likelihood that manual communication will continue to spread to populations other than the deaf.

Hollis and Carrier (1973) in work not reported at the conference examine the work of Premack and Premack and Moores in a framework they have entitled "Prosthesis of Communication Deficiencies," They point out that the learning organism must have the physiological requisites for performance before learning is possible:

> Deaf children require special training to compensate for their inability to perceive and process auditory stimuli. They cannot learn speech and language in the same manner as hearing children. Similarly, there are many communication-handicapped children who may be having difficulty learning speech and language because of other impairments.

The *raison d'être* of the "substitute" systems is the use of visual and tactual systems and a substitute language (in place of a phonological/auditory system): "This eliminates the need for learning speech, or learning speech simultaneously with linguistic principles and opens a whole new vista for teaching the language-deficient."

Section VI, "Early Language Intervention," includes papers by Bricker and Bricker, Horton, and a summary paper by Turton. Turton explains that each of the preceding papers describes intervention procedures which address themselves to generic developmental and environmental issues. The intent of each program is to alter the environment so that the child has an optimal chance to acquire important precursors and early language forms.

Bricker and Bricker are concerned with infants and preschool children who are severely handicapped cognitively, linguistically, and motorically. They attempt to determine the child's status in several important areas of development and then to construct a program of instruction that will stimulate developmental progression. They have attempted to develop a sensorimotor lattice structure which indicates the primary sequential forms of behavior and the prerequisite behavior for each.

They use a test-teach system to cover materials and events that are relevant to the child in the play environment. Their plan is to cover development from the point of certain reflexive responses of infants to intentional and preoperational behavior. The latter is a cognitive level explained in the chapter by Morehead and Morehead (Section II).

The plan developed by Horton includes a home-teaching program for preschool deaf children in which the parents are the agents of change. The plan includes early detection and intensive auditory and linguistic stimulation. The training of parents includes instruction about how to 1) optimize the auditory environment, 2) talk to their child, 3) stimulate the child developmentally, 4) use behavior management, and 5) understand the child's place in the family. The primary training focus is upon receptive language. Parents are taught to optimize their linguistic input to the child.

In summarizing the Bricker and Bricker and Horton programs, Turton highlights the early identification and assessment of handicapped infants and the evaluation of treatment programs and procedures as significant parts of the conference discussion. He also provides an analysis of the prerequisites of an optimal program on early intervention.

Section VII, "Language Intervention for the Mentally Retarded," includes papers by Miller and Yoder; Guess, Sailor, and Baer; and Ruder and Smith, in addition to a summary by Bateman.

Bateman provides a cogent, useful analysis of the complex, extensive nature of the material in Section VII. The reader might want to study Bateman's comments before reading the three papers. In different respects each paper provides extensive coverage of the area of language intervention with the language-retarded.

Miller and Yoder recommend that language intervention strategies should be based upon what is known about normal language development. This knowledge includes the conceptual-semantic bases of language. In addition to the normal acquisition issue, however, they stipulate four other reference points in planning a language program. Their points include realistic "exit behaviors," "normal" interactions, active participation, and a systematic approach to teaching. A prominent feature of the Miller and Yoder program format is the synthesis of cognitive and behavioral principles. Their program "specifies the relationship among form, function, and experience and provides for the shaping of attending behavior and increasing behavior in retarded children." There is considerable similarity between the philosophy of the Miller and Yoder program and that of the Bricker and Bricker program described in Section VI.

The central hypothesis of the Guess, Sailor, and Baer procedures is that "relatively brief instruction along four dimensions of language usage will prove sufficient to produce the beginnings of a fundamental characteristic of normal language—it extends itself further without formal programming." The dimensions are *reference, control, self-extended control,* and *integration* functions of language.

The *reference* functions include things and events which are of constant significance in the child's environment. Thus the child learns that labels are powerful. It is natural then for the child to learn *control* in the form of productive and receptive demands. Further, he learns that to the extent that he knows and uses referents he can control events. This leads to a recognition of the need to learn new referents. Thus, the child is taught to ask questions and to actively seek new labels. This process can be termed *self-extended control.* The fourth dimension, *integration,* involves a continuation of functional contingencies to assure that the child's self-extending efforts result in appropriate storage and later use of the newly acquired labels.

The program described by Ruder and Smith emphasizes 1) the evaluation and selection of a language training program or battery of programs, 2) the content of a language training program, 3) language training procedures, and 4) continuing language assessments. Thus, the program they describe includes a number of issues described in the two previous papers. However, they place primary emphasis upon the syntax of language (content): " . . . an adequate language training program will identify (for training) all and only those structures which are necessary for a particular child's communicative needs."

The points emphasized in each program are further analyzed by Bateman, who also considers the contributions of linguistics, psycholinguistics, and cognitive psychology to the development of language programs. Bateman also highlights several unanswered questions which are subject to empirical investigation. Bateman's summary is a brief, accurate analysis of the current, central issues in intervention research.

A more extensive summary analysis of issues is provided by Staats. He examines the brief history of psycholinguistics, beginning with the publication of *Psycholinguistics* in 1954. Staats' statement highlights the schism that has existed between cognitive and learning approaches and proposes a rapprochement. Staats is especially interested in the theoretical issues of this potentially productive union. Consequently, he advances a neopsycholinguistic system which accommodates each position. He also recommends the utilization of both cognitive and learning approaches in a comprehensive program of language intervention, and he examines the various chapters in relation to their contributions to his basic position.

The book concludes with a brief summary analysis of the content as it relates to intervention strategies. Suggestions are also included regarding issues that can now be synthesized or combined in designing more comprehensive or more definitive procedures.

A DISCUSSION OF LANGUAGE PERSPECTIVES

Effective language intervention with the mentally retarded has a brief history. If the picture is focused upon severely retarded individuals, the span is short indeed. The reason for this delay is that the requisite behavior strategies for effective management were not available before 1960. Rapid progress since that time includes the basic work on the effects of antecedent and subsequent events (Girardeau and Spradlin, 1970; McReynolds, 1970; Risley and Wolf, 1967); on response class concepts (Baer, Peterson, and Sherman, 1967); on sustained attention (Yoder, 1970); on increased or decreased rates of responding (Bradford, 1970; Galloway and Sulzbacher, 1970); on new behavior classes (MacAulay, 1968); on imitation and auditory test functions (Fulton and Lloyd, 1969). This and related behavioral work has established the basis for clinical management for a large number of individuals with limited language (Lovaas, 1966; Bricker and Bricker, 1970; Hartung, 1970; Hewett, 1965). This research has established a behavioral technology for initiating and maintaining language training sessions. Language training has now become a practical reality for virtually all handicapped individuals.

However, many problems remain. These problems fall into two broad classes. First, *what language should be taught?* Should the effort be to teach a functionally normal language system—an awesome undertaking—or to teach critical features of language and otherwise attempt to bring the speaker under the positive control of the natural environment? Should language instruction be undertaken in an experimentally controlled setting or in a natural environment with a wide range of controlling stimuli? Among the environmental issues are the expectations of those with whom the speaker will communicate.

The second broad problem derives from the nature and the complexity of the language system that must be taught and learned. The curriculum for a language instruction program seems to be impossibly complex to many language clinicians and teachers. Research on developmental psycholinguistics has highlighted the complex nature of generative grammar and has raised the possibility of functional relationships between language and environment and between semantic functions and concepts. The relationships among behavioral, linguistic, and cognitive theories are certainly justifiable areas for extensive research.

The primary purpose of the Chula Vista Conference was to formulate a valid basis for teaching language to the mentally retarded and others with language retardation (or disability). However, a number of important subpurposes were served. Each participant probably had more than one purpose for his paper. A number of interests across a range of themes were discussed. A sample list could include:

1. The infant ontogenetic sensory response system
2. The possible existence of innate auditory mechanisms which make the human infant responsive to critical aspects of human speech
3. The role of auditory input in language intervention
4. Semantic features in early language acquisition
5. Concurrent emergence of syntax and semantic functions of language
6. The relationships of receptive and expressive language
7. Special language systems (plastic, manual, and visual)
8. Issues of natural and controlled environments
9. The rationale for language intervention
10. The generative nature of language
11. The general and special purposes of language evaluations
12. The relationship between cognitive and linguistic structures.

The planners of the conference and the book were guided by several preconceptions. First, they felt that there should be a strong emphasis upon receptive language. They felt that the great emphasis that has been placed upon expressive speech for a number of years has failed to reveal the nature of the receptive side of the paradigm. Perhaps we do not know what the stimulus program has been for children, including retarded children. What is the input? What does the child effectively receive and use? Is the natural environment adaptive to the child? Should the instructional environment be patterned after the natural environment? These and many other questions can be answered only if we obtain observational and experimental data about the events to which the child is exposed. We must record these data during the entire development of the child, beginning in early infancy. The research on speech reception must be expanded to include linguistic, semantic, and cognitive material related to the child's response repertoires. The ontogenesis of the receptive process may be especially important to subsequent intervention strategies for the mentally retarded. Speech reception may be constrained by a physiological, programmed device for the detection of speech and with some mechanisms for processing the input cognitively. Does this process mechanism fail to function for some children? Is there a sequential schedule that must be followed for cognitive functioning and subsequent linguistic functioning?

These questions may not be answered (or even answerable). Some may not be entirely relevant for a language teacher. The more direct issue may be: can receptive language functions be taught to children who fail to learn them in a natural (or unnatural) environment? Premack and Premack suggest that language can be taught and used by children who can acquire concepts for symbolic functions. Then the test may be our effectiveness in determining the child's concepts and, further, our success in stimulating additional conceptualization. If concepts and symbolization emerge in somewhat parallel fashion, the teaching process must include an environment where concept development can be accelerated and where language mapping can be improvised. If, as we suspect, the severely retarded child has limited concepts of his environment—including the nature of common objects, the purposes of toys and implements, the intents of adult caretakers, and the purposes of daily constraints and daily activities—he probably will not develop a symbol system congruent with normal persons in his community. Bloom suggests that the adult-child relationship is one that leads to exploration of agent-action-object functions. These functions are linguistically mapped. Her account is strikingly similar to the account of Premack and Premack, and both substantiate the views of Schlesinger about *relational concepts*. Bricker and Bricker seem to agree with all three in devising a concept-training environment for young severely retarded children.

The book also discusses the receptive and expressive processes and functions of children at the early phases of language acquisition. There should perhaps be a heavier emphasis upon the receptive functions of language, at least during the early phases of instruction or until the child develops an obvious range of semantic relationships. However, in light of the recent emphasis upon the transactions described in early language agent-action-object functions, it is difficult to see how the child-adult unit could naturally exclude one or the other. Perhaps expressive and receptive functions emerge together, and the child's speech behavior is shaped out of the same events which produce the receptive functions.

The child's coding abilities in early language development may be strongly influenced by imitative procedures in the natural environment. In the same way (and related to the same doubts and controversies) the imitative modes may be used in teaching early language. Both motor and verbal imitations can be used to sample the child's response capabilities, to focus attention on critical features of speech and language.

The development of concepts is a prominent theme in several papers. The relationship between understanding and speaking is also a prominent part of several papers. Nevertheless, the stages of concept acquisition are even less precisely known than are the linguistic sequences. The careful delineations of

Morehead and Morehead, however, establish a basis for further explorations in this area. The sequences of concept development and/or linguistic development may furnish a basis for planning language training curricula. The basis for programming language training may depend upon our knowledge of the sequences to be taught. A note of caution emerges. Some of the behavioral data show little relationship between success in teaching language features and the sequence in which they are taught.

The possible generative features of language were still another issue. If language is generative, can certain features be taught which will influence the development of other features (presumably of a similar linguistic class)? Likewise, if language emerges sequentially with certain phonological or syntactical features preceding other features, does the teaching of antecedent features stimulate or accelerate the emergence of other classes of linguistic events? These possibilities suggest a comfortable relationship for cognitive, linguistic, and behavioral points of view. However, these possibilities have not been thoroughly researched. Bricker and Bricker; Guess, Sailor, and Baer; and Ruder and Smith have developed language teaching procedures which combine several linguistic-behavioral arrangements or cognitive-linguistic-behavioral arrangements. Other papers suggest the bases for such arrangements. Nevertheless, the full set of possible combinations remains a topic for further study.

SUMMARY

The book is a combination of language information that relates to issues of acquisition, retardation, and intervention. The acquisition issues include infant receptive processes, early development of concepts, early development of receptive language, and the developmental relationship between expressive and receptive language. The intervention issues are covered in three sections dealing with nonverbal communication, early language intervention, and language intervention for the mentally retarded. The book includes several productive controversies that bear upon ontogenetic speech response systems, semantic and syntactic features of early language, relationships between receptive and expressive language, the utility of special language systems, the generative nature of language, the rationale for language intervention, and issues of natural and controlled environments.

Although the book was not designed to contribute to theories of language, cognition, learning, and behavior, Staats provides an analysis of these theoretical systems and discusses a neopsycholinguistics which, in effect, represents a rapprochement of cognitive and behavioral approaches within a modified learning theory. Other sections of the book also provide practical discussions or utilization examples for Staats' formulations.

The design of the book content should be useful to those studying language development and to those who undertake to teach language. The issues for each overlap in each section of the book. The content also highlights the importance of careful operational designs and careful semantic statements in communications about language. Also, the various chapters point up areas of factual omission and potential areas of new research productivity.

REFERENCES

Baer, D. M., Peterson, R. F., and Sherman, J. A. The development of imitation by reinforcing behavioral similarity to a model. *J. Exp. Anal. Behav.*, 1967, *10*, 405—516.

Berger, S. L. A clinical program for developing multi model language responses in atypical children. In J. E. McLean, D. E. Yoder, and R. L. Schiefelbusch (Eds.), *Language Intervention with the Mentally Retarded.* Baltimore: University Park Press, 1972.

Bradford, L. J. The use of operant procedures to reduce rates of reading and speaking. *ASHA Monograph No. 14*, 1970.

Bricker, D. D. Imitative sign training as a facilitator of word object association with low-functioning children. *Amer. J. Ment. Defic.*, 1972, *76*, 509—516.

Bricker, W. H. and Bricker, D. D. A program of language training for the severely handicapped child. *Except. Child.*, 1970, *37*, 101—111.

Carrier, J. K., Jr. Application of functional analysis and non-speech response mode to teaching language. Report No. 7, Kansas Center for Research in Mental Retardation and Human Development, Parsons, Kans., 1973.

Chomsky, C. *The Acquisition of Syntax in Children from 5 to 10.* Cambridge: The MIT Press, 1969.

Fulton, R. T. and Lloyd, L. L. (Eds.) *Audiometry for the Retarded: With Implications for the Retarded: With Implications for the Difficult-to-Test.* Baltimore: Williams & Wilkins, 1969, pp. 57—96.

Galloway, K. and Sulzbacher, S. Deceleration of inappropriate vocal behavior by a hard-of-hearing child. *ASHA Monograph No. 14*, 1970.

Greenfield, P. M., Nelson, K., and Saltzman, E. The development of rule-bound strategies for manipulative seriated cups: A parallel between action and grammar. *Cognitive Psychol.*, 1972, *3*, 291—310.

Hartung, J. R. A review of procedures to increase verbal imitation skills and functional speech in autistic children. *J. Speech Hear. Disord.*, 1970, *35*, 204—217.

Hewett, P. M. Teaching speech to an autistic child through operant conditioning. *Amer. J. Orthopsychiat.*, 1965, *35*, 927—936.

Hollis, J. H. and Carrier, J. K., Jr. Prosthesis of communication deficiencies: Implications for training the retarded and deaf. Working Paper No. 298, Parsons Research Center, Parsons State Hospital and Training Center, Kans., July, 1973.

Lovaas, O. I., Beberich, J. P., Perloff, B. F., and Schaeffer, B. Acquisition of imitative speech by schizophrenic children. *Science*, 1966, *151*, 705—707.

MacAulay, B. D. A program for teaching speech and beginning reading to non-verbal retardates. In H. N. Sloane and B. D. MacAulay (Eds.), *Operant Procedures in Remedial Speech and Language Training*. Boston: Houghton Mifflin, 1968.

McReynolds, L. V. Reinforcement procedures for establishing and maintaining echoic speech by a non-verbal child. In F. L. Girardeau and J. E. Spradlin (Eds.), A functional analysis approach to speech and language. *ASHA Monograph No. 14*, 1970.

Risley, T. and Wolf, M. Establishing functional speech in echolalia children. *Behav. Res. Ther.*, 1967, *5*, 73–88.

Sinclair, H. Sensori-motor action patterns as a condition for the acquisition of syntax. In R. Huxley and E. Ingram (Eds.), *Language Acquisition: Models and Methods*. New York: Academic Press, 1971.

Slobin, D. I. Cognitive prerequisites for the development of grammar. In D. I. Slobin and C. Ferguson (Eds.), *Studies in Child Language Development*. New York: Holt, Rinehart and Winston, 1973.

Trehub, S. E. Auditory-linguistic sensitivity infants. Unpublished doctoral dissertation. McGill University, 1973.

Yoder, D. E. The reinforcing properties of a television presented listener. *ASHA Monograph No. 14*, 1970.

INFANT
RECEPTION
RESEARCH

CHAPTER ONE

INFANT SPEECH PERCEPTION: A PRELIMINARY MODEL AND REVIEW OF THE LITERATURE[1]

Philip A. Morse

Department of Psychology, University of Wisconsin, Madison, Wisconsin 53706

As any investigator of auditory perception in young infants will readily admit, infants are generally quite reluctant to tell us of their perceptual knowledge of acoustics and speech, to say nothing of syntax. But even if they could tell us, what questions would we ask of them concerning the development of receptive language in early infancy? Methodological advances from research in infant learning and perception have recently provided several new paradigms which permit the investigation of young infants' receptive language abilities. The fruits of many years of adult speech perception research have yielded not only several important questions to ask about young infants, but also some of the synthetic stimuli with which to ask these questions. It should be no surprise, therefore, that the initial response of several investigators interested in infant auditory/speech perception was to apply one or another of these new paradigms to the study of the infant's perception of acoustic cues that have been found to be important in adult auditory/speech perception. The majority of the studies to be reviewed below are characteristic of this trend. However, some of the most recent advances in infant (as well as adult) speech perception research suggest that different paradigms impose different information-processing constraints on the subject. Therefore, before any conclusions can be drawn from the existing body of data on infant auditory/speech perception, the findings need to be examined in light of the constraints of the paradigms employed by different investigators.

An understanding of the infant auditory/speech perception literature necessitates a working knowledge of what questions to ask and how to ask them. Consequently, we shall begin with a brief review of the relevant adult speech perception data and with a general description of the procedures and assumptions involved in the two paradigms that have been most frequently

[1] Preparation of this paper was supported by Grant HD 03352-05 from the National Institute of Child Health and Human Development. The author is indebted to Frances K. Graham, Lewis A. Leavitt, James W. Brown, and David B. Pisoni for many stimulating discussions as well as for a critical review of the manuscript.

employed with infants. Finally, before the results of individual studies are examined, a "preliminary model" of the development of speech perception in early infancy will be proposed. It is hoped that this model will provide a framework for 1) organizing *vis-à-vis* development the data on infant auditory/speech perception, 2) assessing these findings in terms of the information-processing constraints of the various paradigms, and 3) considering future research questions about the development of auditory/speech perception.

ADULT SPEECH PERCEPTION

Research on adult speech perception has succeeded in identifying most of the acoustic cues which provide the basis for the perception of segmental (consonant, vowel) and suprasegmental contrasts. Liberman, Cooper, and their colleagues at the Haskins Laboratories have shown that formant transitions, which reflect underlying articulatory maneuvers, provide critical information for the identification and discrimination of stop consonants (see Liberman, Cooper, Shankweiler, and Studdert-Kennedy, 1967, for a review of this literature). Specifically, they observed three things in two formant, synthetic patterns.

1. Changes in the direction and extent of the second-formant (F2) transition are sufficient for the perception of the range of stop consonants which differ according to place of articulation ([b,d,g; p,t,k; m,n,ŋ]). For example, in the syllables [ba, da, ga] the F2 transition either rises to its steady state level ([ba]), falls slightly to it ([da]), or falls rapidly to it ([ga]).

2. Changes in the timing of the onset of the first-formant (F1) relative to that of F2 have been found to be sufficient for the perception of the range of stop consonants which differ according to their voiced-voiceless quality (*e.g.,* [b,p; d,t; g,k]). In English voiced consonants (*e.g.,* [b,d,g]) F1 leads or lags slightly the onset of F2 (negative and small positive values of voice-onset-time, respectively) whereas the voiceless stops ([p, t, k]) are produced when F1 lags the onset of F2 by approximately 30-40 msec or more of voice-onset time (VOT).

3. Research in vowel perception has revealed that changes in the position of the first three formants are sufficient for the perception of the vowel range [i, I, ɛ] (Stevens, Liberman, Studdert-Kennedy, and Oehman, 1969).

Finally, the study of the perception of intonation has indicated that one of its primary cues is the fundamental frequency (F_0) contour of the utterance. Accordingly, Lieberman (1967, 1970) has distinguished between two basic types of utterances or breath groups: a) a normal or unmarked breath group (−BG) which has as an acoustic correlate a terminal fall in fundamental frequency, and b) a marked breath group (+BG) which is signaled by a terminal rise (or nonfall) in F_0. The −BG is characteristic of simple declarative sentences, whereas yes-no questions are generally produced using a +BG in present day English. This by no means constitutes an exhaustive account of all the acoustic cues implicated in the perception of segmental and intonational contrasts, but it does acquaint the reader with those cues which have been investigated most frequently in infant speech perception research.

An investigation of *how* adults perceive the cues for various segmental contrasts has revealed that they often perceive these cues categorically. If we ask adults to label randomly presented stimuli from a given acoustic continuum (*e.g.,* the F2 transition continuum) they will identify the stimuli in categories (*e.g.,* [b, d, g]). If we ask these same subjects to discriminate different stimulus pairs drawn from this continuum, they can only discriminate pairs in which they have labeled the members with different category names. In other words, they are helpless if asked to discriminate two stimuli from the same category; discrimination is therefore no better than identification. This phenomenon, known as "categorical perception," has been observed in the perception of stop consonants, which vary according to place of articulation (F2 transition continuum) and voicing (VOT continuum), whereas vowels are generally not perceived categorically (Fujisaki and Kawashima, 1969; Pisoni, 1971). F2 transitions in isolation and other nonspeech sounds are also not perceived categorically, but continuously; *i.e.,* discrimination is better than identification and there are no peaks in the discrimination function (Mattingly, Liberman, Syrdal, and Halwes, 1971).

The perception of the stop consonants [b,d,g,p,t,k] is not only categorical, but it is further complicated by context effects due to vowel environment and the vocal tract of the speaker. For example, in the syllables [di] and [du] adults perceive an initial stop consonant [d] followed by either the vowel [i] or [u]. Although the initial consonant is perceived as the phonetic segment [d] in both syllables, the acoustic cue for [d] is radically different in the vowel contexts [i] and [u]. In [di] a rising F2 transition is the cue for [d], whereas a falling F2 transition cues [d] in [du]. Conversely, if we hold the vowel environment of [d] constant and vary the vocal tract size of the speaker (from that of a young child to that of an adult male), the same acoustic cue (a given F2 transition value) will be labeled as either [b] or [d] depending on the perceived vocal tract of the speaker (Rand, 1971). In other words, recovery of the phonetic event [d] cannot be accomplished by matching the acoustic signal to a single, stored template in long term memory. Instead, as Liberman *et al.* (1967) have suggested, retrieval of the phonetic event [d] requires that the various acoustic cues for [d] somehow be transformed or decoded by the adult to yield the linguistically appropriate information. It has been argued that this is accomplished through some species-specific "speech decoder."

INFANT DISCRIMINATION PARADIGMS

Heart Rate

The first discrimination paradigm to be applied to auditory/speech perception in early infancy measured the habituation and dishabituation of the cardiac component of the orienting reflex (Clifton and Meyers, 1969; Moffitt, 1968, 1971). According to Sokolov (1963), the orienting reflex (OR) is that normal unconditioned response to a novel stimulus which facilitates the subsequent processing of that stimulus. With repeated presentations of a particular nonsignal stimulus a cortical model of the stimulus begins to develop. Once a match between the cortical model and the incoming stimulus is achieved, the OR habituates. According to theory, the presentation of a novel stimulus produces a mismatch with the previous cortical model, thus causing the OR to be reelicited (dishabituated). One reliable index of the OR is the heart rate (HR) decelerative response (Graham and Clifton, 1966). Since this response is quite easy to record (if not to score) and requires little active participation on the part of the subject (besides remaining awake!), it has been particularly popular with infant researchers. However, although the HR component of the OR is relatively easy to elicit in infants older than 2–4 months, attempts to produce it in younger infants have met with mixed success (see Graham and Jackson, 1970, for a review of the relevant developmental literature). Without an appreciation for the stimulus parameters and state variables which affect the OR in younger infants, the HR habituation-dishabituation paradigm is likely to be of limited value in the study of early infant auditory/speech perception. Many of the findings that have been reported in early infant auditory/speech perception unfortunately support this observation.

Moffitt (1968, 1971) was the first investigator to attempt a study of infant speech discrimination using the HR habituation-dishabituation paradigm. Wisely, he chose infants 5–6 months of age. Since his experimental procedure has been the inspiration for many studies since then, we shall examine it closely. Moffitt presented his subjects with eight discrete trials of synthetic speech syllables. Each trial contained 10 syllables (either [ba] or [ga]); each syllable was 250 msec in duration, and the intersyllable interval was 1 sec. To permit HR response to return to baseline after each trial, a 40-sec intertrial interval (ITI) was introduced between trials. Subjects (S) in stimulus change conditions were given either six trials of the familiarization stimulus ([ba]) followed by two test trials of [ga] (group 1), or seven familiarization trials ([ga]) prior to one [ba] test trial (group 2). Group 3 (the control group) received [ba] on all eight trials. All stimuli had an approximate rise-time of 55 msec and were presented at an intensity of 80 dB against a 60-dB background noise level. Using this procedure, Moffitt observed that all three conditions yielded reliable ORs which subsequently habituated over trials 1–6. As expected, no dishabituation of the OR occurred for group 3 on trials 7 or 8. However, group 1 demonstrated only a marginal recovery to the stimulus change on trial 7, whereas group 2 yielded a reliable recovery of the OR on trial 8. The reason for this difference in dishabituation between groups 1 and 2 is not readily apparent. It seems unreasonable to attribute this difference primarily to the extra habituation trial received by group 2, since groups 2 and 3 both exhibited more rapid habituation by trial 6 than did group 1. Perhaps group differences in the shape of the initial OR may be partly responsible for the marginal dishabituation of group 1 (for group 1 the OR returned to baseline much more quickly than it did for groups 2 or 3). Since group 1 received a [ba-ga] shift and group 2 a [ga-ba] shift, another possibility is that the OR to [ba] is greater than that to [ga]. (Berg's (1971) data suggest to the contrary, however, that the OR to a 1900-Hz tone is greater than that to an 1100-Hz tone.) In any event, Moffitt did successfully demonstrate that the discrete-trial HR habituation-dishabituation paradigm could be applied to the study of speech perception in infants as young as 5–6 months of age.

Nonnutritive Sucking

The other discrimination paradigm to have a major impact on infant auditory/speech perception research is the nonnutritive sucking habituation-dishabituation procedure employed by Eimas, Siqueland, Jusczyk, and Vigorito (1971). In contrast to the relatively passive response measure of the HR paradigm, in this procedure the presentation of the stimulus is made contingent upon the infant's nonnutritive sucking behavior, specifically upon his high amplitude sucking (HAS) response (see Siqueland and DeLucia, 1969, for more details of this paradigm). According to this procedure, as the infant learns that it is his HAS which determines the stimulus event, the rate of HAS (number per minute) increases above a baseline level (during which no stimulus is presented). With the continued presentation of the same auditory stimulus, the rate of HAS decreases (or habituates) as a consequence of the reduction in the reinforcing properties of the stimulus. Once the subject's HAS rate habituates to the original stimulus, a stimulus change occurs (without any interruption in the procedure) and a novel stimulus is now presented contingent upon HAS. If following the stimulus change, the rate of HAS increases relative to that of a control group which continues to receive the original stimulus, we can infer discrimination of the stimulus change. It should be noted, however, that recovery (or dishabituation) of the HAS response depends not only on the infant's ability to discriminate the stimulus change, but also on his finding this change to be reinforcing.

Employing this general procedure, Eimas *et al.* (1971) tested 1- and 4-month-old infants for their categorical discrimination of speech stimuli which differed along the VOT continuum (*e.g.,* [ba] and [pa]). The stimuli were three formant, synthetic syllables with durations and interstimulus intervals (ISIs) of 500 msec. Within each age group Ss received either a between-category shift (+20/+40 VOT, *i.e.*, [ba] *vs.* [pa]), one of two within-category shifts (within [ba]: −20/0 VOT; within [pa]: +60/+80 VOT), or a control shift (following the criterion for habituation subjects continued to listen to the preshift stimulus which consisted of one of the six stimuli above). The results indicated that both age groups demonstrated reliable recovery to the between-category shift, whereas the change in the HAS rate of the within-category Ss did not differ significantly from the control Ss. Eimas *et al.* concluded from these findings that the HAS paradigm had provided evidence that infants as young as 1 month of age cannot only discriminate [ba] from [pa], but do so in a linguistically relevant manner; *i.e.*, with respect to the English categories for [ba] and [pa], they can discriminate between categories but not within.

Heart Rate and Nonnutritive Sucking Compared

Perhaps at this point it would be helpful to indicate some of the relative advantages and disadvantages of the HAS and discrete-trial HR paradigms. Most importantly, both paradigms depend upon an habituated response to the familiar stimulus in order to demonstrate discrimination. The sucking procedure solves this problem by establishing a criterion for habituation. Eimas *et al.* (1971) used a 20% decrement in HAS for 2 consecutive minutes following a 3rd reference minute. In the absence of on-line computer facilities, the investigator who wishes to use the HR paradigm must decide in advance how many trials of the familiar stimulus are likely to produce habituation in his subject population. A casual inspection of the infant visual perception literature will reveal that it is replete with discrimination studies that have yielded negative results because habituation was not obtained. Therefore, it is not surprising that Moffitt (1971) ran two experimental groups (one with six, the other with seven habituation trials); he was perhaps fortunate that the latter group habituated in their alloted seven trials. In contrast to the difficulties which the HR paradigm poses regarding habituation, it does possess at least two distinct advantages: 1) it requires little active participation (or learning) on the subject's part, and 2) the technique is applicable across a wide age range (from infancy to adulthood). The HAS paradigm, on the other hand, does require that Ss evidence "acquisition" and meet a fairly stringent habituation criterion. Although this technique *may* be more sensitive with younger infants than the HR paradigm, its usefulness does not extend much beyond the age of 12 months (although the literature is conspicuously silent regarding the paradigm's applicability to the college sophomore).

Another domain in which the two paradigms would appear to differ involves the need to control the intensity characteristics of the stimulus. In the HR paradigm, stimuli that have a fast rise-time (Hatton, Berg, and Graham, 1970) and/or a high intensity are more likely to elicit not an OR, but rather an accelerative HR response (a defense response). These intensity parameters appear to take on increasing importance the younger the infant is (Berg, Berg, and Graham, 1971). In contrast, some evidence from the HAS paradigm *suggests* that for younger infants, control of intensity parameters may be less important than in the HR paradigm. In the Eimas, *et al.* (1971) version of the HAS paradigm the stimulus onset and offset intensities were tapered such that a rate of two high amplitude sucks per second was required for the stimulus to be at peak intensity (75 dB against a 62-dB background level). Subsequent experiments in which this "conjugate" aspect of the procedure has been eliminated indicate that the resultant abrupt stimulus onset and offset and the reduction in variability of the stimulus intensity do not substantively affect the results obtained with the HAS paradigm (Eimas, in press; Trehub and Rabinovitch, 1972).

Finally, changes in the state of the infant can have important effects on the HR response (Hatton, 1969; Graham and Jackson, 1970). On the other hand, there is some indication that within the limits of the criteria of the HAS paradigm (which involve a minimal number of HAS permitted during baseline and the two habituation minutes) and if state is controlled up to the shift that state changes following the stimulus change may be of less consequence for the demonstration of discrimination using the HAS paradigm (Morse, 1971a). Clearly, before any conclusions can be reached regarding the import of either state or stimulus intensity factors, some of the parametric work that has been done in the HR literature (a distinct advantage for this paradigm) needs to be done with the HAS paradigm. In summary, factors relating to the criteria for habituation and the feasibility of the paradigm with different age populations would seem to be two of the most important procedural differences between the HR and HAS paradigms. A more extensive treatment of some of the differences between the two paradigms *vis-à-vis* habituation and dishabituation will follow in later sections of this paper.

A "PRELIMINARY MODEL" OF THE DEVELOPMENT OF INFANT SPEECH PERCEPTION

To the untutored (and perhaps even to the tutored) observer the data generated in infant auditory/speech perception in the last 10 years may be viewed as a series of findings quite unrelated except for their reliance on a common paradigm or for their use of synthetic or natural stimuli. To such an observer it may also be quite unclear what kinds of research questions should be asked next (aside from perhaps continuing to test the infant's discrimination of the remaining acoustic cues that infant research has inherited from the adult speech perception literature). It would seem, then, that some "preliminary model" of the development of infant speech perception might greatly facilitate the extraction of some semblance of order out of chaos and assist us in organizing the existing body of data in infant auditory/speech perception, in resolving some of the conflicting research findings, and in redirecting our energies in subsequent research.

The particular model to be proposed views the development of infant speech perception as progressing along three dimensions or vectors simultaneously: 1) linguistic coding, 2) microgenetic coding, and 3) ontogenetic age. As the names of the first two dimensions suggest, "coding" is an important concept underlying the entire model. By "coding" we mean the transformation of information from one state into another such that the information at a given state is not related in a 1:1 fashion to that at the previous or subsequent states; *i.e.,* it is related in terms of a code rather than a simple cipher (see Liberman, 1970; Liberman, Mattingly, and Turvey, 1972, for a further discussion of coding and its relation to language).

Linguistic Coding

Recent theories of grammar (*e.g.,* Chomsky, 1965) suggest that syntactical rules serve to relate the deep structure of an utterance to its surface structure. Phonological rules are in turn responsible for transforming the surface structure into a phonetic representation. Liberman (1970) has argued that in a formally analogous fashion, the phonetic structure is transformed or recoded into the final acoustic structure of an utterance by means of the "speech code" or the "grammar of speech." If we disregard the status of the semantic component, according to this composite view of linguistic structure, there are at least three levels of coding which an utterance undergoes: the grammars of syntax, phonology, and speech. Furthermore, according to this view, each of these three grammars in turn consists of an ordered sequence of rules.

If we take this as a model of the adult's linguistic knowledge, how is it acquired? Some have suggested that, in order to account for the rapidity with which the complex grammar of syntax is acquired, the infant must be born with some knowledge of this grammar (*e.g.,* McNeill, 1966). However, one alternative view of early language acquisition which derives from the adult model sketched above is that, in general, the infant acquires the grammars of speech, phonology, and syntax in that order. Furthermore, within each of these grammars, rule acquisition might proceed from the simple to the complex. According to this view of language acquisition, linguistic development in the first few months after birth consists primarily of learning about the rules of the grammar of speech. More specifically, it is suggested that the infant first learns about those rules which involve the least amount of coding in the grammar of speech (low level auditory perception), then he acquires "simple" phonetic rules (*e.g.,* the ability to discriminate the acoustic cues for stops and vowels) followed by an understanding of slightly more complex phonetic rules (*e.g.,* those involved in the categorical discrimination of stops in varying vowel and vocal tract environments). Finally, we would expect to see the acquisition of language-specific phonetic (*i.e.,* phonemic) rules. This sequence of coding levels for the grammar of speech constitutes the "linguistic coding" vector or dimension in our "preliminary model" of infant speech perception. To summarize, the model in its simplest form (Morse and Dorman, 1970) proposes that with development (ontogenetic dimension) the child acquires more and more complex coding rules within the grammar of speech (linguistic dimension).

Microgenetic Coding

One important aspect of the adult's grammar of speech is the categorical perception of stop consonants. The two discrimination paradigms that have been employed most frequently to assess categorical perception in adults are the ABX and oddball procedures. In the first, the *S* hears two different stimuli (A and B) followed by a third stimulus which is identical to either A or B. In the oddball procedure the *S* must report which of three stimuli is the odd one. In both paradigms the *S* must store in memory the first two stimuli presented in order to make a correct judgment upon hearing the third stimulus. If these two paradigms force the *S* to categorize each stimulus for a subsequent stimulus comparison, then the typical finding that adults cannot discriminate within-category differences in stop consonants may be largely an artifact of the information-processing constraints of the paradigms employed. In other words, if the adult has both a short term phonetic memory and a short term auditory (nonphonetic) memory of each speech stimulus presented in a discrimination paradigm (Fujisaki and Kawashima, 1969), then it would be misleading to conclude from the results of a paradigm which may force the *S* to categorize the stimulus phonetically that adults do not have an auditory (nonphonetic) memory for stop consonants. To determine under what conditions adults do have within-category information available about stops and vowels, Pisoni (1971) examined the discrimination of stops and long and short vowels in an ABX paradigm, in a modified signal detection paradigm, and finally, in a delayed-comparison recognition memory task. His findings reveal that at short ISIs information which is available in short term auditory memory permits the within-category discrimination of long vowels, whereas stop consonants are still perceived categorically. The short term auditory memory for short vowels was found to be less than that for long vowels both at short ISIs (short vowels yielded less continuous perception) and at long ISIs (short vowels were perceived categorically, whereas long vowels were not). Pisoni's results demonstrate that the categorical nature of speech perception is intimately tied to the relative contributions of auditory and phonetic short term memory: the short term auditory memory for vowels may facilitate within-category discrimination in vowels (*e.g.,* long *vs.* short vowels), whereas the chance within-category discrimination for stops may be attributed to the relatively poorer short term auditory memory for the stimuli available to the subject in these paradigms.

This intimate tie between memory factors and aspects of the grammar of speech suggests that our understanding of the grammar of speech may eventually have to consider all stages of auditory information processing and how they relate to adult speech perception. Pisoni (1971, 1973) has focused on some of the characteristics of auditory and phonetic short term memory which are important from 250 msec to 2 sec after stimulus offset. Other investigators more concerned with earlier stages in auditory information processing (Massaro, 1972; Dorman, Port, Brady-wood, and Turvey, 1973; Pisoni, 1972) have studied the readout of information from preperceptual memory store (the "tape recorder" stage in which an exact copy of the signal is stored). In many respects, we can conceive of the various stages of auditory information processing (*e.g.,* preperceptual store, auditory and phonetic short term store, and long term store) as successive stages of stimulus decoding very much analogous to the linguistic coding discussed earlier (see Liberman, Mattingly, and Turvey, 1972, for a detailed discussion of the relationship between language and memory codes). Since this auditory information-processing sequence occurs within a matter of seconds or minutes following the reception of an auditory stimulus, rather than over a longer time span (ontogenetic), we refer to it as "microgenetic coding." By including microgenetic coding as a dimension or vector in our "preliminary model" of infant speech perception, we acknowledge developmentally the importance of this intimate link between auditory information processing and the grammar of speech in the adult. Furthermore, the inclusion of this vector or dimension suggests one important way in which conflicting developmental findings in infant auditory/speech perception (that derive from different infant paradigms) may be interpreted and perhaps resolved.

Ontogenetic Age

According to this "preliminary model" of infant speech perception, the infant's speech perception capabilities at a particular age are to be understood by considering both his linguistic and microgenetic coding abilities. Furthermore, with increasing ontogenetic age, the infant is viewed as acquiring both sets of coding abilities. In the development of linguistic coding the infant advances, in general, first within a particular grammar and then from one grammar to another, whereas in developing microgenetic coding skills, the infant obviously does not begin with only preperceptual storage abilities and progress to short term auditory storage abilities at an older age. Instead, developmental changes in microgenetic coding are likely to be seen in such parameters as the decay rate or storage capacity of preperceptual and short term store (Haith, 1971; McBane, 1972). Finally, the term "ontogenetic age" was selected to indicate that this model encourages the investigation of populations of varying chronological and/or mental age as well as gestational and conceptual age.

FINDINGS IN INFANT AUDITORY/SPEECH PERCEPTION

Low Level Auditory Perception

In this first major stage of linguistic coding we are concerned with the infant's ability to perceive some of the primary features of auditory events (*e.g.,* frequency, intensity, duration, and localization) which provide the basis for the extraction of complex phonetic information. Frequency information as represented in a sound spectrogram provides the basis for many of the critical consonant, vowel, and intonation cues. Intensity changes are important in detecting changes in the stress and emotional quality of an utterance. Vowel quality, segmentation, and VOT are signaled by duration information. Finally, localization may be related to the development of lateralization. Strictly speaking, unless we consider the mechanical-neural transformation of information in the ear, features at this level are deciphered more than they are decoded.

Frequency. One of the clearest and earliest demonstrations of frequency discrimination in older infants (5–6 months) is Moffitt's (1971) investigation of F2 discrimination in three formant, synthetic syllables. In Moffitt's study the F2 transitions of [ba] and [ga] started at 846 and 2078 Hz, respectively, and approached a steady state value of 1075 Hz over the course of 55 msec. Using a procedure similar to Moffitt's, Berg (1971) tested 4-month olds for their ability to discriminate 1100- and 1900-Hz pulsed and continuous tones. Stimulus durations (10 sec) and ITI's (40–60 sec) were comparable to those employed by Moffitt (12.5 and 40 sec, respectively). Furthermore, as in Moffitt's first experimental condition, *S*s were presented with six habituation trials and two test trials. In Berg's study a no-change control condition was not run and *S*s were assigned to one of four stimulus-shift conditions: 1) 1100-continuous/1100-pulsed, 2) 1100-pulsed/1100-continuous, 3) 1900-pulsed/1100-pulsed, or 4) 1900-continuous/1100-continuous. Reliable ORs and habituation obtained for all conditions, and, in general, subjects discriminated both the pulsing changes and the 1900–1100 Hz frequency changes. However, a closer inspection of the results indicated that the frequency discrimination was observed primarily in the continuous presentation condition, not in the pulsed condition. In comparing Berg's results to Moffitt's, it should be remembered that Berg's pulsed (400 msec on, 600 msec off) frequency change (group 3 above) is the condition most similar to Moffitt's monosyllabic presentation (250 msec on, 1 sec off). Berg's results are consistent with those of Moffitt's in that pulsed frequency discrimination is difficult to demonstrate in this age range with only six habituation trials (Berg's data suggest, although statistical support for this is lacking in the trend analyses, that the *S*s in the pulsed frequency change condition did not habituate to the familiar stimulus). It seems unlikely that the suggestion of slow habituation to pulsed stimuli in Berg's and Moffitt's data is simply due to a sampling error. Perhaps the slower habituation to pulsed stimuli is related to the larger OR which these stimuli elicit. While evidence for this is only suggestive in Berg's data, Clifton and Meyers (1969) found this difference in OR magnitude to be reliable in 4-month olds. On the other hand, pulsed stimuli may yield slower habituation because, owing to their intermittent nature, the stimulus is perceived as more "complex" and/or it takes more samples of the stimuli within each trial to produce a neuronal model of the stimulus. In any event, Berg's evidence of frequency discrimination in the continuous condition indicates that infants as young as 4 months of age can discriminate 1100 from 1900 Hz with only six habituation trials and ITIs of 40–60 sec.

Attempts to demonstrate frequency discrimination in infants younger than 4–6 months have met with mixed success. Morse (1972) employed the Eimas *et al.* (1971) HAS paradigm to demonstrate that 40- to 54-day-old infants could discriminate combined frequency differences in F2 and F3 transitions (*i.e.,* [ba] *vs.* [ga] as well as differences in the fundamental frequency contour of the syllable ([ba+] *vs.* [ba−]). Since Morse's results indicated that infants at this age found these complex auditory patterns not only discriminable but interesting (*i.e.,* they showed both acquisition and recovery), Brown (1972) reasoned that infants as young as 6 weeks might not only orient to, but discriminate frequency differences in complex nonspeech stimuli. Using the discrete-trial HR paradigm, Brown presented 6- and 9-week-old infants with eight trials (6 habituation, 2 test) of 5-sec continuous, triangular tone sweeps (4 per sec; 1500–2500 Hz *vs.* 150–250 Hz) with ITIs ranging from 30 to 40 sec. Since state factors have been shown to influence significantly the occurrence of the OR in this age range (Hatton, 1969), Brown carefully selected only those *S*s who were alert and nonfussing during testing. Nevertheless, the 6-week-old group failed to demonstrate a reliable OR to stimulus onset, and consequently no significant habituation or dishabituation was evidenced in this group. On the other hand, the 9-week-old group did orient to the complex tone, but their OR failed to habituate, and no significant dishabituation was observed. A number of reasons may be responsible for Brown's failure to obtain evidence of frequency discrimination in 6-week olds, whereas Moffitt (1971) demonstrated it in older infants with the same paradigm and Morse (1972) found it in 6- to 7-week olds with the HAS paradigm. In comparison to Moffitt's procedure, Brown used shorter stimuli (5 sec rather than 10 sec), and he employed continuous rather than pulsed stimuli. Recent evidence has suggested that longer stimuli may be more effective in eliciting the OR in very young infants (Clifton, Graham, and Hatton, 1968), and Berg's (1971) data suggest that at least older infants may respond differently to pulsed and continuous stimuli.

However, assuming that these factors are irrelevant and assuming that Morse's (1972) results are replicable, one reason for the failure of the HR paradigm to reveal discrimination in the 6-week old may have to do with the information-processing constraints imposed by the paradigm. In other words, the ITIs employed not only may be too long for the acquisition of a "neuronal model" in the 6-week old but may also be too long for a novel stimulus to be discriminated from a familiar one. This suggests that the HAS paradigm employed by Morse may have worked with this same age range because it did not constrain the information processing of the 6-week old in this way (*i.e.*, impose such a memory load on the infant during habituation or at the stimulus change). One other explanation for the discrepancy between the Morse and Brown studies is that the maturation of the nervous system may be selective at this age: inadequate for the elicitation of the OR and its habituation, but sufficient for the HAS paradigm to be successful. This explanation is not necessarily ruled out by the existence of some suggestive evidence of the OR in newborns (Kearsley, 1971; Pomerleau-Malcuit and Clifton, 1971; Clifton, 1971; Sameroff, 1973). Only one of these investigators (Kearsley, 1973) observed an OR in awake infants to an auditory stimulus. but only for specific combinations of frequency, intensity, and rise-time.

If 6-week olds (Morse, 1972) as well as 4- to 6-month old infants (Berg, 1971; Moffitt, 1971) can discriminate frequency differences, what about the newborn? Bronshtein, Antonova, Kamenetskaya, Luppova, and Systova (1958) were perhaps the earliest investigators to report that newborns could discriminate frequency changes. However, recent attempts to replicate the basic phenomenon (the Bronshtein effect) employed by these investigators to assess discrimination in the newborn have been far from overwhelmingly successful (see Kessen, Haith, and Salapatek, 1970; Cairns, 1971). The "habituation" of the startle response as measured by cardiac activity and behavioral ratings was employed by Bridger (1961) to assess the discrimination of 400- and 1000-Hz tones in newborns. Bridger reported that 15 out of his 50 subjects evidenced discrimination of the two tones. However, since no control group was run to assess the effects of spontaneous changes in either the dependent measures or the infant's state over the course of the experimental session, his findings are at best suggestive of frequency discrimination in the neonate. Bartoshuk (1962) tested the frequency discrimination of newborns by measuring cardiac acceleration and its habituation and dishabituation to a sequence of changing frequencies. Subjects were presented with a standard stimulus which consisted of a series of 200-msec square pulses, the frequency of which increased monotonically over an 8-sec period from 100 to 1000 pulses per second. Reliable dishabituation was observed in the 10 best habituators (total N = 20). At least two problems arise in interpreting Bartoshuk's findings: 1) no attempt is reported to control or note state changes during the session, 2) since stimulus intensity was not controlled across the frequency range, infants could have been dishabituating to an intensity rather than a frequency change (see Jeffrey and Cohen, 1971, for a more detailed discussion of Bridger's and Bartoshuk's studies). Leventhal and Lipsitt (1964) attempted to demonstrate frequency discrimination in the neonate by measuring changes in respiration, body movements, and leg movements. In two separate studies they failed to obtain evidence of reliable discrimination of 200- vs. 500-Hz or 200- vs. 1000-Hz tones, respectively. Most recently, Siqueland and Lipsitt (1966) have demonstrated that the head-turning responses of newborns could be differentially conditioned with a tone vs. a buzzer as conditioning stimulus. However, since the tone was a 230-Hz square wave presented at 90 dB and the buzzer contained a fundamental of 23 Hz at 80 dB, it is difficult to know what role frequency *per se* played. Nevertheless, the technique is an encouraging one for those interested in investigating the auditory discriminative capabilities of the neonate despite recent complications in replicating aspects of this study (Clifton, Meyers and Solomons, 1972; Clifton, Siqueland, and Lipsitt, 1972). In summary, although the data indicate that by 40–54 days (Morse, 1972) and certainly by 4–6 months (Berg, 1971; Moffitt, 1971) infants can discriminate frequency changes, clear cut evidence for such a capability in the newborn is lacking.

Although the data at present do not reveal that the neonate can discriminate a frequency change, they strongly suggest that the neonate (and perhaps the fetus) can respond differentially over a range of frequencies. Several of these studies suggest that the neonate is particularly sensitive to frequencies within the speech range (the fundamental frequency of adult speech is approximately 120–200 Hz). Hutt, Hutt, Lenard, Bernuth, and Muntjewerff (1968) measured the neonate's electromyographic activity response to 2-sec stimuli (70, 125, 250, 500, 1000, and 2000 Hz sine and square waves. and a male and female recording of "baby"). Their results indicated that in all states of wakefulness the 70-Hz square wave elicited the most startle responses and in awake infants the responses to the 125- and 250-Hz sine and square waves were generally similar to that for "baby" and reliably different from that to all other stimuli. Lenard, Bernuth, and Hutt (1969) reported similar results using the amplitude of the auditory evoked response (N_2; latency: 300–500 msec). Specifically, they found that the female "baby" and the 125 Hz square wave produced a greater response than that to the 1000-Hz square wave, which in turn was greater than that to the 125- and 1000-Hz sine waves. Secondly, they observed a greater N_2 amplitude for the 125-Hz square wave than for broad band noise (200–5000 Hz); the smallest N_2 response obtained for low band (200–500 Hz) and high band (2000–5000 Hz) noise. Lenard *et al.* (1969) concluded that this greater response to the 125-Hz square wave (relative to the broad band noise) indicated that it was not just energy but structure within a frequency range to which the newborn was particularly responsive. Finally, research by Eisenberg and her co-workers (Eisenberg, 1965; Eisenberg, Griffin, Coursin, and Hunter, 1964) has suggested that neonates respond differentially to frequencies above and below 4000 Hz (see Eisenberg, 1970, for a more complete overview of the neonate literature).

Research on fetal responses to sound through the maternal abdominal wall has suggested that the fetus may be responsive to a wide range of auditory or vibratory stimuli (Bernard and Sontag, 1947; Dwornicka, Jasienska, Smolarz, and Wawryk, 1964; Grimwade, Walker, Bartlett, Gordon, and Wood, 1971; Johansson, Wedenberg, and Westin, 1964). Although many of these studies on fetal responses are only preliminary or are beset with numerous methodological/statistical problems, it should not surprise us to learn that the fetus can respond to a range of frequencies if the intensity of the stimulus is great enough: the cochlea and sensory end-organ are presumably developed by the 24th week of gestation (Ormerod, 1960, and Bast and Anson, 1949, both cited in Johansson *et al.*, 1964). This recent research on fetal responses to varying frequencies together with the selective frequency responding of neonates would suggest that the difficulty in obtaining strong evidence of frequency discrimination in neonates may be attributable more to the paradigms employed than to the neonate's capacity.

Intensity and Duration. Although little is known about the infant's capacity to discriminate differences in intensity and duration, a number of investigators have demonstrated that the newborn responded differentially to stimuli of varying intensities or duration. Steinschneider, Lipton, and Richmond (1966) observed that when neonates were presented with a random sequence of intensities ranging from 55 to 100 dB, the magnitude of their motor responses (startle) and cardiac acceleratory responses increased with increases in intensity levels of a broad band noise. A similar relationship between these same intensity values and the magnitude of change in the respiratory responses of the newborn has also been reported (Steinschneider, 1968). Further support for the newborn's sensitivity to a wide range of intensities comes from a study of the auditory evoked responses to clicks in sleeping infants. Barnet and Goodwin (1965) found that the amplitude of a late component in the evoked response varied linearly with the intensity of clicks (range: 35–65 dB above adult waking threshold). Finally, Bartoshuk (1964) has reported that the intensity function for the newborn's cardiac responses to 1000-Hz tones follows Steven's power law. However, recent attempts at replication suggest that this conclusion may be premature.[2]

Research on the infant's response to auditory stimuli of different durations is even less extensive than that on intensity. Nevertheless, two especially important features of the infant's response to duration have been studied. For one, Clifton, Graham, and Hatton (1968) have demonstrated that the newborn's cardiac acceleratory response is an inverted U-function of stimulus duration: for a 75-dB, 300 pps square wave presented at durations of 2, 6, 10,

[2]Harvey and Moffitt, personal communication, Feb. 1973.

18, and 30 sec, the optimal response occurred to the 10-sec stimulus. Whether this optimal duration is constrained by stimulus frequency, stimulus complexity, or the age of the infant has not been investigated. A second major feature of the infant's response to duration is that 4-month olds respond differently to pulsed and continuous tones (Berg, 1971; Clifton and Meyers, 1969). Recent work with younger infants suggests that the cardiac component of the OR may be greater for pulsed than for continuous stimuli in infants as young as 6 weeks of age (Berg, 1972; Brown, 1972; Leavitt, Morse, Brown, and Graham, 1973). Future research with pulsed and continuous stimuli may help to explain Salk's (1962) observation that the sound of the mother's heartbeat (78 beats per min) is particularly soothing to newborn infants, where neonates are conspicuously upset by a galloping heartbeat or a 128 beats per min heartbeat.

Localization. Chun, Pawsat, and Forster (1960) measured head-turning and oculomotor orientations to a buzzer in varying locations around the infant's head. They report that infants older than 26 weeks of age were able to localize a sound source directly in line with either the right or left ear, whereas infants younger than this age were unable to localize the sound source. On the other hand, Wertheimer (1961) observed that within 10 min after birth one subject that he tested showed reliable oculomotor orientation to a toy "cricket" at the left or right ear. Both the Chun *et al.* and Wertheimer studies suffer from a number of inadequacies: 1) no attempt is reported to assess or control for spontaneous variation in the dependent variables, 2) the role of head orientation preferences does not appear to have been considered (Turkewitz, Moreau, and Birch, 1966), and 3) concern for changes in the infant's state during the session was minimal at best (Chun *et al.* do report that their infants were awake and "resting"). Brown (1972) attempted to demonstrate discrimination of a stimulus location change presented through earphones to infants 6 and 9 weeks of age. His failure to obtain evidence of discrimination, as discussed earlier, may be more a result of the information-processing constraints (memory load) imposed by the discrete-trial HR paradigm which he used than of the infant's capacity at these ages. Leventhal and Lipsitt (1964) carried out two studies of sound localization discrimination in newborns using small ear-sized speakers. One important reservation about this procedure is that since small speakers rather than earphones were used and since the tonic neck reflex is quite prominent at this age, infants may have been presented with an intensity as well as a localization change. In their first study Ss were presented with 20 trials of either a 200- or a 500-Hz tone delivered to either the left or right ear, followed by 10 trials of the same tone in the opposite ear. Although habituation occurred, no reliable changes in respiration, leg, or body movements were observed to the stimulus change. In their second experiment, prior to the stimulus location change, half of the Ss were run to a criterion of habituation and half were given 10 trials in which to habituate. The latter group failed to habituate and discriminate the change, whereas the to-crite-rion group habituated and discriminated the shift in location. (In both experi-ments the performance of the shift conditions was compared to that of a no-shift control group.) Although it is somewhat difficult to know exactly what stimulus characteristics these infants responded to (intensity *vs.* localiza-tion) or what the response is that is changing throughout the session (either a change in respiration, leg, or body movements was scored), the difference in the performance of the two shift groups in the second Leventhal and Lipsitt study is consistent with our earlier remarks regarding the importance of using a paradigm tailored to the information-processing capabilities of the infant. In other words, the development of a model of the familiar stimulus prior to shift may require the investigator to present more trials of the stimulus (Leventhal and Lipsitt, 1964, experiment II) or to increase the age of the subjects to reduce the effective memory load imposed by the paradigm (Brown, 1972).

In summarizing the data on low level auditory perception in the infant, we may conclude that the newborn appears sensitive to a variety of auditory stimuli which differ in frequency, intensity, duration, and location in space, whereas the evidence of the young infant's ability to detect a change in any of these "low level" features is far from convincing (if not completely lacking in some instances). Although it is possible that these discriminative abilities develop later in the infant, a much more attractive hypothesis is that our failures or inconsistent successes in discovering these abilities in the newborn or 6-week old may be more a result of the information-processing constraints of the particular habituation paradigm employed (*i.e.,* primarily the memory load imposed on the infant by the ITIs employed). In the case of classical conditioning paradigms, as Sameroff (1971, in press) has suggested, the extent to which the neonate is "prepared" to associate a particular CS to a particular response may also be critical.

Phonetic Cues: Auditory and Linguistic Perception

One other reason for suspecting the information-processing constraints of the paradigms rather than the infant's capabilities for the lack of convincing evidence of low level auditory discrimination in the young infant is that the data at *this* stage in linguistic coding reveal that by 4–6 weeks of age infants can discriminate acoustic cues which are frequency- or duration-based. How-ever, before we examine the data on the development of auditory and linguistic perception of phonetic cues, an important distinction needs to be made. If an investigator demonstrates that infants can discriminate two speech stimuli which differ according to a particular acoustic cue, this does not necessarily imply that these *S*s discriminated the stimuli in a linguistically relevant manner. The latter clearly involves a complex coding of the acoustic cues, whereas the discrimination of the acoustic cues for speech is more directly related to that of "low level" auditory features discussed earlier (Studdert-Kennedy, 1973). If this distinction is considered from an onto-genetic perspective, it suggests that the auditory and linguistic perception of phonetic cues might conceivably constitute separate ontogenetic stages of linguistic coding. However, since the "auditory perception" of phonetic cues does not involve a "code," and in view of the scarcity and redundancy of the developmental data in these two aspects of phonetic cue perception, the data in both areas will be reviewed together.

The investigation of infant auditory and linguistic perception of phonetic features has been limited primarily to three phonetic features: place, voicing, and intonation.

Place. Moffitt's (1971) study, described earlier, constitutes the first ex-amination of the infant's discrimination of a change in the primary acoustic cue for place of articulation: the F2 transition. Employing a discrete-trial HR paradigm, he showed that 5- to 6-month olds could discriminate differences in the F2 transition of three formant [ba]s and [ga]s. He did not demonstrate that infants performed this discrimination in any linguistically meaningful manner. Morse (1972) has subsequently demonstrated that not only can 6-week olds discriminate changes in the acoustic cues for place but they also appear to discriminate them in a somewhat linguistically relevant manner. Morse tested infants using the HAS paradigm for their ability to discriminate differences in 45-msec F2 and F3 transitions in three formant syllables (speech condition: [ba] *vs.* [ga]) or in isolation (nonspeech condition). Discrimination was evidenced in the speech condition by the reliable recovery of HAS following the stimulus shift (relative to a control group). Recovery of the *S*s in the nonspeech condition, however, was bimodally distributed and straddled that of the speech condition; *i.e.,* some *S*s recovered more than the speech condition, whereas the remainder showed less recovery than the speech condition. These results indicate that 6-week olds respond to changes in these acoustic cues differently in linguistic and nonlinguistic contexts; they may even suggest that 6-week olds respond to them in a linguistically relevant manner. Although an analogous bimodal and straddling distribution was observed in the Mattingly *et al.* (1971) nonspeech data on F2 transition discrimination in adults, the demonstration of the categorical discrimination of F2 transitions in a speech context would be more interpretable and persuasive of perception in a linguistically relevant manner.

Despite Brown's failure to obtain even decent ORs from 6-week olds (to say nothing of discrimination), Morse's (1972) success in demonstrating the discrimination of [ba] and [ga] in this age group using the HAS paradigm suggested that the HR paradigm might be successful with the speech stimuli employed by Morse. This suspicion was further buttressed by Moffitt's (1971) success with the HR paradigm using similar stimuli and older infants. In the first of a series of recent studies Morse, Leavitt, Brown, and Graham (in preparation) presented 6-week-old *S*s with [ba]s and [ga]s using the same discrete-trial paradigm that Brown (1972) had employed. The speech stimuli were 500 msec in duration and ISI; each trial consisted of six speech stimuli. Although a sizable OR was observed on the first trial, no habituation or dishabituation obtained. Reasoning that the ITIs in this first study (20–35 sec) may have been too long to produce either habituation or dishabituation in the 6-week old, Morse et al. eliminated the ITIs between stimulus changes in a second discrimination study with the same stimuli. In this experiment 6-week olds were presented with a train of 30 syllables (e.g., [ba]) followed immediately by a train of 30 different stimuli (e.g., [ga]). All ISIs and durations were 500 msec. Each infant received four [ba-ga] changes with a 31- to 45-sec interval between each change block. Once again, a large initial OR to stimulus onset was observed. Infants who remained alert throughout the entire experiment showed significant cardiac acceleration to the change in the first two change blocks and insignificant cardiac deceleration to the third change. While it is difficult to reconcile an accelerative HR response to change with evidence from older infants and adults that HR decelerates with orient-ing, it is possible that the pattern is different in the very young infant or that it requires some exposure to change to develop a neuronal model. Consistent with the latter interpretation is Sameroff's (in press) recent suggestion that a defense response is elicited initially which gives way to an orienting response with increased experience with a particular stimulus (change). This demon-stration of discrimination in 6-week olds with the modified HR paradigm is consistent with our earlier argument that the negative results obtained with the discrete-trial HR paradigm in younger infants may be attributable to the information-processing constraints of the paradigm, not necessarily to the infant's limited linguistic capacity. The HAS paradigm, like the modified HR paradigm employed by Morse et al., permits the infant to compare immedi-ately the familiar stimulus with the novel one, rather than forcing the infant to retain a memory of the familiar stimulus across a 25- to 40-sec interval. Future research in the development of place discrimination in infants needs not only to investigate the categorical discrimination of place cues, but also to continue to focus on the microgenetic aspects of this perception as Pisoni (1971, 1973) has done in adult speech perception.

Voicing. The first investigation of the infant's ability to discriminate differences in the voiced quality of stop consonants was conducted by Eimas et al. (1971). As discussed in more detail earlier, they demonstrated that 1- and 4-month olds not only could discriminate changes in the primary acoustic cue for voicing (VOT) but could make this discrimination in a linguistically relevant manner, i.e., categorically for [ba] and [pa]. No other study in this field has generated as much excitement about the young infant's speech perception capabilities as this demonstration of the linguistic perception of voicing cues by 1 month of age. However, the critics have not been silent. Stevens and Klatt (1974) have suggested that the Eimas et al. results indicate that, in general, infants at these ages cannot discriminate 20-msec differences in VOT and the discrimination evidenced by the between-category shift group (+20 vs. +40) may be attributed to the infant's ability to discriminate the presence vs. absence of an F1 transition. A second question posed by the Eimas et al. results is whether 1-month olds exposed only to English can discriminate categorically other values of VOT which involve a category boundary in languages other than English (e.g., the prevoiced Thai boundary).

Recent attempts by Pankhurst and Moffitt[3] and by Eimas (in press) to investigate infant discrimination at the Thai boundary have produced equivocal results. Pankhurst and Moffitt investigated the VOT discrimination of 5-month olds using the HAS paradigm. Employing the VOT contrasts of −20/−60, 0/−40, 0/+40, +20/+60, they failed to find any evidence of VOT discrimination in their subjects. In view of the Trehub and Rabinovitch (1972) evidence of discrimination with the VOT contrast of +20/+80, the Pankhurst and Moffitt failure to obtain any evidence of discrimination for 0/+40 and +20/+60 is somewhat puzzling. Eimas (in press) reported two attempts to investigate the discrimination of the Thai boundary in 2-month olds. In the first study he examined discrimination for a −20 VOT boundary (as suggested by the adult data collected by Abramson and Lisker, 1970). Although both the between-category (−40/+20) and within-category (−100/ −40) groups recovered to the stimulus shift, a tendency for greater discrimination was evidenced by the −100/−40 condition. Consequently, in a second experiment Eimas examined infant categorical discrimination at the −50 VOT boundary (between: +10/−70; within: −70/−150). The between-category shift evidenced significant recovery, and the within-category group failed to do so. However, since these two conditions failed to differ significantly from each other, we must conclude that strong evidence of categorical discrimination for the Thai voicing category still eludes us. It should be noted that failure to obtain discrimination at the Thai boundary in infants primarily exposed to the English language does not necessarily imply that the Stevens and Klatt (1974) argument regarding the presence vs. absence of the F1 transition is the best explanation of the other infant VOT discrimination studies. Eimas (in press) has recently proposed that the basis for VOT categorization consists of linguistic feature detector mechanisms. The relevant animal literature on feature detectors informs us that experience with a given stimulus category is generally necessary for the activation or structuring of the feature detector response. In the case of the Thai voicing category, experience with category instances may also be a prerequisite for categorical discrimination at the Thai boundary. Perhaps an investigation of the effects of early experience with selected speech categories will provide an answer to this question.

The discrimination of VOT using the HAS paradigm has also been studied by Trehub and Rabinovitch (1972). Infants between 4 and 17 weeks of age

---

[3]Personal communication, Mar. 1973.

were tested for their discrimination of synthetic [ba] and [pa] stimuli, natural [ba] and [pa], and natural [da] and [ta] syllables. Trehub and Rabinovitch found that all three stimulus changes were discriminated relative to a no-shift control group. While it is important to have independent corroboration of some or all of the Eimas *et al.* results, it is not immediately clear what is to be gained by examining the discrimination of natural [ba] and [pa] syllables after one has already demonstrated the discrimination of synthetic [ba] and [pa]. We know that the synthetic stimuli differed solely in their VOT values, but any number of voicing or extraneous cues may have been responsible for discrimination within the two natural speech stimulus pairs.

In our discussion of the frequency and place discrimination findings, we suggested that perhaps the information-processing constraints (primarily memory load) of the discrete-trial HR paradigm are responsible for the different results obtained with the HR and HAS paradigms. If this is correct, we would expect to find that attempts to demonstrate VOT discrimination in young infants using the discrete-trial HR paradigm have also failed, even though the HAS paradigm has provided positive evidence of VOT discrimination (Eimas *et al.*, 1971; Eimas, in press; Trehub and Rabinovitch, 1972). Recent attempts to obtain evidence of VOT discrimination using the discrete-trial HR paradigm are indeed consistent with this hypothesis. Yonas[4] tested 2-, 6-, and 10-month olds on their discrimination of [ba] and [pa] (0/+40 VOT). Although the 10-month olds did discriminate this voicing difference, no evidence of discrimination was found for either the 2- or 6-month olds. Moffitt and Pankhurst[5] have obtained essentially the same results with 2- and 5-month-old infants. Using this same paradigm, they too failed to obtain any evidence of discrimination for [ba] (0 VOT) and [pa] (+40 VOT) in either age group.

Intonation. In his classic review of the early literature on infant speech perception, Lewis (1936) argued that the discrimination of intonation patterns ontogenetically precedes the discrimination of segmental phonetic patterns (*e.g.*, consonants and vowels). However, the data which formed the basis for this claim (Bühler and Hetzer, 1928; Löwenfeld, 1927; Schäfer, 1922) must be interpreted with extreme caution. These studies suffer not only from inadequacies in experimental design and in the definition and appropriateness of the response measure, but more importantly from the inadequate specification of the stimulus. (Most of what we know about speech perception has only been available since the early 1950's.) Since Bühler and Hetzer (1928) and Schäfer (1922) used natural speech stimuli, control over important stimulus parameters was difficult, if not impossible, to achieve. Consequently, we cannot be sure to what aspect of the stimulus their

[4]Personal communication, Feb. 1973.
[5]Personal communication, Feb. 1973.

subjects were responding. The third study (Löwenfeld, 1927) employed nonspeech sounds which consisted of tones and environmental sounds. Such stimuli not only present parameter control problems, but are of questionable relevance to the perception of speech.

Probably the first attempt to investigate the development of intonation perception with any experimental rigor was Kaplan's (1969) recent study of 4- and 8-month olds. Kaplan tested infants for their ability to discriminate rising and falling intonation contours imposed on either a stressed or un- stressed version of the spoken utterance "see the cat." In all stimuli the critical acoustic information was reported to occur in the last 400 msec of the utterance. Utterances were grouped in 5-sec triplets with 5-sec intertriplet intervals. Within each stress condition subjects were presented with a block of 11 triplets of one stimulus (e.g., falling-unstressed) followed by 11 triplets of the change stimulus (e.g., rising-unstressed). Each subject, if cooperative, received five consecutive stimulus shifts, but the data from the first two blocks could not be analyzed. Kaplan's dependent measures consisted of changes in heart rate variability and overt orientations (head-turning and oculomotor responses away from the mother and toward the speaker, which was near the infant's left ear). Only those infants in the 8-month-old stressed intonation condition showed reliable increases in orientation responses and heart rate variability to the stimulus change. Subjects in the 4-month-old stressed intonation condition responded to the change with a decrease in heart rate variability, but Kaplan interpreted this as evidence of habituation, rather than of dishabituation. Kaplan's failure to obtain evidence of the discrimination of rising and falling intonation contours in 4-month-olds (although they did show discrimination of a "male" and a "female" voice using this paradigm) is difficult to interpret for a number of reasons: 1) the underlying processes which are reflected in heart rate variability are not all that clear, especially where scores are not adjusted for initial level, 2) there may be age differences in the extent of heart rate variability, 3) since the stimuli were natural rather than synthetic, we cannot be sure exactly what cues the infants were or were not discriminating, and 4) the length of the stimulus and the imbedded nature of its critical feature may once again have exceeded the information-processing capabilities of the younger infant. Prompted by these interpretive problems as well as by the inadequately tested assertion of Lewis' regarding the earlier processing of intonation in the infant, Morse (1972) employed the HAS paradigm to examine the discrimination of place and intonation in infants 40–54 days of age. Infants were tested for their discrimination of a [ba] with a rising intonation contour (from 120 to 194 Hz) and a [ba] with a falling fundamental frequency (from 120 to 70 Hz); all changes in fundamental frequency were linear over the last 150 msec of the 500-msec stimuli (the place stimuli and results have been described earlier). Both the place and intonation differences were found to be discrim- inable in infants only 40–54 days of age.

Although several authors have echoed Lewis' conclusion that the discrimination of intonation patterns ontogenetically precedes the discrimination of segmental patterns (Fry, 1966; Kaplan and Kaplan, 1971; Lenneberg, 1967), only Kaplan and Kaplan have suggested a specific timetable. The Kaplans have asserted that infants develop the ability to detect intonational information between 5 and 12 months and segmental information closer to 12 months of age. However, the results of Morse's (1972) study, as well as those of Eimas *et al.* (1971), indicate that within the first 2 months after birth infants can discriminate the acoustic cues for segmental and intonational information. Furthermore, infants in this age range respond in a similar manner (*i.e.*, amount of recovery) to changes in either place or intonation (Morse, 1972). It should be noted, however, that neither Morse's nor Kaplan's study demonstrates that intonational cues are perceived by infants in a linguistically relevant manner. The adult literature is not entirely clear as to what linguistically relevant might mean in the case of intonation (see Lieberman, 1967; Studdert-Kennedy and Hadding-Koch, 1971).

Complex Linguistic Perception

So far, we have viewed the development of the grammar of speech in the infant as beginning with the perception of primary auditory features (low level auditory perception), with the subsequent ability to extract from those features the acoustic cues which are important in speech perception, followed by the ability to discriminate differences in these cues linguistically (auditory and linguistic perception of phonetic cues). However, the speech code is much more complex than the categorical perception of [ba] and [pa]. The adult is also capable of identifying a particular consonant in which the relevant acoustic cue differs because of changes in vowel (*e.g.*, [di] and [du]) and/or vocal tract contexts (Liberman *et al.*, 1967; Rand, 1971).

With the exception of a preliminary report by Fodor, Garrett, and Shapero (1970), virtually no data are available which indicate when the infant is capable of these types of complex phonetic perception. According to the brief (15-line) report by Fodor *et al.*, infants 3½-4½ months of age were conditioned (paradigm unreported) to respond to either 1) [pi] and [pa] *vs.* [gu] or 2) [pi] and [gu] *vs.* [pa]. Infants in the first condition learned the discrimination, whereas the infants in the second condition did not. The authors took this as evidence of the infant's ability at this age to perceive the identity of the phone [p] in the two different acoustic contexts. Although it is difficult to appreciate the importance of this report until more detailed information is available, it should be pointed out that the stimuli employed by Fodor *et al.* do not answer the [di]/[du] question; *i.e.*, [pi] and [pa] not only contain the same initial consonant, but they are also similar (and differ from [gu]) in their VOT. It is not clear whether Fodor *et al.* also varied the F2 transitions of their stimuli or if they instead held F2 constant as in the

Liberman, Delattre, and Cooper (1952) study while varying the burst frequency. In any event, no analogous confounding acoustic basis appears to be available for the perception of [d] in [di] and [du]. The [di]/[du] example illustrates an important fact of speech perception. This is that depending upon context the *same* acoustic cue will be perceived as different and *different* acoustic events will be perceived the same. This invariance problem is the basis of the whole issue of complex linguistic perception. It makes speech special and apparently requires the postulation of some specific decoder.

SPECIAL TOPICS IN INFANT SPEECH PERCEPTION

A number of topics to which investigators in infant auditory/speech perception have addressed themselves do not readily fit into the developmental model proposed here. These include the investigation of the "special nature" of speech stimuli, the recognition of the mother's voice, the magnitude of discrepancy hypothesis, and the developmental relationship between speech perception and production.

Is Speech Special?

We know from the adult speech perception literature that categorical perception and laterality differences (hemispheric specialization) suggest that speech is perceived by adults differently than nonspeech signals. Does the young infant also perceive speech in a "special" way? Several recent studies have suggested different ways in which the young infant may be responsive to the "special" nature of speech. Butterfield and Siperstein (in press; Siperstein, 1973) have investigated changes in the neonate's operant nonnutritive sucking when the presentation of vocal-instrumental music is made contingent upon an increase in mean suck duration. If both the vocal-instrumental components or the vocal component alone were presented in this operant paradigm, neonates increased the duration of their individual sucks in order to hear the stimuli, whereas the group that received only the instrumental component did not show a reliable increase in mean suck duration. Although these results provide an impressive demonstration of a new technique for assessing the neonate's discriminative capabilities, they do not specify the features of the speech stimuli that the newborns found particularly reinforcing or how they perceived the speech stimuli differently. Although Morse's (1972) study of speech and nonspeech discrimination of F2 and F3 transitions in infants 40–54 days of age demonstrated that infants at this age discriminate these stimuli differently, it too, fails to tell us how. As mentioned earlier, a study of infant categorical/continuous discrimination of speech and nonspeech stimuli (similar to the Mattingly *et al.*, 1971 study) would be more informative. Although data on the infant's categorical perception of speech *vs.*

nonspeech stimuli may be wanting, a recent dissertation has examined the laterality of the infant's responses to speech and nonspeech signals. Molfese (1972) presented adults, children (4–11 years), and infants (1 week-10 months) with speech ([ba], [dae], "boy," "dog") and nonspeech stimuli (C major chord, 250 Hz-4 kHz noise burst). For all age groups the auditory evoked response (AER) over the left and right temporal lobes revealed a greater AER over the right hemisphere to the nonspeech stimuli and a greater AER over the left hemisphere to the speech stimuli. Whatever it is about speech stimuli which makes them special, the infant brain appears to be receptive to those parameters in a lateralized fashion.

Perception of Mother's Voice

The identification of a particular individual's voice is considerably more complex than "low level auditory perception," but the cues involved are probably not phonetic ones. Although several investigators have examined the infant's ability to identify or discriminate the voice of the infant's mother, they have not succeeded in specifying what it is about the mother's voice that the infant recognizes. Turnure (1971) has shown that with an increase in age (3, 6, and 9 months) infants evidence more motor quieting to mother's voice, to several distortions of the mother's voice, and to the voice of a female stranger. No systematic differences were observed among these stimuli at any given age. In contrast to Turnure's not-too-discriminating subjects, Tulkin (1971) found that 10-month-old infants of "middle class" parents were able to discriminate the mother's *vs.* a stranger's voice, whereas no such discrimination obtained in infants of "working class" parents. If the mother's voice was presented, the middle class infants oriented toward the mother, whereas when the stranger's voice emanated from the speaker, these same *S*s directed their visual attention to the female coder in the room. Most recently, it has been suggested that infants as young as 30 days of age perceive in a speaker's act of vocalizing the unity of auditory and visual space (Aronson and Rosenbloom, 1971). If the locus of the speaker's voice is displaced 90° in space from the perceived speaker (mother or a stranger) who is visible to the infant behind a window, Aronson and Rosenbloom found that infants 30–55 days of age exhibit considerable distress (measured by increased tonguing scores) when compared to the presentation of the speaker's voice at 0° displacement. These three studies represent a small, but important, beginning in our investigation of the infant's knowledge of speaker identity, specifically that of the infant's mother.

Magnitude of Discrepancy Hypothesis

According to this hypothesis, the infant's attention to a novel stimulus (following habituation to a familiar stimulus) is an inverted U-function of the magnitude of the discrepancy between the two stimuli. Although the research which is presumed to support this inverted U-function is far from impressive as well as often difficult to interpret *vis-à-vis* the underlying stimulus dimension, some of the data in infant auditory perception do suggest that infants perceive some stimuli as more discrepant than others (*i.e.,* two points on the inverted U-function). In one study of this hypothesis in which only two levels of discrepancy were employed (Melson and McCall, 1970), 5-month-old girls were habituated to an eight-note tonal sequence and then presented with either a small discrepancy (two notes rearranged) or a large discrepancy (all notes rearranged). Those infants that rapidly habituated to the initial sequence revealed a "greater HR deceleration" on the large discrepancy test trials than on the small discrepancy test trials. An inspection of the data suggests that this effect was due to relatively more habituation of the response to the small discrepancy change during the last two of four test trials. In other words, these infants responded to differing degrees of discrepancy with differential rates of habituation to the new stimuli, rather than with a larger initial OR to the more discrepant stimulus. In a subsequent study McCall and Melson (1970) demonstrated that the amount of recovery in 5½-month-old boys to a discrepant stimulus (the large discrepancy stimulus change of the previous study) increased as a function of the number of habituation trials (4, 8, 12). A more systematic exploration of the infant's response to qualitative as well as quantitative discrepancy has been recently carried out by Horowitz (1972). Following habituation to a sequence of two 5-sec tones (400 and 1000 Hz), infants 6 months of age were given either a change in the initial tone (700 and 1000 Hz), in the final tone (400 and 700 Hz), in the order of the tones (1000 and 400 Hz), or a no-change control which was followed by a change in both tones (600 and 2000 Hz). Dishabituation of the cardiac component of the OR was observed in only the initial change and reversal conditions. In view of the differences in paradigm, stimulus duration, and subject age, it is difficult to know how to reconcile these findings with the demonstration that infants 40–54 days of age can discriminate both initial and final acoustic changes in the stimulus (Morse, 1972).

In summarizing these preliminary findings in the infant's response to differing types of discrepancy, it should be pointed out that each of these three studies represents a different and important aspect of research into the microgenetic development of the infant. One aspect of linguistic coding which is particularly related to this avenue of research involves the infant's discrimination of different phonetic features; *i.e.,* does the infant discriminate some features earlier than others (McCaffrey, 1973, in press) and if so, is this independent of the acoustic differences of the minimal-pairs? A second and related question is whether values of a given feature that are acoustically more discrepant from other values of this feature are perceived as such by the infant. The data collected by Morse (1972) and Eimas *et al.* (1971) would suggest that either the HAS paradigm is not sensitive to between-feature differences or the infant 1–2 months of age discriminates place, voicing, and intonational "features" equally well.

Development of Speech Perception and Production

Distinctive Features. Jakobson (Jakobson, Fant, and Halle, 1952) has proposed that the development of speech can be represented by an ordered sequence of acquired feature contrasts. Although support for this hypothesis derives mostly from data on the development of speech production, McCaffrey (1973, in press) has recently provided data on the perceptual development of coronal *vs.* noncoronal features in infants 3–7 months of age. Employing a modified HR paradigm with natural speech stimuli, he tested the discriminability of various phoneme contrasts involving the consonants [p, t, k, s, n], *e.g.,* [papa] *vs.* [tata]. His findings indicated that infants discriminated more often and at an earlier age consonantal stimuli which differed according to the feature "coronal" ([p/t, t/p, k/t, t/k, k/s, k/n]), rather than features other than coronal ([p/k, k/p, t/s]).[6] Although neither Morse (1972) nor Moffitt (1971) examined the discrimination of coronal contrasts, they both observed that infants 5–6 weeks and 5–6 months, respectively, could discriminate [ba] *vs.* [ga], a noncoronal contrast. The Eimas *et al.* (1971) data suggest an even earlier discrimination of a noncoronal contrast ([ba] *vs.* [pa]).

Perhaps the most productive way in which to interpret the import of McCaffrey's study in relationship to other infant speech perception research (*e.g.,* Eimas *et al.,* 1971; Morse, 1972) is to clarify the distinction between distinctive phonetic features and acoustic features. A distinctive phonetic feature (*e.g.,* coronal) is generally considered to be a relatively abstract concept when contrasted with acoustic features (*e.g.,* VOT, F2 transitions). Although perception of acoustic feature information is necessary for the

---

[6]Although McCaffrey's (in press) approach to the development of infant speech perception (*i.e.,* distinctive feature development) is both refreshing and stimulating, several procedural factors complicate the interpretation of his findings. In the modified heart rate paradigm employed by McCaffrey, infants were presented with up to four different "trials" or stimulus shifts. Each trial consisted of a familiarization stage followed immediately by a change sequence (dishabituation) and a subsequent shift back to the original stimulus. All stimuli were presented with 9-sec ISIs and a 3-minute ITI during which the mother was free to interact with her infant. A stimulus shift occurred when the infant was judged to have habituated by *E* (monitoring the infant's overt behavior) or at the end of 10 stimulus presentations. As McCaffrey has acknowledged, such a procedure does permit experimenter bias to play some role in the data collection. Another factor which may be important in interpreting McCaffrey's findings is the tendency (in subjects receiving both coronal and noncoronal contrasts) for the noncoronal ones to be presented on somewhat later trials than coronal contrasts (this is more pronounced in the younger subjects). If any increase in irritability or drowsiness occurred over trials, (only 2 of the 10 younger subjects tested received all four trials), then the absence of noncoronal discrimination (especially in the younger infants) may be somewhat difficult to interpret. Information (not provided by McCaffrey) about variations in both pretrial initial levels and the number of stimulus presentations necessary for habituation *for each type of trial* might help to dispel some of these concerns.

extraction or construction of a distinctive phonetic feature, the latter need not rely solely on a set of acoustic invariants. In fact, one clear demonstration of the abstract quality of a distinctive feature would be its independence from an acoustic 1:1 relationship. Such a demonstration has two implications for infant research: 1) a paradigm which merely assesses discrimination of stimulus pairs will be inadequate, and 2) in order to eliminate confounding acoustic and distinctive phonetic features, stimuli will have to be employed in which these two levels of features can be separated, *i.e.*, synthetic speech stimuli, rather than natural ones. Since McCaffrey employed natural speech in a discrimination paradigm, his study cannot speak directly to the issue of distinctive phonetic feature perception. Since Eimas *et al.* and Morse also employed discrimination paradigms, their data also fail to speak to the infant's perception of distinctive phonetic features as conceptualized by Jakobson and his colleagues. However, since they employed synthetic stimuli, their data do suggest that at a very early age the infant is able to discriminate important linguistic information in the acoustic features VOT and F2 and F3 transitions. In all fairness to McCaffrey, his study was designed to be but a preliminary investigation of the perception of distinctive phonetic features in infancy. It should now be clear that a more systematic exploration of the development of the relationship between the levels of acoustic feature perception and distinctive phonetic perception (*à la* Jakobson) is an important next step in our understanding of coding in early language development.

Motor Theory. A second aspect of the relationship between infant speech perception and production involves the motor theory of speech perception. The finding that the discrimination of speech contrasts precedes their production raises an interesting issue about adult speech perception. If the speech code of adult speech perception is presumed to be based on motor production rules (Liberman *et al.*, 1967), then is this assumption not false if infants can discriminate in a linguistically relevant manner speech contrasts which they cannot yet produce? A strong version of the motor theory of speech perception (*e.g.*, Allport, 1924) would indeed be embarrassed by the infant perception data. However, an alternative version of the motor theory suggests that "knowledge" about articulatory maneuvers and the human vocal tract is not necessarily acquired ontogenetically but has been phylogenetically acquired. Recent evidence regarding the evolution of the vocal tract (Lieberman, Crelin, and Klatt, 1972) is consistent with this view. However, if the perceptual system is organized phylogenetically with respect to production, *e.g.*, with a "model" of the vocal tract (Morse, 1971b), it becomes somewhat difficult to test such a theory directly by studying infant speech perception (short of single-cell recording). The investigation of the organization of the perceptual system of a phylogenetically related species who possesses an auditory system similar to man's, but who will never possess the production categories of man offers an indirect test of this version of the motor theory.

THE MODEL: PRESENT AND FUTURE

Although our "preliminary model" of infant speech perception has facilitated the organization of a vast body of data on infant auditory/speech perception, do the data really support it as a model? At least two aspects of the literature reviewed suggest that this question may be premature.

1. The discriminative capabilities attributed to the more advanced levels of linguistic coding have not been investigated at all or they have not been studied in very young infants (*e.g.*, 4–6 weeks is the youngest age studied for "auditory and linguistic phonetic perception").

2. The results of those investigations which pertain to the ontogeny of linguistic coding are often difficult to interpret because the microgenetic development of the infant appears to be influencing the results obtained with different paradigms. Consequently, the usefulness of the present model can best be determined by studying these two deficiencies in our understanding of the ontogeny of infant speech perception.

In extending our knowledge of "auditory and linguistic" as well as "complex" phonetic perception, a number of specific studies suggest themselves. Specific cues which need to be investigated involve those for nasality, vowels, and fricatives. For example, since fricatives are relatively less universal among the languages of the world, the acoustic cues which differentiate fricatives might be expected to be discriminated much later by the developing infant than cues which signal universal phonemes. Secondly, since fricatives are less encoded (*e.g.*, show less context-conditioned variability) than stop consonants, their discrimination might reveal more "auditory" than "linguistic" perception in infants. The study of consonant perception in differing vowel (*e.g.*, [d] in [di] and [du]) and/or vocal tract environments, as well as in varying multisyllabic and complex syllabic contexts, will provide us with needed information about the ontogeny of "complex" phonetic coding in the infant.

Our understanding of the concomitant role of microgenetic development can be advanced by at least three related avenues of research. First, the ontogenetic comparison of consonant *vs.* vowel and speech *vs.* nonspeech categorical discrimination (Mattingly *et al.*, 1971; Pisoni, 1971) under varying information-processing constraints (memory loads) will permit us to track the interaction of microgenetic and auditory/linguistic coding in the developing infant. Secondly, a systematic investigation of the nature of the information-processing constraints of at least the HR (discrete-trial and modified versions) and HAS paradigms is badly needed (Graham (1973) provides an excellent review of the HR habituation literature in adults; see Jeffrey and Cohen (1971) for a review of some of the infant habituation literature). Finally, other aspects of microgenetic coding need to be explored as they relate to speech perception. These include a developmental investigation of preperceptual and long term store in the infant.

In summary, this "preliminary model" states that we can better understand the existing data and more intelligently guide our future research in infant speech perception if we consider the development of both linguistic and microgenetic coding in the infant. Furthermore, since it has been suggested by several investigators that retardation may be accompanied by memory deficiencies, any assessment of linguistic retardation in early infancy demands that the development of both linguistic and microgenetic coding be considered together.

REFERENCES

Abramson, A. S. and Lisker, L. Discriminability along the voicing continuum: Cross-language tests. In *Proceedings of Sixth International Congress on Phonetic Sciences, Prague, 1967.* Prague: Academic Publishing House of Czechoslovakian Academy of Sciences, 1970, pp. 569–573.

Allport, F. H. *Social Psychology.* Boston: Houghton Mifflin, 1924.

Aronson, E. and Rosenbloom, S. Space perception in early infancy: Perception within a common auditory-visual space. *Science,* 1971, *172,* 1161–1163.

Barnet, A. and Goodwin, A. Averaged evoked electroencephalographic responses to clicks in the human newborn. *Electroencephalogr. Clin. Neurophysiol.,* 1965, *18,* 441–450.

Bartoshuk, A. K. Human neonatal cardiac acceleration to sound: Habituation and dishabituation. *Percept. Mot. Skills,* 1962, *15,* 15–27.

Bartoshuk, A. K. Human neonatal cardiac responses to sound: A power function. *Psychonom. Sci.,* 1964, *1,* 151–152.

Bast, T. and Anson, B. *The Temporal Bone and the Ear.* Springfield, Ill.: Thomas, 1949.

Berg, W. K. Habituation and dishabituation of cardiac responses in awake, four month old infants. Unpublished doctoral dissertation, University of Wisconsin, Madison, 1971.

Berg, W. K. Cardiac orienting at 6 and 16 weeks. Paper presented at the meetings of the Society for Psychophysiological Research, Boston, Mass., Nov., 1972.

Berg, K. M., Berg, W. K., and Graham, F. K. Infant heart rate response as a function of stimulus and state. *Psychophysiology,* 1971, *8,* 30–44.

Bernard, J. and Sontag, L. W. Fetal reactivity to tonal stimulation: A preliminary report. *J. Genet. Psychol.,* 1947, *70,* 205–210.

Bridger, W. K. Sensory habituation and discrimination in the human neonate. *Amer. J. Psychiat.,* 1961, *117,* 991–996.

Bronshtein, A. I., Antonova, T. G., Kamenetskaya, A. G., Luppova, N. N., and Systova, V. A. On the development of the functions of analyzers in infants and some animals at the early stage of ontogenesis. In *Problems of Evolution of Physiological Functions.* Moscow Academy of Science, 1958. Israel Program for Scientific Translations, 1960, pp. 106–116 (U.S. Dept. of Commerce OTS 60-51066).

Brown, J. W. Orienting responses to repeated auditory stimuli in alert six- and nine-week-old infants. Unpublished master's thesis, University of Wisconsin, Madison, 1972.

Bühler, C. and Hetzer, H. Das erste Verständnis für Ausdruck im ersten Lebensjahr. *Z. Psychol.,* 1928, *117,* 50—61.

Butterfield, E. C. and Siperstein, G. N. Influence of contingent auditory stimulation upon non-nutritional suckle. In *Proceedings of Third Symposium on Oral Sensation and Perception: the Mouth of the Infant.* Springfield, Ill.: Thomas, in press.

Cairns, G. F. The use of a tonal distraction paradigm to study two aspects of auditory processing in the neonate. Unpublished doctoral dissertation, Emory University, Atlanta, 1971.

Chomsky, N. *Aspects of the Theory of Syntax.* Cambridge, Mass.: M.I.T. Press, 1965.

Chun, R. W. N., Pawsat, R., and Forster, F. M. Sound localization in infancy. *J. Nerv. Ment. Dis.,* 1960, *130,* 472—476.

Clifton, R. K. Heart rate conditioning in the newborn infant. Paper presented at meetings of the Society for Psychophysiological Research, St. Louis, Nov., 1971.

Clifton, R. K. Cardiac conditioning and orienting in the infant. In P. A. Obrist, J. Brener, L. DiCara, and A. H. Black (Eds.), *Contemporary Trends in Cardiovascular Psychophysiology.* New York: Aldine, 1973.

Clifton, R. K., Graham, F. K., and Hatton, H. M. Newborn heart-rate response and response habituation as a function of stimulus duration. *J. Exp. Child Psych.,* 1968, *6,* 265—278.

Clifton, R. K. and Meyers, W. J. The heart-rate response of four-month-old infants to auditory stimuli. *J. Exp. Child. Psych.,* 1969, *7,* 122—135.

Clifton, R. K., Meyers, W. J., and Solomons, G. Methodological problems in conditioning the headturning response of newborn infants. *J. Exp. Child Psych.,* 1972, *13,* 29—42.

Clifton, R. K., Siqueland, E. R., and Lipsitt, L. P. Conditioned head turning in human newborns as a function of conditioned response requirements and states of wakefulness. *J. Exp. Child Psych.,* 1972, *13,* 43—57.

Dorman, M., Port, D., Brady-wood, S., and Turvey, M. Forward and backward masking of short vowels. Paper presented at the 85th Meeting of the Acoustical Society of America, Boston, April, 1973.

Dwornicka, B., Jasieńska, A., Smolarz, W., and Wawryk, R. Attempt of determining the fetal reaction to acoustic stimulation. *Acta Oto-laryngol.,* 1964, *57,* 571—574.

Eimas, P. D. Developmental studies of speech perception. In L. B. Cohen and P. Salapatek (Eds.), *Infant Perception.* New York: Academic Press, in press.

Eimas, P. D., Siqueland, E. R., Jusczyk, P., and Vigorito, J. Speech perception in infants. *Science,* 1971, *171,* 303—306.

Eisenberg, R. B. Auditory behavior in the human neonate: I. Methodologic problems and the logical design of research procedures. *J. Audit. Res.,* 1965, *5,* 159—177.

Eisenberg, R. B. The organization of auditory behavior. *J. Speech Hear. Res.,* 1970, *13,* 453—471.

Eisenberg, R. B., Griffin, E. J., Coursin, D. B., and Hunter, M. A. Auditory behavior in the human neonate: A preliminary report. *J. Speech Hearing Res.,* 1964, *7,* 245—269.

Fodor, J. A., Garrett, M. F., and Shapero, D. B. Discrimination among phones by infants. *Quarterly Progress Rep. No. 96,* Res. Lab. Electronics, M.I.T., Cambridge, Mass., 1970, p. 180.

Fry, D. B. The development of the phonological system in the normal and the deaf child. In F. Smith and G. A. Miller (Eds.), *The Genesis of Language: A Psycholinguistic Approach.* Cambridge, Mass.: M.I.T. Press, 1966, pp. 187–206.

Fujisaki, H. and Kawashima, T. On the modes and mechanisms of speech perception. *Ann. Rep. Engin. Res. Inst., Vol. 28,* Faculty of Engineering, Univ. of Tokyo, Tokyo, 1969, pp. 67–73.

Graham, F. K. Habituation and dishabituation of responses innervated by the autonomous nervous system. In H. Peeke and M. Herz (Eds.), *Habituation: Behavioral Studies and Physiological Substrates.* New York: Academic Press, 1973, pp. 163–218.

Graham, F. K. and Clifton, R. K. Heart-rate change as a component of the orienting response. *Psychol. Bull.,* 1966, *65,* 305–320.

Graham, F. K. and Jackson, J. C. Arousal systems and infant heart rate responses. In L. P. Lipsitt and H. W. Reese (Eds.), *Advances in Child Development and Behavior,* Vol. 5. New York: Academic Press, 1970, pp. 54–117.

Grimwade, J. C., Walker, D. W., Bartlett, M., Gordon, S., and Wood, C. Human fetal heart rate change and movement in response to sound and vibration. *Amer. J. Obstet. Gynecol.,* 1971, *109,* 86–90.

Haith, M. M. Developmental changes in visual information processing and short-term visual memory. *Hum. Develop.,* 1971, *14,* 249–261.

Hatton, H. M. Developmental change in infant heart rate response during sleeping and waking states. Unpublished dissertation, University of Wisconsin, Madison, 1969.

Hatton, H. M., Berg, W. K., and Graham, F. K. Effects of acoustic rise time on heart rate responses. *Psychonom. Sci.,* 1970, *19,* 101–103.

Horowitz, A. B. Habituation and memory: Infant cardiac responses to familiar and discrepant auditory stimuli. *Child Develop.,* 1972, *43,* 43–53.

Hutt, S. J., Hutt, C., Lenard, H. G., Bernuth, H. v., and Muntjewerff, W. J. Auditory responsivity in the human newborn. *Nature,* 1968, *218,* 888–890.

Jakobson, R., Fant, C. G. M., and Halle, M. *Preliminaries to Speech Analysis.* Cambridge, Mass.: M.I.T. Press, 1952.

Jeffrey, W. E. and Cohen, L. B. Habituation in the human infant. In H. W. Reese (Ed.), *Advances in Child Development and Behavior,* Vol. 6. New York: Academic Press, 1971, pp. 123–176.

Johansson, B., Wedenberg, E., and Westin, B. Measurement of tone response by the human foetus: A preliminary report. *Acta Oto-laryngol.,* 1964, *57,* 188–192.

Kaplan, E. L. The role of intonation in the acquisition of language. Unpublished doctoral dissertation, Cornell University, Ithaca, 1969.

Kaplan, E. L. and Kaplan, G. A. The prelinguistic child. In J. Eliot (Ed.), *Human Development and Cognitive Processes.* New York: Holt, Rhinehart, and Winston, 1971, pp. 358–381.

Kearsley, R. B. The newborn's responses to auditory stimulation: A demonstration of orienting and defensive behaviors. *Child Develop.,* 1973, *44,* 582–590.

Kessen, W., Haith, M. M., and Salapatek, P. H. Human infancy: A bibliography and guide. In P. H. Mussen (Ed.), *Carmichael's Manual of Child Psychology,* Ed. 3. New York: Wiley, 1970, pp. 287–445.

Leavitt, L. A., Morse, P. A., Brown, J. W., and Graham, F. K. Cardiac orienting in speech and nonspeech stimuli in six-week-old infants. *Pediat. Res.*, 1973, *7*, No. 4. Paper presented at the annual meetings of the Society for Pediatric Research, San Francisco, May, 1973.

Lenard, H. G., Bernuth, H. v., and Hutt, S. J. Acoustic evoked responses in newborn infants: The influence of pitch and complexity of the stimulus. *Electroencephalogr. Clin. Neurophysiol.*, 1969, *27*, 121–127.

Lenneberg, E. H. *Biological Foundations of Language.* New York: Wiley, 1967.

Leventhal, A. S. and Lipsitt, L. P. Adaptation, pitch discrimination, and sound localization in the neonate. *Child Develop.*, 1964, *35*, 759–767.

Lewis, M. M. *Infant Speech.* London: Kegan Paul, Trench, and Trubner, 1936.

Liberman, A. M. The grammars of speech and language. *Cognitive Psychol.*, 1970, *1*, 301–323.

Liberman, A. M., Cooper, F. S., Shankweiler, D., and Studdert-Kennedy, M. Perception of the speech code. *Psychol. Rev.*, 1967, *74*, 431–461.

Liberman, A. M., Delattre, P. C., and Cooper, F. S. The role of selected stimulus variables in the perception of the unvoiced stop consonants. *Amer. J. Psychol.*, 1952, *65*, 497–516.

Liberman, A. M., Mattingly, I. G., and Turvey, M. Language codes and memory codes. In A. Melton and E. Martin (Eds.), *Coding Processes in Human Memory.* New York: Wiley, 1972.

Lieberman, P. *Intonation, Perception, and Language.* Cambridge, Mass.: M.I.T. Press, 1967.

Lieberman, P. Toward a unified phonetic theory. *Linguistic Inquiry*, 1970, *1*, 307–322.

Lieberman, P., Crelin, E. S., and Klatt, D. H. Phonetic ability and related anatomy of the newborn and adult human, Neanderthal man, and the chimpanzee. *Amer. Anthropol.*, 1972, *74*, 287–307.

Löwenfeld, B. Reaktionen der Säuglinge auf Klänge und Geräusche. *Z. Psychol.*, 1927, *104*, 62–96.

Massaro, D. W. Preperceptual images, processing time, and perceptual units in auditory perception. *Psychol. Rev.*, 1972, *79*, 124–145.

Mattingly, I. G., Liberman, A. M., Syrdal, A. K., and Halwes, T. Discrimination in speech and nonspeech modes. *Cognitive Psychol.*, 1971, *2*, 131–157.

McBane, B. Short-term memory and dimensional independence in retardates. Unpublished doctoral dissertation, University of Connecticut, Storrs, 1972.

McCaffrey, A. Phonological universals and natural speech sound differentiation by infants in the first seven months of life. Paper presented at the meetings of the Society for Research in Child Development, Philadelphia, March, 1973.

McCaffrey, A. *Speech Perception in Infancy.* The Hague: Mouton, in press.

McCall, R. B. and Melson, W. H. Amount of short-term familiarization and the response to auditory discrepancies. *Child Develop.*, 1970, *41*, 861–869.

McNeill, D. Developmental psycholinguistics. In F. Smith and G. A. Miller (Eds.), *The Genesis of Language: A Psycholinguistic Approach.* Cambridge, Mass: M.I.T. Press, 1966.

Melson, W. H. and McCall, R. B. Attentional responses of five-month girls to discrepant auditory stimuli. *Child Develop.*, 1970, *41*, 1159–1171.

Moffitt, A. R. Speech perception by infants. Unpublished doctoral dissertation, University of Minnesota, Minneapolis, 1968.

Moffitt, A. R. Consonant cue perception by twenty- to twenty-four-week-old infants. *Child Develop.*, 1971, *42*, 717–731.

Molfese, D. L. Cerebral asymmetry in infants, children and adults: Auditory evoked responses to speech and noise stimuli. Unpublished doctoral dissertation, Pennsylvania State University, University Park, 1972.

Morse, P. A. The discrimination of speech and nonspeech stimuli in early infancy. Unpublished doctoral dissertation, University of Connecticut, Storrs, 1971a.

Morse, P. A. Speech perception in six-week-old infants. Paper presented at the meetings of the Society for Research in Child Development, Minneapolis, April, 1971b.

Morse, P. A. The discrimination of speech and nonspeech stimuli in early infancy. *J. Exp. Child Psychol.*, 1972, *14*, 477–492.

Morse, P. A. and Dorman, M. F. Toward an information-flow model for the development of speech perception. Unpublished paper, 1970.

Morse, P. A., Leavitt, L. A., Brown, J. W., and Graham, F. K. The cardiac orienting response to changes in speech and nonspeech stimuli in six-week-old infants (tentative title), in preparation.

Ormerod, F. C. The pathology of congenital deafness in the child. In A. Ewing (Ed.), *The Modern Educational Treatment of Deafness.* Manchester, England: Manchester University Press, 1960.

Pisoni, D. B. On the nature of categorical perception of speech sounds. Unpublished doctoral dissertation, University of Michigan, Ann Arbor, 1971.

Pisoni, D. B. Perceptual processing time for consonants and vowels. Paper presented at the 84th meeting of the Acoustical Society of America, Miami Beach, Dec., 1972.

Pisoni, D. B. Auditory and phonetic memory codes in the discrimination of consonants and vowels. *Percept. Psychophys.*, 1973, *13*, 253–260.

Pomerleau-Malcuit, A. and Clifton, R. K. Neonatal heart rate responses to tactile, auditory, and vestibular stimulation in different states. Unpublished manuscript, 1971 (cited in Clifton, 1973).

Rand, T. Vocal tract size normalization in the perception of stop consonants. *Haskins Status Reports*, 1971, *SR - 25/26*, 141–146.

Salk, L. Mother's heartbeat as an imprinting stimulus. *Ann. N. Y. Acad. Sci.*, 1962, *24*, 753–763.

Sameroff, A. J. Can conditioned responses be established in the newborn infant: 1971? *Develop. Psychol.*, 1971, *4*, 1–12.

Sameroff, A. J. Learning and adaptation in infancy: A comparison of models. In H. W. Reese (Ed.), *Advances in Child Development and Behavior*, Vol. 7. New York: Academic Press, in press.

Sameroff, A. J., Cashmore, T., and Dykes, A. Heart rate deceleration during visual fixation in human newborns. *Develop. Psychol.*, 1973, *8*, 117–119.

Schäfer, P. Beobachtungen und Versuche an einem kinde in der Entwicklungs Periode des reinen Sprachverständnis. *Z. Pädegogische Psychol.*, 1922, *23*, 269–289.

Siperstein, G. Differential modification of neonatal behavior. Paper presented at the meetings of the Society for Research in Child Development, Philadelphia, March, 1973.

Siqueland, E. R. and DeLucia, C. Visual reinforcement of nonnutritive sucking in human infants. *Science*, 1969, *165*, 1144–1146.

Siqueland, E. R. and Lipsitt, L. P. Conditioned head-turning in human newborns. *J. Exp. Child Psychol.,* 1966, *3,* 356–376.

Sokolov, E. N. *Perception and the Conditioned Reflex.* New York: Macmillan, 1963.

Steinschneider, A. Sound intensity and respiratory responses in the neonate. *Psychosom. Med.,* 1968, *30,* 534–541.

Steinschneider, A., Lipton, E. L., and Richmond, J. B. Auditory sensitivity in the infant: Effect of intensity on cardiac and motor responsivity. *Child Develop.,* 1966, *37,* 233–252.

Stevens, K. N. and Klatt, D. H. Role of formant transitions in the voice-voiceless distinction for stops. *J. Acoust. Soc. Amer.,* 1974, *55,* 653–659.

Stevens, K. N., Liberman, A. M., Studdert-Kennedy, M., and Oehman, S. E. G. Cross language study of vowel perception. *Lang. Speech,* 1969, *12,* 1–23.

Studdert-Kennedy, M. The perception of speech. In T. A. Sebeok (Ed.), *Current Trends in Linguistics,* Vol. 12. The Hague: Mouton, 1973.

Studdert-Kennedy, M. and Hadding-Koch, K. Auditory and linguistic processes in the perception of intonation contours. *Haskins Status Reports,* 1971, *SR-27,* 153–174.

Trehub, S. E. and Rabinovitch, M. S. Auditory-linguistic sensitivity in early infancy. *Develop. Psychol.,* 1972, *6,* 74–77.

Tulkin, S. R. Infants' reactions to mother's voice and stranger's voice: Social class differences in the first year of life. Paper presented at the meetings of the Society for Research in Child Development, Minneapolis, April, 1971.

Turkewitz, G., Moreau, T., and Birch, H. G. Head position and receptor organization in the human neonate. *J. Exp. Child Psychol.,* 1966, *4,* 163–177.

Turnure, C. Response to voice of mother and stranger by babies in the first year. *Develop. Psychol.,* 1971, *4,* 182–190.

Wertheimer, M. Psychomotor coordination of auditory and visual space at birth. *Science,* 1961, *134,* 1962.

CHAPTER TWO

LINGUISTIC PROCESSING OF SPEECH BY YOUNG INFANTS[1]

Peter D. Eimas

Department of Psychology, Brown University, Providence, Rhode Island 02912

A number of studies on the perception of speech by very young infants have led to challenging conclusions not only for developmental psychologists, but also for investigators concerned with constructing a theoretical description of the processes underlying the perception of speech. On the one hand, data from these studies strongly indicate that the processing of the segmental units of speech in a linguistic mode begins at an extremely early age. (As will become apparent shortly, it is more appropriate to speak about the processing of phonetic features rather than segmental units.) This phenomenon occurs at such an early age that Kaplan's question, "Is there such a thing as a prelinguistic child?" (Kaplan and Kaplan, 1971) can most likely be answered in the negative. On the other hand, the data require that theoretical formulations of speech processing, at least at the level of phonetics, be revised so as to include statements describing how the biologically determined structure of the infant is able to accomplish that which was originally believed to be the result of considerable experience and interaction with the linguistic environment.

PERCEPTION IN A SPEECH MODE

As Morse (this volume) has indicated, there is considerable evidence from investigations of adult listeners indicating that perception of speech differs sharply from the perception of nonspeech acoustic signals. Perception of the former events occurs in a linguistic mode, whereas perception of the latter class of stimuli occurs in an auditory mode (but see, for example, Massaro, 1972). The behavioral data for this conclusion come from two major classes of

[1] Preparation of this chapter and the author's research reported herein was supported in part by Grant HD 05331 from the National Institute of Child Health and Human Development. I wish to thank Dr. Franklin S. Cooper for his generosity in making the facilities of the Haskins Laboratories available.

experimental paradigms: 1) studies in which listeners (usually adults) are required to identify and discriminate series of synthetically produced speech sounds that vary along a single linguistic feature, and 2) studies in which listeners (again usually adults) are required to identify dichotically presented speech sounds (either real or synthetic). Data from the former indicate that listeners are extremely consistent in assigning stimuli to phonetic categories. This is particularly true for those features that distinguish the stop consonants: voice onset time (Lisker and Abramson, 1964) which when acoustically varied is sufficient for the perceived distinctions among the voiced and voiceless stops, that is, between [b] and [p], [d] and [t], and [g] and [k], and place of articulation, for which variations in the acoustic representation of this feature are sufficient for the perceived distinctions among the voiced ([b,d,g]) and voiceless ([p,t,k]) stops. Of particular interest, however, are the discriminability functions for the features of voicing and place of articulation. These functions are marked by peaks of discriminability at the region of the phonetic boundaries and very near chance levels of discriminability for within-phonetic-category comparisons. In other words, the discriminability of a given acoustic difference is markedly better when the two speech stimuli are from different phonetic categories than when they are acoustic variations of the same phonetic category. Furthermore, the discriminability functions can be reasonably predicted, with respect to both shape and level, from the extreme categorical assumption that listeners can only discriminate two stimuli to the extent that they can assign differential phonetic labels (Studdert-Kennedy, Liberman, Harris, and Cooper, 1970). This form of perception has been termed categorical (Liberman, Cooper, Shankweiler, and Studdert-Kennedy, 1967), and it is to be contrasted with the nearly continuous form of perception found with nonspeech acoustic stimuli, where discriminability is typically many times better than identifiability (Eimas, 1963; Miller, 1956).

The perception of synthetic steady state vowels is not nearly as categorical as the perception of stop consonants (*e.g.,* Fry, Abramson, Eimas, and Liberman, 1962; Stevens, Liberman, Studdert-Kennedy, and Ohman, 1969), although as conditions more closely approximate real speech (vowels of shorter duration, for example) perception becomes more categorical (Pisoni, 1973; Fujisaki and Kawashima, 1968). For more extensive reviews of related literature, the reader is referred to Liberman (1957; 1970), Liberman *et al.* (1967), Pisoni (1973), Studdert-Kennedy *et al.* (1970), Studdert-Kennedy (1970), and Stevens and House (1972).

Differences between the perception of speech and nonspeech events are further evidenced when the perception of the same acoustic dimension is compared under two conditions: when variations in this dimension signal phonetic distinctions, and when the same variations are present, but in a nonspeech context (see Liberman, Harris, Eimas, Lisker, and Bastion, 1961; Liberman, Harris, Kinney, and Lane, 1961; Mattingly, Liberman, Syrdal, and

Halwes, 1971). Evidently activation of the speech-processing mechanism requires that a sufficient number of the cues for perceived distinctions among phonetic segments must be present. Failure to meet the threshold requirement results in a failure to activate the speech mechanisms, and, consequently, perception in an auditory mode occurs as evidenced by the noncategorical nature of the perception (*cf.* Eimas, Cooper, and Corbit, 1973).

The results from studies of dichotically presented speech signals also provide behavioral evidence that there are specialized mechanisms for the processing of speech. In summary, it has been found that speech signals are better perceived by the right ear (and consequently left hemisphere), whereas nonspeech events are better perceived by the left ear or right hemisphere (*e.g.*, Kimura, 1961; 1964; Studdert-Kennedy and Shankweiler, 1970). Moreover, Studdert-Kennedy and Shankweiler (1970) were able to conclude " . . . that, while the general auditory system may be equipped to extract auditory parameters of a speech signal, the dominant hemisphere is specialized for the extraction of linguistic features from these parameters" (pp. 592–593). Indeed, it would appear that the perception of speech is based upon the ability of listeners to extract phonetic and other linguistic features and that the extraction of linguistic features is a process reserved for the specialized speech processor found in the dominant hemisphere. (For a description of phonetic feature systems, see Jakobson, Fant, and Halle, 1963; Halle, 1964; Chomsky and Halle, 1968.) Moreover, it is because the segmental units of speech are processed with reference to these distinctive phonetic (*i.e.*, linguistic) features that we are able to observe such behavioral effects as categorical perception and the right ear advantage. These effects are the behavioral manifestations of perception in a linguistic mode.[2]

Recently, there have been a number of electrophysiological studies which support the hypothesis that speech signals undergo specialized processing by mechanisms localized within the brain. For example, Wood, Goff, and Day (1971) and Molfese (1972) have shown greater cortical activity on the left side of the brain for speech signals, whereas the right hemisphere is more responsive to nonspeech signals. Of particular interest were the data from Molfese's dissertation indicating lateralization of speech-processing mechanisms in infants as young as 1 week of age. In addition, Dorman (1972) found that the categorical perception of voice onset time may also be evidenced by the electrophysiological measure of averaged evoked potential. The behavioral

---

[2] In retrospect, we can see that, when we speak of the perception of segmental units of speech, we are in fact referring to the perception of distinctive phonetic features. This is especially the case in those studies with synthetic speech that typically presented variations in a single feature (*e.g.*, voice onset time or place of articulation) for identification and discrimination. There is also other evidence for the reality of distinctive features that comes from a number of studies on the short term retention of phonetic segments (Cole, Haber, and Sales, 1968; Cole, Sales, and Haber, 1969; Hintzman, 1967; Sales, Haber, and Cole, 1969; Wickelgren, 1966, 1969, to cite but some of the literature).

and physiological measures were in remarkably close agreement. The data, in summary, appear unequivocal in support of the hypothesis that the segmental units of speech are processed by mechanisms specialized for the analysis and extraction of linguistic information, in this case, the phonetic features.

INFANT STUDIES OF SPEECH PERCEPTION

The goal of many studies of infant speech perception has been to determine the extent to which the infant is capable of perceiving speech by reference to a linguistic or phonetic feature analysis, that is, the extent to which perception of segmental units (phonetic features) could be characterized as being in a linguistic mode.

As Morse (this volume) has noted in some detail, we have used the high amplitude sucking response as the dependent variable. The experimental paradigm can best be described as a satiation and release-from-satiation procedure. After establishing a baseline of high amplitude sucking (*i.e.,* using an amplitude criterion that provides approximately 20–30 responses per minute), the presentation of an auditory stimulus (in our studies a synthetic speech pattern) is made contingent either upon the rate of high amplitude sucking (Eimas, Siqueland, Jusczyk, and Vigorito, 1971) or upon the emission of each high amplitude response. The latter schedule has been used in all of our subsequent studies. What typically occurs is that each individual infant increases his sucking rate shortly after initiation of the contingency. After a variable amount of time, the rate of sucking decreases, presumably because of a loss of the reinforcing properties associated with novel stimulation. When the sucking rate has decreased by 20% or more for 2 consecutive minutes (compared with the conditioned sucking rate for the minute immediately preceding the 1st minute of decrement), the infant is presented with a new auditory pattern without interruption, the presentation of which is again made contingent upon the infant's production of high amplitude sucking responses. After 4 min of exposure to the second stimulus, the experiment is terminated. Control subjects do not receive a shift in stimulation. Their data, however, are fully comparable to those of the experimental subjects in that the point at which a shift in stimulation would have occurred is marked and they are maintained in the experiment for 4 additional minutes. The control listeners provide evidence to counter the argument that any increment in sucking associated with a shift in stimulation is a function of the cyclical nature of the sucking response. Thus, if the experimental listeners show an increment in sucking associated with a change in auditory feedback that is greater than that shown by the control subjects, or if they show a decrement in performance (sucking rate) that is less than that shown by the control subjects, one is able to infer that the difference between the two patterns of stimulation was discriminable.

Discrimination of Voice Onset Time

From this procedure and the logic underlying it, it becomes possible not only to test the infant's ability to discriminate acoustic cues underlying adult phonetic contrasts, but also to obtain evidence regarding the nature of this perception, that is, whether perception is categorical (linguistic) in nature. Thus, in our first experiment, we compared the ability of 1- and 4-month-old infants to discriminate a 20-msec difference in voice onset time under two conditions. In the first condition (D), the two stimuli were from different adult phonetic categories, [b] *and* [p]. In the second condition (S), the two stimuli were acoustic variations of the same adult phonetic category, *either* [b] *or* [p]. Were the infants to indicate greater discriminability for the between-phonetic-category condition and should the within-phonetic-category condition not differ from the control groups, then it would be possible to infer not only that our infants were capable of perceiving differences in phonetic features (phonetic contrasts), but also that perception was linguistic in nature.

Examination of Table 1, which shows the mean recovery data (the mean response rate for the initial 2 min of stimulus shift minus the mean of the response rate for the 2 min prior to the shift in stimulation), reveals that this is exactly what happened. An over-all analysis of variance of these data yielded a significant treatments effect ($p < 0.01$); individual comparisons revealed that group D showed reliably greater amounts of recovery than did either of the other groups, which in turn did not differ from each other. Similar effects are obtained when the entire 4 min of post-shift sucking rates are used. From this Eimas *et al.* (1971) concluded that evidence for perception in a linguistic mode was obtained in listeners " . . . with limited exposure to speech, as well as with virtually no experience in producing the same sounds and certainly with little, if any, differential reinforcement for this form of behavior" (p. 306).

Table 1. Mean Recovery Data (responses per min) for the Initial 2 min after Shift in Stimulation.*

Age	Experimental conditions†		
	Group D	Group S	Group C
mos			
1	8.3	2.8	−4.1
4	12.3	−2.6	−7.1

*Data from Eimas *et al.*, 1971.
†Stimuli were from the [b-p] series.

Shortly after publication of this study we undertook a second study both to establish the reliability of these findings and to extend their generality. In this study, we again investigated the infant's ability to detect differences along the dimension of voice onset time. However, in this instance, voice onset time served to distinguish the voiced and voiceless stops [d] and [t], respectively. The difference in voice onset time was increased to 50 msec in order to determine whether a larger acoustic difference might permit discriminability based on auditory features. Our experimental procedure was similar to that of the first study except that control subjects were omitted, the infants were either 2 or 3 months of age, and presentation of the stimulus was response-contingent rather than rate-contingent; that is, each high amplitude response resulted in one presentation of a 500-msec synthetic speech pattern plus 500 msec of silence.

The results are shown in Table 2. Again the differences between groups S and D were large and reliable. There would appear to be no doubt that infants between the ages of 1 and 4 months are capable of processing voicing information in a linguistic manner.[3] Moreover, when we put all our data together on the infant's ability to detect differences in voice onset time (VOT), a most interesting finding becomes apparent: infant listeners are insensitive to differences in voice onset time, provided that the two stimuli come from different adult phonetic categories. Prior to this study, we had tested a number of infants with stimuli from different voicing categories, in this instance [b] and [p], but where the difference in voice onset time between the two stimuli varied. Groups of 1- and 4-month-old infants were tested with voicing differences of 100 and 60 msec. The results shown in Table 3 give mean changes in sucking rates when the 2 and 4 min postshift are compared with the 2 min prior to shift. We recognize the possible difficulties in comparing groups of infants tested at different times, but the results are worth considering despite the possible pitfalls. It is apparent that the absolute

Table 2. Mean Recovery Data (responses per min) for the [d-t] Series of Stimuli

Recovery time	Experimental conditions	
	Group D	Group S
min		
2	10.4	−5.1
4	9.7	−7.3

[3] This conclusion applies to the voiced-voiceless distinction. Whether infants are also capable of processing the third voicing distinction, prevoicing, which is found in some languages, Thai, for example, has not been unequivocally resolved. For a summary of the evidence on this point, the reader is referred to Eimas (in press) and Morse (this volume).

Table 3. The Mean Increment in Response Rate (responses per min) during the First 2 min or Entire 4 min after a Change in Auditory Feedback

Response measure	Age	Difference in VOT		
		20*	60	100
	mos	*msec*		
Initial 2 min	1	8.3	10.6	7.6
	4	12.3	8.0	14.2
	Mean	10.3	9.3	10.9
Entire 4 min	1	5.6	8.8	5.3
	4	11.5	7.2	13.1
	Mean	8.5	8.0	9.2

*From Eimas *et al.,* 1971.

difference in VOT makes little difference. Indeed, analyses of the data revealed no statistically significant effects due to the absolute difference in voicing between the two stimuli-to-be-discriminated, age, or the interaction of age and magnitude of stimulus difference. The evidence thus indicates that the mechanisms responsible for detecting differences in voicing are sensitive not to absolute differences in voicing, but rather to whether the particular values of voicing being discriminated represent the same or different phonetic feature values.

Discrimination of Place Cues

More recently, we have begun to investigate the infant's ability to perceive the acoustic correlates of variations in place of articulation. Research with adult listeners, spanning the past 2 decades, has revealed a sufficient cue for the perceived distinctions among the voiced and voiceless stop consonants, [b,d,g] and [p,t,k], respectively. This acoustic cue is the second-formant transition. Variations in the starting frequency and direction of this transition correspond to the variations in articulatory movements necessary for the production of bilabial stops ([b,p]) as opposed to apical stops ([d,t]) and for the production of apical stops as opposed to velar stops ([g,k]). As noted above, when a series of synthetic speech patterns that vary continuously in the starting frequency and direction of the second-formant transition are presented to adult listeners for identification and discrimination, the resulting evidence strongly indicates perception that is categorical, and hence linguistic, in nature. In particular, there are discontinuities in the discriminability functions. For a given acoustic difference, discriminability is markedly better when the two stimuli lie on opposite sides of the phonetic boundary than when they are both from the same phonetic category.

In our first study concerned with the ability of infants to discriminate the acoustic correlates of place of articulation, we compared the discriminability of a given acoustic difference under two conditions: 1) when both stimuli were acoustic variations of the same phonetic category, [d] in this instance, and 2) when the two stimuli were from different phonetic categories, [d] and [g].[4] There was also a third condition, the control condition in which, as before, no change in the auditory pattern was introduced after the initial period of satiation. There were 48 infants 2 and 3 months of age who were randomly assigned to the three groups, D, S, and C. The procedural details were identical to those used in our later studies on the perception of voicing contrasts in infants.

Analyses of the postshift sucking rates (mean response rate for the initial 2 min or entire 4 min of postshift stimulation minus the mean response rates for the 2 min prior to the change in stimulation) revealed a reliable effect due to treatments ($0.05 > p > 0.01$), but only when the data for the entire 4 min of postshift stimulation were used. Individual comparisons revealed that group D, which produced a mean increment of 4.1 responses, differed reliably from groups S and C, which in turn did not differ reliably from each other. In both groups S and C, the mean rate of responding declined over the final 4 min, 6.1 responses in the case of group S and 4.3 responses for group C. We are unable to offer any explanation for the relatively slow recovery displayed by group D. However, it appears to be a reliable effect, inasmuch as in a replication of this study with slightly different stimuli, the same pattern of results was obtained; the differences among the three groups did not attain statistical significance unless the data from the entire 4 min of postshift responding were included.[5]

These results, plus those of Morse (1972), strongly indicate that infants by the age of 2 months are capable of perceiving differences in place of articulation in a manner approximating the categorical perception typically shown by adult listeners. Thus, differences in place of articulation, like differences in voice onset time, would appear to be processed by young infants in a linguistically relevant manner. There of course remains the

---

[4] As noted above, variations in the second-formant transition alone are sufficient for the perceived distinctions among either the voiced or voiceless stop consonants. The addition of a third formant with a varying transition results in greater realism. Moreover, the addition of the third formant does not alter the manner in which these stimuli are perceived. Consequently, we, as well as Morse (1972), have used the more realistic, three-formant patterns.

[5] Interpretation of this study with regard to the categorical nature of the perception must be made with some caution. The absolute differences in the starting frequencies of the third-formant transitions were not equated for groups D and S, the difference being greater in group D than in group S. However, given the overwhelming similarity of the two studies with place cues, it seems highly unlikely that the greater recovery by group D was solely a function of the larger acoustic difference in the third-formant transition.

problem of explaining how infants are able to extract phonetic features and to respond in accordance with the values of these features.[6]

THEORETICAL CONSIDERATIONS

In attempting to understand and explain the capabilities of the infant with respect to the perception of speech, it is appropriate to begin our theoretical quest by examining existing models of speech perception—models that were constructed to accommodate the characteristics of speech and of speech perception in the adult listener. However, rather than review all such models, we will concentrate on the analysis-by-synthesis model, offered by Stevens and his colleagues (*e.g.,* Stevens and Halle, 1967; Stevens and House, 1972). The reasons for this decision are, first, that the Stevens position is representative of many theoretical statements on the perception of speech (*cf.* Cooper, 1972; Liberman, 1957; Liberman *et al.,* 1967; Studdert-Kennedy, 1970) and, second, that it is the more explicit and developed theoretical position, especially in its most recent form (Stevens and House, 1972).

The Analysis-by-Synthesis Model

Stevens and House have assumed a number of processing stages prior to the final perceptual experience. Speech signals and nonspeech signals initially undergo a series of transformations by peripheral auditory structures. This peripheral analysis imposes " . . . on the input signal a much more radical transformation than a simple frequency analysis" (Stevens and House, 1972,

---

[6] In a study currently in progress, two groups (D and S) of 2- and 3-month-old infants were presented two-formant synthetic speech patterns that varied only in the starting frequency and direction of the second-formant transition for discrimination. The absolute acoustic difference between the two stimuli was the same for both groups. Two additional groups were presented the same second-formant transitions for discrimination, but now the transitions were presented in isolation, each of which was about 45 msec in duration and was perceived by adult listeners as, for example, a rising "chirp." For greater detail concerning the stimuli, the reader should consult Mattingly *et al.,* 1971. Variations in the second-formant transition were discriminated in a nearly categorical manner, when the stimuli were speech-like. When the same variations were presented as brief chirps, there was no evidence for categorical perception. An over-all analysis of variance of the recovery data for the entire 4 min of postshift stimulation revealed a highly significant stimuli (speech *vs.* chirps) by type of shift interaction. The two groups presented the chirp stimuli did not differ reliably from group D, which was presented with the speech-like stimuli. However, all three of these groups, which incidently showed an increment in the sucking rate during the postshift phase, did differ significantly from group S, with the speechlike stimuli. The latter group showed a continued decrement in the rate of sucking during the postshift period. Evidence of this nature strongly supports the contention that there are two modes for the processing of acoustic events: the auditory and the linguistic. Of greatest interest is the fact that young infants are capable of operating in either mode, which mode being determined by the nature of the acoustic input.

p. 48), although the latter information may also be available (see, for example, Studdert-Kennedy, 1970). Stevens and House further hypothesized that some form of normalization of speech occurs at the periphery, which, in essence, yields highly transformed time segments of normalized auditory patterns. These patterns, stored in a temporary memory buffer, are then analyzed for phonetic features during the second stage of processing, the preliminary analysis. Although speech is a highly encoded message (*cf.* Liberman *et al.,* 1967), there are, as Stevens and House noted, some auditory attributes that bear direct relations with phonetic features; that is, the acoustic-auditory properties do not vary markedly with speaker characteristics or linguistic context. These features might include the presence of voicing, as indicated by periodicities in the signal, or the occurrence of a stop consonant, as indicated by low acoustic energy followed by a rapid energy increment and rapidly changing formant transitions.

The output of the peripheral and preliminary analyses and also lexical and contextual information are all available to the central control component of the speech-analyzing system. On the basis of these data, the control component formulates an hypothesis concerning the portion of the utterance under analysis. This hypothesis, at least a syllable in length, is represented by a string of phonetic segments, each of which in turn is defined by a set of abstract phonetic features. These features underlie the processes of perception and production, inasmuch as during production this hypothesized matrix of distinctive features serves as the input to a set of generative rules that transforms distinctive features into articulatory instructions. In the normal course of speech production, articulatory instructions are further translated into articulatory maneuvers and hence into speech (see also Cooper, 1972; Liberman *et al.,* 1967; MacNeilage, 1970). However, during perception, the generated articulatory instructions serve as the input to the comparator component.

In the latest version of the model, the comparison process involves comparing the stored auditory inputs with the auditory representations previously associated with the articulatory instructions. The speaker-listener is assumed to have acquired with development a "catalog of relations between auditory-pattern attributes and articulatory instructions" (Stevens and House, 1972, p. 53). If a match occurs, then the hypothesized phonetic feature matrix becomes available to higher centers for identification (*i.e.,* perception and comprehension). Mismatches result in new synthesis routines until a suitable match is obtained.

On the basis of this model, it is apparent that the processes of perception and production are directly related: the perception of speech is, in a very real sense, the perception of the listener's generation of the received speech signal. Moreover, the analysis-by-synthesis model is capable of accounting for much of the speech perception data in adult listeners, inasmuch as the critical levels of analyses are primarily linguistic rather than auditory. However, because the levels of analyses are linguistic and demand considerable knowledge on the part of the perceiver, difficulties are immediately encountered when the model is extended to account for the infant's ability to perceive speech in a linguistic mode.

In essence, these difficulties arise when we attempt to attribute synthetic or productive abilities to the infant, especially abilities that include rules which translate abstract phonetic features into articulatory instructions and generate internalized auditory patterns from sets of articulatory instructions. There would appear to be no doubt that these abilities exceed by a considerable degree any acquired competence of the preverbal infant, and to ascribe routines of this complexity to innately determined structures would likewise appear to exceed the usual degree of competencies we are willing to attribute to genetically determined factors. However, these criticisms are not a call to abandon in all respects the theoretical model of Stevens and his associates. Indeed, the model as presently constituted may form a very vital part in the perception of speech by more mature and articulate listeners. Although I do not believe that the synthetic portion of the model is always necessary, it might serve as a periodic check on the processes of perception.

Analysis by Linguistic Feature Detectors

If, as our experimental results indicate, the infant is truly able to detect changes in phonetic features and hence is able to process speech with reference to features (see Table 3 for data that indicate that discriminability is related not to stimulus [acoustic] factors but rather to changes in the phonetic structure of the utterance), then what processes are absolutely necessary to accomplish this behavior? I believe a model of speech perception can be constructed that can account for much of the speech perception data of infants, and, incidently, of adults as well, using only the first two stages of the analysis-by-synthesis model with some modifications: the peripheral analysis and a processing stage analogous to, but more complete than, the preliminary phonetic analysis. The peripheral stage of analysis would operate on both speech and nonspeech signals, yielding transformed auditory patterns, segmented by some unit or units of time. The information in the auditory patterns for speech signals would include a relatively simple frequency analysis, as well as more complex units, *e.g.*, information about the rates of frequency changes; the relation in time between the presence of periodicities and the presence of rapidly changing formant frequencies; and perhaps the relation between formant starting frequencies, rates of change, and the final steady state frequencies. Comparable levels of information in terms of complexity must be extracted from nonspeech signals. However, inasmuch as nonspeech signals are further analyzed by processes different from those to which the speech sounds are subjected, further consideration of the perception of nonspeech sounds will not be undertaken.

During the next stage of analysis for speech sounds, phonetic features are extracted from the auditory patterns by processes and mechanisms that are unique to the speech-analyzing system. The actual mechanisms involved, are, we believe, feature detectors analogous to the detector systems that have been found in the visual system of man and other mammals (*e.g.,* Blakemore and Campbell, 1969; Blakemore and Sutton, 1969; McCollough, 1965) and that are part of the basic perceptual apparatus of man. These detectors, which are certainly very high level analyzers of information, are set in operation merely by the presence of sufficient acoustic-auditory information, which has a direct correspondence with phonetic features. That is to say, the receiver of linguistic information does not have to make an initial, conscious decision that linguistic as opposed to nonlinguistic information has been received and that special processing is required. Rather, activation of the speech-processing system is automatic and unconscious, provided only that a minimal number of linguistic cues are present in the transformed auditory patterns (*cf.* Eimas, Cooper, and Corbit, 1973; Mattingly *et al.,* 1971). If these speech-processing analyzers are part of the inherent structure of the organism and need only adequate or sufficient information for their activation, then there is no reason why these detector systems should not be operative at a very early stage of development. Perception, that is, identification, of a phonetic segment occurs when the pattern of activated detectors matches a stored pattern of features previously associated with a permissible (for that language) constellation of phonetic features. Perception thus involves the operation of innately determined structures as well as linguistic knowledge gained from experience with the individual's language environment. Discrimination of any two segments, on the other hand, need involve only feature-analyzing devices; it would not necessarily require identification of the individual segments. Discrimination of phonetic segments (features) would not seem to exceed the perceptual and/or cognitive capabilities of the very young and inarticulate infant. It is only when identification is required or when production processes are brought into play that higher level processes are involved.

One great advantage of this system is that it permits the infant to be a language-recognizing instrument without benefit of active tuition—an instrument that it has not been possible to create in the laboratory for all possible variations in speech. Thus, the child need not learn that there are two classes of sounds, one speech and the other nonspeech, and that different forms of analyses are required for the two classes of sounds. In not having to acquire this information (if such knowledge could be learned), the processes of language acquisition are markedly hastened.

Two further problems related to the hypothesizing of feature detectors that mediate the perception of speech must be considered: the first concerns the evidence for these mechanisms and the second is related to the problem of acoustic (and presumably auditory) invariance in the speech signal. That is, as noted above, a given acoustic cue often differs considerably with the linguistic context and with the characteristics of the speaker (Harris, 1970; Studdert-Kennedy, 1970; Liberman *et al.,* 1967; Stevens and House, 1972). Whereas we can bring to bear some very direct data to the first issue, at the present time we can offer only our speculations on the second.

Evidence for Linguistic Feature Detectors

In our initial experiments (Eimas and Corbit, 1973; Eimas, Cooper and Corbit, 1973), we attempted to obtain data for the existence of linguistic feature detectors that might mediate the perception of the voiced and voiceless stop consonants. The acoustic dimension investigated was voice onset time. This dimension was selected for a number of reasons, including the categorical nature of its perception by infants and adults, its relative insensitivity to linguistic context, its probable universality, and the uniformity which speakers of diverse languages manifest in utilizing this continuum to produce voicing contrasts. All these factors led us to believe that specialized structures might well exist for the perception of voicing contrasts, each of which was differentially tuned to the acoustic consequences of the different modes of producing voicing distinctions. Our experimental procedures essentially involved selectively adapting our listeners to one or the other of the voicing contrasts found in English by the repetitive presentation of a good exemplar of that voicing mode.

Identification functions were obtained with listeners in an adapted state and compared with the identification functions obtained from the same listeners in an unadapted state. We reasoned that if linguistic feature detectors exist for different voicing distinctions, then repeated presentation of the feature to which a detector is sensitive would fatigue the detector and reduce its sensitivity. As a consequence, the assignment of a series of synthetic stop consonants differing in voice onset time only to phonetic categories would be altered. This is exactly what occurred. After adaptation with a voiced stop, listeners assigned fewer stimuli to the voiced category, especially those stimuli near the original, unadapted phonetic boundary. The converse was obtained when a voiceless stop was used for selective adaptation. Thus, in both cases there was a shift in the phonetic boundary toward the adapted voicing category. Of particular interest was the finding that the adaptation effects were very nearly as robust when the adapting stimulus and the stimuli-to-be-identified were from different series of synthetic stimuli. For example, adaptation with the voiced stop [b] altered the phonetic boundary for the apical series of stops [d,t] nearly as effectively as did adaptation with the apical stop [d]. Thus the evidence strongly indicates that the effects of adaptation were to alter the receptivity of the voicing feature that both the adapting stimulus and identification series had in common, presumably by altering the sensitivity of the feature detector that mediates the adapted voicing contrast.

In the second experiment, Eimas and Corbit (1973) tested the effects of selective adaptation on the discriminability function for a series of bilabial synthetic stops that varied in voice onset time alone. We had reasoned that, inasmuch as discriminability is related to the processes of identification, that is to say, to the manner in which acoustic-auditory attributes are assigned to phonetic feature categories, then after adaptation a shift in locus of the phonetic boundary should be closely paralleled by a shift in the peak of the discriminability function. The data confirmed our expectations: there was a decided shift in the locus of the discriminability peak after adaptation with the voiceless stop [p] that matched the shift in the phonetic boundary after adaptation with the same adapting stimulus.

In a later series of experiments, Eimas, Cooper, and Corbit (1973) found that the locus of the adaptation effect was both central and specific to the speech-analyzing system. Thus, when the adapting stimulus was presented to one ear and the stimuli-to-be-identified were presented to the other ear, the direction and magnitude of the adaptation effects were virtually the same as when the stimuli were presented binaurally. In addition, when the voicing information that was used for adaptation was presented in a nonspeech context, no systematic effects of adaptation on the identification functions were obtained.

From these studies (and see Cole and Scott, 1972), we argued for the existence of two *linguistic* feature detectors, each of which is especially tuned to a restricted range of voice onset time values and mediates the perception of one of the two voicing distinctions found in English and numerous other languages. Whether there is a third detector, underlying the perception of the prevoicing distinctions found in such languages as Thai, remains to be experimentally determined.

As Eimas and Corbit (1973) have demonstrated with a relatively simple model for these feature detectors, it is possible to explain the obtained identification and discrimination functions with and without adaptation. Moreover, Eimas (in press) has shown that these mechanisms are capable of explaining the infant's ability to make essentially categorical discriminations of voicing distinctions, provided only that these detectors are present at or shortly after birth and that merely experiencing human language is sufficient to activate the detectors.

With regard to the perception of place distinctions, Cooper (in press) has demonstrated by means of the selective adaptation procedure that there may very well exist feature detectors that mediate the perception of the three major distinctions along the place of articulation continuum. Using a series of synthetic speech stimuli that varied in the direction and starting frequency of the second- and third-formant transitions, Cooper found that after adaptation there were significant shifts in the phonetic boundaries and in the discriminability peaks. The manner in which these shifts occurred could be accommodated readily by the assumption of three feature detectors, each of which mediated the perception of one of the three place distinctions. The problem, of course, remains as to whether these detectors are sensitive to some as yet unspecified invariant stimulus property or properties associated with place of articulation or whether they are more abstract detector systems, sensitive perhaps to idealized features underlying the production of self-generated signals. Cooper (in press) has assumed the latter to be true, whereas my own predilections favor the former. While the details for either assumption cannot as yet be specified, let us for the moment consider what would be necessary to account for the perception of place distinctions by detectors that respond to invariant acoustic-auditory information, keeping in mind that for at least one level of analysis the sufficient cues for place distinctions vary markedly with the vowel context (but see unpublished manuscript by Cole and Scott for evidence to the contrary). What appears to be necessary is that after the peripheral analysis of the acoustic event the auditory patterns undergo several levels of analysis at the stage where phonetic features are extracted. First, information regarding the direction, starting frequency, and perhaps rate of change of the second- and third-formant transitions must be extracted. Also at this stage of analysis, detector mechanisms would be required to derive information regarding vowel quality (for example, the ratio of the frequencies of the first and second formants[7]). Finally, a set of higher level detectors must respond to the outputs of the lower level analyzers in combination. Moreover, these higher level analyzers, which actually signal place features, must respond to a range of combinations, if parsimony is to be achieved. In this manner, designation of a particular place of articulation is derived not by a single acoustic feature, but rather by several possible combinations of two, three, or more acoustic-auditory attributes. Obviously, this description of the feature detector system for place distinctions is not complete. However, this form of analysis appears, in principle, to be capable of accommodating the acoustic-auditory invariance associated with the cues for place of articulation. Invariance does exist, but at only one level of analysis. At higher levels, invariance is achieved without having to resort to synthetic or generative routines, which, while not beyond the abilities of adults, surpass the cognitive competence of the inarticulate infant.

---

[7] It is known that the steady state volume of the formants, which signal vowel quality, vary with many characteristics of the speaker. As a consequence, when the task is identification, some normalizing procedure must occur prior to the extraction of phonetic features. Given that the vowels [a], [i], or [u] can be used as calibration signals in order to estimate vocal tract size, sufficient information exists in the speech signal for a normalizing procedure (see Lieberman, Crelin, and Klatt, 1970). Although normalization is necessary for identification of vowel quality and undoubtedly for identification of consonantal distinctions, it may not always be necessary when the task is that of simple discrimination, as in our infant studies. This appears more plausible when we consider the fact that the vowel information in the infant speech studies was constant. Hence, we do not as yet need to assume that the young infant is capable of normalizing speech.

It is of interest to note that, in this feature detector model of speech perception, the processes of perception are closely bound to the processes of production. However, the relationship is a consequence of evolutionary development and not of ontogenetic development.[8] What has occurred, in essence, is that over the course of evolution, the processes of speech production, or, to be more precise, the acoustic consequences of articulation, constrained the development of perceptual processes, and conversely. That is, the nature of the developing perceptual apparatus for speech likewise constrained the development of the articulatory mechanisms. Neither the perceptual nor the production systems can be assigned the role of causal agent. Each has determined the course of development of the other. For related discussions on feature detection systems and the nature of the relationship between the mechanisms of speech perception and production, the reader is referred to Abbs and Sussman (1971), Lieberman (1970), and Stevens (1972).[9] As a further consequence of this course of development, the phonetic feature matrices underlying perception and production are comprised of the same phonetic features—but, as emphasized above, the determining events for this characteristic of speech are to be found in evolutionary and not ontogenetic development.

In summary, a feature detector model of speech perception offers a number of advantages. 1) It provides a relatively simple set of mechanisms whereby the infant's (and adult's) ability to perceive phonetic features in a speech mode can be explained. 2) It can accommodate the fact that the infant functions as a speech-recognizing mechanism automatically and without awareness. All that is required for the speech-analyzing mechanisms to be operative is that a sufficient number of attributes, which have some correspondence with phonetic features, be present in the incoming signal. 3) It eliminates the necessity to hypothesize the genetic determination of production routines as would be the case if motor theories of perception were to be extended to explain the infant's ability to perceive speech.

Finally, we recognize that the detector model is in need of additional data: first, it is necessary to describe the higher order invariances, and, second, it is necessary to establish the existence of phonetic feature detector systems for the remaining phonetic features. We are presently directing our research efforts toward these and related problems.

[8] This correspondence between the production and perception of acoustic signals as a consequence of evolutionary development is evidenced in other species, the bullfrog, for example (Capranica, 1965; Frishkopf and Goldstein, 1963).

[9] The close relationship between the processes of production and the processes of perception are further indicated by the following findings. Port and Preston (1972) showed that it is the middle mode of voicing (short voicing lags such as found in the voiced stop of English) that are the first to be differentiated by children. It is this same voicing mode that Lisker and Abramson (1964) found to be present in all of the languages they investigated and that Eimas and Corbit (1973) and Eimas, Cooper, and Corbit (1973) found to be more resistant to the effects of adaptation.

REFERENCES

Abbs, J. H. and Sussman, H. M. Neurophysiological feature detectors and speech perception: A discussion of theoretical implications. *J. Speech Hear. Res.*, 1971, *14*, 23–36.

Blakemore, C. and Campbell, F. W. On the existence of neurons in the human visual system selectively sensitive to the orientation and size of retinal images. *J. Physiol.*, 1969, *203*, 237–260.

Blakemore, C. and Sutton, P. Size adaptation: A new aftereffect. *Science*, 1969, *166*, 245–247.

Capranica, R. R. *The Evoked Vocal Response of the Bullfrog.* Cambridge, Mass.: M.I.T. Press, 1965.

Chomsky, N. and Halle, M. *The Sound Pattern of English.* New York: Harper and Row, 1968.

Cole, R. A., Haber, R. N., and Sales, B. D. Mechanisms of aural encoding: I. Distinctive features for consonants. *Percept. Psychophys.*, 1968, *3*, 281–284.

Cole, R. A., Sales, B. D., and Haber, R. N. Mechanisms of aural encoding: II. The role of distinctive features in articulation and rehearsal. *Percept. Psychophys.*, 1969, *6*, 343–348.

Cole, R. A. and Scott, B. Perceiving speech from invariant cues. Unpublished manuscript.

Cole, R. A. and Scott, B. Phoneme feature detectors. Paper presented at the meetings of the Eastern Psychological Association, Boston, April, 1972.

Cooper, F. S. How is language conveyed by speech? In J. F. Kavanagh and I. G. Mattingly (Eds.), *Language by Ear and by Eye.* Cambridge, Mass.: M.I.T. Press, 1972, pp. 25–45.

Cooper, W. E. Adaptation of phonetic feature analyzers for place of articulation. *J. Acoust. Soc. Amer.*, in press.

Dorman, M. F. Auditory evoked correlates of speech sound discrimination. In *Status Report of Speech Perception*, January-June, 1972. New Haven: Haskins Laboratories, pp. 111–120.

Eimas, P. D. The relation between identification and discrimination along speech and nonspeech continua. *Lang. Speech*, 1963, *6*, 206–217.

Eimas, P. D. Speech perception in early infancy. In L. B. Cohen and P. Salapatek (Eds.), *Infant Perception.* New York: Academic Press, in press.

Eimas, P. D., Cooper, W. E., and Corbit, J. D. Some properties of linguistic feature detectors. *Percept. Psychophys.*, 1973, *13*, 247–252.

Eimas, P. D. and Corbit, J. D. Selective adaptation of linguistic feature detectors. *Cognitive Psychol.*, 1973, *4*, 99–109.

Eimas, P. D., Siqueland, E. R., Jusczyk, P., and Vigorito, J. Speech perception in infants. *Science*, 1971, *171*, 303–306.

Frishkopf, L. S. and Goldstein, M. H., Jr. Responses to acoustic stimuli from single units of the eighth nerve of the bullfrog. *J. Acoust. Soc. Amer.*, 1963, *35*, 1219–1228.

Fry, D. B., Abramson, A. S., Eimas, P. D., and Liberman, A. M. The identification of synthetic vowels. *Lang. Speech*, 1962, *5*, 171–189.

Fujisaki, H. and Kawashima, T. The influence of various factors on the identification and discrimination of synthetic speech sounds. *Reports of the 6th International Congress on Acoustics*, Tokyo, August, 1968.

Halle, M. On the basis of phonology. In J. A. Fodor and J. J. Katz (Eds.), *The*

Structure of Language. Englewood Cliffs, N. J.: Prentice-Hall, 1964, pp. 324–333.

Harris, K. S. Physiological aspects of articulatory behavior. In *Status Report of Speech Perception,* July-September, 1970. New Haven: Haskins Laboratories, pp. 49–67.

Hintzman, D. L. Articulatory coding in short-term memory. *J. Verb. Learning Verb. Behav.,* 1967, *6,* 312–316.

Jakobson, R., Fant, C. G. M., and Halle, M. *Preliminaries to Speech Analysis.* Cambridge, Mass.: M.I.T. Press, 1963.

Kaplan, E. L. and Kaplan, G. The prelinguistic child. In J. Eliot (Ed.), *Human Development and Cognitive Processes.* New York: Holt, Rinehart, and Winston, 1971, pp. 358–381.

Kimura, D. Cerebral dominance and the perception of verbal stimuli. *Can. J. Psychol.,* 1961, *15,* 166–171.

Kimura, D. Left-right differences in the perception of melodies. *Quart. J. Exp. Psychol.,* 1964, *16,* 355–358.

Liberman, A. M. The grammars of speech and language. *Cognitive Psychol.,* 1970, *1,* 301–323.

Liberman, A. M. Some results of research on speech perception. *J. Acoust. Soc. Amer.,* 1957, *29,* 117–123.

Liberman, A. M., Cooper, F. S., Shankweiler, D. P., and Studdert-Kennedy, M. Perception of the speech code. *Psychol. Rev.,* 1967, *74,* 431–461.

Liberman, A. M., Harris, K. S., Eimas, P. D., Lisker, L., and Bastian, J. An effect of learning on speech perception: The perception of durations of silence with and without phonemic significance. *Lang. Speech,* 1961, *4,* 175–195.

Liberman, A. M., Harris, K. S., Kinney, J. A., and Lane, H. The discrimination of relative onset time of the components of certain speech and nonspeech patterns. *J. Exp. Psychol.,* 1961, *61,* 379–388.

Lieberman, P. Towards a unified phonetic theory. *Linguistic Inquiry,* 1970, *1,* 307–322.

Lieberman, P., Crelin, E. S., and Klatt, D. H. Phonetic ability and related anatomy of the newborn and adult human, Neanderthal man, and the chimpanzee. In *Status Report of Speech Research.* New Haven: Haskins Laboratories, 1970, pp. 57–90.

Lisker, L. and Abramson, A. S. A cross-language study of voicing in initial stops: Acoustical measurements. *Word,* 1964, *20,* 384–422.

MacNeilage, P. F. Motor control of serial ordering of speech. *Psychol. Rev.,* 1970, *77,* 182–196.

Massaro, D. W. Preperceptual images, processing time, and perceptual units in auditory perception. *Psychol. Rev.,* 1972, *79,* 124–145.

Mattingly, I. G., Liberman, A. M., Syrdal, A. K., and Halwes, T. Discrimination in speech and nonspeech modes. *Cognitive Psychol.,* 1971, *2,* 131–157.

McCollough, C. Color adaptation of edge-detectors in the human visual system. *Science,* 1965, *149,* 1115–1116.

Miller, G. A. The magical number seven, plus or minus two: Some limits on our capacity for processing information. *Psychol. Rev.,* 1956, *63,* 81–97.

Molfese, D. L. Cerebral asymmetry in infants, children and adults: Auditory evoked responses to speech and noise stimuli. Unpublished Ph.D. dissertation, Pennsylvania State University, University Park, 1972.

Morse, P. A. The discrimination of speech and nonspeech stimuli in early infancy. *J. Exp. Child Psychol.,* 1972, *14,* 477–492.

Pisoni, D. Auditory and phonetic memory codes in the discrimination of consonants and vowels. *Percept. Psychophys.,* 1973, *13,* 253—260.

Port, D. K. and Preston, M. S. Early apical stop production: A voice onset time analysis. In *Status Report on Speech Perception,* January-June, 1972. New Haven: Haskins Laboratories, pp. 125—150.

Sales, B. D., Haber, R. N., and Cole, R. A. Mechanisms of aural encoding: IV. Hear-see, say-write interactions for vowels. *Percept. Psychophys.,* 1969, *6,* 385—390.

Stevens, K. N. The quantal nature of speech: Evidence from articulatory-acoustic data. In E. E. David, Jr., and P. B. Denes (Eds.), *Human Communication: A Unified View.* New York: McGraw-Hill, 1972, pp. 51—66.

Stevens, K. N. and Halle, M. Remarks on analysis by synthesis and distinctive features. In W. Wathen-Dunn (Ed.), *Models for the Perception of Speech and Visual Form.* Cambridge, Mass.: M.I.T. Press, 1967, pp. 88—102.

Stevens, K. N. and House, A. S. Speech perception. In J. Tobias (Ed.), *Foundations of Modern Auditory Theory,* Vol. 2. New York: Academic Press, 1972, pp. 3—62.

Stevens, K. N., Liberman, A. M., Studdert-Kennedy, M., and Ohman, S. E. G. Cross-language study of vowel perception. *Lang. Speech,* 1969, *12,* 1—23.

Studdert-Kennedy, M. The perception of speech. In *Status Report on Speech Perception,* July-September, 1970. New Haven: Haskins Laboratories, pp. 15—48.

Studdert-Kennedy, M., Liberman, A. M., Harris, K. S., and Cooper, F. S. Motor theory of speech perception: A reply to Lane's critical review. *Psychol. Rev.,* 1970, *77,* 234—249.

Studdert-Kennedy, M. and Shankweiler, D. P. Hemispheric specialization for speech perception. *J. Acoust. Soc. Amer.,* 1970, *48,* 579—594.

Wickelgren, W. A. Distinctive features and errors in short-term memory for English consonants. *J. Acoust. Soc. Amer.,* 1966, *39,* 388—398.

Wickelgren, W. A. Auditory or articulatory coding in verbal short-term memory. *Psychol. Rev.,* 1969, *76,* 232—235.

Wood, C. C., Goff, W. P., and Day, R. S. Auditory evoked potentials during speech perception. *Science,* 1971, *173,* 1248—1251.

CHAPTER THREE

DISCUSSION SUMMARY–INFANT RECEPTION RESEARCH[1]

Earl C. Butterfield and George F. Cairns

Ralph L. Smith Mental Retardation Research Center, University of
Kansas Medical Center, Kansas City, Kansas 66103

Morse (this volume) distinguished between investigations
of infants' perception of auditory stimuli, such as the frequency, intensity,
and duration of pure tones, and investigations of infants' discrimination of
speech stimuli, such as synthetically generated consonant-vowel segments like
[ga] and [ba]. He found that studies of auditory stimuli are more numerous
and methodologically varied, but the conferees did not discuss them. Rather,
they devoted most of their attention to studies of infants' speech perception,
the results of which are positive and extremely provocative.

Morse (this volume) also highlighted the fact that two different techniques have been used to study infants' perception of speech: a heart rate
habituation procedure (Berg, 1971, 1972; Moffitt, 1971; Kaplan, 1969) and a
high amplitude suck procedure (Morse, 1972; Eimas, in press; Eimas et al.,
1971, Trehub, 1973; Trehub and Rabinovitch, 1972). Morse observed that
the heart rate habituation (HR) technique has been employed more frequently and has been subjected to a more thorough parametric analysis than
the high amplitude suck procedure (HAS). Nevertheless, the HR procedure
has not been used as systematically as the HAS procedure for the study of
infants' speech perception. Indeed, no HR experiment with speech stimuli,
including recent ones by Morse (this volume), has been replicated. Probably
for this reason, the conferees concentrated on discussing the meaning of the
studies that have employed the HAS procedure to investigate infants' speech
perception.

[1] The preparation of this discussion and the collection of the neonatal data reported in
it were supported by United States Public Health Service Grants HD-00183, HD-02528,
and HD-04756. The authors gratefully acknowledge the assistance of Donna Brahl, Betty
DiRegolo, Gene Hetsel, Peggy Rogers, and Susan Padfield, all of whom contributed
indispensably to the collection of data and preparation of the report. We are especially
indebted to Sandra Trehub, McGill University, Department of Psychology, for allowing
us to use raw data from several of her unpublished experiments in order to clarify
questions about order effects and reinforcing properties of contingent stimuli on older
infants.

Eimas (this volume) has interpreted the findings of HAS experiments. His main interpretation was that speech and nonspeech auditory stimuli are processed differently, that there are special linguistic feature detectors for the processing of speech. While several aspects of this view were considered, the discussion was mainly a consideration of whether any strong interpretation could yet be placed on the findings of the HAS procedures. At times it seems as if some conferees believed that no clear interpretation could be placed on the HAS findings, leading Morse to protest against throwing the baby out with the bath. The eventual consensus was best stated by Baer, who observed that "I wasn't recommending throwing out the baby with the bath. I was recommending delaying his christening until he was cleaner." Baer's metaphor recognized that the HAS procedure has produced replicated findings, but that there are sound reasons for suspending judgment about their precise meaning.

THE FACTS OF INFANT SPEECH PERCEPTION ARE REPEATABLE AND RELIABLE

Findings with the High Amplitude Suck Procedure

In each of the several variants of the HAS procedure, young infants are allowed to suck on a nonnutritive pacifier. Following a brief unreinforced baseline period, a speech stimulus is presented each time the infant emits a high amplitude suck. When the infant's HAS rate falls below an *a priori* response decrement criterion, he is either shifted to a different contingent stimulus or left to experience the same one. Shift is regarded as the experimental condition and no shift as the control. The basic observation has been that infants in the shift condition show a greater increase in rate of high amplitude sucking immediately following the decrement than do infants in the no shift condition.

There seems no doubt that this basic observation is repeatable: certain stimulus shifts result in a repeatably greater increase in sucking rate than do relevant no shift controls. Morse (this volume) and Eimas (this volume) described the results of the HAS experiments they have done. Table 1 summarizes their findings as well as those of Trehub, who is the other chief user of the HAS technique, and those of some other investigators. Table 1 shows 27 shift/no shift comparisons which taken together show the broad limits of the conclusion that the HAS procedure has yielded repeatable results. The first 16 comparisons examined the effects of changing the consonant portion of speech segments, and 10 of the comparisons show shift greater than no shift. This is true for both naturally spoken and synthesized stimuli, when the contrast is in either the first or the second of two syllables, and whether or not the distinction comes from a language foreign to the children's parents. Five of the 6 failures in this group of 16 are understandable. Four of them are between synthetic stimuli which adults do not discriminate.

Table 1. Summary of Shift/No Shift Comparisons: The Stimuli They Contrasted: Whether the Stimuli Were Natural or Synthetic; Whether the Shift Effect was Significant; and the Authors

Stimuli contrasted	Natural or synthetic	Shift > no shift ($p < 0.05$)	Author (s)
Consonant contrasts where shift effect was expected			
1. [ba](VOT+20)/[pa](VOT+40)	Syn.	Yes	Eimas *et al.*, 1971
2. [da](VOT+10)/[ta](VOT+60)	Syn.	Yes	Eimas (in press)
3. [dae]/[gae]	Syn.	Yes*	Eimas (in press)
4. [dae]/[gae]	Syn.	Yes*	Eimas (in press)
5. [ba](VOT-20)/[pa](VOT+80)	Syn.	Yes	Trehub and Rabinovitch (1972)
6. [ba]/[pa]	Nat.	Yes	Trehub and Rabinovitch (1972)
7. [da]/[ta]	Nat.	Yes	Trehub and Rabinovitch (1972)
8. [ba]/[ga][†]	Syn.	Yes	Morse (1972)
9. [za]/[ră]	Nat.	Yes	Trehub (1973b)
10. [aba]/[apa]	Nat.	Yes	Trehub (1973b)
11. [mapa]/[pama]	Nat.	No	Trehub (1973b)
12. [atapa]/[ataba]	Nat.	No	Trehub (1973b)
Consonant contrasts where shift effect was *not* expected			
13. [ba](VOT-20)/[ba](VOT O) [pa](VOT+60)/[pa](VOT+80)	Syn.	No	Eimas *et al.*, 1971
14. [da](VOT-30)/[da](VOT+20) [ta](VOT+50)/[ta](VOT+100)	Syn.	No	Eimas (in press)
15. [dae]/[dae][†] [gae]/[gae][†]	Syn.	No.	Eimas (in press)
16. [dae]/[dae][†] [gae]/[gae][†]	Syn.	No	Eimas (in press)
Vowels			
17. [a]/[i]	Nat.	Yes	Trehub (1973b)
18. [i]/[u]	Nat.	Yes	Trehub (1973b)
19. [pa]/[pi]	Nat.	Yes	Trehub (1973b)
20. [ta]/[ti]	Nat.	Yes	Trehub (1973b)
21. [pa]/[pu]	Nat.	Yes	Trehub (1973b)
Fundamental frequency			
22. Steady/rising	Syn.	Yes	Morse (1972)
Pure tones			
23. 200-Hz/500-Hz sine wave	Syn.	Yes	Wormith (1971)
24. 100-Hz/200-Hz square wave	Syn.	No	Trehub (1973b)
25. 1000-Hz/2000-Hz square wave	Syn.	No	Trehub (1973b)
26. 200-Hz/1000-Hz sine wave	Syn.	No	Trehub (1973b)
27. 100-200/200-100 Hz square wave	Syn.	No	Trehub (1973b)

*Significant for 4 but not 2 postshift minutes.
[†] Second- and third-formant manipulations.

The 5th was from a contrast in the third syllable of three-syllable natural segments which, under the conditions of this experiment, adults may also not have discriminated. The next 5 entries show greater shift effects for natural vowel stimuli, when the contrast is and is not from the language of the childrens' parents, and whether or not the vowel is accompanied by a consonant. Comparison 22 shows that infants changed between steady and rising fundamental frequencies increase their rate more than those who are not shifted. The last 5 contrasts show that most of the time changing between simple tone stimuli does not yield a greater shift effect. We conclude that the phenomenon of greater change for shift than no shift is repeatable across a wide range of speech stimulus manipulations, but not for simple tone manipulations.

Is the Shift Effect Symmetrical?

In view of the repeatability of the shift effect, questions about its statistical reliability are irrelevant. The sole important statistical question seems to be whether the order of presentation of the shifted segments influences the size of the shift effect. If two stimuli are discriminable, then it should make no difference which is presented first. Infants should respond as greatly to the shifting stimuli regardless of their presentation order. Our examination of research reports suggests that investigators have not analyzed their infants' data to determine whether they show this expected symmetry of shift effects, despite the fact that they have always counterbalanced their presentation order and maintained separate no shift controls for each order. Ideally, they would have shown that their shift effects were significantly greater than their no shift effects for both presentation orders. At least, they should have shown unreliable order X condition (shift-no shift) interactions and comparably large effects for both orders.

In order to estimate the frequency of asymmetrical order effects in experiments summarized in Table 1, we asked Sandra Trehub to send us copies of her raw data. Table 2 summarizes the results of our examination of the data from four of her experiments which compared naturally spoken speech segments. Each experiment contained a shift and a no shift condition, and order of stimulus presentation was counterbalanced between groups. Thus, the experiment summarized in the first row of Table 2, which compared the effects of two Czech speech segments employed four groups of infants. The two shift groups ([za/ră] and [ră/za]) and their respective no shift controls ([za/za] and [ră/ră]). The shift was made when the infants reached a decrement criterion of 2 consecutive minutes with fewer than 67% of the number of sucks in the largest preshift minute. The first three columns of Table 2, headed "Orders combined," show the mean change between the last 2 preshift minutes and the first 2 postshift minutes for the combined shift (column 1) and no shift (column 2) groups and the difference between

Table 2. Findings Separated According to Order of Stimulus Presentation from Four HAS Experiments by Trehub (1973b)

	Orders combined			Order I			Order II		
	Shift 1	No shift 2	Δ 3	Shift 4	No shift 5	Δ 6	Shift 7	No shift 8	Δ 9
1. [za]/[rǎ]	17.6	−3.2	20.8*	17.4	1.4	16.0	18.1	−7.8	25.9*
2. [pa]/[ma]	18.2	4.4	13.8*	19.7	8.4	11.3	16.8	−0.5	17.3*
3. [ta]/[ti]	16.8	3.7	13.1*	14.0	6.9	7.1	20.9	0.5	20.4*
4. [apa]/[aba]	18.0	1.9	16.1*	14.3	3.1	11.2	21.7	0.7	21.0

*$p < 0.05$.

these two change scores (column 3). The next three columns, headed "Order I," show the same information for the shift group who received the stimuli in the order listed at the left of the row (column 4), the no shift group which received the first stimulus listed at the left (column 5), and the difference between these two groups (column 6). The next three columns, headed "Order II," show the difference score for the shift group which received the two stimuli in the reverse of their order at the left (column 7), the no shift group which received the second stimulus on the left (column 8), and the difference between the two (column 9). The positive scores in columns 3, 6, and 9 indicate that the shift group changed more than the no shift group in every case.

Analyses of variance for each experiment showed no significant interaction between order and condition. We nevertheless examined the simple effects of condition for each order with t-tests. The asterisks by the differences in columns 3, 6, and 9 of Table 2 indicate which shift and no shift groups differed significantly by these one-tailed t-tests with p set at 0.05. Only three of the eight tests for the different orders were statistically significant, and no experiment yielded significant effects for both orders. By the rule that both orders should show statistical significance, we would be forced to conclude that all four of these experiments show an asymmetry of order. This is probably an unreasonably stringent rule, since the order groups contained only five subjects each. The absolute differences for the two orders in each experiment are all positive, and are rather larger than zero, although for experiments III and IV, the absolute difference for order II is about twice as great as for order I. Judging the importance of this degree of variability is complicated by the small number of subjects involved, but we conclude that experiments with natural stimuli and infants about 2 months old probably have yielded symmetrical order effects.

It seems to us that there are no serious remaining questions about the statistical conventions employed by infant perceptual investigators, and that the basic shift/no shift finding has been repeated so often that we must have confidence in it. We will turn now to how these findings may be interpreted, for it is their interpretation, not their repeatability, from which intervention implications might come.

THE FRAMEWORK FOR INTERPRETING STUDIES OF INFANTS' SPEECH PERCEPTION

To appreciate the problems of interpreting the results of HAS experiments, one must grasp the framework from which they stem. Eimas is the main architect of this framework, though Morse also uses major portions of it. The version presented here has been abstracted from the writings of both men but relies most heavily on Eimas's work.

Studies of infants' speech perception build from the generalization that adults perceive speech differently than they do other auditory signals. The shorthand for this conclusion is that adults' speech perception is linguistically relevant. At least four observations support this conclusion. First, certain acoustic cues, for example, voice onset time (VOT), are used universally, that is, in the spoken forms of all languages. Second, some of the acoustic correlates of speech features, and specifically two of the few that can be generated synthetically by computers, are perceived categorically, unlike either auditory nonspeech or visual cues. Third, identical variations in certain synthetically generated acoustic cues are perceived differently when they are embedded in a speech context and when they are presented in isolation. Fourth, the electrical activity which is evoked by acoustic signals is localized in the left hemisphere of the brain if the signals are correlates of certain speech features, and it is not so localized if the cues are not correlates of those speech features. Dichotic listening experiments also support the notion of lateralized and localized speech perception.

Partly because some acoustic cues are used universally, partly because some speech stimuli evoke hemispherically localized brain potentials, and partly because of his inability to explain how people might learn to segment and discriminate speech stimuli, Eimas concurs with such authors as Mattingly that innate biological structures underlie perception in the speech mode. (The latter phrase is synonymous with linguistically relevant perception.) From this conclusion, he deduced the hypothesis that very young infants also perceive speech linguistically.

This hypothesis might be tested by seeking infant analogues of the four phenomena that support the conclusion that adults perceive in a linguistically relevant manner, but this is impossible with respect to the observation that all spoken languages use similar sets of acoustic contrasts, because infants do not speak. Even if they did, the characteristics of their speech would not necessarily mirror their perceptual capabilities. There are no comparably insuperable barriers to the search in infants for localized brain potentials in response to speech and nonspeech stimuli. According to Morse and Eimas, Molfese (1972) has recently shown that infants who average about 5 months of age show greater left hemisphere potentials for nonspeech auditory stimuli. Morse and Eimas have both conducted experiments to determine whether infants discriminate isolated acoustic cues differently than they do the same ones in speech contexts. Morse's (1972) findings yielded highly equivocal findings, and Eimas' experiment has not been replicated. The hypothesis that infants perceive linguistically thus hangs primarily on the results of the several experiments into whether they perceive categorically.

For adults, categorical perception is established by showing that they do not discriminate between physically different synthetic stimuli to which they attach the same speech label, for example, [ga], but they do discriminate highly accurately between no less physically similar stimuli to which they attach different speech labels. Adults are first asked to categorize a group of stimuli by listening and assigning labels to them. Despite the fact that the stimuli all differ on some acoustic cue, say VOT, adults assign fewer labels than there are stimuli. Those to which they assign different labels are said to vary between categories. Adults are then asked to discriminate between pairs of stimuli which differ equally along the acoustic dimension. For some pairs, both members come from the same category, while for other pairs, the members come from different categories. If the within-category discriminations are made no better than chance and the between-category discriminations are made essentially perfectly, then perception of the underlying dimension is said to be categorical. The more within-category pairs that are not discriminated, and the more abrupt the increase in rate of successful discrimination around the category boundary, the more convincing the demonstration of categorical perception.

It has so far been impossible to secure categorical judgments from infants. Consequently, it has been impossible to make a completely adequate test of whether they perceive categorically, since this requires both categorization and discrimination functions. In order to overcome this limitation, Eimas has assumed that infants would categorize synthetic stimuli precisely as adults do. This assumption allows him to infer categorical perception from infant's discrimination functions alone, if those functions are predicted by adults' categorizations of the stimuli.

Eimas has collected several sets of data which bear on the question of whether adults' categorical functions predict infants' discrimination functions (see Table 1). He has used the high amplutide suck procedure to compare differential responses to members of two within-category pairs and one between-category pair along the VOT dimension in several experiments with infants and found evidence to suggest that the within-category pairs were not discriminated while the between-category pair was, when the VOT boundary was the one used in spoken English. He failed to find such evidence when the VOT boundary was one employed in Thai but not in English, but he argued that the adult Thai's data which he used to select his VOT values may not have accurately identified the categorization boundary. He has also found differences between pairs of stimuli which varied in place of articulation, that is, second-formant transitions, when two pair came from within an adult category and one was composed of items from different adult categories.

Eimas (in press) has previously concluded from his findings that infants perceive at least approximately categorically and therefore in a linguistically relevant fashion. Both he and Morse echoed this conclusion in their papers for this conference, although both failed here to mention the "approximately" part. This is a particularly startling conclusion because it suggested to Eimas a lack of perceptual development between infancy and adulthood, although in this particular, Morse dissented. Nevertheless, Eimas reasoned that since both young infants and adults perceive particular synthetic stimuli in the same (linguistically relevant) fashion, he could conduct experiments with adults to clarify the infants' perceptual processes. Accordingly, he executed a series of adult adaptation experiments from which he has inferred the existence of biologically determined linguistic feature detectors that are tuned to different portions of the various acoustic dimensions which underlie speech cue perception.

This elegant strategy depends centrally upon establishing that infants and adults both perceive linguistically, and to do this it relies heavily upon tests of whether infants' perception is categorical. The consensus of the conferees was that the question of whether infants perceive categorically remains to be answered. Three classes of reasons led the conferees to conclude that we still do not know whether infants perceive categorically and, therefore, linguistically. First, the HAS procedure may not measure discrimination, and the procedure's rationale is suspect. Second, the range and character of the stimulus manipulations in infant experiments precludes attributing the results of the HAS procedure to particular stimulus dimensions or uniquely to speech stimuli. Third, the bridge between infancy and adulthood upon which the interpretation of similar perceptions rests is shaky at both the operational and conceptual levels. The next four sections of this paper treat these three sources of interpretative difficulty.

THE HAS SHIFT EFFECT CANNOT BE CLEARLY INTERPRETED

We believe that the results of any procedure can be clearly interpreted only after the testable portions of its rationale have been validated. The rationale for the HAS procedure comes in two parts: preshift and postshift.

The rationale for the preshift phase of the HAS procedure is that the repeated contingent presentation of an initially reinforcing stimulus, like a synthetic speech segment, leads to the loss of its reinforcing power. Experimenters have tried to demonstrate that the stimulus had reinforcing properties in the first place by showing an increase in rate of responding from a nonreinforced baseline to the minute immediately before the subject met some *a priori* criterion of response decrement. This is an inadequate test on several counts, but the most direct demonstration of this fact is that infants suck significantly more during the minute preceding attainment of a response decrement criterion than during a baseline period when they receive no stimulation. The contingent stimulation does not account for this increase in rate. We have verified this in our laboratory with neonates, and Sandra Trehub has verified it in her laboratory with 6-week olds. The demonstration of loss of reinforcing properties has been that infants show a substantial decrement in response rate at some point following the introduction of the contingent stimulus, but so do infants who receive no contingent stimulation. This has also been shown both in our laboratory with neonates and Trehub's with 6-week olds.

No published report of the application of the HAS procedure to the study of speech perception has employed adequate controls for this first part of its rationale. Either of two controls would show whether the initial stimulus has reinforcing properties. One control is a group of infants who are allowed to suck on the pacifier in the absence of any stimulation for the same amount of time as the group who will experience a stimulus change. This group should show less increase in response rate than the stimulus change group does prior to meeting the response decrement or habituation criterion. A second control would experience the same stimulation as the stimulus change group, but the stimulation would be uncorrelated with the infants' high amplitude sucking. This group, too, should show less response increment. Both of these two groups are also controls for whether the response decrement of the experimental group results from satiation of the reinforcing properties of the initial stimulus or from chance variability or unreliability of sucking rate. If either or both groups meet the habituation criterion as rapidly as the experimental group, then the repeated presentation of the initial stimulus is not the reason for that response decrement. Lacking such controls, the first part of the procedure's rationale is unsupported, and strong interpretation of its results is correspondingly premature. This is particularly true since there are good reasons to wonder about the preshift rationale. Let us turn now to the second part of the rationale for the HAS procedure.

The hallmark of the HAS procedure is its use of an habituation or response decrement criterion. The rationale for the postshift part of the HAS procedure is that a second stimulus, which is introduced for the shift group following attainment of this response decrement, is discriminated from the first stimulus if the introduction of the second leads to an increased rate of responding. The control for "cyclical changes in rate" (Eimas, in press) is to not shift some subjects to the second stimulus following response decrement to the first, but to continue presenting the first stimulus. The problem is to select an appropriate control for the effects of the decrement criterion. The question is whether the no shift condition is the only control required, and we fear that it is not.

Suppose that the criterion response decrement results from a decrease in the reinforcing properties of the initial stimulus, but that decrease does not cease when the reinforcing properties reach zero, i.e., at simple satiation. Suppose that the initial stimulus actually becomes aversive and suppresses sucking below its free-operant level. Then, part, if not all, of the rate increase following shift would be due to removal of the initial, now aversive stimulus rather than from the presence of a discriminably different second or shifted-to stimulus. The appropriate control for this possibility would be to shift, following response decrement, from the initial stimulus to no stimulus or silence. Lacking such a control, the possibility remains that the shift infants did not respond to the difference between the first, preshift and the second, postshift stimulus, but only to the removal of the initial stimulus.

Now, adopt a purely statistical view about whether additional controls are required.[2] The use of an *a priori* criterion of response decrement allows the possibility that infants will meet it by chance alone. If infants did decrease their sucking rate by chance, rather than in response to the repeated presentation of the first stimulus, then the chance expectation following shift would be an increase in rate of sucking. In other words, the pattern of results typically shown by infants in the shift group, rather than infants in the no shift group, would be the chance expectation. To demonstrate this possibility, we collected and then randomly simulated data from a shift condition. Fourteen neonates were shifted from one synthetic phoneme to another, following a response decrement of 25% for 2 consecutive minutes. Half of the infants first heard a stimulus with VOT equal to −20 msec and were then shifted to one with VOT equal to +80 msec. The other half experienced the stimuli in the opposite order. Figure 1 shows their mean number of high amplitude sucks for 3 min before and 3 min after the shift. The pattern of results is highly similar to that obtained by Eimas, Morse, and others from older infants. Following the shift, the infants showed an appreciable increase in their rate of sucking.

We randomly simulated these data by selecting consecutive numbers from a random table. One set was selected for each infant. The only restraints on the numbers were that they had to fall between the maximal and minimal rates of the neonate whose data we were simulating. We selected numbers until we had three more than the number required to meet randomly the

---

[2] While this statistical argument is presented as if it applies only to the HAS procedure, it actually applies to all of the many experiments that rely upon a response decrement criterion to assess when an infant has habituated to a stimulus. Morse and Eimas have used a decrement criterion very much in the established way of infant researchers, and the reader should understand that we are not singling them out for special criticism. Our point is general, and it calls for a reassessment of many findings with infants.

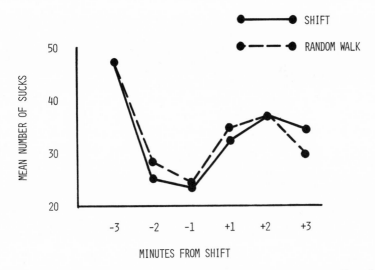

Fig. 1. Data from 14 neonates in an HAS shift condition and a random walk on them.

same response decrement criterion maintained for the infants. The means of these values (random walk) almost precisely duplicate the data produced by the 14 neonates in the shift condition (see Fig. 1). Thus, the no shift control is inadequate to rule out the possibility that rate increases following "habituation" are due to imposing a decrement criterion on the shift group. According to the rationale of the habituation test procedure, that is the sole reason for the no shift control. The problem with this rationale is that it ignores the possibility that the no shift rather than the shift group is the "experimental group," the one which departs from chance expectations. If that is true, then shift effects do not indicate discrimination. Employing a control group which is shifted from the first "habituated" stimulus to silence is the only way to assess this possibility.

We conclude that interpreting the HAS shift effect as evidence of discrimination is premature and must await a test of the procedure's rationale. The results of such a test follow.

AN INVESTIGATION OF NEONATES' SPEECH DISCRIMINATION USING THE HAS PROCEDURE

We had hoped, before we examined the rationale for the HAS procedure, to employ it in our Neonatal Research Laboratory to investigate the discriminative capabilities of human newborns. Our examination convinced us that we should not proceed until we could be more certain that the technique actually tapped infant discrimination.

To reassure ourselves, we compared two synthetic stimuli that Peter Eimas was kind enough to send us. They are his −20 and +80 VOT stop consonants. They were presented contingently, after the fashion of Trehub and Rabinovitch, to shift and no shift groups. We maintained a decrement criterion of 25% below the immediately preceding minute for 2 consecutive minutes. Two shift groups experienced either the −20 followed by the +80, or the +80 followed by the −20 stimuli. Two no shift groups experienced either −20 or +80 throughout the experiment. Each of these four groups was composed of 7 newborn infants. A silence control group of 10 neonates received no stimulation but was carried past the decrement criterion. Another two control groups were first presented with either the −20 or the +80 stimulus. When they attained the decrement criterion, the stimuli were turned off. Each of these shift-to-silence control groups contained 7 newborns.

Evidence about Discrimination

The first purpose of the experiment was to select between two competing hypotheses about how to interpret the observation, which we hoped to replicate, that shift results in a greater postdecrement increase in sucking rate than no shift. The discrimination hypothesis says that the infants in the shift groups discriminate the stimuli which they experience. The pattern of results consistent with this hypothesis is shift > no shift = shift-to-silence. The equality of the last two conditions would indicate that suppression due to the initial stimulus becoming aversive could not account for the greater change in the shift over the no shift group. The aversiveness hypothesis says that the shift infants do not discriminate their two stimuli, but rather their increase is due to the initial stimulus becoming aversive and suppressing the postdecrement rate of the no shift group. This hypothesis would be affirmed by shift-to-silence = shift > no shift.

We decided in advance to pay particular attention to order effects. Thus, we were interested in whether the no shift, shift, and shift-to-silence groups which began with the −20 stimulus showed the same pattern of results as the comparable groups which began with the +80 stimulus. Our reason for this focus will be elaborated later. Table 3 shows the change scores for each of the six stimulated groups in our experiment. These scores were calculated by subtracting the mean of the first 2 postdecrement minutes from the mean of the last 2 predecrement minutes. The table shows that there was a marked asymmetry of order. When −20 was the first stimulus, recovery was far greater for the shift (−20/+80) than for either the no shift (−20/−20) or shift-to-silence (−20/ϕ) groups. When +80 came first, recovery was less for the shift (+80/−20) than for either the no shift (+80/+80) or shift-to-silence (+80/ϕ). The silence (ϕ/ϕ) group recovered about as much ($\overline{M}$ = 3.5) as the other controls. To evaluate the statistical reliability of these findings, we first determined how many infants in each of the six groups which received stimulation fell above and how many fell below the median change (4.0) of all 48 of the subjects. These frequencies are also reported in Table 3. Since there were clearly no differences between the no shift and shift-to-silence

Table 3. Mean and Median Change Scores and Number
of Subjects above and below Over-all Median (Mdn=4.0)
for Each of Six Groups of Neonates

	Shift	No shift	Shift to silence
	−20/+80	−20/−20	−20/∅
Mean change	12.2	2.4	3.0
Median change	14.8	0.5	0.5
Number above Mdn	8	2	3
Number below Mdn	2	5	4
	+80/−20	+80/+80	+80/∅
Mean change	2.9	4.1	5.8
Median change	0	4.5	8.0
Number above Mdn	3	3	4
Number below Mdn	7	4	3

groups, we combined their frequencies and compared each shift group to its own combined control. Fisher exact probability tests showed that the −20/+80 group differed significantly (p = 0.04) from the combined −20/−20 and −20/ϕ control; that the +80/−20 group did not differ (p = 0.29) from its +80/+80 and +80/ϕ control; and that the two shift groups differed significantly (p = 0.035) from each other.

The great similarity of the no shift and shift-to-silence results rules out the possibility that the no shift group failed to recover because the initial stimulus had become aversive to them, and it suggests that chance variability in sucking was not the reason the neonates decreased their rate of responding while the first stimulus was being presented. This suggests that the neonates who received the −20 stimulus first discriminated it from the +80 stimulus, while those who received the +80 stimulus first did not discriminate it from the −20 stimulus. This seems to make neonates different from older infants, who apparently show symmetrical order effects. Moreover, it must cause some uncertainty about interpreting the −20/+80 data as evidence of discrimination. Because of this, we have subsequently replicated the two shift conditions, and once again the −20/+80 group showed a significant postshift recovery, and the +80/−20 group did not. We will return later to why this should be. For now, we conclude that these data provide limited support for the postshift rationale of the HAS procedure.

Evidence about Reinforcing Properties

The second purpose of this experiment was to provide an adequate test of the preshift rationale of the HAS procedure. According to that rationale, the reinforcing properties of the preshift stimulus lead first to an increased rate of sucking, and then, as its reinforcing properties attenuate, there follows a decrement in rate of responding. In practice, investigators have shown that both shift and no shift groups show a significant increase in sucking rate over an unreinforced baseline. But this test misses the mark, because both random walks and unreinforced infants show the same increase provided only that they are required to meet the same response decrement required of shift and no shift infants.

Tests of whether the initial stimulus has reinforcing properties which it loses as a result of repeated presentation were made by comparing preshift rates of responding when a stimulus is contingent on sucking, as in the shift, no shift, and shift-to-silence conditions of our neonate study, to a silence condition in which no stimulus is present. We shall also present comparisons of the preshift behavior of older infants from two experiments by Trehub and from a silence condition which she has conducted. For this purpose, we have selected one experiment of hers that used the natural speech contrast [za/ră] (exp. 1) and one that used 1000- and 2000-Hz square waves (exp. 2).

Backward Plots. If the preshift stimuli are positively reinforcing, then rate of sucking should reach a higher peak for the contingent groups than for the groups which receive no stimulation, and this difference should be most apparent during the 3rd min prior to shift, since most infants' sucking rate is highest then. If the preshift response decrement results from a simple loss of reinforcing properties, then the sucking rate of the stimulation groups should fall to and equal that of the silence group whose sucking is presumably not being reinforced by anything other than feedback from the pacifier. If the initial stimulus actually becomes aversive, rather than simply losing its positive reinforcing properties, the sucking rate should fall below that of the silence infants at minutes −2 and −1. Regardless of whether the decrement reflects a simple loss of reinforcing properties or the action of a newly aversive stimulus, the rationale for the HAS requires that the sucking of infants change differently during the last 3 preshift minutes when stimulation is contingent than when it is absent. Figure 2 shows that no such interaction occurs. For both our neonates and Trehub's older infants in experiment 2, silence leads to more frequent responding during minute −3 than any of the contingent conditions (−20, +80, 1000, 2000). In Trehub's experiment 1, [za] resulted in higher such rates than ϕ, but [ră] resulted in a lower rate during minute −3. All of the contingent groups showed somewhat lower response rates during minutes −2 and −1 than did the silence groups. None of these differences approached statistical significance by any of the numerous tests we employed, even though we relaxed our confidence levels and performed one-tailed tests. We find no evidence for the acquisition and habituation rationale of the HAS procedure in these data.

Forward Plots. It is more difficult to plot HAS data forward from the beginning of the experiment than it is to plot it backward from the point of shift. All infants contribute equally to the 3 min immediately prior to the

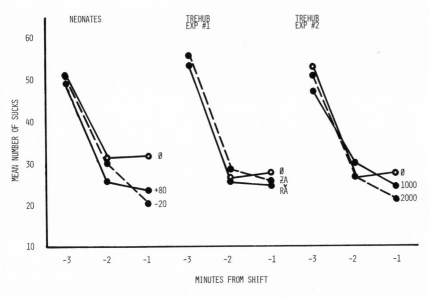

Fig. 2. Comparison of preshift minutes with (−20, +80, [rǎ], [za], 1000, and 2000) and without (φ) contingent stimulation for neonates and Trehub's older infants.

shift, but because of variability in the time to decrement, forward plots must either be restricted to only some of the minutes from the beginning of the experiment or to those infants who take a relatively long time to reach the decrement criterion. Neither is a perfectly satisfactory solution. Moreover, it seems inappropriate to include any of the last 3 preshift minutes in the calculation of forward learning curves, since all 3 are constrained by the decrement criterion. In our experiment, this restriction alone requires the elimination of 5 of 24 neonates who began with the −20 stimulus, and 7 of 24 who began with +80, because this number met the decrement criterion in only 3 min. Several others contributed only 1 min prior to the last 3, and they too must be eliminated because it takes at least 2 min to show changes in rate of responding. In the +80 group, half of the subjects contributed 3 predecrement minutes while half contributed 4 min in the −20 group and 5 min in each of Trehub's conditions. The somewhat longer preshift longevity of Trehub's infants probably stems from the fact that she did not permit either of the first 2 experimental minutes to contribute to the determination of when an infant reached his decrement, whereas we allowed both to contribute to the calculation of the decrement. This speedy attainment of the decrement criterion by itself suggests that none of the stimuli was particularly reinforcing to the infants.

In order to assess the reinforcing properties of the stimuli, we compared the changes in rate across the first few minutes of the experiment for one-half of the infants in each group. Our criterion for whether a stimulus was reinforcing was whether the increase in rate which it produced across these first few minutes was greater than the increase produced by the same age infants under the silence condition. We ruled out the use of the over-all rate, since the presentation of the stimuli might have had some energizing property which would elevate the rate from the beginning of the experiment even though the stimuli had no reinforcing properties. Figure 3 shows the mean number of sucks in each minute from the onset of reinforcement for our experiment with neonates and for Trehub's experiments 1 and 2. Each curve is based on approximately half of the subjects in each condition, and this accounts for the variable number of minutes that are plotted.

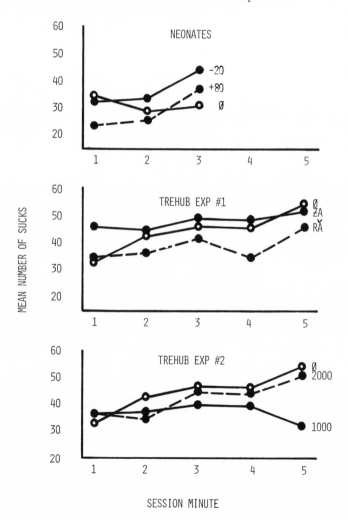

Fig. 3. Number of sucks per minute plotted forward from experimental minute 1 for each of three experiments.

The neonates' data seem to suggest that the −20 and +80 groups both showed a greater increase in rate of sucking across the first 3 min of the experiment than did the ϕ group. That impression is not substantiated by statistical analyses. For example, groups X minutes analyses of variance comparing −20 to ϕ and +80 to ϕ both yielded insignificant minute X group interactions. The only significant difference that was revealed by several analyses of the neonates' data was that the rate for the −20 group was greater over-all than for the +80 group ($F = 6.56, df = 2/52, p < 0.01$). However, the interaction between these groups and minutes did not approach significance ($F < 1.0$). The data from both of Trehub's experiments concur with the implication of neonates' data that contingent stimulation does not affect the rate of increase in number of sucks per minute. The increase of the ϕ group is actually greater than that of any of the four contingent groups: [za], [ră], 1000, 2000. We are forced to conclude that the forward plots, like the backward ones, offer no support for the preshift rationale of the HAS procedure.

Implications for Interpreting the Results of HAS Experiments

The conferees responded to the fact that this experiment yielded no evidence for the preshift rationale of the HAS and only limited evidence for its postshift rationale by concluding that it was a very gentle technique. It is gentle first, in the sense that it does not employ powerful reinforcers, and second, in the sense that one cannot infer an inability to discriminate from a failure to show a postshift recovery of sucking rate. Thus, the conferees implied that the HAS paradigm could not be justified as a conditioning procedure. Eimas, at least, seemed to concur in that the postconference version of his paper (this volume) spoke of it as a satiation technique. Neither Eimas nor Morse concurred with the conclusion that one could not infer a lack of discriminative competence from a lack of discriminative performance, for they both continued to interpret the failure of infants to recover following within-category shifts as evidence for categorical perception. This inference requires that infants, to quote Morse, be "helpless" like adults to make within-category discriminations. It seemed to the conferees that the strongest justifiable interpretation was that infants did not recover as readily following within-category shifts as following between-category shifts. The possibility remains that they may actually discriminate within-category shifts as well as between-category shifts, thereby making the infant quite unlike the adult and not a categorical perceiver. Most conferees agreed that much stronger conditioning procedures would have to be applied to infants before they would conclude with assurance that infants cannot make within-category discriminations.

All of the conferees, including Eimas, agreed with Morse's great emphasis on the importance of exploring further the limits of the HAS procedure. One serious limitation of the technique may be its failure to separate the discriminative and reinforcing properties of the speech stimuli it studies. Postshift recovery depends upon the postshift stimulus having reinforcing properties. If it does not, then the infant will not recover even though he discriminates the postshift from the preshift stimulus. This could account for the failure to recover to within-category shifts. The satiation of the reinforcing properties of the preshift stimulus might generalize more readily to another stimulus from the same category, even though that within-category stimulus remains discriminable from the first stimulus. The reinforcing and discriminative functions of stimuli can be separated by means of a variety of operant discrimination routines, and applying some variant of these routines to infants seems the best way to increase our confidence in the possibility that the within-category failure to recover results from a failure to discriminate rather than from reinforcement effects.

Sooner or later some such converging operations will be required, because, no matter how well we believe we have tested a procedure's rationale, there is always the possibility that we have overlooked some critical process which makes even a replicable result peculiar to our procedure. Until an alternative way of verifying that infants discriminate has been successfully applied, we can only be tentative about whether the failure to observe an HAS shift effect reflects a lack of discrimination. For reasons detailed by Morse, the heart rate habituation technique may be promising as a converging operation. Operant discrimination procedures seem more promising to us, since they have been designed particularly for the investigation of discrimination and to cope with the kinds of ambiguities created by the HAS and the HR procedures.

INTERPRETATIVE DIFFICULTIES RESULTING FROM THE STIMULI USED IN HAS EXPERIMENTS

The conferees' reluctance to conclude that infants perceive categorically also stemmed in part from a recognition of problems with the stimuli used in HAS experiments.

Too Few Within-Category Stimuli Have Been Employed

The conclusion that adults perceive synthetic speech stimuli categorically is based on the observation that their categorizations of stimuli predict accurately their discrimination of the stimuli. The power of this observation is that adult discrimination studies have compared many pairs of stimuli from the dimensions studied, and accurate discrimination has been obtained for only those few pairs that cut across adults' categorical boundaries. Thus, Pisoni (1971) used 13 stimuli from each of the several dimensions he studied. He compared 12 pairs composed of stimuli that were adjacent on each of his continua and 11 pairs that were separated by only 1 intervening stimulus. All of his subjects were asked to judge all 23 pairs, and they succeeded with only those few pairs that cut across the two categorical boundaries encompassed by his 13 stimuli.

It would be practically impossible to perform an HAS experiment using as many stimulus pairs as Pisoni did, since an HAS experiment evaluates only one pair of stimuli per infant. Twenty-three groups of infants would be required to make the relevant comparisons. Elimination of some of the possible comparisons is therefore virtually mandatory for infant experimenters. But Eimas has reduced the number of comparisons to the bare minimum. Each of his experiments used only four stimuli: two pair that cut across an adult categorical boundary and two pair from within adult categories. Consequently, he has been unable to judge whether the discrimination gradients around the category boundary approximate even crudely the steepness of the gradients produced by adults. We suspect that this is why he has always previously concluded that infants' discrimination was *approximately* categorical. In his preconference paper he abandoned his previous qualification, but the conferees judged that his earlier stance was more justifiable. The cure for this problem is to use a few more stimulus contrasts that fall closer to the adult categorical boundary. Until this is done, the evidence that infants perceive categorically is only gross and approximate.

Synthetic Stimuli Are Not Univariate

Categorical perception can only be evaluated with synthetic speech stimuli, because the many acoustic differences between natural stimuli cannot be satisfactorily quantified. It is thus impossible to clearly scale natural stimuli within identification categories. Synthetic stimuli can be quantified and more clearly ordered along objective dimensions. But these dimensions are not univariate. VOT, the dimension that has been studied most often with infants, is particularly complex.

The number of acoustic features that differentiate adjacent stimuli depends upon where they fall on the VOT continuum. Below 0 msec VOT, where the first formant comes on before the second, the dimension is defined by the difference in onset time between the beginning of the first two formants' *transitions.* Above 0 VOT, where the second formant comes on before the first, the first formant's transition is gradually cut back and replaced with a noise source, until at about +30 msec the first-formant transition disappears. Between 0 and +30 VOT, the dimension is defined as the difference in time between the beginnings of the second-formant transition and what remains of the first-formant transition. Moreover, the time between the onsets of the two formants is filled with a noise source that is not present below 0 msec. Above +30, VOT refers to the difference in time between the onsets of the second-formant transition and the *transitionless* first formant. Moreover, the interval from the onset of the second formant until the onset of the first is filled with a noise source. The potential importance of this double confounding along the VOT dimension is highlighted by the fact that infants have been shown to respond to the difference between two VOT stimuli only when one of them falls below +30 and the other falls above +30.

Between them, Eimas (in press; Eimas *et al.*, 1971) and Moffitt (personal communication) have used the HAS procedure to compare 10 pairs of values chosen from the VOT dimension. These values range from −100 to +100 msec. Two comparisons yielded significant shift effects: +20 *vs.* +40; and +10 *vs.* +60. Eight comparisons yielded insignificant effects: −100 *vs.* −40; −60 *vs.* −20; −40 *vs.* 0; −40 *vs.* +20; −30 *vs.* +20; −20 *vs.* 0; +50 *vs.* +100; and +60 *vs.* +80. The only point for which there is evidence of possible discrimination lies between +20 and +40, the range in which the first-formant transition disappears. This raises the question of whether infants perceive differences in VOT, as Eimas has argued, or the presence of first-formant transitions. If it is the former, then the conclusion that infants perceive linguistically is more tenable than if it is the latter. If it is the latter, then the most parsimonious interpretation would be that infants perceive acoustic, not linguistic information. Several arguments bear on the question of whether infants perceive the VOT dimension, and these were reviewed by the conferees.

Establishing That a Dimension Is Perceivable. To establish categorical perception, an investigator must first show that his dimension is perceivable. Not all physical continua are perceivable, and unless the one under investigation is, the failure to discriminate portions of it cannot be taken as evidence of categorical perception. The most satisfactory way to demonstrate that a dimension is perceivable is to show that people discriminate at least two unconfounded points on it. But by this criterion, VOT is not a perceivable dimension even for adults. English speakers discriminate between stimuli that fall above and below +30 msec VOT, but such stimuli confound the presence and absence of the first-formant transition with VOT. Spanish speakers discriminate stimuli that fall above and below a VOT value of approximately 0 msec but such stimuli confound the order of the first and second formant, the absence of a portion of the first-formant transition, and the presence of a noise source with VOT. Thai speakers discriminate between speech segments that fall above and below a value that lies somewhere around −40 msec, and this is the sole discriminable point along the VOT continuum that is apparently not confounded with an alternative acoustic basis for discrimination.

Investigators of neither adults' nor infants' speech perception have employed the most satisfactory demonstration that VOT is a perceivable dimension, yet they agree that it is. The rule that Eimas has employed is that infants show evidence of discrimination at any point on the dimension. He has been relatively unconcerned that that point contains a confound, although he has sought evidence that infants discriminate across the Thai boundary, which is the only unconfounded point that adults discriminate on the VOT dimension. He regards his failure to find this evidence as disappointing, but not as critical to the conclusion that infants perceive categorically. Too few of the conferees commented on this point to allow a statement of a consensus, but we dissent strongly. We believe that the failure to find evidence of discrimination at the Thai boundary must be adequately explained before we can infer from the evidence for discrimination at the English boundary that infants discriminate VOT rather than the presence of first-formant transitions.

The Possible Importance of Prior Experience. Eimas has suggested that English infants may fail to discriminate at the Thai boundary because they have had no prior experience with VOT stimuli that fall near it. If this were true, then his case for categorical perception of the VOT dimension would be much stronger. This proposition has not been tested directly, and it should be. But our findings with neonates bear on the general issue of whether relevant experience is a necessary prerequisite to infants' speech discrimination.

As mentioned above, we decided in advance of our neonatal experiment to pay particular attention to order effects. Thus, we were interested in whether the no shift, shift, and shift-to-silence groups which began with the −20 stimulus showed the same pattern of results as the comparable groups which began with the +80 stimulus. Our main reason for this focus was the possibility it seemed to provide for determining whether neonates were sensitive to VOT or to the presence of first-formant transitions. The −20 and +80 stimuli confound those variables, and we hoped that an examination of order effects might allow us to attribute any observed shift effect to one or the other of them. We took our hope on this point from Eimas's suggestion that discrimination may depend upon prior experience with the discriminated stimuli. Our neonates, who were tested 46 hr after birth, had minimal experience with stop consonants prior to participating in our experiment. Their preshift experimental stimulation was their main experience with the stimuli. If experience is critical to discrimination, and neonates discriminate first-formant transitions rather than VOT, the groups which started with −20 would show a greater shift effect, since only they would have experienced an appreciable number of first-formant transitions. On the other hand, whether or not experience is critical, if neonates discriminate VOT, then the groups which start with −20 and +80 should show comparable shift effects. A symmetrical order effect would support the conclusion that neonates discriminate VOT, while an asymmetrical effect with greater shift for the groups starting with −20 would support the conclusions that neonates discriminate the presence of first-formant transitions and that their discriminations depend on prior relevant experience. A greater effect for the groups starting with the +80 stimulus could not be due to experience but rather would cast doubt on the inference of discrimination even if the shift groups exceeded both the no shift and shift-to-silence groups.

The neonates who received the −20 stimulus first discriminated it from the +80 stimulus, while those who received the +80 stimulus first did not. In order to bolster the possibility that this order effect was related to differential experience with first-formant transitions, we correlated the number of preshift stimulus presentations to the magnitude of the change scores separately for the infants in the −20/+80 and +80/−20 groups. If experience with first-formant transitions triggers the ability to perceive their presence, then the magnitude of the change score should be related to the number of preshift stimulus presentations for the −20/+80 group, but not for the +80/−20 group, since only the −20 stimulus contains a first-formant transition. The correlation between number of preshift stimulus presentations and the change score was 0.60 ($p < 0.05$) for the −20/+80 group and −0.07 ($p >$ 0.25) for the +80/−20 group. We have subsequently replicated this differential correlation. We conclude that the basis for neonates' discriminations of these stimuli is very probably their sensitivity to the presence of first-formant transitions, rather than their sensitivity to VOT, and that this sensitivity is produced by experience with first-formant transitions.

The suggestion of these findings that prior relevant experience is necessary to trigger infants' discriminative capabilities highlights the importance of presenting stimuli near the Thai boundary to infants before testing their discrimination around it. If such prior stimulation is a prerequisite for discrimination, it would greatly strengthen the argument that infants perceive VOT, because there is no apparent confound at the Thai boundary. It would also greatly strengthen the conclusion that prior experience facilitates infants' discrimination. A similar strengthening would result from showing that prior experience with −20 VOT stimuli induced neonates to discriminate in the +80/−20 order.

In view of these considerations, Eimas argued that the conclusion that infants perceive categorically did not depend solely upon studies of VOT discrimination. He pointed out that his experiment on the perception of place of articulation could, by itself, justify the conclusion of categorical perception. We are less sanguine on this point. The vast bulk of the data that have heretofore been cited to justify the inference that infants perceive categorically concerns VOT. Abandoning these data in the face of criticism does not eliminate them, and their problematic aspects need to be explained before we can accept the inference of categorical perception, the data on place not withstanding. Eimas's experiment on place is compelling, particularly because he also showed that place cues are discriminated differently in and out of speech context. But the findings have yet to be replicated. Moreover, place is not a univariate cue either, and the possibility remains that it too, like VOT, may be discriminated acoustically rather than linguistically.

A consensus was found on these issues, and it is that we need to isolate each of the several acoustic cues that comprise the VOT and place continua, and to determine whether each cue is perceived by infants. If the cues are only discriminated in combination, then the argument that infants perceive linguistic dimensions rather than acoustic features would be immeasurably strengthened. Eimas and Morse, as well as other conferees, concurred with this conclusion. They recognized that synthetic stimuli are not univariate, but that fact may be unimportant. Infants may perceive complex dimensions, not simple continua, and the day when we can judge that seems close by.

The Speechlessness of Synthetic Stimuli

Our present knowledge of how adults and infants perceive speech signals depends heavily, if not wholely, upon experiments with synthetic stimuli. It seems strange, therefore, that these stimuli should sound so little like natural speech. Experimenters who use such stimuli regularly are clearly not bothered by this fact, while researchers who are not experienced with synthetic stimuli are bothered by it. This issue was not discussed rationally at the conference, but it clearly was an issue. Some of the conferees simply could not bring themselves to believe that stimuli which sounded more like telephone busy signals than fluent English could be used to study speech perception. Others, like Morse, could not bring themselves to believe that anything but synthetic stimuli could yield precise understandings of speech perception. In between were people who felt that the synthetic stimuli that have so far been studied fail to capture most of the contrasts that are functional in oral discourse.

The conferees failed to sort out the ways in which synthetic stimuli facilitate and the ways in which they limit perceptual research with infants. The chief value of synthetic stimuli is that their properties can be specified precisely. The chief disadvantage of them is that their characterization as speech depends upon the judgment of experienced listeners. Infants are not experienced listeners. The infant experimenter who uses synthetic stimuli must, therefore, depend upon adults to establish that his stimuli are speech-like. The purpose of most infant researchers is to discover how infants divide and apprehend their world. This purpose recognizes that infants may perceive different dimensions than adults. Unless the infant researcher is careful, the use of adults to judge his stimuli may strangely defeat the basic purpose of his perceptual research on infants by delimiting inappropriately the stimuli he presents to children. The danger is that relying solely on synthetic stimuli may cause the infant investigator to miss the opportunity to observe that infants perceive features adults do not.

THE UNBRIDGED GAP BETWEEN INFANCY AND ADULTHOOD

The use of adult-defined stimuli is not the most important way in which Eimas' work attempts to bridge the gap between infancy and adulthood. His research strategy depends centrally upon establishing that infants and adults perceive similarly, that is, linguistically. Indeed, the most remarkable interpretation of his infant research is that there is no important development between 1 month and adulthood in the perception of phonemic stimuli. He does not deny that learning occurs, because infants obviously do not have the same speech labels that adults do, but he does assert that infants and adults both rely upon innate linguistic feature detectors to perceive speech. Ultimately this view may be sustained, but it certainly is not justified yet.

So far, the main evidence that Eimas' view may be correct has to do with whether infants, like adults, perceive categorically. We have already advanced several reasons for withholding judgement on this issue. Here, we will consider additional methodological and conceptual reasons for doubting that Eimas has yet to bridge adequately the gap between infancy and adulthood.

The Minimal Evidence for Categorical Perception Cannot Yet Be Obtained from Infants

Studdert-Kennedy, Liberman, Harris, and Cooper (1970, p. 236) have unequivocally prescribed the minimal acceptable evidence that perception is categorical:

> From the foregoing it should be clear that the degree to which perception is categorical or continuous can only be unequivocally determined from an examination of both identification and discrimination data. Identification functions alone are not enough: clear-cut categories are characteristic of categorically perceived stimuli, but may also be yielded by any continuum of which the stimuli selected for testing lie far enough apart. Discriminative peaks and troughs alone are not enough: they must be appropriately correlated in level and position along the continuum with identification categories, the peaks occurring at category boundaries, the troughs within categories.
>
> What is needed, therefore, is a procedure for comparing identification and discrimination functions and determining the degree to which they are related.

What is needed cannot be obtained from infants, because there is yet no way to determine how they identify the stimuli which they are subsequently asked to discriminate. Not even half of the data required to establish that infants perceive categorically is available. We need, in addition to the incompletely specified discrimination functions obtained by Eimas, both infant identification functions and a determination of the degree to which these relate to their discrimination functions.

Eimas has attempted to circumvent the need for infant identification functions by using those of adults. He has, in this way, established a provocative relationship between adult identification and infant discrimination. But this strategy is completely inadequate to establish that infants perceive categorically as adults do, because Eimas has no independent evidence for his assumption that infants categorize stimuli as adults do. In fact, there is reason to doubt that infants categorize stimuli at all, in which case they must not perceive categorically.

If Identification Underlies Discrimination, Then Infants Cannot Perceive as Adults Do

In order for Eimas to conclude that infants and adults perceive stop consonants similarly, he must conclude that adults' identification functions result from their inability to discriminate within-category VOT differences. He must reject the possibility that adults' discrimination functions arise from their having learned to attach the same linguistic label to stimuli that they are competent to identify as physically different. Infants cannot attach the same labels to the stimuli that adults do, since the labels have to be learned. Therefore, the comparable basis for the discrimination of infants and adults must be based on innately determined discriminative capacities, and adults must come to identify stimuli similarly because they are constitutionally incapable of discriminating them.

The method by which adult discrimination is assessed makes it at least possible that differential identification underlies discrimination performance, not *vice versa* as Eimas requires. The procedures that have been used to investigate adults' speech discrimination require that they retain one of the stimuli in memory for later comparison to another stimulus. The question is, how do adults store the first stimulus, and the answer is very probably that they store it phonetically. They very probably identify and assign a phonetic label to the stimulus when it is presented and compare that label to the phonetic label which they subsequently assign to the next presented stimulus. In other words, these discrimination tests very probably assess whether adults identify stimuli similarly, not whether they discriminate them on the basis of some auditory cue. Thus, the methods that have been used to study categorical perception by adults raise serious questions about the possibility, upon which Eimas bases his entire theoretical account, that infants and adults use similar processes to discriminate VOT. This may not invalidate his notion of innate feature detectors, but it surely causes us to question the most compelling reason for hypothesizing them, namely, that infants and adults discriminate in the same fashion.

WHAT DO STUDIES OF INFANT SPEECH PERCEPTION SAY ABOUT HOW TO FACILITATE LANGUAGE DEVELOPMENT?

Neither Morse nor Eimas claims that his work is relevant to training language development. Eimas has only once suggested that how infants perceive speech is relevant to how their language develops. He argued on logical grounds that infants must be able to segment the speech stream in order to interpret its meaning. While he does not speculate on the matter, we doubt that very many infants fail to learn language because they cannot segment and discriminate features of the speech stream. Morse proposed only an indirect relationship between speech perception and language development, namely, that since mentally retarded people have memory deficiencies, any study of their linguistic retardation must be performed in light of the fact that memory processes affect the outcomes of the methods we use to study linguistic processes. These men did not claim that their work was relevant to language deficiency or its remediation, and so it was left to the conferees to decide if it was.

The conferees found that the HAS shift effect was reliable and replicable, but that it was not clearly interpretable. Before the shift effect can be interpreted clearly, the rationale for the HAS procedure must be clarified and validated. Moreover, at least one set of converging operations must be employed. Once these problems of response measurement are remedied, questions stemming from stimulus characteristics must be eliminated before confident conclusions can be drawn about categorical perception. More pairs of stimuli must be compared, and evidence for discrimination must be found at points on at least the VOT and place continua that are not confounded by acoustic variations such as the disappearance of formant transitions. Ways must be found to bridge more satisfactorily the gap between infancy and adulthood before all of these other prerequisites will allow confident inferences about the categorical perception of infants. Before it can safely be concluded that infants perceive linguistically, more evidence must also be adduced to show that infants perceive acoustic cues differently in speech and nonspeech contexts, and it must be shown conclusively that speech evokes lateralized brain potentials at a very early age. No clear sentiment was expressed about how likely we are to meet all of these prerequisites to strong interpretation of Eimas' and Morse's findings. However, there was a strong sense that these men had adduced provocative evidence that was worth pursuing.

Even though the conferees could not conclude that infants' perception is either categorical or linguistically relevant, they were willing to conclude that young infants could discriminate a wide variety of speech stimuli. By 2 months of age, infants somehow discriminate between vowels, between fundamental frequency contours, and between different sequences of vowels and consonants (see Table 1). They show no comparable evidence of discriminating pure tones, but this may well be due to the limited sensitivity of the HAS procedure. The basis for these various speech sound discriminations is unclear, because in many cases the stimuli have been natural rather than synthetic. The possibility remains, therefore, that the apparently different discriminations are mediated by a small number, perhaps only one, characteristic of speech. But this seems unlikely. The more likely possibility is that normally developing infants achieve a wide range of speech discriminations at a very early age. There is some evidence from our study with neonates that this development has important experiential determinants, but this possibility needs further testing.

By themselves, these interpretations of the findings on infant speech perception have very little to say to those who would like to improve the language development of abnormal infants. Before they will speak to interveners, we will have to determine whether there are significant individual differences in speech perception. Do any infants lack these discriminative capacities? Do any develop them only much later in life? The only data that bear upon this question have been collected by Sandra Trehub, and their utility is extremely difficult to assess. She has reported that infants who are reared in orphanages from birth do not show the shift effects which she has demonstrated so repeatedly with infants reared at home. The problem with this observation is that it could be due to any of a host of irrelevant confounded variables, such as the temperature and ambient noise level of the orphanage. Nevertheless, this lone observation suggests that it might be useful to search for individual differences in speech perception and their correlates. The question is, how shall we look for such differences? The HAS procedure suffers the grave liability of working with half or fewer of the infants to whom it is applied, and these are in many senses a select group of infants. Morse's (1972) experiment illustrates this point best: only 10% of the infants whose mothers were motivated enough to bring them to his laboratory completed his experiment. He rejected infants for "state" during the experiment by observing them. Trehub (1973) has noted that he might have succeeded in eliminating all of his subjects if he had used a more sensitive physiological index of the infant's state! This example is admittedly extreme, but it highlights the fact that the HAS procedure, while it is the best available for its purpose, does not adapt well to the search for individual differences. Those infants who are most likely to have language problems by reason of perceptual problems are more likely than the routine experimental infant to fail the minimal requirements of the task. Some conferees felt that these problems might become less formidable if infant experimenters adopted individual subject designs and saw infants more than once.

If individual differences could be found, and if they were associated with abnormal language development or risk thereof, then language interveners might justifiably try to train speech discrimination of infants who were at risk for language abnormalities. The question then would be, how does one train such discriminations? The only evidence that bears on this issue is our observation of an order effect with neonates, and this is not very helpful. It suggests only that relevant stimulation might somehow trigger discriminative capacities. But what is relevant, and would such stimulation help infants who have discriminative deficits? No one ventured a confident answer to this question. What did seem clear to a number of the conferees was that we needed infant experiments designed to assess the impact of environmental interventions on their perception. Data of that sort seemed likely to tell us whether language intervention programs could benefit from trying to train speech discrimination.

102Butterfield and Cairns

REFERENCES

Berg, W. K. Habituation and dishabituation of cardiac responses in awake, four month old infants. Unpublished doctoral dissertation, University of Wisconsin, Madison, 1971.

Berg, W. K. Cardiac orienting at 6 and 16 weeks. Paper presented at the meetings of the Society for Psychophysiological Research, Boston, Nov., 1972.

Eimas, P. D. Speech perception in early infancy. In L. B. Cohen and P. Salapatek (Eds.), *Infant Perception.* New York: Academic Press, in press.

Eimas, P. D., Siqueland, E. R., Jusczyk, P., and Vigorito, J. Speech perception in infants. *Science,* 1971, *171,* 303–306.

Kaplan, E. L. The role of intonation in the acquisition of language. Unpublished doctoral dissertation, Cornell University, Ithaca, 1969.

Moffitt, A. R. Consonant cue perception by twenty- to twenty-four-week-old infants. *Child Develop.,* 1971, *42,* 717–731.

Molfese, D. L. Cerebral assymmetry in infants, children and adults: auditory evoked responses to speech and noise stimuli. Unpublished doctoral dissertation, Pennsylvania State University, University Park, 1972.

Morse, P. A. The discrimination of speech and nonspeech stimuli in early infancy. *J. Exp. Child Psychol.,* 1972, *14,* 477–492.

Pisoni, D. B. On the nature of categorical perception of speech sounds. Unpublished doctoral dissertation, University of Michigan, Ann Arbor, 1971.

Studdert-Kennedy, M., Liberman, A. M., Harris, K. S., and Cooper, F. S. Motor theory of speech perception: A reply to Lane's critical review. *Psychol. Rev.,* 1970, *77,* 234–249.

Trehub, S. E. Auditory-linguistic sensitivity infants. Unpublished doctoral dissertation, McGill University, Montreal, 1973a.

Trehub, S. E. Infant's sensitivity to vowel and tonal contrasts. *Develop. Psychol.,* 1973b, *9,* 91–96.

Trehub, S. E. and Rabinovitch, M. S. Auditory-linguistic sensitivity in early infancy. *Develop. Psychol.,* 1972, *6,* 74–77.

Wormith, J. S. Pure tone discrimination in infants. Unpublished masters thesis, Carleton University, Northfield, Minn., 1971.

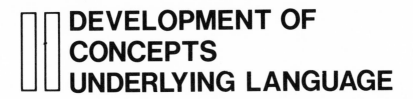

DEVELOPMENT OF CONCEPTS UNDERLYING LANGUAGE

CHAPTER FOUR

SOME ASPECTS OF THE CONCEPTUAL BASIS FOR FIRST LANGUAGE ACQUISITION[1]

Eve V. Clark

Committee on Linguistics, Stanford University, Stanford, California 94305

Language does not develop *in vacuo;* it develops with the function of representing thoughts, percepts, and feelings. It is a communicative system, designed to convey what X might think, feel, or see, to Y. For this reason, language is inextricably linked to the conceptual factors that underlie it. This chapter explores some aspects of the conceptual basis for language acquisition and use and, in particular, examines some of the perceptual-cognitive skills that the child brings to the complex task of learning what language means and what the relationship is between his experience and the words used to convey it to another person. This will necessarily involve some consideration of the relation between language development and cognitive development (*e.g.,* Sinclair-de Zwart, 1967) and hence of the relationship between cognitive and semantic complexity (Slobin, 1973; Clark, 1973b). Throughout this chapter, the terms "cognitive" and "conceptual" will be used to refer to the interpretive system(s) into which different kinds of input have to be mapped, *e.g.,* perceptual input from the visual or the tactile modality. Language also constitutes input to such an interpretive system, and therefore it is assumed that the semantics of language is isomorphic with the cognitive interpretive system so as to allow mapping between the two. This is a basic requirement, given that language is used to talk about all kinds of input to the system.

The study of language acquisition by children has long been of interest to both psychologists and linguists (Blumenthal, 1970), and, in the early sixties, Chomsky's work in linguistics provided a new impetus for research on this topic (Chomsky, 1959, 1965). Most of this research, until recently, has been concerned primarily with the acquisition of syntax: grammatical markers such as articles and inflections, word order, and the underlying grammatical

[1] This research was supported in part by National Science Foundation Grant GS-30040. I thank Jonathan Baron for his comments on an earlier version of this chapter, and Herbert H. Clark for his helpful discussion of the issues. The present chapter also benefitted from comments made at the conference itself.

relations such as "subject-of" and "verb-of" (*e.g.*, McNeill, 1970). This bias toward syntax in language acquisition research was a natural consequence of Chomsky's influence. However, it has led many investigators to overlook, or more probably, assume as given, the cognitive phenomena that underlie language. The child who is learning language, though, has to find out exactly what aspects of his experience (his percepts, his feelings) can be represented in words. He is faced with the puzzle of assigning *meaning* to words at a point when he still knows very little about the language he is learning and at a stage where his world knowledge is still rather limited compared to the adult's. This situation gives rise to a number of questions, some of which will be considered in the present paper. For example, is the assignment of a meaning to a word dependent on prior perceptual-cognitive factors? Does the child use strategies of interpretation based on his previous experience when faced with a "new" word? To what extent does the child's first meaning for a word coincide with the adult one? Does the child's meaning change over time as he learns more, both about his surroundings (world knowledge) and about his language?

Slobin (1973) recently proposed the general hypothesis that the child will first learn those aspects of language that are within the scope of his current cognitive development, so that as the child develops cognitively, he will gradually learn to use more complex linguistic formulations. In other words, cognitive development provides the basis for language acquisition, and the order in which certain linguistic distinctions will be acquired can be predicted on the basis of their relative cognitive complexity. Moreover, if a bilingual child, for example, should mark a distinction like plurality correctly (*i.e.*, just as the adult would) in one language, but not in the other, the cognitive basis hypothesis could be used to arrive at some conclusions about what constitutes formal linguistic complexity. The bilingual situation shows that the child does know the distinction because he marks it correctly in one language. The fact that he omits it or uses it incorrectly in the other allows us to infer that the linguistic forms used to mark that distinction in the second language have some formal complexity over and above their cognitive complexity. Slobin pointed out that the assumption of invariance in the order of acquisition of cognitive distinctions, *e.g.*, of the kind studied by Piaget, allows one to ask detailed questions about the kinds of strategies (operating principles) and cognitive processes children bring to the task of acquiring language. The focus of the present paper will be on the role played by such factors in the basic process of assigning meaning to words.

Many words can be ostensively "defined" by someone's pointing out an appropriate exemplar of the category referred to. Wherever concrete referents are available, it could be claimed that this is all that is necessary for the child to infer what the adult word means. However, ostensive definitions (particularly when based on few exemplars) do not *per se* provide one with much information about the set of criterial features of the category named (Clark, 1973b). To say: "That's a doggie [pointing]. Say 'doggie'," does not tell the child whether he should be paying attention to the dog's shape, the dog's size, the texture of its coat, the way it moves, all of these, or only one or two of them. This problem can be seen more clearly perhaps if it is posed in terms of how one would describe to a Martian the basis for setting up a category named "dog" in such a way that the Martian could determine whether the object he came across was an exemplar of that category or not. The child, in trying to map his percepts into language is faced with much the same problem, despite the help that ostensive definition may provide along the way. The child has to decide which is the relevant factor of the many features he can see. If he decides that everything is relevant, no doubt he might treat "doggie" as a proper name, unique to that one animal; in other words, the child would have set up a smaller category than the adult one. This hypothesis would be upset almost immediately, though, upon the adult's pointing out another exemplar, so the child would have to start again, and make a new decision about what the word "doggie" was really referring to. In fact, the data available suggest that the child picks out only one or two features as criterial to begin with and gradually adds in the others used by the adult until his meaning for the word eventually matches the adult meaning (Clark, 1973b). Many words in language, though, do not have tangible referents because instead of naming objects, they name relations between objects or between events, or else they name properties that are variable and tend to be assessed relative to some standard which itself may also vary, *e.g.*, words like "under," "after," "in front of," "big," "wide." Such words do not offer the adult the possibility of simply pointing in order to identify the referent of the word, although in a few cases he might try to demonstrate through his actions, *e.g.*, with words like "under" or "in front of." Nonetheless, the child manages to learn the meanings of words for tangible referents and words for relations during the course of learning language. This chapter will explore some of the perceptual and cognitive skills that seem to play a role in the process of learning such word meanings. I shall argue that one very important aspect of the conceptual basis that the child draws on in acquiring language is his use of hypotheses and strategies of interpretation when mapping his percepts into language.

I shall deal first with nonrelational words, those words whose meanings may be defined ostensively, and consider what kinds of perceptual skills the child has already developed at the point where he begins to work on language. Secondly, I shall discuss some of the recent work that has been done on relational words. In particular, I shall concentrate on the role of certain non-linguistic strategies in the acquisition of the meaning of spatial prepositions like "in" and "under" and dimensional adjective pairs like "big-small" and "long-short."

WORD MEANINGS AND PERCEPTS

Theories about the development of semantic knowledge during language acquisition have to deal with two central questions: what meaning does the child attach to a particular word, and what relation does the child's meaning bear to the adult's? The hypothesis put forward by Clark (1973b) is that the child learns the adult meaning of words gradually. When the child first begins to use a word with some consistent semantic content, he cannot be expected to know the full (adult) meaning because his experience and general knowledge are still very rudimentary compared to the adult's. However, because of the overlap in experience at the perceptual level (the child can see, touch, and listen to things just as the adult can), the content of the child's early lexical entries will correspond to some extent to some of the features of meaning found in the adult's lexical entries. There is, therefore, sufficient overlap to allow for a certain amount of communication from the very beginning. Another way to talk about this early state of affairs is to say that the child begins by identifying the meaning of a word with only one or two of its semantic components on features of meaning, rather than with the complete combination of components used by the adult (Clark, 1973b; Bierwisch, 1967, 1970).

Once the child has attached *some* meaning to a word, however incomplete, it obviously *has that meaning* for him and is used accordingly. Whatever components or features of meaning the child has picked out as the meaning of the word (its lexical entry) will be criterial in deciding whether it can be applied or not in a particular situation. If the word meanings are incomplete, one would predict that the child should make noticeable misapplications of words from the point of view of the adult. For instance, he might call a large variety of objects "x," where the adult has two or more different categorizations, and therefore uses two or more different words. Such misapplications on the child's part have been called "overextensions" (Clark, 1973b).

The phenomenon of overextension is the result of the child's picking out less than the full set of features as the meaning of some word. The child's choice presumably depends on what is available to him as a potential meaning. Since perceptual input provides a primary source of information for the child, one can argue that it is the perceptual attributes of an object, *e.g.,* shape, that are most immediately available to provide a meaning for a new word. Furthermore, given that the child and adult systems of meaning have to interlock at some point of common understanding, it would seem very plausible that the child's interpretation of some perceived characteristic(s) would coincide with the adult's. Indeed, overlap at the perceptual level within the semantic system seems much more likely to occur in the earliest stages than, say, overlap due to one's knowledge of function or of cultural factors. This is because the child would have to have much more knowledge of the world before he would know what functions an object could have, whereas, to know its perceptual attributes, he has merely to look. Later on, obviously, the function of an object may prove to be as important as (or even more important than) its perceptual characteristics in deciding what it should be called in a particular situation in a particular culture.

Just as an object may have a number of perceptual attributes, which, *combined,* characterize that category, so a word meaning is made up of components or features of meaning which are combined to form the lexical entry for the word. These elements of meaning may be considered to be drawn from a universal set, such that languages differ from each other mainly in terms of which semantic components are used and how they are combined to form the meanings of words (Postal, 1966; Bierwisch, 1967). This assumption of universality is dependent on another factor also. It is assumed that among the components or features of meaning used in semantic analysis one will eventually be able to identify a set of semantic primitives, the universality of which is the result of their being directly related to the cognitive and perceptual functioning of *homo sapiens* (Bierwisch, 1967; Clark, 1973b; H. Clark, 1973). Ideally, therefore, one could assume that the initial feature or features of meaning picked out by the child are necessarily the same as some of the adult's for a particular word meaning. However, at present, there is no positive way of identifying particular features as semantic primitives. It is therefore simply assumed that there is some correspondence between the adult and child perceptual features and that it is this correspondence that allows communication in the first place when the child begins to use words with some consistency.

The phenomenon I have called overextension is perhaps best illustrated by a brief account of some of the observations made in various diary studies. Several diarists kept very detailed records of children's use of words and even performed small experiments in order to find out more about the early meaning children seemed to have for certain words. For example, Major (1906) related that he took his son, aged 2:0 years, to visit a zoological museum. While there, he asked him what different stuffed animals were called. The child freely named most of the animals on demand as follows: he called most of them "mum" (namely, hippopotamus, opossum, peccary, guinea pig, tiger, wolf); in addition, he called the monkey "babie" [baby] and referred to bird's eggs in a nest and a set of snail shells as "balls." Major had also found that in an informal picture-identifying task (given shortly before the museum visit), the child seemed to use "mum" for any four-legged animal for which he had no name already. The "meaning" of "mum," then, could be narrowed down to a feature of the form [four-legged X].[2] Major later followed up these observations by taking the child back to the same

---

[2] This should not be taken as a claim that features like [four-legged] are in any way simple or primitive. They merely represent a subset of the criterial perceptual attributes that have been interpreted by the child as being the meaning of a particular word.

museum 11 months later (aged 2:11), with the result that the child now refused to name any unfamiliar animals except the hippopotamus and the peccary ("pigs"), and the emu, which he called a "chicken." Instead of naming, he insisted that his father tell him what each animal was called. (Elsewhere, interestingly, Major noted that at about this time the child had begun to ask questions with much greater frequency, using mainly "what" and "where" interrogatives.)

Another investigator, Perez (1892), observed a very similar phenomenon and also followed it up. His child also seemed to have a general word for animals, and Perez found that when he presented the child with indeterminate drawings of a horizontal line with four downward projections, the drawings also elicited the general animal word and no other. This would appear to give striking confirmation to the inference that the child was using some feature like [four-legged].

Lastly, Stern (1930) found that his own children would freely name schematic drawings at about age 1:10, but some 8 months later (aged 2:6 and upwards) they apparently failed to recognize what such schematic drawings represented and therefore could no longer name them.

One interpretation of these data is that these children's early words were minimally specified in the sense that they had only one or two percept-based features in their lexical entries. At the same time, these few features happened to coincide with the perceptual features of the schematic drawings shown to them by Perez and Stern. But, by the time Stern's children were some 8 months older, they had added more features to the meanings of the words in their vocabulary, so that there was no longer any simple match between the children's lexical entries and the components in the schematic drawings—hence their failure to "recognize" what the drawings represented.

These naturalistic manipulations by Major, Perez, and Stern provide us with some insights into the perceptual basis for the overextensions used by very young children. In a survey of the extensive diary literature (Clark, 1973b), I found that the majority of the features first used by children in overextensions seemed to be directly derived from their perception of the object named. Overextensions such as those described above have been reported in the speech of children from a wide variety of language backgrounds, including Danish, English, Estonian, French, Georgian, German, Hungarian, Russian, and Serbian. Furthermore, there is great consistency in the ages for which such overextensions are reported. Young children seem to use noticeable overextensions between the ages of 1:1 and 2:6, and the period of noticeable use rarely lasts for more than a year. This reliance on a limited set of perceptual attributes for categorization, therefore, seems to be operative primarily during the 1st year of learning to use language.

A few of the more detailed diary studies implicitly relate the phenomenon of overextension to vocabulary growth. The end of the period of overextension is generally marked by a large increase in questioning activity (of the "what(s) that" type) combined with a rapid growth in vocabulary. The most striking element common to all these reports, though, is that the features or components of meaning that the child appears to be using criterially in order to produce these overextensions are derived from the perceptual input to the child—whether it be tactile, visual, olfactory, or auditory in nature (see Table 1). The perceptual basis for overextensions also explains the consistency of such reports for the acquisition of different languages. Indeed, it may also explain the highly similar overextensions observed by the Gardners in the early use of signs by the chimpanzee Washoe (Bronowski and Bellugi, 1970).

The principal criterial characteristics that form the basis of overextensions can be sorted into six categories: those based on *shape,* on *movement,* on *size,* on *sound,* on *taste,* and on *texture* (Clark, 1973b). The perceptual modality employed for the different categories of overextension can be listed as follows, with visual perception playing the primary role in normal children: 1) shape: visual, tactile; 2) movement: visual, auditory; 3) size: visual, tactile; 4) sound: auditory; 5) taste: gustatory, olfactory; 6) texture: visual, tactile.

Since the child undoubtedly uses perceptual information in first assigning meanings to words, it is possible to delve deeper and try to find out what types of perceptual information the child has successfully interpreted and organized by the time he starts to work overtly on language. Such organized perceptual knowledge may constitute a large part of the conceptual basis for early language use. Rather than review perceptual development according to the modality used by the child, I shall take up in turn those aspects of perceptual development relevant to each of the main categories of overextension, *viz., shape, size, movement, sound,* and *texture.* (*Taste* will be omitted here for two reasons. First, such overextensions are rare, and all pertained to sweet things only. Secondly, there is little research on the infant's capacity to taste things, although some mother-infant studies do suggest that the infant very early learns to recognize familiar smells.)

Shape

There is a certain amount of controversy over how one determines whether the very young infant can perceive form (Hershenson, 1967; Bond, 1972). However, newborns (1–5 days old) can evidently see differences in brightness (Hershenson, 1967). Kessen, Haith, and Salapatek (1965) found some evidence that vertical contour detectors are present in the young infant, and further work by Salapatek and Kessen (1966) showed that infants had a preference for looking at the vertices of a figure. This result, however, may be confounded with the brightness contrast. Since lines and edges in particular orientations are known to stimulate maximally certain cells in the visual cortex (Hubel and Weisel, 1962; Sutherland, 1963), it is perhaps not surprising to find the newborn paying attention to lines and vertices (Gibson, 1969). Furthermore, Fantz (1961a, 1963) found that infants aged 1–15 weeks

Table 1. Some Examples of Overextension in Young Children's Speech*

Category	Word	First referent	Domain of overextension	Language
Shape	[mooi]	moon	→ cakes → round marks on windows and in books → round shapes in books → tooling on leather book covers → postmarks (round) → letter O	English
	[buti]	ball	→ toy → radish → stone spheres at park entrance	Georgian
	[kotibaiz]	bars of cot (crib)	→ large toy abacus → toast rack with parallel bars → picture of building with columns on facade	English
	[tick-tick]	watch	→ clocks → all clocks and watches → gas-meter → fire-hose wound on spool → bathroom scales with round dial	English
Size	[fly]	fly	→ specks of dirt → dust → all small insects → his own toes → crumbs of bread → small toad	English
	[bébé]	baby	→ other babies → all small statues → figures in small pictures and prints	French
Movement	[bird]	sparrows	→ cows → dogs → cats → any animal moving	English
Sound	[fafer]	sound of train (chemin de fer)	→ steaming coffee pot → anything that hissed or made a noise	French
Taste	[cola]	chocolate	→ sugar → tarts → grapes, figs, peaches	French
Texture	[va]	white plush dog	→ muffler → cat → father's fur coat	Russian

*Table based on Clark, 1973b.

preferred complex patterns over simple ones. He interpreted these data to mean that some degree of form perception is actually innate. Further evidence of the infant's attention to contour comes from the studies of preferences for "real" faces over "scrambled" representations of faces (Fantz, 1961a; Ahrens, 1954). Bower (1966, 1967a, 1967b) reported a series of studies which seem to provide further evidence that young infants, in their first few months, can perceive certain properties of shape or contour.

Other research suggests that infants have some perception of the three-dimensionality of objects. Fantz (1961b; Fantz and Nevis, 1967) found that infants between 1 and 6 months old preferred to look at a solid sphere rather than a circle if there was an observable difference in pattern due to the texture and contour shading of the solid. Bower, Broughton, and Moore (1971a) found that infants aged 16–24 weeks expect a perceived object to be solid, and they expect it to be there when they grasp it. This expectation was demonstrated when a virtual object was projected in front of the infant. The virtual object elicited the same grasping response as a real object, but the infant's inability to actually grasp what he saw evoked a strong startle response and even distressed crying. In another study (Bower, Broughton, and Moore, 1971b), Bower demonstrated that as early as 2 weeks old, infants exhibit avoidance behavior with approaching objects when sitting in an upright or semiupright position. Avoidance responses (pulling back of head, raising of hands, distressed crying) were specific to approaching objects. No reaction was evoked by stationary or departing ones. This suggests that as early as 2 weeks of age, the infant has some perception of both distance and movement.

While the degree to which the infant's perceptions are the same in some sense as the adult's remains a fairly open question, the research outlined above makes it clear that the child has already developed a number of perceptual skills even before the age of 6 months, and possibly earlier. These include the perceptual skills that appear to be called on when the child starts to represent his percepts symbolically with language.

Finally, several studies of slightly older children provide some information on the early use of shape (*vs.* other attributes) in sorting tasks. Ricciuti (1963, 1965) found that children aged 12–24 months used shape as their main criterion in free sorting tasks. Brian and Goodenough (1929) found that children below the age of 3:0 years preferred shape or form (80% of choices) to color in the grouping of "similar" stimuli. In fact, 56% of the younger *S*s matched only on form even in nonperseverating responses. Kagan and Lemkin (1961) also found that form (shape) was preferred in paired comparisons over both color and size. Indeed, when presented with situations where form was not available as a basis for matching, over 20% of their subjects (aged 3:9–8:6) said they didn't know the answer. Baley and Witwicki (1948) reported a similar preference for form, in form *vs.* size comparisons. Engel

(1935) also reported an exclusive interest in form (*vs.* color) in children below the age of 3:6. Lastly, Huang (1945) found that form was always predominant for matching real objects for kindergarten children. However, the relative salience of the dimensions used in these tasks may not be a completely reliable guide to the general importance of certain dimensions.

The dominance of form over color in younger children may be the explanation of why no overextensions are found based on color. Furthermore, the emphasis on form where form or size provides a basis for matching objects seems to parallel the proportions of overextensions based on shape *vs.* those based on size that have been reported in the diary literature (see Clark, 1973b).

Movement

The infant's attention to motion has been considered in several developmental studies of perception (*e.g.,* Bower, 1967b; Bower, Broughton, and Moore, 1971b). Motion appears to be detected by the infant as young as 2 weeks old, as shown by their avoidance of approaching objects. However, very young infants may fail to recognize as the same an object in motion *vs.* the same object at rest. Bower, Broughton, and Moore (1971a) also showed that young infants will follow an object in motion and, for example, will anticipate the reappearance of moving objects that vanish behind a screen. One view of the role of motion in perception is that motion makes an object more perceptible against its background. Motion helps the child detect edges and contrasts that might otherwise escape him.

In the case of overextensions based on movement, it is either the motion itself that attracts the child's attention, or else the motion associated with a characteristic sound (*cf.* Clark, 1973b).

Size

While Bower's earlier work (1965a, 1965b) presented some evidence relative to size constancy in the infant as early as 8 weeks of age, few other studies in the development of perception have taken up this issue. There is some research, though, on the infant's perception of depth and of distance (Gibson, 1969). In tasks with older children where preferences for matching on various dimensions were studied (generally a choice between shape, size, and color), size seems to play a negligible role. Kagan and Lemkin (1961) found that size was rarely used in judging similarity. Form was always preferred to both size and color, and if form was not involved, color tended to be chosen over size. Baley and Witwicki (1948) also found that form was preferred to size, but when size and color were the options, the younger Ss (3:0–4:0 years) tended to choose color while the older ones (5:0–6:0) tended to choose size.

This is not to say that size, or rather relative size, is ignored by the young child. Indeed, comparative size may well be used where a factor like shape does not differentiate between objects. It is perhaps rare, though, that size is the only differentiating feature, and that could be the reason why size is less frequently used as the basis for overextension than a property like shape.

Sound

Wertheimer (1961) showed that the infant will respond to auditory stimulation within a few moments of birth. Young infants also appear to distinguish early among sounds that differ in frequency, intensity, duration, and location in space (Spears and Hohle, 1967). By the age of 2 weeks, the infant distinguishes between voices and other sounds such as bells, whistles, and rattles (Wolff, 1966). Several observers have also noted the effectiveness of the human voice in eliciting smiles and vocalization from the infant (*e.g.,* Champneys, 1881; Preyer, 1890; Nakazima, 1966). By 4 weeks, the infant responds differentially to affective qualities, *e.g.,* angry *vs.* friendly voices (Wolff, 1966). Wolff (1963) also found that infants of this age seemed to distinguish between familiar and unfamiliar voices. By 4 months, they can also distinguish male from female voices (Kaplan, 1969). Lastly, several recent studies have shown that the infant very early shows the ability to discriminate between different speech sounds (*cf.* Moffitt, 1968; Eimas, Siqueland, Jusczuk and Vigorito, 1971; Morse, 1972, this volume).

The overextensions based on sound are mainly based on characteristic nonspeech sounds, *e.g.,* the sound of a train. However, there has been much less research on the child's ability to identify or recognize these kinds of sound than there has been on speech sounds.

Texture

Texture is one of the visual cues to whether an object is two- or three-dimensional. Fantz (1963, 1965) showed that infants between 1 and 6 months old prefer to look at a solid sphere (3-D) over a circle (2-D) as long as there is an observable difference in pattern due to the texture and shading of the solid. Texture, though, is not only perceived visually; it can also be explored tactilely. Many observers (*e.g.,* Piaget, 1954, 1962) have noticed how much time infants spend exploring new and old objects with their hands and mouths as well as their eyes (see also Bower, Broughton, and Moore, 1970). The modality of touch is a distinct source of information about texture, *e.g.,* whether an object is smooth or rough, cold (metallic), or warm (wooden, woolen), etc.

The overextensions based on texture seem to be of both sorts: some are based on visual information about texture while others seem to be based mainly on touch (*cf.* Clark, 1973b).

The preceding outline of what the child learns early in life, from the perceptual viewpoint, provides us with a fairly broad view of the kind of conceptual information that the child could probably derive from his percepts. The extent of the child's perceptual knowledge is not surprising given that he spends the 1st year of his life exploring his surroundings through all his senses. The more detailed problem that will require much further research is the exact matching up of perceptual features and semantic features at the interpretive level.

HYPOTHESES AND STRATEGIES

Implicit in the foregoing discussion of the child's perceptual skills and his use of overextensions in the early stages of language acquisition is the assumption that the child starts out with certain hypotheses about what a "new" word might mean. In the case of the overextensions reported in the diary literature, these hypotheses could be characterized very generally in the following terms:

A word refers to some identifiable (perceptually salient) characteristic of the object pointed to.

Given such an hypothesis, the child can then adopt the following strategy to guide his own use of words:

Pick out whatever seems to be the most salient characteristic(s) perceptually, and assume [until given counter-evidence] that that is what the word refers to. Act on this assumption whenever you want to name, request, or call attention to something.

Such an hypothesis and concomitant strategy would account very well for the large number of overextensions observed during the 1st year or so of speech. However, these noticeable overextensions then disappear. The reason for this is most probably that the children have received sufficient negative feedback about their initial hypothesis to have realized that it was wrong. At the same time, they have learned much more vocabulary. They therefore adopt a more cautious approach in the matter of naming categories and actively solicit information about the words for new objects by asking numerous questions of the "what(s) that" variety.

Such hypotheses and their derived strategies provide a plausible account of the processes involved in the acquisition of a word meaning that refers to some tangible referent. Further research, in fact, suggests that young children use the same approach—constructing an hypothesis and deriving strategies from it—in the acquisition of the meanings of relational words as well (Clark, 1973c). On some occasions, of course, the child's hypothesis may coincide with the adult meaning of the word in question so that the child would appear to understand the word correctly. Under other circumstances, however, it can be shown that the child's hypothesis differs considerably from the adult meaning, and, as a result, the child makes consistent *errors* in his interpretations. These errors can be accounted for by the postulation of cognitive strategies that are used by the child prior to the acquisition of semantic knowledge. The strategies used with respect to both nonrelational words like "doggie" and relational words like "in" or "under" appear to be derived primarily from the child's prior percept-based knowledge of "the way things are" in the world around him. Since these strategies are ones used in the initial assignment of meaning to a word, they seem in some sense to be more basic and more directly dependent on cognitive factors than the kinds of parsing strategies for the analysis of grammatical relations discussed by Bever (1970).

As an illustration of the kind of hypothesis-and-strategy approach the young child appears to apply during the acquisition of relational terms, I shall give a brief account of some recent studies of the locative terms "in," "on," and "under" (Clark, 1972a, 1973c) and of certain dimensional adjective pairs (Klatzky, Clark, and Macken, 1973).

Locative Terms

In the first study, children (aged 1:6–5:0) received instructions of the form "Put the x in [on, under] the y," where x was a small toy animal and y was one of six different reference points (RPs) or loci. The RPs consisted of a box on its side, a tunnel with a flat top, a tip-truck, a crib, a table, and a bridge. Thus, each RP allowed two of the three spatial relations named by the prepositions. For example, x could be either in or under the crib. When the children's responses were scored according to adult criteria for semantically appropriate responses, the majority of the children over 3:0 got all three prepositions correct. However, there were significant differences among the three younger groups because of the general increase in percentage correct with age. Furthermore, each preposition produced a different pattern of improvement. These data are shown in Table 2. The order in which the three locatives were acquired appeared to be "in" first, then "on," then "under."

Table 2. Percentage of Semantically Correct Responses*

Group	N	Mean age	In	On	Under	Mean
		yrs:mos	*% correct responses*			
I	10	1:9	94	61	4	53
II	10	2:3	98	72	57	76
III	10	2:9	96	80	98	91

*Each percentage based on 80 data points. Table based on Clark, 1973c.

The actual errors made by each child were very consistent. For example, if the RP offered a choice between "in" or "on" as the spatial relation, the young children would always choose "in." In other words, instructions with "in" and instructions with "on" were both treated as if they contained the word "in." Instructions with "in" and "under" were treated in the same way, as if both contained "in." Lastly, where "on" and "under" were the two possible relations, both kinds of instruction were treated as if they contained "on." The responses from the youngest children therefore produced the following error pattern (the errors are starred):

1. RP allowing "in" or "under"   a. instruction "in" → in
                                     b. instruction "under" → in*
2. RP allowing "in" or "on"   a. instruction "in" → in
                                     b. instruction "on" → in*
3. RP allowing "on" or "under"   a. instruction "on" → on
                                     b. instruction "under" → on*

Thus, "in" appears always to be interpreted correctly, and "on" is interpreted correctly unless the RP is a container such that the relation "in" is a possibility. "Under" is rarely, if ever, correct because the other options—"in" or "on"—are generally chosen by the youngest children. These errors could be the result of applying two simple, ordered rules based on the child's perception of what will be called normal or canonical spatial relations (Clark, 1973c):

Rule 1: If RP is a container, x is inside it.
Rule 2: If RP has a horizontal surface, x is on it.

These rules are strictly ordered in the sense that rule 1 is always applied, but if it "fails," then rule 2 is applied next. Rule 1 then predicts the error of "on" going to "in" and of "under" to "in," while rule 2 predicts the error of "under" going to "on" where rule 1 fails to apply.

These rules suggest an alternative approach to the comprehension data reported in Table 2. It is quite possible that the very young children do not understand "in," "on," and "under." Therefore, more of their data should be accounted for by the use of rules 1 and 2 than by the adult semantics criteria used in Table 2. The data accounted for by the strategies represented as rules 1 and 2 are shown in Table 3. A comparison of the two tables shows that initially, the child's strategies accounted for most of the responses given (89%). This percentage had decreased to 54% for group III (aged 2:6–2:11). In fact, the minimum that could be accounted for by the strategies is 50% since the scoring criteria for strategies *vs.* semantic knowledge cannot separate the responses to instructions containing "in" or half the responses to instructions containing "on" (see further Clark, 1973c). Concomitant with the decrease in the amount of data accounted for by rules 1 and 2, there is an increase from 53% (near the minimum possible) to 91% of the data accounted for by semantic knowledge (Table 2). Thus, the child starts out depending simply on his strategies, but these give way to semantic knowledge as the child gets older.

The youngest child's dependence on strategies such as those in rules 1 and 2 was further explored in a setting where the child had to copy the configuration of object and RP presented by the experimenter. The configurations either did or did not conform to the strategies. It was predicted that, if the younger children made any errors, they would only make them on those configurations not conforming to the strategies, *e.g.*, *x* placed under the crib or *x* placed beside an upright glass. The findings fitted the predictions in that the errors that occurred were on the predicted configurations. The exact form of error made in each instance was also predicted accurately in 84% of the instances (see further Clark, 1973c).

In further experiments carried out on children's acquisition of the meanings of spatial prepositions where none of the RPs were containers and therefore offered no opportunity for the use of a rule 1 strategy, the youngest children consistently applied rule 2 when they did not understand the word used (Clark, 1973c and unpublished data). For example, instructions containing "at the bottom," "below," "in front," and "in back" all produced as semantic "errors" the placement of *x* on the topmost or largest horizontal surface available for the particular RP. These data constitute more extensive support for the use of the rule 2 strategy.

The strategies represented by rules 1 and 2 depend on some very general perceptual properties of objects in the world, namely whether they are containers or not, and whether they have any horizontal surface space. The strategies themselves are derived from the hypotheses the child has constructed on the basis of his prior knowledge. In the case of spatial relations, the child's hypotheses depend heavily on his perception of the normal or expected spatial relations that may hold between objects in the world. For example, containers normally hold things and are therefore normally oriented with their opening upwards. This knowledge is exemplified by the younger children's manipulations of boxes, glasses, and other containers to move them

Table 3. Percentage of Responses Accounted for by Use of Ordered Rules 1 and 2*

Group	Instruction			
	In	On	Under	Mean
I	94	79	96	89
II	95	72	43	69
III	96	62	3	54

*Each percentage based on 80 data points.
Table based on Clark, 1973c.

from a nonupright position to one in which the opening always faced upwards, as well as by their insistence that objects could only go in, not under, RPs such as the crib.

The order of acquisition of the three terms, "in," "on," and "under," therefore, seems to be the result of an interaction between the child's initial hypotheses about what the words mean and what these words actually mean. In the case of the term learned earliest, "in," the child's strategy coincides with the adult meaning, and so the child will receive little or no negative feedback. With "on," the child is sometimes right and sometimes wrong if he simply follows rules 1 and 2. He therefore has to adjust his use of such rules and learn when not to apply them. The same tack has to be followed for "under," but in this instance neither rule will ever produce a semantically correct response and so the child has to learn to disregard these strategies altogether (Clark, 1973c). These data seem to provide further corroboration of Slobin's (1973) hypothesis that relative cognitive complexity—here the degree of correspondance between strategies and adult semantics—is the basic determinant of order of acquisition. Moreover, the identification of such strategies should enable one to measure complexity more precisely and to make detailed predictions about order of acquisition across languages as well as within a particular language.

Dimensional Adjectives

The notion that children initially set up hypotheses about what words mean and then derive strategies for interpretation is also compatible with some work that has attempted to account for the asymmetry that has been observed in the acquisition of positive dimensional adjectives, e.g., "big," "tall," "wide," and their negative counterparts, e.g., "small," "short," "narrow." Children acquiring their first language consistently learn to use and understand positive terms before negative ones. Dimensional adjective pairs such as "high-low" or "long-short" are used asymmetrically. The positive terms (here "high," "long") not only denote comparatively greater extent on the dimension named, but are also used to name the dimension itself (e.g., "height," "length"), to indicate the dimension used in measure phrases (e.g., 10 meters high, 3 meters long), and to ask "neutral" questions (e.g., "How high/long is it?"). In contrast, the negative terms (e.g., "low," "short") are only used to denote relative lack of extent on the dimension in question (Bierwisch, 1967; Greenberg, 1966; Sapir, 1944; Vendler, 1967). Such adjective pairs have also been called unmarked-marked pairs (e.g., Greenberg, 1966). The positive term is regarded as unmarked because of its neutral uses. For example, the positive question "How high is it?" sets up no particular expectation about the kind of answer the inquirer might be given. This contrasts with the question "How low is it?" in which the inquirer obviously starts out with the expectation that the object lacks height.

Such asymmetries in usage result in the positive members of such adjective pairs being more frequent than their negative forms. At first glance, this difference in frequency could be used to account for the acquisition data. However, the asymmetry could equally well be due to an underlying asymmetry at the cognitive level where perception of greater and lesser extent is interpreted. The asymmetry in favor of the positive adjectives (greater extent) could result from a strategy of picking the object with greater extent. Such a strategy, of course, would not differentiate between different adjective pairs where different sets of conditions of application have to be learned as well (Bierwisch, 1967; Clark, 1972b). Indeed, the differences between adjective pairs such as "big-small" and "tall-short," for example, may be still further complicated by the fact that there seems to be a built-in preference for paying attention to the vertical dimension (Ghent, 1961; Braine, 1972) which would presumably confound experimental manipulations designed to get at the difference between "big" and "tall." However, the child using a strategy based on choice of an object with relatively greater extension would be correct more often for the positive pole adjectives than for the negatives because his strategy would coincide with that aspect of the word meaning. In a natural language context, though, it is impossible to eliminate the frequency of the words themselves as an explanatory factor.

Klatzky, Clark, and Macken (1973), therefore, designed a study which attempted to differentiate between an adult usage/frequency explanation for the asymmetry and an explanation based on a conceptual asymmetry. Young children were given a concept-learning task in which nonsense syllables (CVCs) replaced the English words for both the positive and the negative poles of four dimensions: *size, height, length,* and *thickness.*

Since CVCs were substituted for English words in the concept-learning task, there should be no effect of asymmetries in adult usage. This means that if the asymmetry in acquisition is due to the greater frequency of the positive terms, there should be no asymmetry between the positive and negative CVCs. However, if the asymmetries are due to some underlying cognitive asymmetry, then one should find the same positive-negative differences with CVCs as with natural language terms.

The learning data for the CVCs showed that the syllables for the positive end of each of the four dimensions required significantly fewer trials to criterion and produced significantly fewer errors during learning. These data are shown in Figure 1. The asymmetry in the learning of positive and negative CVCs is compatible with the conceptual mechanism explanation but not with the usage/frequency one. Furthermore, neither translation nor mediation seemed able to provide viable explanations of the data (see Klatzky, Clark, and Macken, 1973).

It was therefore proposed that the asymmetry found between positive and negative adjectives and positive and negative CVCs was due to an

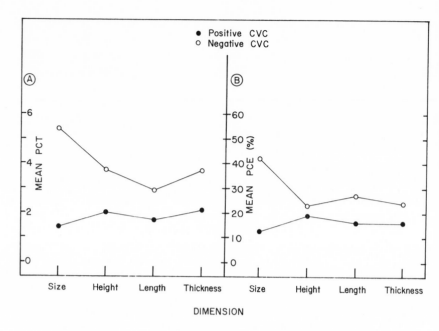

Fig. 1. Precriterion trials (PCT) and precriterion errors (PCE) in the acquisition of positive and negative CVCs. Based on Klatzky, Clark, and Macken, 1973.

underlying conceptual mechanism that could deal with extension or relative extension on a dimension more easily than with relative lack of extension. Extension can be most clearly represented in terms of two reference points: the origin from which extension has to be measured, and the standard being used (implicit or explicit). The simplest situation would be one in which only the first is relevant, where one simply observes that some object has extension. However, wherever one is considering comparative positive extension, the instances in which there is a standard present are in fact analogous to the simple case where no comparison is involved. This is because one has only to select the item with the greatest extension from the origin, and this may be done by treating the standard itself as an origin and then picking the item with extension. This contrasts with the situation in which one is looking for an item that has a relative lack of extension *vis-à-vis* the standard. Here one necessarily uses both reference points: the origin and the standard. One has first to decide which item has most extension from the origin, then make this item the standard, and, in a sense, double-back in order to find an item with extension, but with less extension than the standard.

A mechanism with those properties would predict that there should be a response bias in favor of the item(s) with greater extension during the period of acquisition. Such a bias has been observed in both production and comprehension in natural language acquisition. For example, Donaldson and

Wales (1970) reported that children aged 3:6–5:0 rarely use negative adjectives in their spontaneous speech to describe the relations between objects that differ on various dimensions (see also Wales and Campbell, 1970). Furthermore, Farnham-Diggory and Bermon (1968) found that when children explained how objects differed on one dimension, they nearly always (over 80% of the time) mentioned the object with greater extent first; that is, they described the larger of the two items as "taller," "longer," "bigger," etc. with respect to the other which served as the standard. Comprehension studies such as Donaldson and Balfour (1968) and Palermo (1973) have shown that children also consistently appear to understand positive terms before they can understand negative ones during acquisition. One could argue further that it is this cognitive asymmetry that provides the explanation for the asymmetries found in adult usage and frequency.

The studies that have been described provide convincing evidence that conceptual factors, and in particular the interpretation of one's percepts, play an important and probably crucial role in the acquisition of language. In examining some aspects of this role, I have concentrated primarily on the problem of what meaning the child attaches to individual words, and how his early meanings might be accounted for in terms of certain hypotheses and the strategies derived from them. I have not, however, considered the issue of what further meaning is conveyed by the combination of different words in early utterances (*cf.* Slobin, 1970; Schlesinger, 1971, this volume; Bloom, 1970, 1973).

CONCLUSION

This chapter has concentrated on one aspect of the conceptual basis of language acquisition: the relation between cognitive-perceptual factors and the acquisition of word meanings. However, there are also many other aspects of language that depend on a conceptual substratum. For example, an utterance may be used to make an assertion in one context and to convey a request in another. It is particularly difficult to identify the child's communicative intent in making a particular utterance. There is some preliminary research available on the kinds of functions used by the young child. Both Gruber (1973) and Antinucci and Parisi (1973) have proposed that the child's earliest utterances fall into two classes: requests and descriptions (*cf.* also Dore, 1973). Gruber (1973) suggested that the earliest of these two functions to develop is the request-type utterance (see also Ingram, 1971). Schlesinger (1971, this volume), from a slightly different standpoint, has also proposed that the child's communicative intention in producing an utterance is crucial to its interpretation and (syntactic) analysis by the adult.

A related approach has been taken to the analysis of the syntactic function-in-context of early utterances by investigators such as Brown

(1973), Bowerman (1973a, 1973b), and Bloom (1970). In their analyses, they looked at the structural properties of the utterances and the context of occurrence in an effort to classify utterances of two words or more as locative (*e.g.,* "baby highchair"), demonstrative (*e.g.,* "that boat"), attributive (*e.g.,* "ball red"), possessive (*e.g.,* "daddy cup"), and so on. A somewhat similar approach to relating the child's choice of utterance-form in the case of more complex utterances to the linguistic or the external context was also taken by Clark (1973a).

Bloom (1973) also tried to relate cognitive-perceptual factors directly to the acquisition of syntactic structure via the mapping of perceived roles such as "agent" or "object of action" into language. She proposed that the child first has to learn to interpret a role-like agency at the perceptual-cognitive level and that he then looks for a consistent representation of such a role in the surface forms of language. In other words, the child notices the participants and their relations to each other within particular contexts and then listens to see how these are described by the adult. In the process of learning how the perceived situation gets encoded linguistically, the child comes to realize that a role like "agent" is often encoded (syntactically), let us say, as the initial nominal of the adult utterance (*i.e.,* as the surface subject). From this, the child infers that agents are generally sentence subjects. While this example is greatly oversimplified, it does suggest that the acquisition of syntactic structure by children may not require the postulation of strong linguistic universals of the sort proposed by Chomsky (1965) and McNeill (1970). It is first necessary to explore the limits of the relationship between general cognitive capacities and the ability to acquire language. One basic issue for those doing research in acquisition is therefore the identification of the cognitive mechanisms being used, their role in determining order of acquisition, and their relation to complexity in language.

REFERENCES

Ahrens, R. Beiträge zur Entwicklung des Physionomie und Mimikerkennes. *Z. Exp. Angew. Psychol.,* 1954, *2,* 412–454, 599–633.

Antinucci, F. and Parisi, D. Early language acquisition: A model and some data. In C. A. Ferguson and D. I. Slobin (Eds.), *Studies of Child Language Development.* New York: Holt, Rinehart & Winston, 1973, pp. 607–619.

Baley, S. and Witwicki, T. Barwa, Ksztalt i Wielkosc w Spostrzezenui Dzieci. *Psychol. Wzchow.,* 1948, *13,* 1–23.

Bever, T. G. The cognitive basis for linguistic structures. In J. R. Hayes (Ed.), *Cognition and the Development of Language.* New York: Wiley, 1970, pp. 279–352.

Bierwisch, M. Some universals of German adjectivals. *Found. Lang.,* 1967, *3,* 1–36.

Bierwisch, M. Semantics. In J. Lyons (Ed.), *New Horizons in Linguistics.* Harmondsworth, Mddx.: Penguin Books, 1970, pp. 166–184.

Bloom, L. M. *Language Development: Form and Function in Emerging Grammars.* Cambridge, Mass.: M.I.T. Press, 1970.

Bloom, L. M. *One Word at a Time: The Use of Single Word Utterances before Syntax.* The Hague: Mouton, 1973.

Blumenthal, A. L. *Language and Psychology: Historical Aspects of Psycholinguistics.* New York: Wiley, 1970.

Bond, E. K. Perception of form by the human infant. *Psychol. Bull.,* 1972, *77,* 225–245.

Bower, T. G. R. Stimulus variables determining space perception in infants. *Science,* 1965a, *149,* 88–89.

Bower, T. G. R. The determinants of perceptual units in infancy. *Psychonom. Sci.,* 1965b, *3,* 323–324.

Bower, T. G. R. Slant perception and shape constancy in infants. *Science,* 1966, *151,* 832–834.

Bower, T. G. R. Phenomenal identity and form perception in an infant. *Percept. Psychophys.,* 1967a, *2,* 74–76.

Bower, T. G. R. The development of object permanence: Some studies of existence constancy. *Percept. Psychophys.,* 1967b, *2,* 411–418.

Bower, T. G. R., Broughton, J. M., and Moore, M. K. The coordination of visual and tactual input in infants. *Percept. Psychophys.,* 1970, *8,* 51–53.

Bower, T. G. R., Broughton, J. M., and Moore, M. K. Infant responses to approaching objects: An indicator of response distal variables. *Percept. Psychophys.,* 1971a, *9,* 193–196.

Bower, T. G. R., Broughton, J. M., and Moore, M. K. Development of the object concept as manifested in change in the tracking behavior of infants between 7 and 20 weeks of age. *J. Exp. Child Psychol.,* 1971b, *11,* 182–193.

Bowerman, M. F. *Early Syntactic Development: A Cross-linguistic Study with Special Reference to Finnish.* Cambridge: Cambridge University Press, 1973a.

Bowerman, M. F. Structural relationships in children's utterances: Syntactic or semantic? In T. E. Moore (Ed.), *Cognitive Development and the Acquisition of Language.* New York: Academic Press, 1973b, pp. 197–213.

Braine, L. G. The apparent upright–Implications for copying and for perceptual development. Paper presented at XXth International Congress of Psychology, Tokyo, 1972.

Brian, C. R. and Goodenough, F. L. The relative potency of color and form perception at various ages. *J. Exp. Psychol.,* 1929, *12,* 197–213.

Bronowski, J. and Bellugi, U. Language, name and concept. *Science,* 1970, *168,* 669–673.

Brown, R. W. *A First Language.* Cambridge, Mass.: Harvard University Press, 1973.

Champneys, F. Notes on an infant. *Mind,* 1881, *6,* 104–107.

Chomsky, N. Review of B.F. Skinner: *Verbal Behavior. Language,* 1959, *35,* 26–58.

Chomsky, N. *Aspects of the Theory of Syntax.* Cambridge, Mass.: M.I.T. Press, 1965.

Clark, E. V. Some perceptual factors in the acquisition of locative terms by young children. *Papers from the Eighth Regional Meeting, Chicago Linguistic Society,* 1972a, pp. 431–439.

Clark, E. V. On the child's acquisition of antonyms in two semantic fields. *J. Verb. Learning Verb. Behav.,* 1972b, *11,* 750–758.

Clark, E. V. How children describe time and order. In C. A. Ferguson and D. I. Slobin (Eds.), *Studies of Child Language Development*. New York: Holt, Rinehart & Winston, 1973a, pp. 585–606.

Clark, E. V. What's in a word? On the child's acquisition of semantics in his first language. In T. E. Moore (Ed.), *Cognitive Development and the Acquisition of Language*. New York: Academic Press, 1973b, pp. 65–110.

Clark, E. V. Non-linguistic strategies and the acquisition of word meanings. Cognition, 1973c, *2*, 161–182.

Clark, H. H. Space, time, semantics and the child. In T. E. Moore (Ed.), *Cognitive Development and the Acquisition of Language*. New York: Academic Press, 1973, pp. 28–64.

Donaldson, M. and Balfour, G. Less is more: A study of language comprehension in children. *Brit. J. Psychol.*, 1968, *59*, 461–472.

Donaldson, M. and Wales, R. J. On the acquisition of some relational terms. In J. R. Hayes (Ed.), *Cognition and the Development of Language*. New York: Wiley, 1970, pp. 235–268.

Dore, J. The development of speech acts. Unpublished doctoral dissertation, City University of New York, New York, 1973.

Eimas, P. D., Siqueland, E. R., Jusczyk, P., and Vigorito, J. Speech perception in infants. *Science*, 1971, *171*, 303–306.

Engle, P. Über die Teilinhaltiche Beachtung von Farbe und Form; Untersuchung an 800 Schulkindern. *Z. Pädagogische Psychol.*, 1935, *36*, 202–214, 241–251.

Fantz, R. L. The origin of form perception. *Sci. Amer.*, 1961a, *204*, 66–72.

Fantz, R. L. A method for studying depth perception in infants under six months of age. *Psychol. Rec.*, 1961b, 27–32.

Fantz, R. L. Pattern vision in newborn infants. *Science*, 1963, *140*, 296–297.

Fantz, R. L. Visual perception from birth as shown by pattern selectivity. *Ann. N. Y. Acad. Sci.*, 1965, *118*, 793–814.

Fantz, R. L. and Nevis, S. Pattern preferences and perceptual cognitive development in early infancy. *Merrill-Palmer Quart.*, 1967, *13*, 77–108.

Farnham-Diggory, S. and Bermon, M. Verbal compensation, cognitive synthesis and conservation. *Merrill-Palmer Quart.*, 1968, *14*, 215–227.

Ghent, L. Form and its orientation: A child's-eye view. *Amer. J. Psychol.*, 1961, *74*, 177–190.

Gibson, E. J. *Principles of Perceptual Learning and Development*. New York: Appleton-Century-Crofts, 1969.

Greenberg, J. H. *Language Universals*. The Hague: Mouton, 1966.

Gruber, J. S. Correlations between the syntactic constructions of the child and the adult. In C. A. Ferguson and D. I. Slobin (Eds.), *Studies of Child Language Development*. New York: Holt, Rinehart & Winston, 1973, pp. 440–445.

Hershenson, M. Development of the perception of form. *Psychol. Bull.*, 1967, *67*, 326–336.

Huang, I. Abstractions of form and color in children as a function of the stimulus object. *J. Genet. Psychol.*, 1945, *66*, 59–62.

Hubel, D. H. and Weisel, T. N. Receptive fields, binocular interaction and functional architecture in the cat's visual cortex. *J. Physiol.*, 1962, *160*, 106–154.

Ingram, D. Transitivity in child language. *Language*, 1971, *47*, 888–910.

Kagan, J. and Lemkin, J. Form, color and size in children's conceptual behavior. *Child Develop.*, 1961, *32*, 25–28.

Klatzky, R. L., Clark, E. V., and Macken, M. Asymmetries in the acquisition of polar adjectives: Linguistic or conceptual? *J. Exp. Child Psychol.*, 1973, *16*, 32–46.

Kaplan, E. L. The role of intonation in the acquisition of language. Unpublished doctoral dissertation, Cornell University, Ithaca, 1969.

Kessen, W., Haith, M. M., and Salapatek, P. The ocular orientation of newborn infants to visual contours. Paper presented at the Psychonomic Society Meeting, Chicago, Oct., 1965.

McNeill, D. *The Acquisition of Language: The Study of Developmental Psycholinguistics.* New York: Harper & Row, 1970.

Major, D. R. *First Steps in Mental Growth.* New York: Macmillan Co., 1906.

Moffitt, A. R. Speech Perception by Infants. Unpublished doctoral dissertation, University of Minnesota, Minneapolis, 1968.

Morse, P. A. The discrimination of speech and non-speech stimuli in early infancy. *J. Exp. Child Psychol.*, 1972, *14*, 477–492.

Nakazima, S. A comparative study of the speech development of Japanese and American English in childhood. 2. The acquisition of speech. *Stud. Phonol.*, 1966, *4*, 38–55.

Palermo, D. S. More about less: A study of language comprehension. *J. Verb. Learning Verb. Behav.*, 1973, *13*, 211–221.

Perez, B. *Les trois premières années de l'enfant.* Paris: Alan, 1892.

Piaget, J. *The Construction of Reality in the Child.* New York: Basic Books, 1954.

Piaget, J. *Play, Dreams and Imitation in Childhood.* New York: Norton, 1962.

Postal, P. M. Review article: André Martinet, *Elements of General Linguistics. Found. Lang.*, 1966, *2*, 151–186.

Preyer, W. *The Mind of the Child.* New York: Appleton, 1890.

Ricciuti, H. N. Geometric form and detail as determinants of similarity judgments in young children. In *A Basic Research Program on Reading.* Final Report, Cooperative Research Project No. 639, U.S. Office of Education, 1963, pp. 1–48.

Ricciuti, H. N. Object grouping and selective ordering behavior in infants 12 to 24 months old. *Merrill-Palmer Quart.*, 1965, *11*, 129–148.

Salapatek, P. and Kessen, W. Visual scanning of triangles by the newborn infant. *J. Exp. Child Psychol.*, 1966, *3*, 155–167.

Sapir, E. Grading: A study in semantics. *Philos. Sci.*, 1944, *11*, 93–116.

Schlesinger, I. M. Production of utterances and language acquisition. D. I. Slobin (Ed.), *The Ontogenesis of Grammar: A Theoretical Symposium.* New York: Academic Press, 1971, pp. 63–101.

Sinclair-de Zwart, H. *Acquisition du langage et développement de la pensée: Sous-systèmes linguistiques et opérations concrètes.* Paris: Dunod, 1967.

Slobin, D. I. Universals of grammatical development in children. In G. B. Flores d'Arcais and W. J. M. Levelt (Eds.), *Advances in Psycholinguistics.* Amsterdam: North-Holland, 1970, pp. 174–186.

Slobin, D. I. Cognitive prerequisites for the development of grammar. In C. A. Ferguson and D. I. Slobin (Eds.), *Studies of Child Language Development.* New York: Holt, Rinehart & Winston, 1973, pp. 175–208.

Spears, W. C. and Hohle, R. H. Sensory and perceptual processes in infants. In Y. Brackbill (Ed.), *Infancy and Early Childhood.* New York: The Free Press, 1967, pp. 51–121.

Stern, W. *Psychology of Early Childhood.* New York: Holt, 1930.

128   Clark

Sutherland, N. S. Shape discrimination and receptive fields. *Nature,* 1963, *197,* 118–122.
Vendler, Z. *Adjectives and Nominalizations.* The Hague: Mouton, 1967.
Wales, R. J. and Campbell, R. On the development of comparison and the comparison of development. In G. B. Flores d'Arcais and W. J. M. Levelt (Eds.), *Advances in Psycholinguistics.* Amsterdam: North-Holland, 1970, pp. 373–396.
Wertheimer, M. Psychomotor coordination of auditory and visual space at birth. *Science,* 1961, *134,* 1692.
Wolff, P. H. Observations on the early development of smiling. In B. M. Foss (Ed.), *Determinants of Infant Behavior,* Vol. II. New York: Wiley, 1963.
Wolff, P. H. The natural history of crying and other vocalizations in early infancy. In B. M. Foss (Ed.), *Determinants of Infant Behavior,* Vol. IV. London, Methuen, 1966.

CHAPTER FIVE

RELATIONAL CONCEPTS UNDERLYING LANGUAGE [1]

I. M. Schlesinger

Hebrew University of Jerusalem and Israel Institute of Applied Social Research, Jerusalem, Israel

In her chapter Eve Clark discussed how meanings of individual words develop. She went only briefly into the problem of what meaning may be conveyed in addition by the combination of words in early utterances. It is the latter issue which is the subject of this chapter. We shall be concerned here with the relations holding between words (or a word and its affix). When the child acquires a grammar, he masters concepts pertaining to these relations, such as the agent concept (or, according to another view, the subject concept). We shall call these "relational concepts" (or "relations," for short). A point to be remembered throughout this chapter is that this term, as used here, does *not* refer to concepts referred to by words like "under," "in," "on," etc., which were dealt with in Eve Clark's chapter, but rather to certain semantic or syntactic concepts. The problem will be discussed whether relational concepts are specifically linguistic or whether they coincide with general cognitive categories, and to what extent one is justified in inferring from linguistic concepts to more generally cognitive ones.

SYNTACTIC *VERSUS* SEMANTIC RELATIONAL CONCEPTS

In recent theories of first-language acquisition there have been two approaches to relational concepts. Under the influence of the newly emerged school of transformational grammar, investigators first held that the child learning language must master those structures and rules specified by the grammar. This meant transformational grammar of the Chomskyan type in 1965, when this view was promulgated by its most prominent spokesman, David McNeill (1966). The relational concepts underlying the child's language

[1] This paper was prepared within the framework of a study supported by the Human Development Center of the Hebrew University, Jerusalem. I am indebted to several persons who have made valuable comments on a draft of this paper, in particular Yehoshua Bar Hillel, Charles Greenbaum, Sidney Greenbaum, M. Mordecha, Lila Namir, and Edy Veneziano. In writing the final version of this paper I have also benefited from comments made at the conference, notably by Melissa Bowerman.

are, according to McNeill, the concepts of the deep structure as specified in Chomsky's grammar, *i.e.,* such syntactic concepts as "subject"–which is the noun phrase directly dominated by "sentence" in the deep structure–and "object," which is the noun phrase of the verb phrase. These are specifically linguistic concepts, and the fact that they are not exhibited in the surface structure of adult speech raised the problem of how they can be learned. The answer to this was the famous and much debated postulate that certain aspects of deep structure are not learned at all but are innate.

In 1967 Schlesinger suggested that the relational concepts underlying child speech are semantic in nature and reflect the way the child perceives the world (Schlesinger 1971b,c). Learning grammar takes place by observing how the adult expresses these relations in speech. While McNeill and others held that the input to the child's language acquisition device is merely the linguistic productions of adults, Schlesinger pointed out that these are paired with the situation which the adult talks about and which is perceived by the child in terms of certain semantic categories. The situation is directly accessible, and learning the grammar involves finding out how the situation connects with adult sentences referring to it. There are, then, according to this approach no specifically linguistic relational concepts hidden away in the deep structure, which, as mentioned, pose a severe problem for learning theory. Instead, there are semantic relational concepts, such as agent and action, possessor and possessed, location of object, etc., in terms of which the child perceives his environment. The attainment of these is dependent on the child's general cognitive development and not on any innate syntactic concepts.

It has been argued that by positing relational concepts which are semantic in nature the link connecting child grammar with adult grammar is broken, because the latter is formulated in terms of syntactic categories. But in principle this presents no problem. It should be remembered that the deep structure of Chomskyan grammar is interpreted by a so-called "semantic component," which, roughly speaking, assigns meaning to it. Thus, in certain sentences, the noun phrase dominated by "sentence" in deep structure (*i.e.,* the subject) and the main verb may be interpreted as standing in the agent-action relation. In the classic transformational model we have two systems of rules: one mapping deep structures into their semantic interpretations and one mapping the same deep structures into surface structures. In principle one can formulate for each pair of rules applying to a given deep structure–one rule from each of the above two systems–a single rule connecting the semantic structure with the surface structure directly. It is therefore possible that the grammar underlying the child's speech as well as that underlying adult speech consists of such rules mapping semantic relations directly into surface structures. In this connection, it should be noted that some recent models of generative grammar in fact posit a base which is semantic in nature.

This, then, is one way of viewing the relationship between the child's grammar and that of the adult: both are basically similar in that they are formulated in terms of semantic relational concepts. Another possibility has been proposed by Melissa Bowerman (1971). Bowerman critically evaluated the two rival claims concerning the nature of the concepts underlying child language. She pointed out that a syntactic concept like "subject of"—in deep structure—does not coincide with any one semantic concept, but rather subsumes a number of these. Experiencers of states, agents of actions, and instruments can all be deep structure subjects, as in "John wants bread," "John cuts bread," and "The knife cuts bread," respectively. The usefulness of the "subject" category is that it permits us to subsume under one rule linguistic phenomena pertaining to sentences expressing all the above semantic relations. "It is bread that John wants," and "It is bread that John—or the knife—cuts,"—are synonymous with the above sentences. There is a virtue, then, in not disposing of syntactic concepts as far as adult grammar is concerned, according to Bowerman. On the other hand, she concluded, after examining child speech for categories like "subject of," that there is no evidence that such syntactic relations are operative.

Bowerman therefore advanced the following solution. The child learning language operates at first with semantic concepts. These he learns to express verbally. For instance, he learns that (in English) the word for the initiator of an action precedes the word for the corresponding action, as in "Danny runs." Somewhat later he learns that the word for person affected precedes the verb describing how the person is affected, as in "Danny wants . . .," and, similarly, the "instrument" precedes its action ("The knife cuts."). Eventually he comes to realize that the nouns expressing these semantic relations follow similar rules in respect to position in the declarative sentence and to transformational possibilities. This leads to the abstraction "subject" which henceforward functions in his system of rules. A similar pattern may be followed for some other syntactic categories.

This is a very plausible account of how the child may acquire "abstract" syntactic relational concepts. It elegantly solves the problem of preserving the simplicity of the rule system made possible by syntactic concepts without paying the price of forgoing a learning approach in favor of innate knowledge. There is, however, an alternative solution to the problem of simplicity which does not necessitate the assumption that the child abandons semantic relational concepts for more abstract syntactic ones.

It seems possible that in the course of learning language the child restructures his cognitions so that one semantic concept is taken to be a special instance of another. For instance, when the child realizes that "Danny wants," "Fred sees," and similar constructions involving persons affected follow the same rule as the previously learned one for the agent-action construction ("Danny runs," "Fred plays"), he comes to regard "want" and "see" as denoting a kind of action. And the fact that in active sentences the words for the instruments, like those for agents, precede the words for the corresponding actions ("the knife cuts," like "the dog barks") leads him to treat instruments as a kind of agent. It is this extended agent concept which in the more mature system of adult rules plays a role parallel to that of what the linguists call "subject."[2] It is by no means only the terminology which is at issue here, because the postulation of an extended agent has empirical consequences. It implies that when the person affected appears in subject position, it is in some sense viewed as having the character of an agent. Likewise, by subjectivizing the instrument it receives some connotations of an instigator of an action. Nothing of the sort follows if person affected and instrument are subsumed, together with the agent, under the higher order concept "subject." These are therefore empirically meaningful alternatives.

Is there any evidence for such an assimilation of person affected and instrument? There seems to be some support, at least in the case of the instrumental. This comes from the observation that instruments cannot always be subjectivized. Thus we have:

> The brush paints flat surfaces.
> The brush scratches the picture.

but not

> The brush paints the picture.

The reason seems to be that when the instrumental is subjectivized it is invested with characteristics of the instigator of an action. It then seems possible to regard the brush somewhat metaphorically as scratching or painting flat surfaces on its own. However, where a work of art is concerned this would mean stretching the notion of an agent too far: painting a picture requires an artist who holds the brush. In general, when the action requires deliberation, the instrumental cannot function as subject.[3] Thus it would be strange to say:

[2] Of course, there is a limit beyond which no such restructuring of the concept of agent is possible. Suppose that in some language the location of an action were always expressed before the action, and all transformations applying to agents were to apply also to the locations. Even so, it would still be highly unlikely that the speaker of this language would conceive of locations as some kinds of agents.

[3] This seems to be yet another instance of surface structure influencing meaning. It is not clear how Fillmore (1968) would deal with this restriction on the subjectivization of instrumentals. Constraints on the transformation rules would have to be rather complex to account for this, since they would have to be defined over subject, verb, *and* object. This is because both "the brush paints" and "the brush . . . the picture" are acceptable. One might try to base the constraints on the verb and specify that some verbs, like "sketch" and "embroider," do not permit subjectivization of the instrumental. This would neccesitate two entries for "paint"–one for the application of coloring and one for the creative act–and similarly for "write." But then what should one make of "illustrate," which permits

> An example illustrates the idea.

but not

> Paper and pencil illustrate the idea.

There cannot be two entries for "illustrate," because we have

> Charles illustrates the idea with an example by means of paper and pencil.

This pen writes poetry.
The pencil sketches the plan.
Ivory pieces play chess.

Compare this to:

This pen draws thin lines.
The pencil draws a circle.
Ivory pieces move on the chess board.

This goes to show that the subject partakes of the nature of an agent, as in the above sentences. What apparently happens is that the concept of the instrumental is absorbed into that of the agent. Thus one can coordinate not only agents and agents or instruments and instruments, as *e.g.*,

The area was ravaged by floods and by storms.
The area was ravaged by mercenaries and by guerilla forces.

but in certain cases, also agents and instruments, as in

The area was ravaged by floods and by guerilla forces.

(Quirk, Greenbaum, Leech, and Svartvik, 1972, p. 325).

This assimilation of the concept of instrument to that of the agent seems to occur in the ontogenesis of grammar as well as in phylogenesis. The case of ontogenesis has been argued above: the child forms extended agent concepts. As Greenfield, Nelson, and Saltzman (1972) showed, the 11-month-old child wielding a cup views it as an extension of his own hand, and somewhat later "by connection with the child's hand the cup becomes 'animate' and therefore an actor. . . ." As for phylogenesis, the above examples seem to show that the agent concept at some point in the development of the English language came to accommodate the instrumental. There seems to be a very general principle at work here. Semantic relations create a syntactic mold, and subsequently other semantic relations are cast into it, but not without a certain amount of reinterpretation. The agent-action relation may have been an example of this. A certain sentence structure was made to serve this relation, and the instrumental was later viewed as a special kind of agent. Consequently, it could be expressed by means of the existing structure.

Similar processes may have been at work when other cases are realized as subjects. Thus, "see," "hear," and "receive" may be treated as actions of agents, just like "look," "listen," and "accept," respectively. In fact, it is not easy to convince college students that "see" is not an action in the usual sense (Sidney Greenbaum, personal communication). Sentences with some verbs which appear to be not at all like actions cannot be passivized, *e.g.*,

The truck weighs five tons.
The bottle contains vinegar.
He had a good time.

Here one of Bowerman's principal motivations for positing a subject category does not apply.

It remains to be seen whether the subject category is completely dispensible in a semantically based performance model. It may turn out that several semantic categories, in addition to the agent, may serve as subjects (see also footnote 2). If so, simplicity considerations might prescribe the reinstitution of the subject category, as suggested by Bowerman. Presumably the subject could then figure in the rule system which maps deep structures consisting entirely of semantic relations into sentences (*cf.* Fillmore's system where "subject" is a surface structure notion). One thus would not have to assume that semantic relations are *replaced* by syntactic ones, but rather that the rule system is augmented by the latter. Note that, even if one were to assume that a development occurs in the deep structure with syntactic relations taking the place of semantic ones, the latter would still have to function in the semantic component.

The discussion in the following sections will be based on the assumption that relational concepts underlying language are semantic in nature. The next question to be dealt with concerns ways in which such concepts can be inferred.

INFERRING THE CHILD'S RELATIONAL CONCEPTS

Several studies have recently been made of small children acquiring various languages. In a review of this work Slobin (1971) listed available material in 30 languages. For some of these, data have been recorded in sufficient detail to permit a comparison of the semantic relations underlying children's speech in various languages. Crosslinguistic universals of language acquisition have recently come into the focus of interest, and there have been interesting attempts to formulate such universals (Slobin, 1971). In a comparison of the acquisition of four unrelated languages—English, Finnish, Samoan, and Luo—Bowerman (in press) found a number of semantic relations occurring in the speech of all the children studied in what she called early stage I (*i.e.,* MLUs of up to 1.30–1.50). Bowerman's list of universal relations is as follows (some of the terms here differ from those she used):

1. agent-action (*e.g.,* "Mommy push")
2. action-object (*e.g.,* "bite finger")
3. possession (*e.g.,* "aunt car")
4. demonstratives (also called introducer + X, ostensive sentences, nomination, *e.g.,* "there cow")
5. attribution (sometimes called modifier + noun, *e.g.,* "big bed"). Bowerman reported that only constructions in which an adjective serves as

modifier are found in all speech samples and those in which nouns are modifiers, like "animal book," appear only in some of them.

In addition, some relational concepts occurred in some, but not all, speech samples, and are therefore probably not universal:

6. agent-object (*e.g.,* "Kendall spider," with "looked at" implied). Not all writers would agree that this is a separate relation but would rather view these constructions as the result of applying a deletion transformation to more complex deep structures (Bloom, 1970). This problem will be taken up below.

7. location of object ("car garage") and of action ("sit bed")

8. negation

9. recurrence (*e.g.,* "more nut")

10. notice (*e.g.,* "hi spoon")

In late stage I (*i.e.,* MLUs up to 2.00 morphemes) three-word strings appear, combining two of the above relations, *e.g.,* agent-action-object or agent-action-location. Negation appears in all samples, and in addition there is one new relational concept:

11. dative (or recipient of action, *e.g.,* "show me book")

Brown (1973) identified yet another relational concept in early child speech:

12. affected person (or: experiencer), state, and source (*e.g.,* "hear horn," "Adam see that," "I like jelly")

While the linguistic expression of this relation is like that of the agent-action-object relation, it should be distinguished from the latter, because verbs like "want," "like," "see," and "hear" do not refer to actions instigated by agents. Relation 12 appears in late stage I of all five children included in Brown's analysis.

It is noteworthy that while locations (7) are among the first relational concepts realized in the child's speech, temporal modification appears much later. This is true already at the one-word stage. Greenfield, Smith, and Laufer (forthcoming) reported one-word utterances expressing location of actions and objects, but none referring to time of occurrence. In fact, when the children they studied first used words describing actions, these were locational (or directional) words: "down" and "up." Jespersen (1964) stated that in the child's questions "where?" appears earlier than "when?" (incidentally, "why?" appears in between). Similarly, comprehension of temporal questions develops late, and up to the age of 3 the child tends to answer: "when?" questions as if they were "who?" or "where?" questions (Ervin-Tripp, 1970). Location is apparently easier to grasp than time. An interesting parallel are words like "before" and "after" which, in English, and similarly in many other languages, were originally spatial and are now used to refer to temporal concepts, whereas the reverse occurs much less frequently (Seiler, 1970).

To return to the above list of relations, it seems to raise some questions. Why, for instance, should (1) and (2) be both represented here as dyadic relations, whereas (12) is expressed as a triadic relation? Could one not just as well say that there is one agent-action-object relation, or else an affected person-state alongside a state-source relation? Should (7) be considered as one relational concept, location, or as two different ones, location of object and location of action?

One way of dealing with questions such as these is by referring to the child's speech which exhibits these relational concepts. If two items in a list of possible relations begin to appear in children's speech simultaneously, and if they use the same syntactic patterns to express these, there is good reason to regard them as belonging to one and the same underlying relational concept. According to this test one may be reasonably confident about treating (1) and (2) as separate relational concepts, and (7) as a single one. On the other hand, I am uncertain about the status of (12). Clearly, many problems remain even with these criteria for defining relations. In a later section we shall return to them.

Another approach is to deal with the child's relations within the framework of a grammar. In contrast to Bloom (1970) and Schlesinger (1971b,c), who inferred semantic relations from corpora on an intuitive basis, most recent analyses of child speech have followed more or less closely one of the semantically based grammatical models: Fillmore's (1968) case grammar (e.g., Bowerman, 1973) or generative semantics (e.g., Antinucci and Parisi, 1973). Such analyses seem to be on somewhat firmer ground, although the question is still open which is the best grammar for the representation of child language. Even if it were settled which grammar is more elegant and simple by linguistic criteria, this would not necessarily mean that the same grammar is operative in the child acquiring language. In the last section of this chapter I shall attempt to show that inferring from adult grammar to that of a child may indeed lead to incorrect analysis of his speech.

Perhaps the most reliable conclusions would be those based not exclusively on the child's corpus of utterances, but also on what is known independently about his cognitive development. Some attempts in this direction have already been made. Both Brown (1973) and Sinclair (1971) have argued that early language is based on the achievements of the sensorimotor period.

Brown suggested that the ability to recognize objects acquired in the sensorimotor period is a precondition for the child's expressing demonstratives—(4) above: "this . . .," "that . . ."—and recurrence, (9): "more. . . ." When the 4- to 8-month-old child sees a familiar object, he sometimes performs the habitual action schema in abbreviated form (e.g., when he sees a rattle he "shakes" his hands), and this may be regarded as the nonverbal precursor of demonstratives (and, we may add, of "notice"–(10) above). At this period the child also develops procedures to make interesting sights last, which forms the basis for the verbal expression of recurrence.

Further, Brown argued, the child's ability to express nonexistence ("all gone . . .," "no more . . ."–subsumed in the above list under negation) presupposes his ability to anticipate objects on the basis of signs and notice when anticipations fail to be confirmed, and this ability is also attained in the sensorimotor period. Finally, object permanence is required for the child's posing questions about location ("where . . ."): the child now knows that an object does not cease to exist when it disappears from sight.

Sinclair (1971) has argued that there is a similarity between certain aspects of Chomskyan deep structures and those structures which, according to Piaget, are the outcome of the sensorimotor period. At the end of the sensorimotor period the child can: 1) order temporally and spatially, which corresponds to concatenation of elements in base structure; 2) use a whole category of objects for the same action, which corresponds to categorization of major categories in the base, (e.g., noun-phrase, verb-phrase); and 3) embed one action pattern into another, which corresponds to the recursive rules of embedding in the base.

A more elaborate study of the underpinnings of early child language has been carried out by Veneziano (1973). On the basis of Piagetian theory she attempted to trace the development of agent and action schemas and their expression at the one-word stage. Lack of space prevents summarizing Veneziano's intriguing theory here.

An experimental approach which seems to hold much promise for the investigation of the cognitive basis of linguistic development is that of Greenfield, Nelson, and Saltzman (1972). In an experiment on the manipulation of cups they found a developmental sequence of strategies which has a parallel in the developmental sequence of two linguistic structures: conjunction of sentences by "and" and sentences with relative clauses. They concluded that it is the same cognitive organizations which make possible motor behavior and linguistic behavior.

TRENDS IN THE DEVELOPMENT OF RELATIONAL CONCEPTS

The manner in which the child categorizes experience undergoes many changes in the course of his development. These manifest themselves among others in the way he uses words to refer to concepts. Eve Clark (this volume) provided an extremely interesting discussion of the phenomenon of overextension: the child uses words for a wider range of reference than the adult does. Gradually a process of differentiation sets in and he ceases to call all animals "doggie" and all men "daddy."

At a still later stage the opposite occurs, and more abstract and general concepts are attained and names learned for them. Brown (1968) has discussed at length the problem of what determines the level of abstraction at which the child starts out. But even at the first stages of learning to speak there are cases not only of overextension, like those discussed by Eve Clark, but also of overrestricted use of words. Leopold (1949, pp. 105–151) stated that this is less common than overextension. His examples are "hot" used for hot objects but not for hot weather, and the German word "weiss" for snow but not for other white things. An example was quoted by Werner and Kaplan (1963, p. 160) of a 25-month-old child who had two words for "milk"—one for milk in a bottle and one for milk in a cup. Lewis (1959, pp. 126–139) also gave examples of such overrestricted use of words. Segerstedt (1947) gave a mixed example of overextension and overrestriction: a 16-month-old child who used "cake" for any food that can be taken through the mouth by the child himself and "eat" for all other food. More recently, Saltz, Soller, and Sigel (1972) have shown overrestriction to be predominant in 5- to 6-years olds and then to decrease with age. In the development of relational concepts, overrestriction (rather than overextension) seems to be the rule. Let us examine the available evidence for overrestriction in the relational concepts of child language.

Child grammar begins at the one-word stage according to Greenfield, Smith, and Laufer (forthcoming). These authors argued convincingly that the "sentential" character of the single word at the holophrastic stage does not inhere in the word, but in the combination of the word with some situational element. To quote one of their examples, when the child says "gone" when his mother leaves him, he is expressing verbally the action of the agent-action relation, whereas the agent (mother) is given in the situation. In their monograph Greenfield *et al.* presented material which enables us to trace the development undergone by the concepts of agent, action, and object at the one-word stage. Seven of the relations treated by them are relevant to these concepts. These are presented in Table 1 roughly in the order of their appearance in the children studied, together with representative examples. Moreover, an interpretation has been attempted in Table 1 of each of Greenfield's relations in terms of the types of agent, action, and object involved. The interpretation has been guided by the examples provided by the writers and their explanations, and while I have gone beyond the latter, I believe I have not misrepresented the data thereby. In each case only one of the concepts is verbally expressed, and this concept has been italicized. It will be seen that at first words for objects are uttered, only later those for actions, and lastly for agents.

As the table shows, there is a progressive extension of the agent concept. At first it is only the child himself which functions as agent. Then other animate beings can be agents, and at last actions are ascribed also to inanimate agents. As mentioned, the agent is at first only given in the situation and left verbally unexpressed. When the agent is first expressed (in the last relation in Table 1, "agent of action"), it is typically animate. As for the action concept, demands are expressed before other actions (referred to by "acts" in the table). However, there seems to be no comparable development of the object concept, since inanimate objects seem to appear very shortly after animate objects in the earliest stages of one-word speech.

The gradual widening of the child's concepts may be graphically represented by means of concentric half-circles (see Fig. 1, which is based on the information contained in Table 1.) The left-hand side of Figure 1 describes the development of the agent concept and the right-hand side that of the action and object concepts. The child moves from the center of the circle outward, and just as each larger half-circle includes each smaller one, so each stage of conceptual development adds to the preceding one and includes it. For instance, at the time the child talks about inanimate agents, he can also talk about animate ones.

Table 1. Relations in Greenfield *et al.*'s Study Involving Agents, Actions, and Objects

		Underlying concepts		
Relation	Example	Agent	Action	Object
Vocative	"Mommy," when requiring something	I	Demand	*Animate*
Object of demand	"Milk," while reaching for it	I	Demand	*Inanimate*
Action performed by agent	"Gone," when mother leaves him	Animate	*Acts*	
Inanimate object of action	"Spoon," when mother takes out spoon	Animate	Acts	*Inanimate*
Action of inanimate object	"Gone," after mother says: "The record is up here."	Inanimate	*Acts*	
Experiencer (affected person)	"Mommy," when giving her something	Animate	Acts	*Animate*
Agent of action	"Mommy," handing knife to mother after trying unsuccessfully to cut with it.	*Animate*	Acts	?

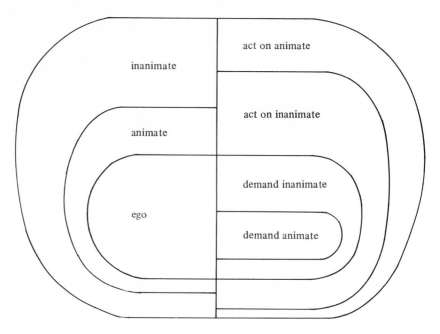

Fig. 1. Schematic representation of the development of agent, action, and object concepts, after Table 1.

These data, then, show an extension of relational concepts. That the agent-action relation develops from overrestricted use through gradual extension has also been suggested by Melissa Bowerman (1971), who proposed that rules involving this relation may have been generalized from more primitive rules " . . . for each verb specifying that the name for the one who initiates the particular action of the verb, such as eating or driving, precedes the name for the action." Possibly, said Bowerman, the abstractions about agents and actions may be arrived at *via* some intermediate levels of abstraction. A further example is that of the agent concept which—according to the interpretation advanced in the first section—comes to include instruments as well as agents.

In addition to overrestriction of relational concepts I have also come across one instance of overextension, the phenomenon described by Eve Clark for word concepts. Greenfield *et al.* (forthcoming) reported that at exactly the time the child begins to use people's names for their possessions he points at a location and names the person or object that belongs there. At this stage the child probably has no precise notion about possession. Instead he perceives some kind of belongingness between two things, as when he says "shoe" on seeing an adult's bare feet. Greenfield *et al.* therefore proposed an "associative case" which includes both possession and habitual location. (Witness the child who insists that something is "his" when he just holds it.)

INFERENCES FROM SPEECH TO COGNITIVE DEVELOPMENT

The discussion in the preceding section of the development of relational concepts suggests that we have here an instrument for studying the child's cognitive development. If the child first talks about himself as agent, later about animate beings and only lastly about inanimate objects, this seems to be a reflection of his gradually widening world view. And if he at first fails to distinguish between possession and habitual location in his speech, this seems to be evidence that this distinction is lacking in his cognitive structure. That the child's language can be taken as an indication of his perception of the world is indeed implied by Greenfield *et al.*'s (forthcoming) treatment of one-word speech and seems to be taken for granted by several other writers. However, a note of caution seems in order here.

As far as adult language is concerned, it is generally recognized that, as Sapir put it, "it would be naive to imagine that any analysis of experience is dependent on pattern expressed in language" (Sapir and Swadesh, 1964). English has a word for dead people and for dead animals but not for dead plants, but this and similar lexical gaps do not indicate a corresponding lack of concepts in the cognition of speakers of the language. The fact that a primitive language may be " . . . capable of expressing a multiplicity of *nuances* which in other languages must be expressed by clumsy circumlocutions" (Jespersen 1964, p. 427) is in itself no evidence of parallel differences in the ability to conceptualize the world. Some deaf people use a language of signs in which the subject and the object of the sentence can usually not be distinguished by grammatical means, but this lack certainly does not incapacitate them from dealing with the world (Schlesinger, 1971a). It is possible, then, to perceive relations which are not incorporated in the grammar of a language. There seems to be no reason why this should not be true also of child language. If it were not, we would have to conclude that structurally ambiguous utterances in child speech invariably reflect a lack of distinction between the relations in question. For instance, when a noun + noun sequence is used for indicating possession ("Mommy sock" = Mommy's sock) as well as agent and object of the action ("Mommy sock" = Mommy puts on the sock) (*cf.* Bloom, 1970, pp. 1–14), this would indicate that the child confuses the notion of a possessor with that of the agent of an action. But this seems to be quite implausible. Imagine how the child would react if mother would put on her sock instead of handing it to the child!

While conclusions drawn from a lack of distinction in child language as to the immaturity of his cognitions often seem to be compelling, one should never accept unquestioningly the evidence of child language alone. There seem to be three factors which may cause linguistic development to lag behind cognitive development:

1. Complexity of the linguistic expression. This factor has been stressed by Slobin (1971), who has formulated the principle that "new functions are first expressed by old forms." When a child has matured to the point that he wishes to express a semantic intention for which he as yet has no linguistic means, he uses existing forms until he gradually acquires those accepted in adult language. The order of acquisition of linguistic forms is dictated in part by their relative complexity and hence may be out of pace with the maturing of concepts the child is ready to express. Slobin cited the case of a bilingual child who verbalized certain locative relations in Hungarian while failing at the same time to express them in Serbo-Croatian. In the latter language the linguistic realization is more complex.

2. Communicative needs. The factor of complexity is obviously irrelevant to Greenfield's data on one-word speech discussed in the previous section. What may be relevant, however, is immaturity of communicative needs, which may have restricted the relations expressed in his speech. Certain relational concepts may remain unexpressed, because it is not important for him to communicate about them or because there are others which are more important. For instance, "vocative" and "object of demand" are among the first relations appearing in one-word speech, according to Greenfield *et al.*'s findings. The reason for this may be not that the child is unable to conceive of any agent except himself or any action except demands, but rather that calling Mother and asking for satisfaction of his needs are of such all-inclusive importance that the child, a newcomer to language, talks about nothing else.[4]

3. Saliency. This factor is closely related to that discussed in 2. Owing to the limitations on length of utterance, the child will presumably tend to express only the most salient features of the situation. That he omits mention of others does not imply that he is unaware of them or unable to deal with them conceptually. Bowerman (in press) wondered why the instrumental does not appear in early child language despite the obvious importance of this relation for the child, although he uses spoons and playthings to reach, hit, and otherwise act on other things. The reason may be that it is usually the effect attained by the use of these tools which is most salient to the child and not the tools themselves. As mentioned, the

[4] Admittedly, such explanations are *ad hoc,* and to an extent even circular. They seem to indicate, however, that caution should be exercised in inferring from speech to cognitive structure. The extrapolation from Greenfield's data in Figure 1 may show no more than what the child talks about, not how he perceives his environment. It should be noted, furthermore, that in determining which relational concepts—or "cases" in their terminology—are exibited in the child's speech, Greenfield *et al.* rightly apply linguistic criteria. These they state to be: 1) "related semantic functions which emerge at the same time are classified as a single case"; 2) "if a semantic function does not achieve productivity . . . it cannot be a separate case"; and 3) "a case cannot be defined in terms of a small number of lexical items." These criteria would be much less justified if their primary objective had been to ascertain how the child structures his picture of the world, rather than to describe what underlies his linguistic output.

latter may be perceived as an extension of the child's hand (Greenfield *et al.*, 1972).[5]

These, then, are possible reasons why the child may fail to express relational concepts which are operative in his cognition. Occasionally the reverse situation may hold: the child expresses linguistically relations which are left unexpressed in adult language. The difference between durative and nondurative actions is not invariably and unequivocally grammatically marked in English, but some children have been reported to use—for some time—the present tense for the former while reserving the past tense for the latter; *e.g.,* "wash" on the one hand, and "broke" or "dropped" on the other, irrespective of the time the action took place (Huxley and Ingram, 1971, pp. 75–76). Further, many children go through a stage of combinations of two nouns the first of which refers to the agent of an action and the second to its object. It has been suggested that they may thereby express an agent-object relation, since often "the agent and the object seem to be in direct inter-action; a person initiates movement in a thing" (Brown, 1973; for alternative explanations of this construction see Bloom, 1970, and Schlesinger, 1971b). No such relation appears in adult grammar of English. In the course of subsequent linguistic development the child learns to funnel the perceived relations into linguistically appropriate constructions.

COGNITIVE STRUCTURES AND I-MARKERS

The above considerations lead to the conclusion that cognitive structures must be distinguished from the deep structures which underlie the production and comprehension of sentences. We are capable of organizing the world around us in innumerable ways, perceiving any number of relations between objects, attributes, states, actions, etc. We are also capable, in principle, of talking about any one of these perceived aspects. But many of them are not linguistically relevant; *i.e.,* the grammar provides no rules for tying them to surface structures of sentences. For instance, the durative-nondurative distinction mentioned above is one which the speaker of English may be aware of, but it is not a distinction made in the grammar of his language. It would be a mistake to assume that any relation perceived must *ipso facto* figure in the deep structure underlying the sentence pertaining to this situation. Some of the relations are provided for by the grammar and many more are not.

It has been useful to employ the term "I-marker" for those relations which figure in the grammar and are expressed in speech (since they represent

---

[5] Bowerman also raised the question of the scarcity of datives (indirect objects) in the earliest stages. But datives apparently do occur in many of the children studied (see Brown, 1973). Perhaps their relatively low frequency reflects the fact that the small child more often receives than gives—and just as he usually omits to mention himself as agent, he tends not to mention himself as receiver.

semantic *i*ntentions and serve as *i*nput to the sentence production mechanism). The term is intended to distinguish these structures from underlying P-markers, which are not formulated in semantic terms (Schlesinger, 1971b,c).

Our cognitive structures, then, are infinitely richer and more variegated than the I-markers which function in language.[6] Given sufficient verbal skill, one can talk about everything which appears in the cognitive structures, but grammar does not always pave the way for us. Which aspects of cognitive structures are represented in the I-markers depends on the particular language. Some of them, like the agent-action and the action-object relations, appear in the I-markers of the speakers of almost all languages (see, however, Schlesinger, 1971a), but others, like the durative-nondurative distinction, only in some languages.

It follows, then, that the child must learn which of the multifarious aspects of the world around him are included in the I-marker, and hence expressed in speech. However, I-markers are not acquired as an independent system. Rather, the child learns the system of I-markers together with its relationships with syntactic constructions. As already pointed out, this does not present an unsurmountable obstacle for a learning approach, since I-markers are part and parcel of the child's cognitive structure.

The distinction between cognitive structures and I-markers made here also provides a basis for answering a question posed by Brown (1973) concerning relational concepts. Brown argued that "ultimately *each* utterance expresses a distinct relation which is the meaning of that utterance." This raises the question as to the criteria for categorizing these relations, or, in Brown's words: "How finely should they be sliced?" As far as cognitive structures are concerned, this question certainly stands: these may contain infinitely many relations, and at present there even seems to be no evidence for the psychological reality of any classification of these relations. But if the question is asked about I-markers, the answer may be suggested that there should be as many relations as are necessary to account for the rules which map them into surface structures. In other words, a relation in an I-marker is one which makes a difference, linguistically.

To illustrate this principle, take the development of negation in child speech, as described at length by Bloom (1970). She discussed three categories of negation: nonexistence, rejection, and denial. Intuitively it seems clear that when the child utters a negation, he intends *either* nonexistence *or* rejection *or* denial: cognitively there is presumably no confusion among these categories (although one might well ask whether there are not still finer cognitive distinctions to be made). The question examined by Bloom is

---

6 "Cognitive structures" in this paper refers to structures operative at the time an utterance is made and leading to it, and *not* the more permanent aspects of cognitive organization.

whether these categories are differentially expressed in the child's speech. She concluded that at first all three categories are expressed by the same syntactic structures, and only subsequently are different semantic categories of negation expressed differentially. In the above terminology, in the first stages there is no distinction between types of negation in the child's I-markers and only subsequently is such a distinction attained. Here, too, cognitive structures mature before I-markers.

In the above we have seen that when deep structures are assumed to be semantic in nature there is no need to postulate that the child is born equipped with specifically linguistic structures. It might be argued, however, that this is a spurious advantage, because all that is achieved thereby is to push the problem of innateness one step back since now semantic relations must be assumed to be innate. This is incorrect according to the above view of the relationship between I-markers and cognitive structures. The question of how much innate structure there is in cognitive is left entirely open. The soundest approach would be to make as few assumptions as possible, *i.e.*, to impute to the child's cognition at the outset as little categorization of relations as possible. He probably comes into a world which is a booming and buzzing confusion, rather than into one which is neatly parceled into agents, actions, and so on. At first he perceives only that his mother takes him up, his father takes him up, his mother moves away, etc., and he does not lump all this together into one agent-action relation. Relational concepts gradually become crystallized. The child forms I-markers which are the schematic representation of a motley world.[7] Language presumably plays a major part in this. By hearing sentences in which all agents are treated the same way, he acquires the agent concept with rules for realizing it in speech. It is of course true, but trivial, that the capability for forming such concepts must be innate.

In contrast to "cognitive determinism" which postulates a one-way influence from cognitive to linguistic development, I propose therefore an interactionist approach. Language builds on the developing cognitive repertoire and in turn shapes it. In regard to the development of words and concepts such a view of a two-way effect has long since been well known: by learning the meanings of words the child learns how to categorize the entities these words stand for. It seems plausible that the learning of sentence structures similarly leads to a certain manner of "slicing up" experience.

However, the acquisition of I-markers does not imply that previously existent distinctions in cognitive structure are obliterated. The child as well as

[7] Stemmer (in press) has advanced a behavioristic theory of learning of grammar which seems to be based on the first stage where only different actions are operative and no general agent-action relation (see also Bowerman, 1971). Stemmer saw no need to assume that the child moves on from there to the abstraction of agent-action. It seems implausible to me that language learning can proceed without such an abstraction. Quite a different account of the emergence of the agent-action relation has been given by Veneziano (1973).

the adult may continue to be aware of relations not expressed in the I-markers of his language. Examples are the above-mentioned distinction between durative and nondurative and the instrumental case discussed in the first section. The instrumental is of course a relation in cognitive structure notwithstanding the fact that its linguistic expression in English and in some other languages is by means of that surface structure which is commonly used for the agent-action relation, *e.g.,* "The knife cuts bread" like "The boy cuts bread." One way of putting this is that the same I-marker is operative in the two cases.[8] By viewing two relational concepts, like the agent and the instrument, as similar in some way, they can be treated identically in the I-marker. Consequently they are expressed identically in the surface structure. This is one way of formulating the principle discussed in the first section, that different functions are perceived as similar so that they can be expressed in the same linguistic form.

Now it is most plausible that not only at the stage when the child's language develops, but also later, a two-way process is operative. Two relational concepts are viewed as similar and treated indiscriminately in the I-marker, and the lack of differentiation in the I-marker leads in its turn to the similarity between these concepts being more salient. Consider the example of the affected person-state relation ("John likes music." "John hears music."). Some similarity perceived between this relation and the agent-action relation may have been the reason why both came to be expressed by the same syntactic constructions, in English, and in many other languages. However, this cuts both ways, because, as Waisman (1962) suggested, the fact that "I see the tree" is constructed like "I cut the tree" " . . . makes it appear as if the seeing was a sort of action directed at the tree." Similarly, in "The tree is seen by me" " . . . it almost looks as if something *happened* to the tree. . . ." It is possible therefore, that the system of I-markers affects the system of nonlinguistic cognitions. Most probably this does not manifest itself in a complete elimination of distinctions in cognitive structure, but only in a tendency to play down the differences and emphasize similarities. The fact that only meagre experimental support has been forthcoming for such Whorfian notions (*e.g.,* Carroll and Casagrande, 1958) does not mean that we can afford to dismiss them summarily. The possibility is to be kept in mind.

TWO FALLACIES

The distinction between cognitive structures and I-markers discussed in the preceding section seems to be especially important in the investigation of child language. It implies, on the one hand, that one should not infer without

---

[8] And a different I-marker is operative when uttering "Bread is cut with a knife." There is obviously also the possibility that different I-markers may be expressed by the same surface structure. The decision between these two explanations must await a more comprehensive theory.

further evidence from immature features of a child's speech to a comparable immaturity of his cognitive development. On the other hand, it is also possible to fall into the opposite error of inferring from the child's cognitive development to the development of his I-markers. This is the first fallacy to be dealt with here: attributing relations presumably existing in a child's cognitive structures to his I-markers without independent confirmation from the child's speech.

Related to this is what one might call the anachronistic fallacy, namely, that of viewing the child's linguistic development from the vantage point of adult grammar. In much recent research on child language the goal has been an explanation of how the child acquires adult grammar. This approach may result in a tendency to work backward from adult grammar and credit the child with as much of it as possible. The child's speech is interpreted in terms of relations which are known to be represented in adult grammar. It is sounder methodology to ascribe as little as possible to the child's I-markers and to show how he builds these up by gradually augmenting them.

While writers in the field have not been completely blind to the danger of incurring these fallacies, they have sometimes not been sufficiently aware of it. Let us exemplify this with a mild case of affliction due to the joint operation of both the above fallacies: a recent analysis of child language by Antinucci and Parisi (1973 and in press).

Antinucci and Parisi (AP) presented an interesting approach to the description of child language, which leans heavily on notions taken from generative semantics. They are the first to have introduced the concept of *performative* into the field of language learning. The "semantic configurations" which they impute to the child at the stage when he utters his first two- or three-word sentences are impressive in their complexity. Thus, when Italian-speaking Claudia says "mamma da" (= mommy give), commenting on the fact that mother gave her something, the semantic representation, according to AP, contains:

1. A proposition stating that (a) for something (b) mother (c) causes this something to be close to (d) Claudia.
2. A "descriptive" performative expressing the fact that by making this utterance something is described or stated. When the same two words are uttered in order to ask mother to give her something, the performative is "requestive."

All this, AP argue, must be in the structure realized by the child, because she obviously understands all this. Although Claudia utters only the two words standing for the agent—"mamma"—and for the action—"da"—she obviously knows that she herself is the recipient and that the intention of the utterance is "descriptive" rather than "requestive."

AP are undoubtedly right about the child's understanding, but what their argument establishes is that this information is contained in the child's cognitive structures, and not that it is represented in his I-markers. The latter, by definition, contain only what the child expresses in his speech. It seems that at that stage Claudia did not express all the information contained in (1) and (2) above. By inferring directly from what the child "obviously knows" to her grammar, AP commit the first fallacy. The distinction between I-markers and cognitive structures insisted upon above is designed to guard against this error.

AP point out that "da" is a three-place verb (X gives Y to Z). To argue that therefore all three arguments, X, Y, and Z, must be represented in the child's grammar would be to commit the anachronistic fallacy, unless it can be shown that not only adult grammar but also the child treats it as a three-place verb. In fact, Claudia at this stage never mentions all three arguments in a single utterance. AP, however, believe that they can prove that "da" functions as a three-place verb by showing that through adequate prompting the various elements can be brought to the surface one at a time (*e.g.,* Claudia: "doll;" Mother: "Where is the doll?" Claudia: "here-is") or two at a time (*e.g.,* "eat Mummy" and then "eat noodles"). They conclude therefore that the semantic structure is all there, and the child lacks only the ability to express more than part of it.

But does this really follow? Could it not be that the child attends only to one or two aspects of the situation at a time and tries to realize these verbally? The effect of prompting might be merely to induce the child to change his focus from one aspect to another. To return to "da," it is possible that in the child's I-marker it appears on one occasion with the agent only, on another with the object only, and on the third with the recipient. It was pointed out above that the agent-object construction observed in many children may express that the agent interacts with the object; *i.e.,* only the agent and the object and no action appear in the I-marker. To argue otherwise on the grounds that there are no such constructions in adult grammar (and no such I-markers in adult speech) would be to commit the anachronistic fallacy. The same applies to the agentless passive and to transitive verbs without the appropriate object,[9] which occur in child language and apparently result from I-markers different from those of the adult. The possibility cannot be ruled out that an I-marker may contain elements which are not realized in the utterance. But in each case evidence for such a claim would have to be based on linguistic behavior.

AP do not distinguish between I-markers and cognitive structures, and as shown here, this lack of distinction may lead to certain fallacies and distortions in the description of child language. It might still be thought that their

---

[9] It should be noted that a verb may require an object in one language whereas its translation equivalent in another language requires no object. Thus, "repair" requires an object in English, but in Hebrew one may say "He repairs" simply, without object. And the same holds for some other verbs.

semantic configurations give an adequate account of cognitive structures, though not necessarily of I-markers. But this is also questionable; in fact, it seems doubtful whether at this stage of our knowledge cognitive structures can be formally described at all.

Consider that on the above occasion when Claudia says "mommy gives," mother may have been smiling while giving the pencil, or whatever it was, that she was in the kitchen wearing a green dress, and that Claudia was crying. Claudia may have been attending to all this when saying "mommy gives." But AP would not for a moment maintain that the semantic representation underlying her utterance is the same as that underlying, say, "In the kitchen mother, dressed in a green dress, smilingly gives a pencil to crying Claudia." In fact they expressly distinguish between the agent, recipient, object, and action, on the one hand, which do appear in semantic representations of the child's early utterances, and "adverbials" and other optional structures, which make their appearance only later (Antinucci and Parisi, in press).

Now note that the distinction between obligatory and optional structures is justifiable only in adult grammar, where utterances omitting the action and in some cases also the agent, recipient, or object, are ungrammatical.[10] There is no reason why one should credit the child with this distinction, before he has learned it as part of the rules of grammar. Therefore, AP's approach of not distinguishing between I-markers and cognitive structures, if followed consistently, would require that everything the child notices be included in the semantic representation. Consequently, their semantic representations would have to be indefinitely large and be dependent on a host of motivational factors, and hence they would be almost useless for describing child language. This shows once again that the only meaningful way of representing the child's underlying structures must be based on what he actually utters, not on what he may be assumed to know to be the case.

ENVOI

In this chapter I have touched upon various methodological issues in the investigation of relational concepts underlying children's language. The discussion revolved mainly around the relation between linguistic and cognitive

---

10 AP also state that such optional structures as adverbials and noun modifiers are not realized in the child's early utterances. But the available data show this to be incorrect at least for one kind of adverbial: the locative. Even in the one-word speech of the children reported by Greenfield *et al.* (forthcoming) the location of an action or object was verbalized before the agent of an action. As far as adverbials and noun modifiers of the example given above are concerned, they certainly do not appear to be beyond the child's cognitive capacities. Presumably he may say: "mommy smile" and "Claudia cry." In any case, the absence in the child's speech of certain concepts can never in itself prove that these are nonexistent in his cognitive structures, as pointed out above.

development. After a period of attempts to study the development of the grammatical rule system without relating it to the child's general development, and even without viewing his utterances in relation to the situation in which they occur, there has recently been growing recognition of the close links between the child's linguistic and cognitive structures. The error now to be guarded against is insufficient distinction between these structures. In the future, a careful examination of their interaction may be expected to lead to a better understanding of child development.

REFERENCES

Antinucci, F. and Parisi, D. Early language acquisition: A model and some data. In C. A. Ferguson and D. I. Slobin (Eds.), *Studies of Child Language Development.* New York: Holt, Rinehart and Winston, 1973.
Antinucci, F. and Parisi, D. Early semantic development in child language. In E. and E. Lenneberg (Eds.), *Foundations of Language Development: A Multidisciplinary Approach,* in press.
Bloom, L. *Language Development: Form and Function in Emerging Grammars.* Cambridge, Mass.: M.I.T. Press, 1970.
Bowerman, M. *Early Syntactic Development.* London: Cambridge University Press, 1973.
Bowerman, M. Structural relationships in children's utterances: Syntactic or semantic? Paper presented at the University of New York at Buffalo Summer Linguistic Institute, 1971.
Bowerman, M. Cross-linguistic similarities at two stages of syntactic development. In E. and E. Lenneberg (Eds.), *Foundations of Language Development: A Multidisciplinary Approach,* in press.
Brown, R. How shall a thing be called? *Psychol. Rev., 1968, 65,* 14–21.
Brown, R. *A First Language.* Cambridge, Mass.: Harvard University Press, 1973.
Carroll, J. B. and Casagrande, J. B. The function of language classification in behavior. In E. E. Maccoby, T. Newcomb, and E. L. Hartley (Eds.), *Readings in Social Psychology,* Ed. 3. New York: Holt, Rinehart and Winston, 1958, pp. 18–31.
Ervin-Tripp, S. Discourse agreement: How children answer questions. In J. R. Hayes (Ed.), *Cognition and the Development of Language.* New York: Wiley, 1970.
Fillmore, C. J. The case for case. In E. Bach and R. T. Harms (Eds.), *Universals in Linguistic Theory.* New York: Holt, Rinehart and Winston, 1968, pp. 1–90.
Greenfield, P. M., Nelson, K., and Saltzman, E. The development of rule-bound strategies for manipulating seriated cups: A parallel between action and grammar. *Cognitive Psychol., 1972, 3,* 291–310.
Greenfield, P., Smith, J. H., and Laufer, B. *Communication and the Beginnings of Language: The Development of Semantic Structure in One-word Speech and Beyond,* forthcoming.
Huxley, R. and Ingram, E. (Eds.). *Language Acquisition: Models and Methods.* London: Academic Press, 1971.

Jespersen, O. *Language: Its Nature, Development and Origin.* New York: Norton, 1964.

Leopold, W. F. *Speech Development of a Bilingual Child: A Linguistic Record.* Vol. 3, *Grammar and General Problems in the First Two Years.* Evanston, Ill.: Northwestern University Press, 1949.

Lewis, M. M. *How Children Learn to Speak.* New York: Basic Books, 1959.

McNeill, D. Developmental psycholinguistics. In F. Smith and G. A. Miller (Eds.), *The Genesis of Language: A Psycholinguistic Approach.* Cambridge, Mass.: M.I.T. Press, 1966, pp. 15–84.

Quirk, R., Greenbaum, S., Leech, G., and Svartvik, J. *A Grammar of Contemporary English.* New York: Harcourt and Brace, 1972.

Saltz, E., Soller, E., and Sigel, I. E. The development of natural language concepts. *Child Develop.,* 1972, *3,* 1191–1202.

Sapir, E. and Swadesh, M. American Indian grammatical categories. In D. Hymes (Ed.), *Language in Culture and Society.* New York: Harper and Row, 1964, pp. 100–110.

Schlesinger, I. M. The grammar of sign language and the problem of language universals. In J. Morton (Ed.), *Biological and Social Factors in Psycholinguistics.* London: Logos Press, 1971a, pp. 98–121.

Schlesinger, I. M. Learning grammar: From pivot to realization rule. In Huxley and Ingram, 1971, pp. 79–89.

Schlesinger, I. M. Production of utterances and language acquisition. In D. I. Slobin (Ed.), *The Ontogenesis of Grammar.* New York: Academic Press, 1971c, pp. 63–101.

Segerstedt, T. T. *Die Macht des Wortes: Eine Sprachsoziologie.* Zürich: Pan Verlag, 1947.

Seiler, H. Semantic information in grammar: The problem of syntactical relations. *Semiotica,* 1970, *2,* 321–334.

Sinclair, H. Sensorimotor action patterns as a condition for the acquisition of syntax. In Huxley and Ingram, 1971.

Slobin, D. I. Developmental psycholinguistics. In W. O. Dingwall (Ed.), *A Survey of Linguistic Science.* College Park: University of Maryland, 1971.

Stemmer, N. *An Empirical Theory of Language Acquisition.* The Hague: Mouton, in press.

Veneziano, E. Analysis of wish sentences in the one-word stage of language acquisition: A cognitive approach. Unpublished master's thesis, Tufts University, Boston, 1973.

Waismann, F. The resources of language. In M. Black (Ed.), *The Importance of Language.* Englewood Cliffs, N. J.: Prentice Hall, 1962.

Werner, H. and Kaplan, B. *Symbol Formation: An Organismic-Developmental Approach to Language and the Expression of Thought.* New York: Wiley, 1963.

CHAPTER SIX

FROM SIGNAL TO SIGN: A PIAGETIAN VIEW OF THOUGHT AND LANGUAGE DURING THE FIRST TWO YEARS

Donald M. Morehead and Ann Morehead

Department of Child Development, California State University, Hayward, California 94542 and City College, San Francisco, California 94112

In the late 1950's the rediscovery of Piaget and the introduction of Chomsky's general theory of linguistics brought attention to the young child as the source for understanding universal mental abilities in humans. Both theorists emphasized the considerable intellectual and linguistic achievements of the child during the first 5–7 years of development. While Freud was probably the most influential modern theorist to point to the importance of early development for the understanding of behavior, the parallel traditions of developmental biology and ethology also focused on the early years as basic and formative periods.

These traditions are exemplified in the theories of Piaget (1971) on cognitive development and Bowlby (1969) on social attachment. Following the lead of early work in embryology and ethology, development is viewed as an *interaction* among genetic programming; physical maturation; environmental influence, including social transmissions; and self-regulation—the last functioning as an internal system of feedback (and feedforward) between the entire organism and his environment. The importance of regulated interaction among genetic inductors, physical maturation, and environmental influence without social transmission has been well documented in studies on embryology (Kuo, 1967) and imprinting (Bateson, 1966). Piaget (1971) and Bowlby (1969) are both interested in social transmission as a factor in development and, quite naturally, focus on the human child.

From a developmental view, the first 2 years are almost exclusively concerned with the child's initial freeing of himself from the universal constraints of evolution, maturation, gravity, time, space, and fixed action patterns. One of the more important aspects of this "distancing principle" is the development leading to and the onset of symbolic or representational behavior (Werner and Kaplan, 1963; Piaget, 1962). Just as walking frees the child's upper body from gravity, so representation frees the child from the immediate present (*i.e.*, perception and actions) and allows him to re-present reality (*i.e.,* deferred imitation, imagery, symbolic play, language, etc.) and to evoke the past or anticipate the future. Inherent in the capacity to release from the immediate present is the ability to release from the immediate self—a social condition prerequisite to the acquisition of a collective representational system such as language and, ultimately, shared rational thought (Piaget, 1962). This position suggests that language functions primarily as a social system (Levi-Strauss, 1966).

Since the young infant is initially neither social nor linguistic, it is of considerable heuristic value to consider the development of these behaviors from the position of a theory of universal mental development such as that offered by Piaget (1970a). Piaget's (1952, 1954, 1962) detailed description of early development provides a general outline of apparently universal behaviors that may prefigure and, in some instances, even operate as direct precursors to the eventual linguistic development and socialization of the child (Brown, 1973). Encouraged by the striking uniformities in the development of cognition, researchers are now attempting to determine universal operating principles that the child may use in constructing the relationships between form and content in cognition and language (Ervin-Tripp, 1973; Slobin, 1973; Sinclair, 1971a, 1973).

This chapter will provide a structural view of thought and language during the first 2 years. First, Piaget's genetic theory including a brief comparison with some aspects of Chomsky's general theory of language will be presented. This comparison will be followed by a somewhat more detailed description of the structure of Piaget's theory of cognitive development. It will provide the base for an account of mental development that may prefigure or function as a precursor to linguistic development appearing in the 2nd year. Finally, recent studies which consider linguistic development prior to and including the onset of syntax will be discussed within a Piagetian frame.

PIAGET AND CHOMSKY—A STRUCTURAL APPROACH

According to Piaget (1971), all mental development (including language) is an extension of biological organization and adaptation. This does not imply that he assumes an innate position. He postulates that what is inherited is a set of functional invariants—processes basic to all biological adaptations which reflect sensitivities to internal as well as external functions. Organization refers to the formation of structured systems which are internally or self-regulated.

Adaptation, a predisposition of all living systems, has two complementary processes called assimilation and accommodation. In assimilatory processes, reality is modified to match internal organization (or structure) in the brain. In accommodatory processes, internal structures are modified in accordance with environmental influences. The former guarantees that reality is not passively copied, and the latter assures that cognitive structures do have some correspondence to the real world. Assimilation in its extreme form is best seen in fantasy and symbolic play, which are more responsive to the internal structures of the child than to environmental factors. Accommodation, on the other hand, is best exemplified in imitation, which is maximally responsive to environmental influence and can function relatively independently of inner structures. Imitation, then, is a kind of hyperadaptation while play signifies relaxations from the demands of adaptation. Assimilation is the process which incorporates objects or events into actions and their existing knowledge. That is, new knowledge is always first interpreted by reference to existing knowledge. When there is a moderate discrepancy between new knowledge and existing knowledge, an element of the existing knowledge is modified or accommodated to the new knowledge, and a structural change occurs. Under conditions where structural change is less likely to occur, the child may opt for one of two relative conditions. If no element of existing knowledge is modified, then assimilation maintains primacy over accommodation and there is play. In the converse condition, if accommodation maintains primacy over assimilation, then existing knowledge is adapted without utilization of the new knowledge—hence no concomitant change in the structure of the existing knowledge. Thus, existing knowledge cannot be accommodated beyond itself, which is the reason that children cannot imitate much beyond what they know.

Between the two functional invariants and their extremes as manifested in symbolic play and imitation is logic (intelligence), which in adult thinking is relatively free from either internal or external forces. In logical thought, reality is viewed not only as a series of states but also as a series of relations or transformations between states. These transformations characterize the changes that take place during transitions from one state to another or changes in the relations between states. For example, if from two relations (A > B and B > C) an unknown relation is derived (A > C), then new information is achieved which does not require changes in elements A, B, or C during assimilation or the modification of our own cognitive structures during accommodation. Logic, then, operates on transformations and wholes rather than on states or elements and as such represents a relative balance between assimilation and accommodation. The term "balance" in this case refers to the notion of equilibrium or self-regulation. For Piaget, then (1970b, 1970c, and 1971), logic is central and has its source neither in perception nor in linguistic organization but in action on the environment, specifically sensorimotor actions that are coordinated and then internalized, becoming thought (albeit prelogical) during the latter part of the 2nd year. Thus, thought is not *for* action but *is* action.

Through the processes of assimilation, accommodation, and self-regulation, cognition proceeds through stages of structural reorganization with each stage incorporating the previous stage and being qualitatively different from it. Moreover, these distinct periods of development are postulated to be universal, and each child goes through an invariant sequence or succession of stages. It is important to note that the universality of stage development is not singularly due to the invariant functions of organization and adaption but also to an experienced world that has its own universal structure (Piaget, 1970c). For Piaget, there are four stages of development beginning with infancy and extending through 12–14 years of age. For the purposes of this discussion, only the first stage–the sensorimotor stage (0–24 months) and the transition to the preoperational or representational stage (2–7 years)–will be presented.

Chomsky (1965, 1968) makes similar claims regarding language. Syntax is central, and its base component can exist independent of phonology or semantics in much the same way that logic exists independent of assimilation (play) and accommodation (imitation). Implicit in the concept of centrality of syntax or logic are the complementary aspects of surface *vs.* deep structure in language and states *vs.* transformations in thought–one relating to superficial aspects and the other to underlying aspects of a system. Moreover, it seems probable and there are some data which support the notion that the properties and relations in the base component, which are central to language much as logic is central to thought, also do not become fully operational in the sense of logic until 7 years, when complex relations in transformational rules are clearly established (Sinclair, 1969, 1971a; de Villers and de Villers, 1972). Further, Chomsky (1968) also proposes a self-regulatory function of grammars that, once structured, allows the creation of novel utterances which never go beyond the system and preserve the rules of that system.

Although language for Chomsky (1966) has its roots in reason rather than *vice versa,* his position is not, as often cited, extreme nativism. For example, he clearly implies that during successive stages of language acquisition "more detailed and highly structured schemata are applied to the linguistic data," *i.e.,* base cognitive functions (Chomsky, 1965, p. 202, note 19). Moreover, that his position is very close to the position of Piaget is obvious in the statement that "[what is needed] is the detailed study of the actual character of stimulation and the organism–environment interaction that sets the innate cognitive mechanisms into operation" (Chomsky, 1968, p. 76).

An essential difference between the theories of Piaget and Chomsky is that Piaget is attending to processes and stages of construction (structures) in intelligence while Chomsky attends primarily to rules of construction (structures) in language. In other words, Chomsky offers a competence model while Piaget offers both a competence and a base performance model.

PIAGET'S GENERAL THEORY OF COGNITIVE DEVELOPMENT

Piaget (1963, 1970b) has long maintained the primacy of logic (action) or, more precisely, of logical-mathematical structures over perceptual and symbolic structures (including language) as the primary contact with and orga-nizer of reality.[1] Although perception is seen as an active process, it deals primarily with states rather than transformations between states in reality. To know reality, it is necessary to act upon or transform it. In the process of manipulating reality (first through sensorimotor actions and later by mental operations—internalized actions which around 7 years become reversible), it is transformed from an existing state to an alternative state, and, as a result of transformations, the child discovers the properties and relations of objects and events in reality. The child derives properties of objects in reality not from actions alone but from the specific objects themselves. For instance, the child can derive the property of enclosure only from objects that allow that action (*e.g.,* a mouth or a cup but not a table). The relations between objects are derived from coordinating actions on the objects—a logic of actions that does not require particular objects. For example, enclosure can also be relational in the sense that all objects with that quality can enclose all other objects of appropriate dimension.

Piaget (1970a, 1970b, 1971) makes a distinction between two aspects of intelligence, the operative and the figurative. The operative aspect is the more basic of the two. It includes innate know-how (roughly instinct), logical-mathematical knowledge, and physical knowledge. The relationship among the three is complex and need only be outlined here to emphasize the importance of logic as the base organizer of experience.

Innate know-how operates primarily as reflexive behavior and is predomi-nant only during the 1st month of infancy, but it is crucial to understand that the organism is not a *tabula rasa* at birth but is already organized by genetic regulation in the form of reflexes.

A gradual shift to early prelogical-mathematical structures begins between the 2nd and 4th month and dominates organization at 2 years although thought remains prelogical until around 7 years of age. Piaget (1971) refers to this shift as the transition from genetic or programmed regulation of behavior to constructive regulation, keeping, however, the inherited func-tional invariants of all living forms—organization and adaptation. Logic (intel-ligence), then, replaces genetics as the source of self-regulation or equilibrium. It is for this reason that logic, founded in early direct coordinations of actions (*via* regulation of assimilation and accommodation), is central in Piaget's theory of intelligence.

Physical knowledge, which may be attributive or functional, is derived from both actions and the properties of objects. For physical knowledge to be interrelated between objects and, hence, form classes, it is necessary that it be assimilated to the already organized logical-mathematical structures and for these structures to accommodate themselves to those object relations. The

---

[1] Pribram (1971) offers a similar view based on recent work in neuropsychology.

operative aspect of intelligence is seen as being basic and the only aspect of intelligence that can make contact with and organize a dynamic, transforming reality.

Operative activities have been described as activities which transform reality so that its properties and relations can be assimilated to existing cognitive structures and thus conferred with meaning. A second aspect of intelligence is concerned not with transforming the environment but with presenting or re-presenting the environment as it appears and as such is primarily accommodatory behavior. Piaget (1970a) refers to this aspect of intelligence as the figurative aspect, which is seen in rather pure form in perception but also found in imitation and imagery. These activities, until coordinated and thus structured by operative thought, deal with 1) reality as it appears in its momentary, static configurations (i.e., perception); 2) the extreme adjustment or accommodation to immediate reality within the limits of the existing cognitive structures (i.e., imitation); and 3) the representation of what is perceived or cognitively known in the absence of immediate perception or ongoing action (i.e., imagery).

Perceptual mechanisms and activities, some of which are well organized at birth or very early and change little with age (i.e., primary illusions; Bower, 1966), are described by Piaget (1969) as being essentially static rather than transformational until they are partially coordinated with the operative aspect at around 7 years of age. As such they can only deal with the moment-to-moment appearance of reality rather than its constantly changing characteristics. However, perception is seen as an active rather than a passive process as indicated in the following primary functions: 1) reorganization of sensory data to disambiguate static figures in figure-ground relations, 2) integration of parts into unified wholes with neither parts nor wholes losing their identity, and 3) strategies involving exploration of a perceptual field (Elkind, 1969). Perception differs from imitation (deferred) and imagery in that the latter two can come to represent reality when it is not present. For Piaget (1962) it is the function of representing reality when it is not immediately available to the senses or present in immediate action that indicates the onset of the symbolic or semiotic function which includes not only language but also deferred imitation, imagery, symbolic play, drawing, and dreaming. This function is the capacity to represent an object, event, or cognitive structure (the significant) by an image, gesture or word (the signifier). Thus, the symbolic function releases thought from actions (knowing from the immediate present) and in so doing facilitates thought but is still structured by it.

THOUGHT AND LANGUAGE–THE FIRST TWO YEARS

We have briefly described the two primary aspects of Piaget's theory of intelligence. One, the operative aspect, deals with the early reflexive organization of the brain (instinct or innate know-how), knowledge of objects and their attributive as well as functional properties (physical knowledge), and knowledge of the relations between objects (logical-mathematical knowledge). The other, the figurative aspect, deals with objects or events as they appear in static form (perception), the adjustment of existing organization or cognitive structures to objects or events immediately present (imitation), and the representation of objects that are absent or events that are not immediately available to perception (deferred imitation and imagery). It is from the figurative aspect of intelligence that the symbolic function, necessary for representational or preoperational intelligence which dominates mental behavior between 2 and 7 years, will evolve.

Piaget's (1962) most significant insight into the relationship between thought and language and language to other mental behavior was to postulate that language is part of a larger system or function, namely the symbolic function. As stated earlier, the symbolic function includes all mental behavior capable of re-presenting reality when it is not immediately present, including deferred imitation, imagery, symbolic play, language, drawing, and dreaming. As we shall see later, language is special since unlike other aspects within the symbolic function such as imagery it is, save in the very early stages, social and communicable rather than individual and private and, in this sense, shares these features with thought.

Since logic (action) is central to Piaget's theory of intelligence, any behavior which does not act to transform or change an object or event into an alternate state and thereby discover its properties and relations is seen as accommodatory behavior. Behavior that is primarily accommodatory deals with reality in its present, static state (perception), attempts to produce its present form (imitation), or evokes the object or event when it is not present (deferred imitation and imagery). To see how these accommodatory behaviors (particularly imitation) relate to intelligence or thought and provide the source for the symbolic function, it is necessary to begin with the first imitative behaviors appearing in the context of general sensorimotor development.

Substage 1–Birth to Two Months

The sensorimotor period, the first of four major developmental periods, extends from birth to the end of the 2nd year and consists of six substages. In the first substage or birth to the end of the 1st month, the infant is completely fused with his environment. Assimilation and accommodation show little differentiation, and sensory and motor systems, aside from reflexive connections, lack coordination (Piaget, 1952). Nevertheless, this first substage is important because reflexive behavior begins to undergo change as a result of interaction with the environment—a change that marks the beginnings of the transition from genetically regulated behavior to behavior regulated by the gradual construction of logic (intelligence). Secondly, from the beginning, the infant is active and attempts to apply existing action schemas (stable patterns of movement) to the environment. The tendency to use or apply a cognitive structure if it is available is early assimilatory activity, while modification of reflexes as a result of use is early accommodatory activity which itself leads to new assimilations. Imitation during substage I, like other less extreme forms of accommodation, is not clearly manifested except that reflexive behavior can be set off by certain external stimuli, amply demonstrated in studies of classical conditioning.

Substage II—Two to Four Months

In substage II, which extends from 2 to 4 months, several important changes occur in general sensorimotor development. First, if when exercising an action schema, results occur which were not anticipated, the infant will attempt to recapture the result by repeating the action over and over again. This action is called the primary circular reaction and is the very foundation for early adaptations since, in the course of repeating action schemas, one or more repetitions of a schema are altered (structural changes occur) by first applying the schema (assimilation) and then modifying it as a result of environmental circumstances (accommodation). Next, the spiral of adaptation is set up by incorporating new accommodations into the action schemas themselves and then applying them in subsequent assimilatory activity.

Secondly, the sensory schemas of reflexive seeing, hearing, touching, etc. and the reflexive motor schemas of sucking, crying, closing the hand, etc. begin their coordination first within and then between one another. For example, instead of hearing, the infant soon begins to listen and shortly after coordinates looking and listening, listening and vocalization, and so on. This is a vital first step toward the acquisition of intelligence for it is in this stage that the external world begins to have coherence. By the end of the substage he can look while listening, grasp while looking, vocalize while listening and, of course, *vice versa.*

These coordinations are also crucial for the onset of imitation, which in the second substage is sporadic and limited to a small repertoire of actions such as vocal and articulatory movements, visual following, and grasping or prehension. The most common forms of imitation to occur during this substage are what Piaget (1962) calls vocal contagion, mutual imitation, and sporadic imitation. In the first, the infant vocalizes in the context of vocalizations from other sources with no attempt at imitation. Vocal contagion marks the beginning of vocal imitation. During mutual imitation, the infant will imitate another person *if* that person imitates the infant at the very moment he is producing an articulate sound sequence (implying more than mere vocalizations as in vocal contagion). Piaget (1962) describes mutual imitation in the following observations:

At 0;2 (11) after he had made the sounds *la, le,* etc. I reproduced them. He repeated them seven times out of nine, slowly and distinctly. The same day, I reproduced the sounds he usually made when he himself had not made them for half an hour. He smiled silently, then began to babble, and stopped smiling. He did not produce each individual sound, but uttered sound under the influence of my voice when I confined myself to sounds with which he was familiar (Piaget, 1962, p. 9, Obs. 2).

In the case of sporadic imitation, the infant will imitate a previously known articulate sequence produced by another person even though the infant has not uttered it *immediately before* the model's production. It is not frequent in this substage, but its appearance at the end of the substage sets the pattern for substage III.

The most significant observation of this period is that the infant will only imitate that which he is already capable of producing. The model's activities or movements are simply assimilated to the infant's own action schema, and the repetitive or circular character of these actions allows immediate imitation. Thus, imitation is not an extension of perception that later acquires a motor response *via* association with a movement, but rather it is an attempt to prolong something that is perceptually familiar but only recognized by reproducing it at the same time it is perceived.

With the appearance of sporadic imitation at the end of substage III, the infant shows the first clear indication of what Piaget (1962) would call a prelinguistic act. From the latter part of this period until the end of the 1st year (substage IV), all movements (including vocal), both of the infant and of other persons or objects, can potentially act as *signals* which are assimilated to existing action schemas. The concept of the signal is borrowed from the classical conditioning paradigm. The signal can be defined as any indicator which elicits an action schema and in which there is no differentiation between the form of the action (signifier) and its content (significant).

In the evolution from the signal to the true sign during the 2nd year, the infant learns first to respond to certain indicators (signal); next, to utilize the similar or shared properties between his own action schemas and those of other persons and objects as a way of knowing their actions (index); then, to represent an object or an event by other objects or events that have similar features (symbol); and, finally, to use words as designators of cognitive structures or thought that represent the object or event and to derive novel meanings from new relations between words (true sign). Thus, the signal represents the first step in the development of the symbolic function while the word is not a true sign until it designates thought and draws meaning from novel relations.

Early information exchange is also affected by the restricted function of the signal. Such exchanges between the infant and other persons are fixed (by the available repertoire of action schemas) rather than mobile (allowing anticipation or reconstruction that goes beyond immediate perception). However, the successful use or "exercising" of these action schemas is important since it, in part, determines the rate of development toward mobile schemas and, hence, alternative communication modes (Bell and Ainsworth, 1972).

Substage III—Four to Eight Months

An important development in substage III (4—8 months) is the infant's ability to free himself partially from gravity and begin to crawl and pull himself up. As a result, along with the further coordination of vision and grasping, circular reactions are no longer primary (*i.e.*, focused on his own bodily activities) but become secondary in that he is now interested in the environmental effects of these activities. The infant now strikes, shakes, rubs, and swings objects rather than simply looking, grasping, listening, and touching. That is, he begins to act on objects and attends to the effects of his actions. As a result, primary circular reactions are gradually integrated into secondary circular reactions that attend to the environmental consequences of actions. This transition has important implications for the development of early physical knowledge and logical-mathematical knowledge. Objects now begin to form primitive classes as instruments to shake and listen to, swing and see motion, etc. Relational knowledge is seen in more subtle distinctions made between the action schema and the object to which it is applied. However, the infant still persists in applying action schemas without clear intention, and as a result his behavior remains circular in that he first acts (ends) and then applies various action schemas (means which are now more coordinated) to keep the interesting object or event under control.

With a new interest in the effects of his actions on objects and events, the infant makes considerable progress in the formation of the object concept—a concept which characterizes his eventual realization that he is an object within a universe of objects. For instance, if an object is dropped, the infant will look for it, showing an initial trust in the permanency of reality. The development of the object concept and later of causal relations is an important metric for following the child's differentiation between himself and reality, then between his actions and reality, and finally between objects and events in reality. This separation lays the foundation for distinguishing between the subject of the action and the object of the action—a crucial distinction for the development of logic (subject-object) and language (subject-predicate) (Piaget, 1970c). However, as Chomsky (1965) and recently Watt (1970) have emphasized, it is important to distinguish cognitive principles which underlie sentences from grammatical principles which specify sentences. Each set of principles may follow its own peculiar laws (Piaget, 1962; Slobin, 1973; Brown, 1973).

Imitation in substage III is still confined to vocal and articulatory behavior that the infant has produced previously and is capable of auditorily monitoring. For hand and other body movements there are similar constraints in that these movements must not only have been previously made but also seen during any imitative attempts. However, it is now possible to explain why the infant's imitation is confined to his previously performed action schema. The infant in substage III only knows his movements (vocal or otherwise) by reference to his actions (*i.e.*, tactile and kinesthetic feedback). Thus, vocal and articulatory imitation is possible only if the infant has an auditory schema which can be continued by its corollary in ongoing action (vocal and articulatory movements). Likewise, imitation of hand and body movements is possible only if the infant has previously produced the movement and his own imitative attempt of a model can be seen. What is illustrated here is the dependence of visual or auditory perception of an action, which is itself temporary, on previously produced actions, since only by incorporating these temporary actions or events into the circular reaction are they given some permanence. Similar behavior is seen in attempts to find an object that has disappeared by continuing to repeat the action previously performed on the object while visual search is taking place.

Substage IV—Eight to Twelve Months

It was stated earlier that much of the information exchange between the infant and other persons was restricted or fixed by the focus on self and actions as well as the availability of schemas of action. At substage III, the infant has built up a larger repertoire of action schemas by attending to their effects on the environment (secondary) rather than to the actions themselves (primary). As a result, in substage IV (8–12 months) these action schemas are generalized (freed from old content) and coordinated in novel ways to develop new forms or action schemas. In the process, several old action schemas are applied (means) until the infant finds one that works (end or goal) rather than accidentally discovering a goal and then repeating the action schema (means) that was successful, as was done in substage III. Means now precede the end or goal, and the infant knows what he wants to do and applies action schemas to achieve that end. This "practical intelligence" is clearly seen in the following observation:

> If Jacqueline, at 0;8 (8) has shown herself capable of removing a hand which forms an obstacle to her desires [obtaining a toy duck] she has not delayed in making herself capable of the inverse behavior pattern: using the other person's hand as an intermediate in order to produce the coveted result. Thus at 0;8 (13) Jacqueline looks at her mother who is swinging a flounce of material with her hand. When this spectacle is over, Jacqueline, instead of imitating this movement, which she will do shortly thereafter, begins by searching for her mother's hand, places it in front of

the flounce and pushes it to make it resume its activity (Piaget, 1952, p. 223, Obs. 127).

Thus, the infant's behavior becomes mobile (intentional and anticipatory behaviors which go beyond the immediate present) by coordinating action schemas that include spatiotemporal relations. In the first part of the above example, early logical-mathematical knowledge is reflected in knowing that the object (hand) *in front of* the object desired (toy duck) must be removed *before* the desired object can be grasped. Physical knowledge is seen in the specific action applied to the objects. For example, the hand was pushed while the duck was grasped. An important change seen in the second part of the example is that the infant sees persons and objects other than himself as sources of action or, as Piaget (1954) puts it, "endowed with causality." Similar changes have taken place with regard to the object concept. If objects are dropped out of sight, the infant no longer continues the previous action while looking for the object. He now actively searches for it or engages someone else to assist.

The newly developed intentionality and anticipation have important implications for the development of imitation and an emerging communication system. As Bell and Ainsworth (1972) have recently shown, it is in this substage that the infant uses new means (other than crying or other expressive signals) to communicate, particularly if prompt attention from the primary caretaker has allowed this "practical intelligence" to function (*i.e.,* allowed the infant to achieve his goal or end). It is the new coordination of action schemas (*e.g.,* vocalizing while shaking the side of the crib) that effectively allows the replacement of expressive signals such as crying as the primary communicative contact.

A second and more significant development coming out of new coordinations of action schemas is the *index* which substantially replaces the expressive signals whose form is tied to the immediate context or content. With the appearance of the index, we see the first clear separation of form from content or an action schema from its immediate context. The index, like other behavior at this stage, is mobile (*i.e.,* anticipatory and intentional) rather than fixed as in the case of expressive signals and, as such, provides a structure in which the relationship between a signifier (*i.e.,* form—image, symbolic play, word) and its significant (*i.e.,* meaning or content—object, event, concept) can eventually function.

Even though the signifier and the signified are relatively fused at this stage in the sense that the occurrence of one depends upon the occurrence of the other, the mobility of the index allows "the anticipation of the immediate future and the reconstruction of the recent past" (Piaget, 1962, p. 42). The index functions in a general way during substage IV. For example, a door opening (signifier) implies a person entering (signified), or a mother putting on her coat (signifier) implies that she is leaving (signified). This anticipatory and reconstructive behavior is clearly pre-representational and thus functions as a necessary prerequisite to representational or symbolic behavior (including language). To appreciate its importance and the way it functions, the index will be described in the context of imitation, particularly imitations of vocal and articulate sequences.

Beginning in substage I there has been a gradual differentiation between the infant, his actions, and the environment as seen in the development of the object concept and in this substage, substage IV, the realization that other persons or objects can also be a source of action (*i.e.,* causality). This distinction between the actions of self and those of others is obviously important for imitation and, moreover, the ultimate socialization of thought and language (Piaget, 1954). A parallel development of differentiation between assimilation and accommodation has also been taking place. It is this gradual differentiation of assimilation (applying action schemas) and accommodation (modifying action schemas as a result of their application) that allows the infant to free himself from the direct assimilation of a model to his own circular action schemas, with little or no concurrent modification in the schema itself. Assimilation mediated by indices with definite accommodations to the model now takes over. The mediating index functions, then, to establish a correspondence between the actions of the infant and those of the model and aids in the coordination of action schemas developed independently during substage III. Listening has already been coordinated with its corresponding tactile-kinesthetic movements during babbling, and looking has been coordinated with corresponding tactile-kinesthetic feedback from hand to body movements. But these coordinations themselves must now be fully coordinated for the imitation of actions not in the infant's repertoire to occur—a process that allows the infant to move from babbling to the onset of true speech. Babbling is primarily an assimilatory activity while early speech necessarily involves accommodation. The coordination of listening with looking or secondary action schemas through the mediating function of the index can be seen in the following observations:

In the case of T. there was no reaction to movements of the mouth or eyes until about 0;9. At 0;9 (21) however, he looked at me attentively when I opened and closed my mouth (without making a sound) and then said *tata* and *papa* (neither had assigned meaning). Obviously, the reason for this reaction was that he recognized the movement I made when I myself said *papa* (he had imitated the sound on the preceding day) and thus assimilated this movement of my lips to the familiar vocal schema. At 0;9 (29), when I opened my mouth (still without making any sound) T. again said *papa,* but this time in a whisper. He did not, however, imitate any movement related to the tongue, eyes or nose.

At 0;9 (30) he again said *papa* or *tata* in a whisper when I opened my mouth, but when I put out my tongue, he opened his mouth again without making a sound. The same day, when I again began to open and close my mouth, he imitated me correctly, no longer making any sound.

At 0;10 (21) he correctly imitated the following movements: opening the mouth (silently), putting out the tongue (almost silently) and putting his finger in his mouth. He imitated the last of these at the first attempt, without the sound as index and without any previous spontaneous reaction. (Piaget, 1962, p. 40, Obs. 30).

In the previous substage (substage III) the infant could only imitate the actions of the model when the model produced actions that the infant had just made, and, secondly, the infant could only imitate movement which was under some control of its corresponding monitoring system. These restrictions are due to the general lack of coordination between the secondary action schemas as mentioned earlier. Moreover, the restrictions create an interesting paradox in that until substage IV the infant is unable to imitate vocal or articulate sequences for the very reason that his own productions are known to him only through their corresponding auditory and tactile-kinesthetic schemas and are not visible (*i.e.*, coordinated with visual schemas). In the observations given above, the infant comes to imitate the opening and closing of the mouth (which is not visible to him and hence not immediately present to him) by assimilating the model's behavior to a familiar action schema (in this example, "tata" and "papa") and then adjusting or accommodating this schema to the mediating index or salient properties shared between the model and the infant's own actions. Other persons and objects now have actions that the infant recognizes as separate from his own activity but do not exist independently of it. After the index has served its function of bridging the gap between his behavior and the unknown behavior of the model, it drops out. The infant can now immediately imitate the model's opening and closing of the mouth without the index. Thus, the salient properties or distinctive features of familiar action schemas or forms are used to establish a correspondence between the infant's behavior and the behavior of the model or new content.

The types of mistakes that the infant makes in attempting to establish a correspondence between his own actions and those of the model also suggest "understanding" in terms of the shared features or properties of the two actions. For example, when one of Piaget's children first observed him opening and closing his eyes, she first opened and closed her mouth, then her hands, then hands and mouth, and finally assigned the features of open-closed to her eyes. This correspondence of shared features in imitation is also seen in attempts to reproduce new articulate sequences. In response to "gaga" (which Jacqueline had not previously produced), Piaget observed the following effort: "mama," "aha," "baba," "vava," and finally "papa" in that order (Piaget, 1962, p. 146, Obs. 32). Thus, in imitating speech the infant appears to use indices or shared features as mediators between the new behavior of the model and his own familiar action schemas.

Imitative behavior during substage IV appears to be systematic and functions "as though he [the infant] tried out various hypotheses and then finally decided on one of them" (Piaget, 1962, p. 45). Once the infant grasps a correspondence in behavior between himself and the model, it is sudden rather than exponential or gradual as predicted in classical learning theory, which is the reason Piaget (1962) calls the index an early sign of intelligent behavior. As the reader will have observed, there are striking similarities between what Piaget describes in early imitation and both the motor theory of speech perception and Jakobson's distinctive feature theory in the acquisition of phonology (Liberman, Cooper, Shankweiler, and Studdert-Kennedy, 1967; Jakobson, 1968). It is not surprising, then, that "mama" and "papa" and similar forms occur first for the simple reason that they are visible as well as audible and thus, can be more easily assimilated to the shared properties of known action schemas. It is interesting to note that blind children apparently produce first words later than sighted children (Wundt, 1971). Talking for the infant early in this substage may signify no more than the opening and closing of someone's mouth and a keen interest in knowing what is happening inside it. That is, early speech behavior appears to deal with the observable or surface forms rather than with the nonobservable or underlying forms of adult speech.

Substage V—Twelve to Eighteen Months

Substages III and IV were dominated by behavior that was conservative and "practical." In substage III, once the infant happened on a desired end or goal, he repeated the action schema which was initially successful. With the freeing of action schemas from their usual content (generalization) and the more complex coordination of action schemas (mobility), the infant in substage IV could choose an end and, if available, the means to achieve it. Substage V (12–18 months) is somewhat less practical because the child can now develop new means with no fixed or set ends other than active experimentation. Piaget (1952) describes the behavior of this period as being dominated by the tertiary circular reaction (still repetitive though less so and, hence, circular) the primary aim of which is the pursuit of novelty or active experimentation. This emphasis on the novel can be seen in the active exploration of different states of objects to discover their properties (physical knowledge) by varying the actions and observing their relations and effects (logical-mathematical knowledge). The gradual change in focus from actions to their environmental effects which began in substage IV is now nearly complete, owing in part to the child's increased mobility in space (*i.e.,* walking).

Exploration of an object through "experiments in order to see" necessitates a more distinct separation of accommodation of action schemas from the application of action schemas (assimilation) in order that action schemas may be modified depending on the properties of the object and its relations to other objects. The child also considers other persons and objects to be sources of action independent of his activity so that rather than pushing a person's arm, he will now put the object in the person's hand and expect action. He now conceives of himself as the source or subject of actions as well as the recipient or object of actions (Piaget, 1954). The object concept also advances, as seen in the accurate location of an object dropped if its journey to the ground is at least partially visible. If it is not visible, the child will generally fail to find the object since he will only look in the place where the object was last seen. The following observations provide a vivid example of the reaction at this stage:

> At 0;10 (11) Laurent is lying on his back but nevertheless resumes his experiments of the day before. He grasps in succession a celluloid swan, a box, etc., stretches out his arm and lets them fall. He distinctly varies the position of the fall. Sometimes he stretches out his arm vertically, sometimes he holds it obliquely, in front of or behind his eyes, etc. When the object falls in a new position (for example on the pillow), he lets it fall two or three times more on the same place, as though to study the spatial relation; then he modifies the situation. At a certain moment the swan falls near his mouth; now he does not suck it (even though this object habitually serves this purpose), but drops it three times more while merely making the gesture of opening his mouth (Piaget, 1952, p. 269, Obs. 141).

There is a serious attempt to discover the properties of objects and their functional relations by varying the actions applied to them. Early in the period the relationship between an object and its functions (determined from knowing its properties or physical knowledge) is not entirely clear. However, by the end of substage V, actions become more appropriate to the object being used. For example, the child may pet his bottle or dust a doll's face. Relations between himself and other objects and between two or more objects are dictated more by his actions or the properties of objects than by knowing how they go together. By the end of the period, relational knowledge will reflect "adultomorphisms" with objects being used in a way that is recognizably similar to adult usage. That is, the pail is used for carrying water, the brush for brushing hair, etc. The significant advances in physical and logical-mathematical knowledge during this period are due to the child's ability (mobility) to discover new means in the process of experimenting with various ends. Actions become more "distant" and less central as persons and objects begin to be used as tools or instruments of discovery, each with its own independent system of causes and effects. The child is now very close to considering himself as an object within a world of objects. For example:

> In her bath, Jacqueline engages in many experiments with celluloid toys floating in the water. At 1;1 (2) and days following, for example, not only does she drop her toys from a height to see the water splash or displace them with her hand in order to make them swim, but pushes them halfway down in order to see them rise to the surface (Piaget, 1952, p. 273, Obs. 147).
>
> At 1;3 (30) Jacqueline holds in her right hand a box she cannot open. She holds it out to her mother, who pretends not to notice. Then she

transfers the box from her right hand to her left, with her free hand grasps her mother's hand, opens it, and puts the box in it. The whole thing has occurred without a sound. This type of behavior pattern is common around 1 ;4.

So, also during the next days, Jacqueline makes the adult intervene in the particulars of her games, whenever an object is too remote, etc.: she calls, cries, points to objects with her finger, etc. In short, she well knows that she depends on the adult for satisfaction; the person of someone else becomes her best procedure for realization. Furthermore, her grandfather being the most faithful of her servants, she says "Panama" (grandpapa) as soon as her projects fail and she needs a causal instrument which is not defined or present as such in the context of her field of action (Piaget, 1954, p. 311, Obs. 152).

Imitation during substage V, as in the previous substages, follows closely the changes in general sensorimotor development. The discovery of new means by extensive coordination of action schemas through active experimentation allows more systematic and exact imitation of new models. However, imitations are still governed by controlled trial and error. Nevertheless, the child begins to imitate words or actions in adult behavior as well as the movements of objects that are not identical to his own spontaneous production. The close scrutiny of shared properties or features between self and others (including objects) is more actively pursued in imitative attempts as seen in the following observation:

At 1;2 (6) L. looked for my tongue on her own accord, opening my mouth (which was closed) with her fingers. She touched my tongue and then at once touched hers, definitely making a long and careful comparison. She did so again the next day. I then tried opening and closing my eyes. She immediately reproduced the movement, keeping her eyes half closed and puckering her nose, as if she had just understood the difference between the eyes and the mouth as a result of the previous imitation (Piaget, 1962, p. 59, Obs. 50a).

Imitation at substage V involves active discovery and systematic attempts to modify the action schemas in order that more exact correspondences exist between the child's behavior and the behavior of the model. The modifications or accommodations during the early part of the substage are still dependent on the model's action being present during imitative attempts. In this sense, imitation in the beginning of this substage is still dependent on overt actions for adjusting the behavior of the child to the behavior of the model through shared or corresponding properties. The shared features continue to function as indices between the model and initial attempts to duplicate the model's behavior. Thus, early in the substage the signifier (the child's imitative attempts) must be interpreted through the index (shared properties) and at the same time coexist with the signified (the model's behavior). As a result, the signifier and the signified are still basically undifferentiated in that they have to coexist temporally and spatially.

Continual differentiation during this substage is necessary if the child is to use the symbol (more differentiated than the index but still requiring physical or functional similarity between the signifier and the signified). At the end of substage V and the beginning of substage VI, the signifier and the signified separate and, thus, are differentiated; that is, they no longer need to co-occur in time and space and thus can exist somewhat independently. It is for this reason that in the final substage of sensorimotor development the most direct precursors to the symbolic function in general and language in particular will be found.

Substage VI—Eighteen to Twenty-four Months

During substage V, new means were discovered by varying the action schemas applied to objects through active experimentation with objects. As a result, by the end of the substage, the child has come to know a good deal about objects and their possible relations as evidenced in "adultomorphic" behavior. That is, the child acted on objects in a more appropriate way with the salient and functional properties of objects now dictating his behavior rather than applying the already existing action schemas somewhat indiscriminately as in substage IV. Substage VI is the final substage in the sensorimotor period. As such, it is an important transition period when the child—formerly dependent on action schemas (direct physical experience) for knowing reality—will come to utilize action schemas that are internalized and appear in the form of representation and invention. Representation makes its first appearance in substage VI and indicates the child's ability to evoke his now internalized action schemas that were previously coordinated in imitation during substage V. Invention is the spontaneous reorganization of the internalized action schemas derived from physical and logical-mathematical knowledge. This spontaneous reorganization now occurs prior to action and in the absence of immediate perception. Thus, the first indication of mental recombinations or thought freed from actions appears in substage VI. The child now manipulates reality internally prior to acting on it, a skill also known to the great apes as demonstrated in the studies of insight by Kohler (1925). The following rather lengthy observation captures the essence of this important transition.

    Another mental invention, derived from a mental combination and not only from a sensori-motor apprenticeship was that which permitted Lucienne to rediscover an object inside a matchbox. At 1;4 (0), that is to say, right after the preceding experiment, I play at hiding a chain in the same box used in Observation 179. I begin by opening the box as wide as possible and putting the chain into its cover (where Lucienne herself put it, but deeper). Lucienne, who has already practiced filling and emptying her pail and various receptacles, then grasps the box and turns it over without hesitation. No invention is involved of course (it is the simple application of a schema, acquired through groping) but knowledge of this behavior pattern of Lucienne is useful for understanding what follows.

Then I put the chain inside an empty matchbox (where the matches belong), then close the box leaving an opening of 10 mm. Lucienne begins by turning the whole thing over, then tries to grasp the chain through the opening. Not succeeding, she simply puts her index finger into the slit and so succeeds in getting out a small fragment of the chain; she then pulls it until she has completely solved the problem.

Here begins the experiment which we want to emphasize. I put the chain back into the box and reduce the opening to 3 mm. It is understood that Lucienne is not aware of the functioning of the opening and closing of the matchbox and has not seen me prepare the experiment. She only possesses the two preceding schemata: turning the box over in order to empty it of its contents, and sliding her finger into the slit to make the chain come out. It is of course this last procedure that she tries first: she puts her finger inside and gropes to reach the chain, but fails completely. A pause follows during which Lucienne manifests a very curious reaction bearing witness not only to the fact that she tries to think out the situation and to represent to herself through mental combination the operations to be performed, but also to the role played by imitation in the genesis of representation. Lucienne mimics the widening of the slit.

She looks at the slit with great attention; then, several times in succession, she opens and shuts her mouth, at first slightly, then wider and wider! Apparently Lucienne understands the existence of a cavity subjacent to the slit and wishes to enlarge that cavity. The attempt at representation which she thus furnishes is expressed plastically, that is to say, due to inability to think out the situation in words or clear visual images she uses a simple motor indication as "signifier" or symbol. Now, as the motor reaction which presents itself for filling this role is none other than imitation, that is to say, representation by acts, which, doubtless earlier than any mental image, makes it possible not only to divide into parts the spectacles seen but also to evoke and reproduce them at will. Lucienne, by opening her mouth thus expresses, or even reflects her desire to enlarge the opening of the box. This schema of imitation, with which she is familiar, constitutes for her the means of thinking out the situation. There is doubtless added to it an element of magic-phenomenalistic causality or efficacy. Just as she often uses imitation to act upon persons and make them reproduce their interesting movements, so also it is probable that the act of opening her mouth in front of the slit to be enlarged implies some underlying idea of efficacy.

Soon after this phase of plastic reflection, Lucienne unhesitatingly puts her finger in the slit, and instead of trying as before to reach the chain, she pulls so as to enlarge the opening. She succeeds and grasps the chain.

During the following attempts (the slit always being 3 mm wide), the same procedure is immediately rediscovered. On the other hand, Lucienne is incapable of opening the box when it is completely closed. She gropes, throws the box on the floor, etc., but fails (Piaget, 1952, pp. 337–338, Obs. 180).

From the above example, it can be seen that early representations are a continuation of behavior also observed in the use of the index, yet in important ways differing from it. It was stated earlier that the index replaced expressive signals whose form (action) was undifferentiated from its content (context). With the appearance of the index in substage IV, the infant begins to vary the form imitation takes by attempting to establish a correspondence with the behavior of the model. As a result, the index (shared properties) functions as a mediator between the child's known schemas and the object or the model's behavior.

The index marks the first clear appearance of a relationship between a signifier (imitative attempts) and the signified (object or model's behavior), though they are still undifferentiated since they both must co-occur in close proximity in time and space. For example, in observation 30 (above) the infant at substages IV and V considers persons other than himself as a source of action and interprets their actions by comparing the shared features of his own behavior ("papa" and "tata"–actions previously known) with those of the other person or model (opening and closing mouth). However, in observation 180 (above), the child uses opening and closing the mouth to represent or motorically symbolize the intention to open the lid of the box further–prior to acting on it. Thus, in substage VI, the signifier (opening and closing of the child's mouth) can now exist prior to the signified (further opening of the lid of the box) just as representations of actions can exist prior to actions and, as such, indicates the use of a *symbol* rather than an index. Piaget (1962) follows the classic definition of the symbol in that the signifier and the signified, even though they may function separately, must have some physical or functional resemblance to each other.

With the appearance of representation and the symbol, objects and events now become totally permanent since they can be recreated by representation. Further, relational knowledge (causal relations) can now be loosely inferred if either the cause or the effect is given. That is, if the child observes the cause, he can anticipate the effects, or, if only the effects are available, he can reconstruct the cause.

Representation or the appearance of the symbolic function is also seen in imitation at substage VI. For the first time, the child can imitate the behavior of a model or other objects without their being immediately available to perceptual activities. Piaget (1962) calls imitation in the absence of the model "deferred imitation." Imitations that do co-occur with the model's behavior are immediate (with little or no trial and error or overt accommodation) and are now more exact. These changes in imitation are exemplified in the following observations:

> At 1;4 (3) J. had a visit from a little boy whom she used to see from time to time, and who, in the course of the afternoon got into a terrible temper. He screamed as he tried to get out of a play-pen and pushed it backwards, stamping his feet. J. stood watching him in amazement, never having witnessed such a scene before. The next day, she herself screamed in her play-pen and tried to move it, stamping her foot lightly several times in succession. The imitation of the whole scene was most striking. Had it been immediate, it would naturally not have involved representa-

tion, but coming as it did after an interval of twelve hours, it must have involved some representation or pre-representative element (Piaget, 1962, p. 63, Obs. 52).

At 1;4 (0) J. watched me quickly crossing and uncrossing my arms and hitting my shoulders (the movement one uses to get warm). She never before tried to imitate this action, which I had recently suggested to her two or three times. She succeeded, however, in giving a correct imitation at the first attempt. Her movement was rather short, but perfectly produced (Piaget, 1962, p. 62, Obs. 51).

At 1;4 (8) J. said *in step* as she was walking, although she had never uttered these words and they had not been said in her presence immediately before. It was a case of virtual imitation becoming a real imitation in an active context (Piaget, 1962, p. 63, Obs. 54).

The ability to re-present objects or events and their related action schemas is for Piaget the onset of symbolic behavior (Piaget, 1962). The development of the index through imitation during substages IV and V is the source or the primary precursor to the symbolic function. In substage IV, imitation provides the infant with his first signifiers that allow the actions of the model that are no longer immediately available to preception to be re-presented (*i.e.*, "papa" and "tata" functioned as signifiers for the opening and closing of the model's mouth). Moreover, with representation at substage VI the actions no longer have to co-occur with the child's immediate imitative attempts, a condition that was necessary for imitation during substage IV and the early part of substage V. Thus, once an action schema is acquired, in this case through imitation, it is applied. However, the continued application of an action schema is dependent on its being conferred with meaning, *i.e.*, related to a preconcept or internalized actions (thought).

Imitation in its deferred form is the first indication of internalized accommodation or representation, in the same way that mental combinations or inventions are the first signs of internalized action schemas. Moreover, internalized accommodation or representation forms the basis of the image which functions to designate objects or events not immediately available to perception. Thus, the image is not derived from perception but rather from imitative attempts which provide a correspondence between the child's actions and those of the object or event. The covert image rather than the overt imitation now becomes the signifier of the objects or events to be designated or signified. However, the image is reproductive or limited to evoking objects or events that have previously been perceived and, as such, remains static and does not become transformational until it is coordinated with operational thought at about 7 years (Piaget and Inhelder, 1971). Once coordinated, images become anticipatory in that, without prior observation, the child can evoke an image of an object and envision transformations or changes in the imagined object.

Since accommodatory behaviors or signifiers (deferred imitation and imagery) do not function independently of assimilation or the signified, the signifiers can be assimilated to existing cognitive structures (preconcepts) with concomitant accommodation and thereby be conferred with meaning, or they can be assimilated without accommodation and result in symbolic play (Piaget and Inhelder, 1971). With the appearance of this option, assimilation and accommodation fused at substage I are now clearly separate and can function somewhat independently since thought, rather than action schemas (preconceptual), now anchors both assimilation and accommodation.

Play, like imitation and imagery, has its own development (Piaget 1962) but does not become symbolic or capable of using symbols until imitative actions are internalized and representation appears. The first signs of representation in play also appear in substage VI and are seen in make-believe or pretend behavior. Pretending necessitates the ability to evoke a signifier (image or symbolic gesture) which designates the real object or event. In the following observations the child first designates the act of sleeping by producing salient features of actual sleeping and then allows that the stuffed animals "pretend" to be asleep.

> " . . . make-believe" first appeared at 1;3 (12) in the following circumstances. She saw a cloth whose fringed edges vaguely recalled those of her pillow; she seized it, held a fold of it in her right hand, sucked the thumb of the same hand and lay down on her side, laughing hard. She kept her eyes open, but blinked from time to time as if she were alluding to closed eyes. Finally, laughing more and more, she cried "no no." The same cloth started the same game on following days. At 1;3 (30) it was the tail of her donkey which represented the pillow! And from 1;5 onwards, she made her animals, a bear and a plush dog also do "no no" [sleep] (Piaget, 1962, p. 96, Obs. 64).

The use of the symbol in play and imagery has important implications for the general development of the symbolic function as well as intelligence itself since the child soon comes to substitute objects or events (signifiers) for other objects or events (the signified). For example, when a child uses a piece of paper to cover a doll or stuffed animal and a fountain pen replaces a bottle during "feeding," he is demonstrating *double or symbolic knowledge* about objects, a function that has considerable significance for the development of preconceptual thought and words in language (Furth, 1969). Double or symbolic knowledge is used in play and allows the child to know objects in more than one way by coordinating, as in the index, shared properties of correspondence between the evoked or absent object and the object symbolized. However, deferred imitation, imagery, and symbolic play, though important in the initial separation of form from content and, thus, in establishing a structure for signifier-signified relations, remain individual and private. They function primarily to designate objects or events rather than to communicate (Piaget and Inhelder, 1971).

The child's first words are intermediate between the private symbol seen in symbolic play and the shared *sign* found in social thought and language.

The true sign is social and general in that there is a more abstract relationship between the signifier (word) and the signified (concept). Words, like images, function to designate but they designate preconcepts and, later, concepts rather than objects or events (Piaget and Inhelder, 1971). However, it is necessary that the image also be assimilated to the preconcept or the concept in order to be conferred with meaning. It is the preconcept or concept, derived from the operative aspect rather than the figurative aspect of intelligence or the symbolic function, that allows interpretation and comprehension. Since the word marks cognitive distinctions rather than objects or events, it functions in a way that is quite different from other symbolic behavior such as imagery, symbolic play, etc., and therefore is an important aid in the socialization of thought or the formation of general classes. Thought and language share certain properties that lead to their eventual socialization. That is, unlike sensorimotor action schemas, they are general rather than private, social rather than individual, abstract rather than concrete—in short, thought and language are both communicable. Because it shares these features with thought, language is viewed as a special but not a separate function of more generalized symbolic behaviors found in deferred imitation, imagery, symbolic play, drawing, and dreaming (Piaget, 1962).

As stated earlier, early representations and inventions are evoked action schemas previously coordinated during the sensorimotor period and internalized during the transition to the preoperational period. These newly internalized action schemas initially retain their private and individual quality and thus interfere with attempts to communicate them. As a result, during the early part of this second major developmental stage the child is literally tied to his own representations in a way not unlike that in which the infant is tied to his own circular reactions. The behaviors associated with the symbolic function (except for language) such as imitation, imagery, symbolic play, dreaming, and drawing are of little help in decentering these representations or the child's own world view since they are themselves individual and private. It is left for language to act as a catalyst for decentering both operative as well as figurative representations by providing data from the social world. However, language remains subordinate to thought and not fully coordinated with it until adult thought appears around 12 years of age. Piaget (1926) has long maintained that language does not take the form of real dialogue until thought is basically socialized at about 7 years of age. The following observations exemplify the initial phase of these transitions beginning with the first verbal schemas.

T. at 1;0 (0) said *tata* for all successful actions, e.g., getting hold of a toy with a string on it, or finding an adequate response to an attempt at imitation.

At 1;2 (23) he said *daddy* to J. who held out her arms to him like his father. The same day he used *daddy* in reference to a male visitor and to a peasant who was lighting his pipe (though he never referred to him thus in the usual way). For several weeks after 1;3 (2) *mummy* was used as *pavene* (grandfather) in the case of T., to indicate he wanted something. At 1;4 (4), for example, he said *mummy* as he pointed at something he wanted, even when he was referring to his father or to some other person. Also at 1;6 (23) he said *mummy* to his father as he pointed to a lamp that he wanted to light and put out (although it was only his father that ever played this game with him). At 1;4 (10) however, he said *mummy* when he gave his mother a piece of paper and also when he saw her clothes in a cupboard. Similarly, he said *daddy* at 1;4 (23) when he saw his father shaving, also a few days later when his father was serving him and then when he saw his father's ruck sack. At 1;4 (29) when one of my friends was there, and I asked him "who is it?" he replied *daddy* pointing to him. At 1;5 (19) *daddy* referred to any man who was fifteen to twenty yards away and at 1;5 (25) to men in general.

At 1;5 (19) *no more* meant going away, then throwing something on the ground, and was then used for something that was overturning (without disappearing). He thus said *no more* to his blocks. Later *no more* merely meant that something was at a distance from him (outside his field of prehension), and then it referred to the game of holding out an object for someone to throw back at him. At 1;6 (23) he even said *no more* when he wanted something someone was holding. Finally, at 1;7 *no more* became synonymous with begin again (Piaget, 1962, pp. 217–18, Obs. 102).

In the above observations, a general principle is operating that is found in cognition and language. New forms are first used to express old content while new content is first expressed through old forms (Piaget, 1962; Slobin, 1973). In establishing relationships between form and content, the child always "starts from the surface" (Piaget, 1962, p. 283). As described in the development of intelligence (logic), the child is initially fused with his environment and only applies circular actions to the surface aspects of reality. Once the child begins to differentiate himself from his actions and from objects or events, he begins to coordinate actions and then internalizes them as thought capable of being used free of overt actions, a process necessary for forming schemas which interpret and comprehend (operative function). Intelligence thus described does not appear before substage VI.

Since the operative aspect of intelligence, derived from sensorimotor action schemas, functions to interpret and confer meaning, the first verbal schemas, which will be discussed in some detail in a later section, should reflect general cognitive functioning during substage V and substage VI and the beginnings of the preoperational period (Piaget, 1962; Brown, 1973; Slobin, 1973). Slobin (1973) has proposed a general principle derived from cross-cultural data that suggests that while all children may have certain cognitive distinctions available at about the same age, certain languages allow some distinctions to be more easily marked than others. Within a given language there is some evidence that specific cognitive functions such as spatial concepts dictate the order of appearance and use of locatives (Johnston, 1973).

Just as the child is fused and undifferentiated from his actions and objects or events, so sound (signifier) and meaning (signified) in language first appear as fused and undifferentiated, as clearly seen in the functions of expressive signals and the early use of the index during the first 8 months in infancy. During substage IV the index replaces expressive signals and the child establishes the first relationship between his own spontaneous productions (babbling) and adult language. At this substage, the relationship is simply a vague connection, mediated by shared properties or features between the child's opening and closing of his mouth and similar actions occurring in the model. Through the use of the index (shared properties) the child soon begins to produce recognizable forms made by the model that co-occur or follow closely in time with his own productions.

The first transition from operating on behavior observed on the surface to operating on some aspect of an underlying form may be no more than the infant's attempt to replicate what goes on inside someone else's mouth. Thus, it appears unlikely that the child begins with the underlying structural base of a sentence, as proposed by McNeill (1970) and Ingram (1971), during the production of single words any more than he begins with an analogous underlying base for logic, *i.e.,* internalized actions.

PIAGET'S THEORY AND RECENT STUDIES IN EARLY LANGUAGE DEVELOPMENT

Recent work in early language development provides evidence that is remarkably consistent with Piaget's (1962) general position on the development of the symbolic function. Bloom (1973) has provided convincing evidence from the study of single words that the child begins with surface, rather than deep structure (grammatical) aspects of language. Single words that function as single words rather than "word sentences" support the view that sound and meaning by substage IV are differentiated but like all representational functions must await the appearance of mental combinations before they are relational. Since form and content are fixed prior to substage IV, there is no reason to assume that sound and meaning, derived from them, would begin as mobile and differentiated. Moreover, the differentiation beginning in substage IV is gradual and follows a pattern similar to that described earlier for assimilation and accommodation. By the end of substage V and the beginning of substage VI, both assimilation and accommodation and sound and meaning are differentiated and, as a result, thought (preconceptual) and syntax (pretransformational) make their first appearance.

The first recognized word forms usually appear during substage IV with the appearance of the index and the awareness that actions can exist in other persons or objects separate from the infant's actions but not totally independent of them. As a result, first words follow closely the functions of imitation during this substage. It will be recalled that indices, unlike expressive signals such as crying and vocalization, were mobile rather than fixed in that form could now exist separate from immediate context or content. That is, the infant could only imitate (form) the actions of the model (content) through the mediative functions of the index (shared properties). The index soon drops out and the infant can imitate the form directly. For example, Bloom (1973) states that Allison's first use of "away" at 10 months followed repeated statements of the general form, "Let's throw it away," when she began playing with or mouthing objects her mother had not intended for her. The general form "away" was always used in the same general context and Allison soon began to use it appropriately to refer to the disappearance of objects or people. Aside from her early forms, which included "mama," "dada," "mimi," and "baby" (all highly visible!), Allison did not continue to use the index (shared properties) but moved quickly on to word forms derived from early deferred imitation which pairs the child's recognition of shared properties with familiar contexts rather than with the model or object. It is interesting to note that some children continue to rely heavily on imitation, and, moreover, as Bloom (1973) has noted, degree of imitation may be a good predictor for the kind of strategy utilized in forming early syntactic constructions. That is, the child who imitates a good deal usually starts with function plus substantive forms (*e.g.,* "more milk") rather than two substantive forms which can take on several meanings (*e.g.,* "mommy sock").

During what appears to be substage V, Allison used two classes of words. The first class (substantive words) initially included objects and persons and somewhat later actions or events. Forms such as "chair," "book," "back," "tumble," which made up the object and action terms, appeared and disappeared, and then reappeared, sometimes changing their forms, with some regularity. As Bloom (1973) puts it, these forms had a "high mortality rate." This high mortality rate is predictable since the child has not yet internalized action schemas that allow representation and is dependent on contextual recognition that is static and momentary. With the appearance of representation, the child has the more permanent preconcept which the substantive words can consistently designate or mark. Even with the appearance of preconcepts which are relatively stable compared to perception, imitation, or imagery, the actual phonetic (form) and semantic (content) aspects of new words apparently continue to be unstable for some time (Morehead, 1971; Oller, 1973; Clark, 1973). Person forms were more stable than object or action forms since they referred to highly familiar people in the child's milieu. These forms included "mama," "dada," "mimi," and "baby."

The second class of words used by Allison are called function words and refer primarily, as do early substantive words, to "orders and expressions of desire" (*i.e.,* intentionality, which begins in substage V, Piaget, 1962, p. 222). They included the forms "stop," "no," "more," "up," "away," etc. Function words and, as mentioned earlier, person words appear to stabilize early since once they appear they are continued in the child's production. The early stability of function words is no doubt related to the fact that substage V is still action-based and that these lexical items refer to functional rather than attributive aspects of physical knowledge. Objects or events now have some permanency, and the child behaves as though they exist in a continuous state that does not change significantly except to appear, disappear, reappear, or cease to function. It is apparently these functional aspects of knowing objects or events such as disappearance, recurrence, cessation, etc. to which function words such as "away," "more," "stop," etc., refer (Brown, 1973; Bloom, 1973). As mentioned earlier, person words probably stabilize because of their repeated occurrence in highly familiar contexts. Function and person words also dominate the lexicon until the onset of substage VI.

Descriptive terms such as adjectives that refer to the attributes of objects did not appear except on rare occasions. As noted earlier, with the appearance of representation at substage VI, words mark preconcepts (internalized actions). Apparently, objects are not initially coded in terms of perceptual attributes alone but rather are derived from shared properties found in known actions and familiar contexts (Bruner, 1971). For example, color which obviously cannot be derived from actions is notably missing from the list of properties Clark (1974) has postulated young children use in applying early form (words) to content (objects and events). The properties include movement, shape, size, sound, texture, and taste, all of which have tactile-kinesthetic correspondences that can mediate between the object or event and perception.

In contrast to Piaget (1970a), Clark (1973, 1974) assumes that perception rather than actions mediates between first words and the objects or events to which they indirectly refer. The relatively unimportant role given to perception by Piaget is clear from his definition of a sensorimotor schema. The schema is defined as " . . . stable patterns of movement together with a perceptual component geared to recognition. . . ." Perception, then, is necessary only for recognition while actions are necessary for understanding or meaning (Piaget and Inhelder, 1964, p. 14). For Clark (1973, 1974) intelligence is apparently derived from perception rather than actions, and thus perceptual attributes rather than known actions, familiar contexts, or preconcepts provide the source of "meaning" for early words. There is considerable evidence that the grouping of members into a class (extension) according to the defining attributes of that class (intension) does not occur until the emergence of class inclusion at 7 years when the child finally frees himself from perceptual constraints and surface representations (Piaget and Inhelder, 1964; Furth, Youniss, and Ross, 1970). Moreover, Piaget (1962), Brown (1973), and Bloom (1973) have observed that children frequently use early single words to refer to the entire object rather than a single attribute or to ongoing actions or events which are presumably cued by the shared properties (initially mediated by tactile-kinesthetic correspondence as seen in the index) in familiar contexts.

As mentioned earlier, at the end of substage V children begin to use objects in an "adultomorphic" way. The child plays with objects according to their surface functions. Brooms are used to sweep, blankets to cover, dolls to hold, etc. It is interesting that both Allison and notably Gia in Bloom's studies (1970, 1973) also began to use "adultomorphic" forms longer than one word—a kind of nonsense talk often noted in children's speech patterns at this substage. This process is similar to imitating opening and closing the mouth at substage IV, in that it involves little or no understanding and focuses on salient surface manifestations. For example, Gia talked in long unintelligible sequences and Allison used a nonsense form "weda," which acted as a "pivot" following substantive and function forms. Bloom (1973) interprets this phenomenon as further evidence that children at this substage deal with language in a rather superficial way.

Additional evidence for the position that children during substage V (18–24 months) use single words rather than "word sentences" could reasonably come from the analysis of the child's general level of sensorimotor behavior and the use of the symbol; that is, it is unlikely that the child will use syntactic forms prior to the appearance of mental combinations and representation.

With the appearance of internalized actions (preconcepts) and the symbol, "adultomorphic" behavior markedly decreases. Objects are no longer treated as though they have a continuous state of existence; the surface or functional characteristics of objects can now serve symbolic functions, and the superficial imitation of adult speech patterns fails as an artificial form of communication. During this transition the child comes to know that objects (including persons) and events are capable of action independent of his activity—a new source of action that also reflects lax causal relations (*i.e.,* global notions of cause and effect). Moreover, he begins to have *double knowledge;* objects or events can now function not only in one continuous state but also in different states as long as each state maintains shared properties of physical or functional similarity to the reference state (*i.e.,* the symbol). Double knowledge reflects the characteristics of the symbol and can be used even if the object or event is absent since the image is now capable of evoking objects or events in their absence. For example, the child uses make-believe or pretense (signifier—*i.e.,* pretend sleeping) to symbolize the real act (signified—*i.e.,* the act of sleeping); substitutes an object with similar physical or functional properties for another object (*i.e.,* a fountain pen for a doll bottle); and single words like "stick," "fish," and "bird," may reflect several aspects of a preconcept while marking the same object (stick) in different rather than continuous states. Shvachkin (1973) observed a child who referred to the object stick as "stick" when it was on the ground, as "fish" when it was floating on water, and as "bird" when it was in the air. The first clear indication of Allison's use of double knowledge appeared when "mama," "dada," etc. ceased to refer only to adult persons but began to refer also to objects associated with them. For instance, when noticing her mother's glove, she would say "mommy" rather than "glove" (Bloom, 1973).

Although "adultomorphic" behavior obviously continues, objects and events can now symbolize or function in the place of other objects or events. As a result, the child has at least doubled what he knows and can represent regarding objects or events and their relations. It is for this reason that the symbol has such important implications for lexical entries and primitive groupings in early language and thought. With the appearance of double knowledge at the end of substage V, the naming explosion to which Lenneberg (1967) refers generally occurs. It is at this point that many substantive words for objects (including persons) and events began to appear in Allison's lexicon simultaneously with the appearance of double knowledge since she now had preconcepts reflecting this expanded knowledge that words could consistently mark. Thus, the mortality rate of substantive words decreases and the lexicon, like the object before it, shows signs of some permanency. Finally, the use of the symbol reflected in double knowledge moves the child away from dealing with only surface forms of objects and events to their more general characteristics that can have a correspondence or relation to other objects or events. This transition is exemplified by Allison's use of "mommy" to mark the objects related to the person such as glove, coat, etc., as well as the person. It is important to point out that children do not conserve an object such as a stick in transformation between states nor the form that designates its corresponding concept until near 7 years (Elkind, 1969). Imagining or symbolic play also decreases with the ability to conserve objects in different states by following the transformation from one state to another and back again to the original state (*i.e.,* reversibility) (Piaget, 1970a).

To reiterate, the child at the beginning of substage VI is capable of representation and invention. The action schemas which were coordinated during substages IV and V are now internalized and their patterns can be re-presented before action in the child as well as anticipated in other objects or persons. Moreover, these internalized actions can be combined in novel ways as seen in invention or insight. During the first half of this substage, Allison, Eric, and Gia began to use successive single words which marked early preconcepts corresponding to the previous, actual, or intended states of objects or events (Bloom, 1973). For example, Allison said "daddy," "peach," "cut" while handing her father a peach and a spoon, indicating that she knew the intended state (cut) of the object and that another person (daddy) was capable of acting independent of her activities. Moreover, implicit in the verbal sequence was the global and juxtaposed causal relationship between the act of cutting (cause) and the cut peach (effect). That is, she knew the intended end (cut peach) and was able to request from persons other than herself the means (act of cutting) to that end. Even though representation and invention are obviously more coordinated, as seen in this example, the movement of these coordinations is still slow. Piaget (1952) likens early imagery and mental representation at the beginning of substage VI to a motion picture being displayed one frame at a time. This analogy captures the essence of successive single words. Their intonation contours fall at the end of each word. Each word has relatively equal stress, and there is a definite pause between them (Bloom, 1973). Further, the order is determined by the order in representation which may not have a one-to-one correspondence with the order in reality or the order reflected in adult grammatical relations. Thus, prior to the onset of syntax, the child must have internalized coordinated action schemas so that relational aspects of the referent can be represented prior to talking and in the absence of the referent and, secondly, he must have double knowledge or know a referent in more than one way in order that he can begin a stable lexicon with differentiated feature markings. The description given for substage V—particularly the slow movement in imagery and mental representation and the lack of a fixed order in successive single words—would also appear to characterize the linguistic accomplishments of the chimpanzee Washoe trained in American sign language (Gardner and Gardner, 1969).

The latter part of substage V and the early part of substage VI set the stage for the appearance of syntax or the child's first sentences. Syntax, like other mental development, emerges from what has gone before. Bloom (1970, 1973), Schlesinger (1971), and Brown (1973) have found that early syntax appears in two distinct forms. One form appears to derive from physical knowledge which underlies primarily function words while the other derives from logical-mathematical knowledge which provides the base primarily for substantive forms. The first form is represented by early two-word constructions in which either word is capable of marking the same preconcept. Thus, they represent a closed semantic set having to do with reference, rather than relations. According to Bloom (1970), Schlesinger (1971), and Brown (1973), these forms include the nominative or existence (*e.g.*, "that ball"), recurrence (*e.g.*, "more milk"), nonexistence (*e.g.*, "no mommy") rejection (*e.g.*, "no doggy"), and denial (*e.g.*, "no cry"). In addition to successive one-word utterances, Washoe is also apparently capable of signing constructions that are analogous to these referential forms save their fixed word order.

The second form, which derives from logical-mathematical or relational knowledge, differs from the first in that neither word in two-word constructions marks the preconcept. Rather, it is the relation between the two that designates the preconcept. These relational forms almost always follow a definite order as did the reference forms—something that was missing in successive single words and apparently, in Washoe's sign combinations, suggesting that the chimpanzee may lack logical-mathematical knowledge (Brown, 1970). Examples of the second form include agent-action (*e.g.,* "daddy walk"), action-object (*e.g.,* "mommy sock"), possessive (*e.g.,* "mommy sock"), locative (*e.g.,* "sweater chair," "go store"), and the attributive (*e.g.,* "big ball"). Thus, it appears as though early syntactic forms directly parallel those aspects of operative intelligence—knowledge of objects and events and their properties and knowledge of the relations between objects or events—which Piaget (1962) postulates they designate or mark.[2]

Finally, when the child marks the global aspects of a preconcept rather than shared properties in action (*i.e.,* index) or familiar contexts (*i.e.,* symbol), he is capable of using the *sign.* " . . . that is to say, it [the word] is no longer part of the action, but evokes it [by representation] " (Piaget, 1962, p. 222). Relational forms (*e.g.,* "mommy sock") appear to be less closely tied to action and objects than reference forms (*e.g.,* "more milk") in that they designate relations rather than actions or objects; thus, relational forms mark the onset of syntax just as juxtaposed "and-constructions" in preoperational thought mark early preconcepts or prelogic. That is, early syntax appears to proceed as does prelogic from particular to particular with definite though syncretic relations between elements.

In summary, during the first 2 years, the child moves through a series of substages that carry him from reflex to preconcept and from signal to sign. The essence of this movement is the base separation of assimilation from accommodation which allows the emergence of intelligence (logic)—a state of relative balance or equilibrium between assimilation and accommodation. As a result of this separation, form is differentiated from content, allowing sound and meaning to be distinguished and, as a result, the emergence of relational syntax. Soon after the onset of relational syntax, the child begins to ask his first questions (*e.g.,* "what that?"), indicating an initial awareness that the language of others (*i.e.,* social world) can be a source of information separate from his own actions—a natural outgrowth from the child's earlier knowledge that other persons besides himself are sources of actions. For Piaget (1962) the appearance of the first question forms indicates a significant movement toward the formation of concepts or socialized thought and communication or socialized language. However, the two do not fully coordinate until logic (thought) becomes propositional at around 12 years of age. Finally, even after complete coordination, Piaget finds language to be subordinate to thought in that "these superstructures [of propositional logic] go beyond the language of the subject and cannot even be formulated by means of the current language alone" (Piaget, 1963, p. 58).

---

[2] Brown (1973) and Sinclair (1971b, 1973) describe additional parallels between sensorimotor intelligence and the onset of syntax.

PIAGET'S THEORY AND EARLY LANGUAGE TRAINING[3]

There has been considerable controversy over whether or not Piaget's theory of cognitive development implies training. The details of the controversy are fully discussed elsewhere and for the purposes of this section need not be reviewed (Kohlberg, 1968; Engelmann, 1971; Kami and Derman, 1971). We will assume that the theory provides an excellent base for deriving new and promising methods of assessing and habilitating language-deficient children. We will begin this section with general concepts in Piaget's theory that are particularly relevant to the development of a base linguistic system and later provide examples of how training for part of the developmental sequence described in this chapter might be implemented.

The first general notion that is crucial for the acquisition of a base system of language is the concept of interaction between the child and his environment. For mental structures which are spontaneously learned in their natural settings such as logical-mathematical and linguistic structures, mass generalized experience provides the data necessary for their development and, once developed, their reorganization, *i.e.,* learning. A central issue in language training, then, is whether the quality and extent of interaction can significantly change the rate of acquiring linguistic structures. Recent studies of the quality and extent of the interaction between the child and the primary caretakers suggest that these factors are of considerable importance. For example, Bell and Ainsworth (1972) found that the promptness of a mother's response to an expressive signal such as crying and vocalization determines the rate at which the child develops alternative uses of the signal (*i.e.,* its mobility). Whitehurst, Novak, and Zorn (1972) reported that training the mother in the quality and extent of verbal interaction had dramatic effects on a severely language-delayed child. These studies suggest that the scope of training should be broadened considerably beyond the frequently used short training sessions to include changes in the total quality and extent of linguistic interaction.

Language was described earlier as part of a more general representational system that evolved out of one aspect of intelligence, the figurative aspect, and gradually coordinated itself during the first 12 years with the more basic aspect of intelligence, the operative aspect. This view of language emphasizes the crucial point that language learning is normally an integral part of mental development and that language should not be isolated in training from its broad developmental context. Even though language is an integral part of mental growth, language and related symbolic functions do not organize experience; rather they serve cognition by freeing the child from direct sensory and physical experience which dominates the sensorimotor period

[3] Written in collaboration with Judith Johnston.

and, as a result, allow the development of representation and the exchange of social experience. It is cognition that organizes experience and thus confers meaning on linguistic and symbolic functions. However, the dependency of language on cognition is not unilateral and the two systems achieve full coordination at the level of propositional logic appearing during early adolescence.

This view of a continuing relationship between language and thought has recently received some attention in developmental research. For example, Sinclair (1969) demonstrated the dependence of language on cognition in her study of comparative structures. She found that children at the preoperational stage of logical development had great difficulty in learning the coordinated comparative structure of "longer but thinner" vs. "this one is long, that one is thin." Those children who did learn to produce this syntactic structure generally showed no concomitant growth in operativity. Furth's (1966) work with deaf children also suggests that although some children with severe language deficiencies develop normally in some areas of intellect well into the middle childhood years, eventually intellectual growth is impaired. The initial effects of language deficiency may be minimized since these children have the use of private nonlinguistic symbols and/or because only certain aspects of intelligence depend upon the conventional inguistic systems. However, both Piaget's theory and Furth's work with the deaf argue that the child must thoroughly coordinate complex intellectual and linguistic systems if adult intellectual competence is to evolve by 12–14 years.

The coordination of representational systems with advancing intellect should be central to language training even during the earliest stages of development. General coordination of systems seems to be an important operating principle found in both cognition and language—new forms first designate old content while new content initially appears in old forms. Normally the child uses a new word or linguistic rule to represent a preconcept or notion he already has; as his cognitive structures become more differentiated and coordinated and as he receives social feedback about the appropriateness of his language use, these first word meanings are refined. Although a child may be taught to imitate a word or linguistic rule, unless these language forms are appropriate to his level of cognitive development, they will not enter into the integrated processes of mental growth. Instead, they will remain imitative tricks, restricted to the specific context in which they were acquired. Many "carry-over" problems could be avoided by increased attention to the normal interaction of intellectual and linguistic growth.

There is some evidence that language-deficient children who are not markedly retarded have a general deficiency in all representational functions (Morehead and Ingram, 1973). It is also possible that some manipulation of nonlinguistic symbols is prerequisite to language and, moreover, may facilitate the rapid growth of language in the normal child between 16–18 months and 37–40 months. If so, this relationship has important implications for language training. For children with high level language (postsyntactic or two or more words per utterance), supportive training in other nonlinguistic representational systems—symbolic play with objects, role playing, imagery, and drawing—could be implemented. Programs could be developed to facilitate such behavior in the same way that experiences are structured in attempts to facilitate the learning of language forms (Miller and Yoder, this volume).

For a child with low level language development (prelinguistic, single or successive single word utterances), Piaget's theory represents one of the few attempts to provide a detailed account of the successive development of prelinguistic and linguistic behavior prior to the onset of syntax (Piaget, 1962). Since prelinguistic and early linguistic behavior develops in the context of general sensorimotor development, it is first necessary to establish the particular substage of the child and then to ascertain the level of prelinguistic or early linguistic functioning. Several tests are available for determining sensorimotor substages (Uzgiris and Hunt, 1966; Mehrabian and Williams, 1971), and this chapter provides a description of presyntactic development and the order of successive appearance beginning with the signal and ending with the true sign.

Language training could begin as early as the appearance of a stable expressive signal during substage III. For example, if a child were found to be functioning at sensorimotor substage IV and yet showed few alternate uses of the signal other than crying and some vocalizations, the research of Bell and Ainsworth (1972) on the conditions under which other modes of signaling or early communication develops could easily be adapted for training purposes.

At the level of the index, training would focus primarily on imitation, first in immediate, then deferred form. To exemplify, consider a child who is found to be at substage IV or the early part of substage V according to one of the sensorimotor tests given earlier. The child will only imitate the actions of persons or objects that are visible to him and which he can see his own body reproduce. This restriction, of course, precludes vocal imitations including speech. The baseline prelinguistic behavior would be the imitation of familiar, *visible* movements. The goal, developmentally determined, would be to imitate familiar actions in other persons or objects but that are nonvisible in his own actions. For example, facial movements which the child has been seen to produce (known actions) should be selected such as chewing, opening the mouth, licking lips, blinking eyes, and wrinkling the nose. This action would be presented as a model for imitation in its simplest context, in this example, immediately after the child has spontaneously produced it. Supportive information would also be provided to help the child isolate the relevant variables by incorporating additional natural indices such as those associated with the concomitant auditory cues of smacking when chewing, sniffing when wrinkling the nose, and then phasing these indices out. Finally, the imitation model should be presented as often as possible and in a variety of instances of the same class of behavior, waiting for the successful imitation of many different nonvisible actions before moving on to the next goal of deferred imitation. In these ways the child's natural progress in imitation can be optimized, bringing him closer to using the imitative gesture as a symbol.

In the case of employing the symbol in training, symbolic play and its underlying function of double knowledge of persons, actions, objects, and events are extremely useful. If training were continued with the child trained on familiar but nonvisible actions and deferred imitation and the training was successful, our new goal determined from the normal developmental sequence would be the symbol. Our baseline behavior would be the inability to substitute one action, object, or event for another action, object, or event with similar functions—to use a different verbal label ordinarily assigned to a specified and known person or object in a particular state for the same person or object in another state and through the use of successive single words, to comment on agent-action-object sequences whose order is determined by their appearance in cognition rather than grammatical order. We would assume the child was at a presymbolic level since substitution on the basis of shared properties or double knowledge was absent. Training could begin with the substitution of actions for a referent or significant such as rhythmical vocal patterns replacing music while dancing. All three behaviors would have to be familiar to the child prior to training, new information being derived first from the reorganization of old knowledge. Next, objects or events could be played with in the absence of objects or events that usually elicit certain behaviors, i.e., blocks of wood for cars, boxes for doll beds, etc. Then, we would want to train the child to differentially label objects in different contexts or states, such as a ball or balloon with a mop head for hair and a face drawn on one of its vertical surfaces. Finally, we would encourage the child to mark verbally ongoing actions or events beginning with his own action sequences, without prescribing any particular grammatical order.

In the developmental sequence of prelinguistic and early linguistic behavior, the true sign follows the symbol. We earlier defined the sign as the designation of a cognitive distinction (preconcept) by a word or the derivation of novel relations between words to mark new cognitive distinctions. Moreover, the sign also indicates that the child now views other persons as sources of information that go beyond his own direct experience. Defined in this way, the word is not a true sign until the onset of syntax and the appearance of the question form which follows soon after. With the appearance of syntax and the question form, the use of the word or sign now necessitates the functions of referential syntax such as nomination, recurrence, etc., and the functions which mark agent, action, and object relations.

Miller and Yoder (this volume) have developed assessment and training procedures for this period of early linguistic development based on recent research in child language development.

REFERENCES

Bateson, P. The characteristics and context of imprinting. *Biol. Rev.*, 1966, *41*, 177–220.

Bell, S. and Ainsworth, M. Infant crying and materal responsiveness. *Child Develop.*, 1972, *43*, 1171–1190.

Bloom, L. *Language Development: Form and Function in Emerging Grammars*. Cambridge, Mass.: The M.I.T. Press, 1970.

Bloom, L. *One Word at a Time: The Use of Single-Word Utterances before Syntax*. The Hague: Mouton, 1973.

Bower, T. G. R. The visual world of infants. *Sci. Amer.*, 1966, *215*, 80–92.

Bowlby, J. *Attachment and Loss*. Vol. 1, *Attachment*. New York: Basic Books, 1969.

Brown, R. *A First Language*. Cambridge, Mass.: Harvard University Press, 1973.

Brown, R. The first sentences of the child and the chimpanzee. In R. Brown (Ed.), *Psycholinguistics*. New York: The Free Press, 1970.

Bruner, J. Competence in infants. Paper presented to the Society for Research in Child Development, Minneapolis, 1971.

Chomsky, N. *Aspects of the Theory of Syntax*. Cambridge, Mass.: M.I.T. Press, 1965.

Chomsky, N. *Cartesian Linguistics*. New York: Harper and Row, 1966.

Chomsky, N. *Language and Mind*. New York: Harcourt Brace Jovanovich, 1968.

Clark, E. What's in a word? On the child's acquisition of semantics in his first language. In T. E. Moore (Ed.), *Cognitive Development and the Acquisition of Language*. New York: Academic Press, 1973.

Clark, E. Some aspects of the conceptual basis for first language acquisition. This volume.

De Villiers, P. A. and De Villiers, J. G. Early judgements of semantic and syntactic acceptability by children. *J. Psycholing. Res.*, 1972, *1*, 299–310.

Elkind, D. Developmental studies of figurative perception. In L. P. Lipsitt and C. C. Spiker (Eds.), *Advances in Child Development and Behavior*, Vol. IV. New York: Academic Press, 1969.

Engelmann, S. Does the Piagetian approach imply instruction? In D. Green, M. Ford, and G. Flamer (Eds.), *Measurement and Piaget*. New York: McGraw-Hill, 1971.

Ervin-Tripp, S. Some strategies for the first two years. In T. E. Moore (Ed.), *Cognitive Development and the Acquisition of Language*. New York: Academic Press, 1973.

Furth, H. *Thinking without Language: Psychological Implications of Deafness*. New York: Free Press, 1966.

Furth, H. *Piaget and Knowledge: Theoretical Foundations*. Englewood Cliffs, N. J.: Prentice Hall, 1969.

Furth, H., Youniss, J., and Ross, B. Children's utilization of logical symbols:

An interpretation of conceptual behavior based on Piagetian theory. *Develop. Psychol.,* 1970, *3,* 36–57.

Gardner, R. A. and Gardner, B. T. Teaching sign language to a chimpanzee. *Science,* 1969, *165,* 664–672.

Ingram, D. Transitivity in child language. *Language,* 1971, *47.* 888–909.

Inhelder, B. and Piaget, J. *The Early Growth of Logic in the Child.* London: Routledge and Kegan Paul, 1964.

Jakobson, R. *Child Language, Aphasia, and Phonological Universals.* The Hague: Mouton, 1968.

Johnston, J. Spatial notions and the child's use of locatives in an elicitation task. Paper presented at the Stanford Child Language Research Forum, Palo Alto, 1973.

Kamii, C. and Derman, L. The Engelmann approach to teaching logical thinking: Findings from the administration of some Piagetian tasks. In D. Green, M. Ford, and G. Flamer (Eds.), *Measurement and Piaget.* New York: McGraw-Hill, 1971.

Kohlberg, L. Early education: A cognitive-developmental view. *Child Develop.,* 1968, *39,* 1013–1063.

Kohler, W. *The Mentality of Apes.* New York: Harcourt Brace, 1925.

Kuo, Z. *The Dynamics of Behavior Development: An Epigenetic View.* New York: Random House, 1967.

Lenneberg, E. *Biological Foundations of Language.* New York: Wiley, 1967.

Levi-Strauss, C. *The Savage Mind.* Chicago: University of Chicago Press, 1966.

Liberman, C., Cooper, F., Shankwieler, D., and Studdert-Kennedy, M. Perception of the speech code. *Psychol. Rev.,* 1967, *74,* 431–461.

McNeill, D. *The Acquisition of Language: The Study of Psycholinguistics.* New York: Harper and Row, 1970.

Mehrabian, A. and Williams, M. Piagetian measures of cognitive development up to age two. *J. Psycholing. Res.,* 1971, *1,* 113–126.

Miller, J. and Yoder, D. An ontogenetic language teaching strategy for retarded children. This volume.

Morehead, D. Phonological processing in young children and adults. *Child Develop.,* 1971, *42,* 279–289.

Morehead, D. and Ingram, D. The development of base syntax in normal and linguistically deviant children. *J. Speech Hear. Res.,* 1973, *16,* 330–352.

Oller, D. K. Instability in child phonology. Unpublished paper, University of Washington, Seattle, 1973.

Piaget, J. *The Language and Thought of the Child.* New York: Harcourt, Brace, 1926.

Piaget, J. *The Origins of Intelligence in Children.* New York: Norton, 1952.

Piaget, J. *The Construction of Reality in the Child.* New York: Norton, 1954.

Piaget, J. *Play, Dreams and Imitation in Childhood.* New York: Norton, 1962.

Piaget, J. Le language et les operations intellectuelles. In *Problemes de psycholinguistique: Symposium de l'association de psychologie scientifique de langue francaise.* Paris: Presses University France, 1963.

Piaget, J. *The Mechanism of Perception.* New York: Basic Books, 1969.

Piaget, J. Piaget's theory. In P. Mussen (Ed.), *Carmichael's Manual of Child Psychology.* New York: Wiley, 1970a.

Piaget, J. *Genetic Epistomology.* New York: Columbia University Press, 1970b.

Piaget, J. *Structuralism*. New York: Basic Books, 1970c.

Piaget, J. *Biology and Knowledge*. Chicago: University of Chicago Press, 1971.

Piaget, J. and Inhelder, B. *Mental Imagery in the Child*. New York: Basic Books, 1971.

Pribram, K. *Languages of the Brain: Experimental Paradoxes and Principles in Neuropsychology*. Englewood Cliffs, N. J.: Prentice-Hall, 1971.

Schlesinger, I. M. Production of utterances and language acquisition. In D. I. Slobin (Ed.), *The Ontogenesis of Grammar*. New York: Academic Press, 1971.

Shvachkin, N. The development of phonemic speech perception in early childhood. In C. A. Ferguson and D. I. Slobin (Eds.), *Studies in Child Language Development*. New York: Holt, Rinehart and Wilson, 1973.

Sinclair, H. Developmental psycholinguistics. In D. Elkind and J. H. Flavell (Eds.), *Studies in Cognitive Development*. New York: Oxford University Press, 1969.

Sinclair, H. Acquisition of language, linguistic theory and epistemology. Paper presented at the International Colloquium on Problems in Psycholinguistics, Paris, 1971a.

Sinclair, H. Sensorimotor action patterns as a condition for the acquisition of syntax. In R. Huxley and E. Ingram (Eds.), *Language Acquisition: Models and Methods*. New York: Academic Press, 1971b.

Sinclair, H. Language acquisition and cognitive development. In T. E. Moore (Ed.), *Cognitive Development and the Acquisition of Language*. New York: Academic Press, 1973.

Slobin, D. I. Cognitive prerequisites for the development of grammar. In C. A. Ferguson and D. I. Slobin (Eds.), *Studies of Child Language Development*. New York: Holt, Rinehart and Winston, 1973.

Uzgiris, I. and Hunt, J. McV. An instrument for assessing psychological development. Urbana: University of Illinois, Psychological Development Laboratory, 1966 (mimeo).

Watt, W. C. On two hypotheses concerning psycholinguistics. In J. R. Hayes (Ed.), *Cognition and the Development of Language*. New York: Wiley, 1970.

Werner, H. and Kaplan, B. *Symbol Formation*. New York: Wiley, 1963.

Whitehurst, G., Novak, G., and Zorn, G. Delayed speech studied in the home. *Develop. Psychol.*, 1972, *7*, 169–177.

CHAPTER SEVEN

DISCUSSION SUMMARY–DEVELOPMENT OF CONCEPTS UNDERLYING LANGUAGE [1]

Melissa F. Bowerman

Bureau of Child Research, and the Department of Linguistics, University of Kansas, Lawrence, Kansas 66045

Until about 6 years ago, studies of the child's acquisition of syntactic knowledge focused primarily on formally defined categories and relationships. Only recently have the cognitive bases for the development of language begun to be extensively explored. In considering the old but still challenging problem of the causal relationship between linguistic and cognitive development, recent investigators of language acquisition have tended to stress the primacy of cognitive growth (*e.g.,* Antinucci and Parisi, 1973; Bloom, 1970, 1973; Bowerman, 1973a, b; Brown, 1973; Schlesinger, 1971; Sinclair-de Zwart, 1969, 1971, 1973a,b; Slobin, 1973). For example, Slobin (1973, p. 184) has postulated that "the pacesetter in linguistic growth is the child's cognitive growth, as opposed to an autonomous linguistic development which can then reflect back on cognition."

The current emphasis on cognition and the postulation of some specific ways in which cognition and language are related allows a cautiously optimistic answer to the question, posed in this conference by Menyuk, of whether there may be "prerequisites to the teaching of language" to retarded and language-delayed children "which would help the learning of language when you got there."

The following discussion is organized around five major themes which figure prominently in recent literature on the relationship between linguistic and cognitive development and which were dealt with in this section of the conference. The contributions of the Clark, Schlesinger, and Morehead papers, the discussions they engendered, related materials, and implications for intervention are presented within this framework. The first three topics to be considered are related in that they all derive from the postulate that language is deeply rooted in more general cognitive abilities and from its corollary that an adequate explanation of language acquisition must take into

[1] The preparation of this paper was partially supported by Grants NS-10468-01 from the National Institute of Neurological Disease and Stroke and HD 02528-08 from the National Institute of Child Health and Human Development.

account the development of the relevant cognitive structures and processes in the child. Briefly, the topics are:

1. The hypothesis that language is only one manifestation of a very general ability to represent or symbolize experiences which may not be perceptually present.
2. The hypothesis that for given linguistic structures or operations there are analogous or formally equivalent nonlinguistic structures and operations, and that it is the achievement of the more general cognitive skills which makes acquisition of those aspects of language possible.
3. The hypothesis that children use consistent or rule-governed strategies in processing language to arrive at the relationship between meanings and the linguistic structures by which meanings are expressed, and that these strategies may in many instances derive from the child's nonlinguistic interactions with and understanding of the world.
4. Attempts to determine what concepts, categories, and relational or structural meanings are functional or "psychologically real" in children's early linguistic rule systems.
5. How the relationship between language and cognition should be handled in giving formal representation to children's knowledge of linguistic structure.

LANGUAGE AS A MANIFESTATION OF THE SYMBOLIC FUNCTION

Much of the recent interest in the cognitive underpinnings of language can be attributed to the "discovery" of Piaget by developmental psycholinguists, who are increasingly appreciating the implications of his work for a theory of language development. Thus, many of the ideas discussed in this paper either can be directly traced to his theories, or are in large measure compatible with his views on linguistic and cognitive development.

In their paper, Morehead and Morehead outline Piaget's view of language development as closely linked to the emergence of the symbolic function in the child's development. This refers to the ability to make something stand for or represent an object or event which may not be perceptually present. The symbolic function is manifested not only in language but also in several other behaviors or processes which begin to appear at about the same time, such as deferred imitation, symbolic play, drawing, mental imagery, and gestures.

The ability to represent one thing with another can be regarded as one of the most fundamental cognitive prerequisites for language acquisition. A child who has trouble with the basic process of symbolizing must inevitably experience difficulties with language. Several studies have indeed indicated that the problems of at least some language-delayed children can be related to a general deficiency in representational ability (e.g., Morehead and Ingram, 1973). In particular, some children with language difficulties were found to do poorly in tasks involving imagery, while their basic intellectual or logical development appeared adequate (Inhelder, 1966; Ajuriaguerra, 1966).

In discussion, Morehead observed that when one views language development as rooted in a general representational ability, one is led to the investigation of methods for the diagnosis and treatment of language delay which focus not on the child's language ability itself but upon related abilities such as symbolic play and imagery. In this connection, he noted that many children with little or no speech seem unable to play symbolically; they are unwilling to substitute one play item for another, *e.g.,* a shoebox for a doll bed (see Morehead, 1972). One such child, an autistic boy, was given training strictly on symbolic play. At the same time that he began to use objects symbolically to represent cars, he began to use the word "car," previously restricted to a single toy, to refer to a variety of carlike objects.

According to Piaget, the symbolic function does not appear suddenly in final form but rather builds gradually upon the achievements of the sensori-motor period. In view of this, it would be important to investigate a language-deficient child's level of functioning with regard to possible preconditions for the acquisition of the representational ability. Mehrabian and Williams (1971) have developed a cognitive developmental scale designed to allow one to identify and assess the preverbal skills most directly related to representation, such as the concept of object permanence, the ability to imitate actions, etc. As Morehead and Morehead note in their paper, such tests can aid in determining, for a particular child, where to enter into the development sequence leading to the symbolic function in order to help the child reach this goal.

FORMAL SIMILARITIES BETWEEN COGNITIVE AND LINGUISTIC STRUCTURES AND PROCESSES

The development of the symbolic function, or the ability to symbolize, is an important precondition for the acquisition of language, but this general cognitive ability cannot in itself account for the structure of language or for how language is acquired. In this section and the next, some efforts to specify more closely the cognitive structures and processes involved in the "what" and "how" of language acquisition are investigated.

Clark's proposals about the existence of cognitive strategies for acquiring language touched off much discussion among conference participants, with the debate focusing primarily on the method by which children acquire language and how it can be investigated. However, Clark (1973), along with several other investigators of child language, has argued that there is a close relationship between what is learned—the structure of language—and the way in which it is acquired. What follows in this section is a consideration of the possibility that the formal structure of language is ultimately derived from more basic cognitive structures and processes. It is provided to put the subsequent discussion of cognitive strategies for acquiring language into a broader perspective.

The possibility that the structural characteristics of language can be traced to the characteristics of more fundamental cognitive abilities is an intriguing one. Lenneberg (1971) has recently argued that "man's language ability is due to a more general, deep-seated cognitive ability characteristic of the species," which also underlies mathematical ability. The basic elements common to both language and mathematics are processes of *relating;* these processes combine into integrated systems. Piaget approaches the problem from a different perspective, but has come to a similar conclusion. According to Sinclair-de Zwart (1973a), who summarizes his position, Piaget believes that during the first 2 years of life children establish "very general cognitive structures composed of systems of actions." These constitute the basis for many different types of more specific cognitive structures like those which underlie both logicomathematical thinking and ideas about aspects of the physical world such as force, movement, time, and causality. Thus, "there are links between knowledge in one field and that in another." Piaget has suggested that linguistic structures themselves "may well be yet another symptom of the very general universal cognitive structures" (Ferreiro, 1970, quoted in Sinclair-de Zwart, 1973a).

Although little is yet known about the nature of these hypothesized deepest and most basic cognitive structures, there have been some proposals concerning the relationship between language and better understood aspects of cognition such as the practical intelligence acquired during the sensorimotor period. For example, as Schlesinger notes in his paper for this conference, Sinclair-de Zwart (1971) has argued that certain abilities which are achieved by the end of the sensorimotor period are reflected in Chomskian deep structures. The ability to order temporally and spatially corresponds to the concatenation of deep structure elements; the ability to classify in action by using a whole category of objects for the same action schema or a whole category of action schemas for the same object corresponds to syntactic categories like noun-phrase and verb-phrase; the ability to embed action patterns into each other corresponds to recursive rules for sentence embedding in deep structure; the ability to apprehend relations among objects and actions corresponds to basic grammatical relations; the child's first concept of invariance, that objects have continuing existence across a variety of perceptual conditions, corresponds to the concept of deep structures which preserve meaning despite the application of transformational operations which can result in surface structures which are superficially unlike each other.

There exists a small amount of experimental evidence for the cognitive foundations of particular linguistic structures. For example, Sinclair-de Zwart (1969) found that the far-reaching cognitive restructuring which takes place with the establishment of the first concrete operations (*e.g.,* conservation of liquids and seriation) is paralleled by striking linguistic developments in the use of certain lexical items and syntactic structures. (She also presented evidence that the cognitive advances are not caused by the linguistic developments.)

In an experimental study, Greenfield, Nelson, and Saltzman (1972) explicitly explored Piaget's hypothesis that there is a "general isomorphism between language and other forms of cognition" by looking for a direct formal parallel between action and grammar. They found three distinct strategies for making constructions with nesting cups which seem formally similar to certain grammatical structures. Moreover, the cup strategies and the acquisition of the grammatical structures are developmentally ordered in the same way. For example, the ability to treat a single cup as an acted upon object and then as an actor in the same structure is acquired later than the ability to make multicup constructions in which each cup plays a single role, just as the ability to form relative clauses in which a single noun phrase functions in dual grammatical roles as both object and subject follows the ability to use "and" to coordinate sentences or noun phrases within sentences. The authors do not view the cup strategies as causing the corresponding linguistic capacities or *vice versa,* but rather view both as "behavioral manifestations of underlying internal forms of organization which may have many other concrete applications as well."

Working outside a Piagetian framework, H. Clark (1973) has argued that there is a formal parallel between linguistic and cognitive structures in another domain, one which is directly relevant to E. Clark's (this volume) proposal that children use cognitively based strategies in hypothesizing about the meaning of spatial terms (*e.g.,* dimensional adjectives and locative prepositions). According to H. Clark's analysis, the properties of spatial terms in English and probably all languages correspond directly to man's nonlinguistic structuring of the space around him. More specifically, man's biological endowment, including in particular his perceptual apparatus, leads him to develop a particular kind of "perceptual space" which is characterized by (among other things) a concept of man's canonical or normal position, three reference planes, and several associated directions which have naturally definable positive or negative values: 1) a plane at ground level with upward positive; 2) a vertical left-to-right plane through the body with forward from the body positive; 3) a vertical front-to-back plane with leftward and rightward both positive. H. Clark argues that these properties of the nonlinguistic structuring of perceptual space coincide exactly with the properties of English spatial terms. He hypothesizes that the child acquires spatial terms by learning how to apply them to his prior understanding of perceptual space, with the order of acquisition determined by the cumulative complexity of the spatial information they encode (*e.g.,* location words like "in" and "on" being learned earlier than location-plus-direction words like "into," "onto"), and possibly also by the order in which the child learns the properties of perceptual space.

STRATEGIES FOR LANGUAGE ACQUISITION DERIVED FROM THE CHILD'S COGNITIVE STRUCTURING OF THE WORLD

With the above sketch of certain proposals concerning the relationship between linguistic and cognitive structures, we are in a better position to consider some related hypotheses about strategies for language acquisition.

The term "strategy" has appeared in a number of articles in recent years (*e.g.*, Bever, 1970; Slobin, 1973; Ervin-Tripp, 1973; Greenfield *et al.*, 1972; Sinclair and Bronckardt, 1972) with somewhat varying meanings. Most frequently, it is used to indicate either consistent methods children use in processing sentences to arrive at their meanings or, more generally, consistencies in the way in which children go about mapping language onto their nonlinguistic understanding of the world, *i.e.*, the way in which they construct a linguistic rule system for both producing and interpreting speech.

Strategies relevant to a number of different aspects of language processing have been proposed (see especially Bever, 1970; Slobin, 1973). Following Clark's lead, we shall be concerned here with a particular subset of these. Clark, along with Sinclair-de Zwart (1973a,b) and (within a more restricted domain) Greenfield *et al.* (1972), has hypothesized that in interpreting speech and constructing linguistic rule systems children employ strategies derived from their prelinguistic or general cognitive experiences with and understanding of the world.

In Clark's view (this volume), much of the cognitive basis for early language consists of the *perceptual* information which the child "has successfully interpreted and organized by the time he starts to work on language." In particular, she proposes that in acquiring the meanings of words, children employ strategies based on their perceptual understanding of the world. In learning the meaning of ostensively definable words like "doggie," children attend to salient perceptual attributes involving shape, movement, size, sound, and texture. For inherently relational lexical items such as locative prepositions and dimensional adjectives, they rely on their nonlinguistic interpretation of perceptual space. Because the properties of space encoded by spatial terms correspond closely to the child's nonlinguistic organization of space (see H. Clark, 1973 and above), his hypotheses will often be correct. For example, in making hypotheses about the meanings of locative prepositions such as "in" and "on," the child initially refers to his perception of the usual or canonical spatial relations which hold between objects in the world and thus will make few errors in normal situations.

Sinclair-de Zwart and Greenfield *et al.* differ from Clark in emphasizing not perception but rather *action* as the source for interpretive strategies. For example, in their discussion of developmentally ordered strategies for combining nesting cups, Greenfield *et al.* (1972) speculate that "the existence of action structures formally similar to grammatical structures may provide a cognitive base for language learning itself. A known action pattern could provide a strategy for decoding a linguistic description of that action."

Arguing in a more general way, Sinclair-de Zwart suggests that the child's construction of grammar is linked to his previous construction, through action on the environment, of sensorimotor or practical intelligence. In her view, the structural properties of sensorimotor intelligence (or, more accurately, of the "universal cognitive structures" underlying both sensorimotor intelligence and language) provide the child with a set of basic assumptions about the structural properties of language (1973a, b). The process by which the cognitive structures are initially constructed through action converts, in some as yet unspecified way, into a "heuristic model for language learning" which gives rise to basic strategies for building up knowledge of language structures (Sinclair-de Zwart, 1973b).

In formulating these proposals, Sinclair-de Zwart (1973a) follows Piaget's postulates that "higher-level knowledge involves a reconstruction of already acquired concepts and patterns," and that the formation process is "isomorphic to that by which earlier knowledge was acquired." Thus, she hypothesizes that the acquisition of particular linguistic structures parallels on the representational level the way in which the relevant sensorimotor cognitive structures were initially constructed on the action level. She has presented some experimental evidence which appears to support this view (Sinclair-de Zwart, 1973a,b). Young French-speaking children were asked to act out anomalous sentences representing all possible permutations of two nouns and a verb or two verbs and a noun. The children interpreted them according to consistent patterns, different for different ages; these patterns suggested that the sequence in which a child builds up links between linguistic elements representing agent, action, and object mirrors the sequence in which he previously differentiated on the action level between actions and objects acted upon and between himself as agent and others as agent.

Although Clark emphasizes perception rather than action as the source of the child's linguistically relevant cognitive knowledge, she, like Sinclair-de Zwart, has suggested that in acquiring a given aspect of language the child in a sense recapitulates the developmental sequence he went through in establishing the nonlinguistic knowledge underlying it. She cites evidence that in the development of perception the child progresses from attending to individual features (*e.g.*, high contrast edges, spots, moving parts) to attending to configurations or bundles of features (such as define a face). This progression in perceptual development from the use of single features to sets of features appears to be repeated, she observes, when children begin to interpret their perceptual input in order to use it in attaching meanings to words (Clark, 1973).

In the discussion of Clark's paper for this conference, Morehead noted the difference between Clark's position and the Piagetian one on the relative importance assigned to perception as a source of word meaning. He observed that according to Piaget, perception alone cannot be the basis for early word meanings because it is too transitory, too dependent upon temporary conditions, to confer meaning. In Piaget's view, the acquisition of word meaning depends upon the prior establishment of relatively stable internalized representations of the referents, and these representations or "preconcepts" which the early words mark are internalized *actions* rather than perceptual images. In an effort to reconcile Clark's data on the way in which children overextend words with Piaget's theory, Morehead pointed out that the particular perceptual attributes which appear to serve as the source of early word definitions have "tactile-kinesthetic" correlates which may in fact contribute to the formation of the relevant preconcepts.

Morehead's observation in this regard suggests a way in which we may be able to resolve the apparent differences between Clark's and Sinclair-de Zwart's positions on perception *vs.* action as the source of language processing strategies. In Piaget's view, the perceptual model of the world which the child has attained by the end of the sensorimotor period is neither a "given" nor an autonomous development. Rather, it is constructed by the child out of his actions and interactions in the world. Thus, perceptual concepts such as "shape," "size," "canonical position," and "extent," which Clark has shown may be relevant for the acquisition of various ostensively definable words and relational words, are perhaps acquired through the child's action upon objects rather than by passive observation, and it might be that strategies for acquiring word meanings are based primarily on the way in which the child's organization of perceptual input is build up rather than on the final characteristics of the organization itself. The proposals by H. Clark mentioned above, on determinants of the order in which spatial terms are acquired, suggest some lines along which this hypothesis might be elaborated.

In considering Clark's proposals about cognitively based strategies for language acquisition, several conference participants wondered whether the various response patterns found in Clark's experiments and taken by Clark as evidence of cognitive strategies could not be explained in some other way. Menyuk, for example, suggested that the construct of "cognitive strategy" may actually be made up of a number of variables. One is *perceptual saliency.* The perceptual cues children use in classifying are evidently hierarchically organized, such that while children may initially tend to use color or shape in classifying, they are able to use function as well, provided that the former two criteria are blocked. Another set of variables involves *motivation.* For example, Mehler and Bever (1967) found that certain children who gave nonconserving responses when faced with two rows of clay pellets of different lengths were able to assess amount accurately when clay was replaced by M&Ms and the children were told to select one of the rows and eat all the M&Ms in it. A third factor which may influence the behavior which has been ascribed to cognitive strategies is the *task variable,* which involves how the child's apparent understanding of a situation or a sentence may be affected by the materials present in the testing situation.

A different approach to the question of how Clark's data should be interpreted was pursued by Premack and Baer. They suggested that Clark's study of the way in which children comprehend "in," "on," and "under" might actually be a developmental study of a shift in *preferences* rather than of the acquisition of word meaning. As Premack elaborated it, Clark's study involved looking at the probability that subjects would respond in certain ways. Response probabilities have a number of determinants, only one of which is language, *i.e.,* the instruction to the child. If, *prior* to linguistic instruction, the possible responses (*e.g.,* putting something into as opposed to on top of an object) have different probabilities of occurring, then it is impossible to determine the role of language. Thus, for example, children could start out with strong preferences for dealing with objects in certain ways. Even if they understood an instruction like "put the doll *on* the glass," their preference, or response bias, for using things as containers whenever possible might lead them to ignore the instruction and follow their own desires.

The crucial question, then, said Premack, is "to what extent does the existing response bias *compete* with the language instruction?" Clark's data could be accounted for by saying that children at first have strong preferences and later none. Thus, at some point the language instruction begins to compete actively with the existing response biases and the child will do as he is told, thus appearing to have just learned the meanings of the words, even though in fact he may have known them earlier. Premack acknowledged that in principle his interpretation of Clark's data as due to preferences and hers as due to cognitive strategies were not incompatible. Thus, a child might have an initial preference and use it as the basis of a strategy for word interpretation. However, his point was to demonstrate that in the experiment, alternate interpretations were confounded.

Clark felt it was unreasonable to assume that an 18-month-old child really understands all the instructions but has simply decided to please himself rather than the experimenter. She noted that the children she worked with had been in several other experiments, appeared to be very cooperative, and were upset if they got negative feedback. Baer observed that even under these circumstances, children don't necessarily prefer to win the experimenter's approval over the opportunity to put something into something else.

Various methods of getting around the problem were considered. Staats suggested that one could overcome the initial response biases and get the child to attend to instructions by reinforcing him for doing so. Clark noted that one cannot give feedback on correct and incorrect responses in studies of what the child knows semantically, since this might change his response to particular terms in the course of the experiment and thus defeat the purpose of the experiment. Premack felt that it is impossible to answer questions about responses to language instructions in young children unless initial response probabilities are equal. Since this is evidently not the case for "in," "on," and "under," questions about the acquisition of comprehension cannot be answered for these words. Chapman wondered whether the confounded variables could not be separated even when response biases are unequal by determining what the biases are in advance. Premack answered that in such a situation, only a special kind of outcome, that which goes *against* the known probabilities, would be interpretable. Most outcomes would not be interpretable.

In this section and the last, we have examined studies of the possibilities that 1) particular linguistic structures may depend upon more basic underlying cognitive structures which are in some sense ismorphic to them and 2) the child may make use of either the characteristics of his existing cognitive structures or the developmental process he went through in acquiring them in deriving strategies for the interpretation of linguistic data. Investigations like these may lead to new tools for diagnosing and treating children who do not acquire language normally.

First, it is clearly relevant to find out how far along in the sensorimotor construction of reality a language-delayed child is, and, if necessary, to intervene to help him acquire the requisite nonlinguistic structures. The language intervention program outlined by Bricker and Bricker in this conference looks promising in this respect: they investigate a child's functioning in a number of linguistically relevant cognitive areas such as object permanence and the functional motoric classification of objects, and train where necessary.

Second, and more difficult, is the need to investigate a linguistically deviant child's methods of analyzing linguistic input. Studies of strategies for language acquisition highlight the fact that it is not enough for a child to control the cognitive structures or basic meanings which are prerequisites for language; he must also have methods of determining the relationship between meanings and the linguistic structures by which meanings are encoded in his language. The deficits of some children may be primarily in this area rather than in that of the basic sensorimotor cognitive structures. Such a child could perhaps be aided to acquire language with training situations specifically designed to help him notice formal similarities between linguistic structures, on the one hand, and action patterns, perceptions, and the like, on the other, and on this basis to formulate hypotheses about what aspects of language might correspond with what aspects of experience. Beyond this, as Clark pointed out in discussion, we need to find out more about how children who have adopted a given hypothesis go about determining whether or not it is correct.

WHAT ARE THE FUNCTIONAL CONCEPTS AND CATEGORIES UNDERLYING EARLY MULTIWORD UTTERANCES?

In an influential 1971 paper (originally circulated in 1968), Schlesinger proposed that the basic concepts underlying sentence construction are not syntactic relations like subject, predicate, and direct object, but rather semantic notions like "agent," "action," "object," and "location." He hypothesized that children acquire language by learning "realization rules," such as those for ordering elements within the sentence, which map underlying semantic concepts directly onto surface structures.

Schlesinger's suggestion that a fairly small set of relational meanings such as "agent action" and "action-object" can account for the large majority of children's early word combinations has since been supported by data from children in many different language communities (Brown, 1973, p. 182; Slobin, 1970, p. 175; Bowerman, 1973a). Brown accounts for the apparent universality of these basic semantic meanings by reference to the child's accomplishments during the sensorimotor period which immediately precedes word combination (see Schlesinger's paper).

Brown (1973, p. 173) cautions, however, that the kinds of semantic concepts discussed by Schlesinger (and others) may be nothing more than convenient categories for data reduction, analysis, and comparison. They may or may not actually correspond to aspects of the structural knowledge which enables children to produce and comprehend utterances.

In his present paper, Schlesinger has undertaken the important task of trying to characterize more exactly the relational concepts which are psychologically functional for children and adults. The problem is not a purely theoretical one. It has empirical consequences in that the breadth and makeup of the categories upon which rules operate are important determinants of the way in which the child will use his rules in new situations, and thus what kinds of novel utterances are available to him. For example, if the child follows a rule such as "agent precedes action" in producing utterances like "Johnny ride" and "mommy go," he should be able to apply the rule immediately to any previously unknown action word and produce appropriately ordered agent-action strings involving that word. It is possible, however, that early sentences classifiable as "agent-action" strings are produced with a number of different rules based on the individual lexical items involved (*e.g.*, "the name for one who rides (goes, jumps) precedes the name for the action of riding (going, jumping)." In other words, the child might see no similarity among the initiators of diverse actions and make no use of the agent concept at all. In this case, upon learning a new word for an action, the child would be unable to use it in combination with a name for the initiator of the action until he had specifically learned a new rule for that purpose. Still another possibility is that the child has a nonlinguistic concept of agent, but that this does not figure explicitly in his linguistic rule system.

In considering the nature of the functional relations underlying sentence production and comprehension, Schlesinger has somewhat modified the position he took in his 1971 paper. In his conference paper and the discussion of it, he clarified his present view on the relationship between cognitive and linguistic development as basically interactional. Whereas earlier he had proposed that the concepts underlying the early utterances do not reflect specifically linguistic knowledge but rather are determined by the "innate cognitive capacity" of the child, or the way in which the child views the world regardless of whether he acquires language or not, he now felt that the child's initial cognitive structures might be rather amorphous and develop not only through experience with the world of objects and events but also through linguistic experience. The way in which various concepts are treated linguistically suggests to the child what belongs together and influences the formation of given cognitive concepts. For example, a child may not begin language acquisition with a clear cut agent-action concept. He may instead have only an understanding of specific instances of the relationship, such as that between one who throws something and the act of throwing or between one who cuts something and the act of cutting. But his language, by giving identical formal expression to all such relationships between initiators of specific actions and the actions initiated, would lead the child to collapse these varied concepts into the more abstract concept of the relationship between agent and action. Alternatively, a child might initially form an overextended agent concept in which animate agents and instruments like knives are regarded as equivalent, and gradually, through observation of the way these are treated linguistically, he would differentiate agent and instrument into two separate concepts.

Premack was dubious about the influence of language upon basic "case grammar" concepts like "agent," "action," and "location." He felt that an understanding of the relationship between agent and action, for example, comes built-in and does not need to be learned through language. However, he agreed with Schlesinger that linguistic and cognitive development interact at points. He suggested that not only does language influence cognitive development in some ways, but also that there may in fact be some linguistic distinctions such as those made by the logical connectives ("and," "either-or," etc.) which simply lack nonlinguistic counterparts (*e.g.*, do not admit of visual representation) and are therefore introduced into the cognitive structure solely through language. The reason for this speculation, said Premack, was that he had found it virtually impossible to devise nonlinguistic tests for the existence of such concepts, whereas other concepts such as perceptual categories and the notion of "different" can easily be tapped by language-free techniques. Schlesinger noted that difficulty in constructing language-free tests for the presence of cognitive concepts underlying the logical connectives does not necessarily mean that the concepts are absent. He suggested that this was a technical problem. Some concepts are more easily represented in one medium than another. However, Premack still felt that the problem might be one of substance rather than simply technical.

Bowerman observed that Clark's approach to the way in which children assign meanings to particular lexical items could provide information essential to the accurate specification of the nature of the concepts functional in children's early rule systems. Words like "want," "need," "see," and "hear," as they are understood by adults, are not actions and thus do not take agents in the role of subject but rather experiencers or "persons affected" (*cf.* Fillmore's (1968) dative case). It is possible, though, that children do not understand "want" and the like as adults do, but rather define them essentially as actions such that "want" might be equivalent to the adult's "demand" or "give," "see" to "look," "hear" to "listen," and so on. If so, children who purely on the basis of the lexical items they use in sentences might appear to control a semantic notion like "person affected" and rules for ordering it may in fact be producing utterances like "Johnny want cookie," and "mommy see dog" with the same linguistic mechanisms used in producing sentences with agents. While Schlesinger also suggests that the agent concept may absorb concepts which are really not agents, such as persons affected and instruments, Bowerman's proposal differs from his. In Schlesinger's view, the agent concept may be overinclusive for adults as well as for children, whereas, according to Bowerman's suggestion, this would be true only for children as a result of their incomplete lexical entries. Once children acquired the adult understanding of verbs like "want," sentences including them could no longer be generated by rules based on the concept of agent.

A second possibility suggested by Clark's work is that just as an adult understanding of lexical items appears to develop gradually, feature by feature, items in a child's "vocabulary" of functional relational concepts may develop over time. It has been suggested that Fillmore's case roles can be defined in terms of combinations of semantic features such as "cause," "instigator," "intent," "control," "goal," etc. (McCoy, 1969, cited in Cook, 1972). In establishing a linguistically relevant semantic concept like "agent," a child may initially attend to only one or two features rather than the entire set of features which define the concept for an adult; the features he attends to may or may not be criterial for the adult. As in the case of the child's use of single words, a lack of correspondence between the adult's concepts and those of the child would be revealed in overextensions or other inappropriate usages. For example, the childish version of the adult agent concept might be defined only by the feature "that which is capable of independent movement." This would result in the child's treating cars, machinery, and the like as agents. Alternatively, he might form an agent-like concept defined by the feature "that which physically interacts with an object." Such a concept would exclude some things considered agents by adults, such as the subjects of "sit" and "run," but include other things which adults may distinguish from agents, such as instruments.

Theoretical debates about the relational meanings of early sentences and the nature of the linguistic knowledge underlying the production of these sentences have important implications for language intervention. Miller and Yoder (1972, this volume), for example, have constructed a language training program around the premises that 1) the content of a program should be taken from normal developmental data in an effort to approximate *what it is* that normal children learn in acquiring language and 2) what is learned appears to be how to express various semantic concepts or functions. Miller and Yoder derived their list of semantic functions to be taught from recent studies which make use of familiar terms such as "agent," "action," "location," "recurrence," etc.

While this is a promising starting point, the above discussion should make it clear that such terms may or may not actually correspond to constructs in the normal child's own rule system. As our methods of investigation become more ingenious, it should be possible to specify more closely the concepts which are actually functional for the normal child early in linguistic development and how these change over time. This will provide training programs such as Miller and Yoder's with a more principled guide for grouping utterances to be trained and sequencing these groups in such a way as to engage the child's own sense of what constitute meaningful concepts at various stages of linguistic development. This should facilitate the child's induction of general rules for sentence production and comprehension.

REPRESENTING CHILDREN'S KNOWLEDGE OF LINGUISTIC STRUCTURE

A generative grammar written for a language is in essence a hypothesis about the native speaker's internalized rule system, or his knowledge of language structure (Chomsky, 1968, p. 23). Hence, speculations about the nature of the knowledge children draw upon in comprehending and producing utterances lead naturally to questions about the best method for formally representing this knowledge in grammars.

Much discussion was devoted to the way in which the relationship between language and cognition should be handled in linguistic representations. Schlesinger emphasized that in writing grammars for children, general knowledge about the world should be carefully distinguished from linguistically relevant knowledge. At the time of speech, the child may know a great deal about the nonlinguistic situation, but only part of his understanding comes into play in his linguistic production. Schlesinger's concept of the

I-marker, or intention-marker, was developed to represent those aspects of the child's cognitive structure which not only are present at the time of speech but also are used in the formulation of the utterance. Unlike cognitive structures, which may be rather elaborate and elusive, I-markers are probably a finite and fairly small number of categorized relations, those relations which make a difference linguistically.

There was much discussion of whether Schlesinger's system of I-markers and the realization rules by which the child learns to link I-markers to surface structures provide an adequate account both of what is learned and of the learning process itself. Cromer questioned whether syntactic deep structures can be dispensed with in favor of semantic I-markers in a theory of language acquisition. He noted that the reason deep structures were postulated in the first place was to represent aspects of language which are abstract and cannot be explained solely by reference to surface structures. But because I-markers are linked to surface structures by purely associative mechanisms, they are not abstract and thus cannot account for certain features of language structure. If many aspects of language are abstract, moreover, it is impossible to account for language acquisition by stimulus/response theory, because much of what the child must acquire is never directly observable in speech (*cf.* Bever, Fodor, and Weksel, 1965). And there is developmental evidence, Cromer noted, that children do acquire abstract structures rather than simply picking up aspects of the surface structures they hear—for example, the way in which negation is acquired. In the light of these arguments, Cromer felt that Schlesinger's theory was unable to account for either the abstractness of the system which is acquired or the way in which it is acquired.

Schlesinger responded that while indeed I-markers can be linked to surface structures by associative principles, this does not imply a one-to-one relationship such that for each I-marker there is one surface structure. The system does admit of abstract rules mapping I-markers into surface structures. Many of the things children say which are errors from the standpoint of adult surface structures result from their wrong application or overgeneralization of these rules.

Nevertheless, added Schlesinger, the theory of I-markers is not simply a terminological revision of deep structures. Unlike deep structures, I-markers are formulated in semantic terms. In addition, they do not posit an abstract underlying order for sentence elements. Finally, they are not universal but can develop differently in different languages. For these reasons they seem more accessible to experience than deep structures.

As for the proposal that learning theory is incapable of accounting for language acquisition because much of what must be acquired is abstract, Schlesinger considered it to be based on faulty arguments. In actual language-learning situations, he pointed out, deep structures are not abstract in the sense that Bever *et al.* posited because they are tied to the situation. The child witnesses the event, *e.g.,* Johnny giving a ball to daddy, and hears a sentence describing it. Thus, he can code the elements of the event into an I-marker, a deep structure, and associate it with the observed sentence.

Cromer broached a different line of inquiry into the adequacy of I-markers by asking whether they had to be entirely semantic or whether they might not contain some purely linguistic elements. He thought that the latter might be necessary to account for the difference between the ability to entertain certain concepts or meanings nonlinguistically and the ability to express those meanings in language. He added that if I-markers do contain any specifically linguistic mechanism, this might be disturbed or damaged in some children. Schlesinger replied that the I-markers could be considered linguistic in a sense, in that experience before language does not come parceled into agents, actions, instruments and so on. Rather, experience with language itself teaches the child that these things go together in the I-markers. Beyond that he was uncertain about any purely linguistic properties of I-markers.

A related line of thought, pursued by Bowerman, was whether Schlesinger's attempt to describe the kinds of concepts underlying speech production and comprehension in purely semantic terms was psychologically accurate. She noted that the subjects of many sentences resist interpretation as agents, or even as extended agents which might include instruments and persons affected—for example, "the situation justifies taking drastic measures," "caution outweighed the need for action," "health legislation continues to be a problem," "John benefited from the assignment," "the boat trip resulted in several deaths," etc. It is difficult to pinpoint specific cognitive concepts (aside from whatever nonlinguistic correlates the meanings of the specific lexical items have) which could serve as the structural components to which rules for ordering and other operations could apply. To achieve any kind of economy in the rule system, it would seem to be necessary to depart at points from a purely semantic specification of structural relations. Possibly some children experience problems with language not because they lack the requisite underlying cognitive concepts which language encodes, but because they are unable to perform the feats of abstraction necessary to arrive at an understanding of the purely formal linguistic relationships which hold between parts of sentences (such as subject-predicate, verb-direct object) and which cannot be mapped directly onto underlying semantic concepts.

SUMMARY

The variety of approaches to the cognitive prerequisites for language which have been discussed in this chapter and the three preceding ones point strongly to the conclusion that cognition plays multiple roles in the acquisition and use of language. Accordingly, delays in acquiring language might have as their source deficits in one or more of a number of different cognitive abilities. To recapitulate briefly, the following kinds of nonlinguistic knowledge and skills were suggested, each one having an associated potential for deficit. This is by no means an exhaustive list of all the cognitive factors which are involved in language acquisition:

1. The general ability to use symbols to represent objects and events which may not be perceptually present.
2. The development of basic cognitive structures and operations which are in some sense prerequisites to and isomorphic with specific aspects of language structure (e.g., the ability to order spatially and temporally, the ability to classify in action, the ability to embed action patterns into each other, the establishment of concepts of basic invariance underlying superficial changes of state (object permanence, conservation), the ability to assign dual roles to an object in a single action sequence, the construction of a model of perceptual space with certain properties).
3. The ability to derive strategies for processing linguistic material from general cognitive structures and processes which are isomorphic to aspects of language structure, and/or from the developmental sequence in which language-relevant cognitive knowledge is acquired on the nonlinguistic level.
4. The ability to formulate appropriate concepts or categories to serve as the structural components upon which linguistic rules such as those for ordering sentence elements can operate. Neither the exact nature of the early categories nor the way in which they change over time is as yet known. In particular, it is unclear whether, as Schlesinger suggests, relational semantic concepts like "agent" (or "extended agent") are the basic building blocks of the linguistic knowledge not only of children but also of adults, or whether instead semantic concepts must eventually be supplemented with or supplanted by an understanding of more abstract syntactic relationships which hold between parts of sentences and which can be defined solely in linguistic terms.

The cognitive abilities represented above are clearly not independent of one another, but their relationships are complex and little understood. In addition, the abilities are not unitary but can be broken down into a number of components. Nevertheless, even a rough outline such as this of some of the major ways in which cognitive factors appear to figure in the acquisition of language may suggest lines along which the development of language intervention procedures might profitably progress. Implicit in such listing is the notion that it may be possible to develop diagnostic techniques sensitive enough to detect deficiencies in particular language-relevant cognitive abilities and to design training programs specifically aimed at improving certain target nonlinguistic skills.

REFERENCES

Ajuriaguerra, J. de. Speech disorders in childhood. In C. Carterette (Ed.), *Brain Function: Speech, Language, and Communication,* Vol. III. Los Angeles: University of California Press, 1966.

Antinucci, F. and Parisi, D. Early language acquisition: A model and some data. In C. A. Ferguson and D. I. Slobin (Eds.), *Studies of Child Language Development.* New York: Holt, Rinehart and Winston, 1973.

Bever, T. G. The cognitive basis for linguistic structures. In J. R. Hayes (Ed.), *Cognition and the Development of Language.* New York: Wiley, 1970.

Bever, T. G., Fodor, J. A., and Weksel, W. On the acquisition of syntax: A critique of "contextual generalization." *Psychol. Rev.,* 1965, *72,* 467–482.

Bloom, L. *Language Development: Form and Function in Emerging Grammars.* Cambridge, Mass.: M. I. T. Press, 1970.

Bloom, L. *One Word at a Time: The Use of Single-Word Utterances before Syntax.* The Hague: Mouton, 1973.

Bowerman, M. *Early Syntactic Development: A Cross-linguistic Study with Special Reference to Finnish.* Cambridge, England: Cambridge University Press, 1973a.

Bowerman, M. Structural relationships in children's utterances: Syntactic or semantic? In T. E. Moore (Ed.), *Cognitive Development and the Acquisition of Language.* New York: Academic Press, 1973b.

Brown, R. *A First Language: The Early Stages.* Cambridge, Mass.: Harvard University Press, 1973.

Chomsky, N. *Language and Mind.* New York: Harcourt, Brace, and World, 1968.

Clark, E. V. What's in a word? On the child's acquisition of semantics in his first language. In T. E. Moore (Ed.), *Cognitive Development and the Acquisition of Language.* New York: Academic Press, 1973.

Clark, H. H. Space, time, semantics, and the child. In T. E. Moore (Ed.), *Cognitive Development and the Acquisition of Language.* New York: Academic Press, 1973.

Cook, W. A. A set of postulates for case grammar analysis. Georgetown University Monogr. Series on Language and Linguistics, Working Papers, No. 4, 1972.

Ervin-Tripp, S. Some strategies for the first two years. In T. E. Moore (Ed.), *Cognitive Development and the Acquisition of Language.* New York: Academic Press, 1973.

Ferreiro, E. *Les relations temporelles dans le language de l'enfant.* Geneva: Droz, 1971.

Fillmore, C. J. The case for case. In E. Bach and R. T. Harms (Eds.), *Universals in Linguistic Theory.* New York: Holt, Rinehart and Winston, 1968.

Greenfield, P., Nelson, K., and Saltzman, E. The development of rulebound strategies for manipulating seriated cups: A parallel between action and grammar. *Cognitive Psychol.,* 1972, *3,* 291–310.

Inhelder, B. Cognitive development and its contribution to the diagnosis of some phenomena of mental deficiency. *Merrill-Palmer Quart.,* 1966, *12,* 299–319.

Lenneberg, E. H. Of language knowledge, apes, and brains. *J. Psycholing. Res.,* 1971, *1,* 1–29.

McCoy, A. M. A case grammar classification of Spanish verbs. Unpublished Ph.D. dissertation, University of Michigan, Ann Arbor, 1969.

Mehler, J. and Bever, T. G. Cognitive capacity of very young children. *Science,* 1967, *158,* 141–158.

Mehrabian, A. and Williams, M. Piagetian measures of cognitive development for children up to age two. *J. Psycholing. Res.,* 1971, *1,* 113–126.

Miller, J. F., Yoder, D. E. A syntax teaching program. In J. E. McLean, D. E. Yoder, and R. L. Schiefelbusch (Eds.), *Language Intervention with the Retarded: Developing Strategies.* Baltimore: University Park Press, 1972.

Morehead, D. M. Early grammatical and semantic relations: Some implications for a general representational deficit in linguistically deviant children. In D. Ingram (Ed.), *Papers and Reports on Child Language Development.* Stanford: Stanford University, 1972.

Morehead, D. M. and Ingram, D. The development of base syntax in normal and linguistically deviant children. *J. Speech Hear. Res.,* 1973, *16,* 330–352.

Schlesinger, I. M. Production of utterances and language acquisition. In D. I. Slobin (Ed.), *The Ontogenesis of Language.* New York: Academic Press, 1971.

Sinclair-de Zwart, H. Developmental psycholinguistics. In D. Elkind and J. H. Flavell (Eds.), *Studies in Cognitive Development.* New York: Oxford University Press, 1969.

Sinclair-de Zwart, H. Sensori-motor action patterns as a condition for the acquisition of syntax. In R. Huxley and E. Ingram (Eds.), *Language Acquisition: Models and Methods.* New York: Academic Press, 1971.

Sinclair-de Zwart, H. Language acquisition and cognitive development. In T. E. Moore (Ed.), *Cognitive Development and the Acquisition of Language.* New York: Academic Press, 1973a.

Sinclair-de Zwart, H. Some remarks on the Genevan point of view on learning with special reference to language learning. In L. L. Hinde and H. C. Hinde (Eds.), *Constraints on Learning.* New York: Academic Press, 1973b.

Sinclair, H. and Bronckart, J. P. S. V. O. a linguistic universal? A study in developmental psycholinguistics. *J. Exp. Child Psychol.,* 1972, *14,* 329–348.

Slobin, D. I. Universals of grammatical development in children. In G. B. Flores D'Arcais and W. J. M. Levelt (Eds.), *Advances in Psycholinguistics.* Amsterdam: North-Holland Publishing Co., 1970.

Slobin, D. I. Cognitive prerequisites for the development of grammar. In C. A. Ferguson and D. I Slobin (Eds.), *Studies of Child Language Development.* New York: Holt, Rinehart and Winston, 1973.

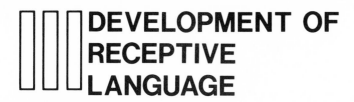

DEVELOPMENT OF RECEPTIVE LANGUAGE

CHAPTER EIGHT

EARLY DEVELOPMENT OF RECEPTIVE LANGUAGE: FROM BABBLING TO WORDS

Paula Menyuk

School of Education, Boston University, Boston, Massachusetts 02215

The reception of language can be viewed as a two-sided linguistic performance. One aspect is perceiving the structural properties of the language which are used to categorize a sentence, word, and speech sound and to differentiate among items belonging to these classes. The second aspect is understanding the communicative functions of these structural properties. Although these two aspects are clearly related and interdependent, studies of the development of the reception of language have not always reflected this interdependency. This has been due, in part, to the difficulty in assessing early receptive language, and in part to varying definitions of the comprehension of language. For example, when an infant distinguishes between falling and rising intonational contours, does this reflect his ability to distinguish between statements and questions or only his ability to distinguish acoustic events? When a child's utterances contain phonological sequences that seem to be words, are marked prosodically, and are used in a context which implies the expression of a semantic relationship, has he categorized each C and V of this sequence in terms of the distinctive features of the segments or made observations about syllabic and morpheme structure or sentence structure, or is he only generating speech events as whole items without differentiating their parts? Presuppositions about the infant's knowledge of the communicative function of linguistic structural properties which classify sentences, words, and speech sounds have to be validated by data. However, questions of the kind posed earlier are, for the most part, unanswered.

If the infant does accomplish the structural and functional categorizations which are similar to those of adults in kind if not in content during his first 18 months, then the rapidity with which he develops basic knowledge of the grammar and how to use it is partially explained. However, most observations of language development during these early months have only been concerned with describing the structural properties of utterances produced. Thus, data on the infant's perception of linguistic structural properties and his comprehension of the function of these properties are still largely missing. Some recent studies have addressed themselves to these aspects of early receptive language development. The data they provide is rather sparse to lead to any conclusions about the infant's receptive language abilities. These few studies do, however, point to the directions that further research might take in order to obtain more complete answers to the questions. These studies of early perception and production of aspects of the language will be reviewed and examined to see if some tentative conclusions can be reached about the infant's early perception of linguistic properties and his comprehension of their communicative function. Data on mother-child communicative inter- actions will be examined to determine tentatively the effect of this interac- tion on the acquisition of linguistic categorizations and concepts of the communicative functions of language and the effect of this development on later development. Possibly fruitful areas for further research will be dis- cussed throughout.

PERCEPTION AND PRODUCTION OF LINGUISTIC PROPERTIES

Before Babbling

The changes in the structure of the utterances produced from 0 to 6 months seem to be primarily a reflection of the child's increasing ability to control parts of the vocal mechanism (Truby, Bosma, and Lind, 1965). This seems to be due to maturation of the vocal mechanism and to the development of body posture. Thus both cry and noncry vocalizations become stabilized during this period, and the sudden changes in pitch and amplitude which occur in utterances during the early part of this period no longer occur in the latter part. However, most of the utterances produced during this period are vocalic in nature. Transcriptions and spectrographic analyses indicate that complete closure of the tract to produce sounds is a rare occurrence, usually associated with some physiological act such as coughing or gurgling. Tongue height changes and lip protrusion, rounding, and contraction occur, which result in the production of different vowel-like sounds such as [w]. True consonantal production, or babbling, begins after this period.

At a very early stage in this same period of development (0–6 months) experimenters have found that infants discriminate not only between vowel- like sounds (Eisenberg, 1969), but also between acoustic parameters that distinguish some consonants (Eimas et al., 1971; Morse, 1973) and rising and falling (see Morse chapter of this book for a detailed discussion of these) fundamental frequency contours. However, the infant's ability to differentiate between the voicing onset time characteristics of [pa] vs. [ba], for example, is not clearly reflected in his production of speech even at the end of the 1st year. Stop consonants babbled by infants at this age tend to fall in the middle range of voicing onset time; that is, there is no clearly differ- entiated group of voiced vs. unvoiced consonants (Preston and Yeni-

Komshian, 1967). Although infants aged 2 months differentiate between the rising and falling contour of a syllable, it has been found (in a study of the vocalization of 30 infants) that utterances marked by final rising fundamental frequency in contrast to those having a final falling fundamental frequency contour do not appear until the 7th month of life (Tonkova-Yompol'skaya, 1969).

These contrasting data on the perception and production of distinctive parameters of the speech signal can be viewed in two different ways. One is that perception of the structural properties that distinguish certain aspects of the speech signal long precedes the realization of these properties in the production of speech. That is, distinctions that are perceived are much later mapped into the production of utterances. The second is that although the infant can make these distinctions they are not used by him until some later stage of development. He might then have to rediscover them as he begins to produce them in different linguistic contexts. It is the case that neonates behave differentially to rising and falling tones (Eisenberg, 1969) and 40- to 54-day-old infants respond to changes between [ba] with falling and [ba] with rising fundamental frequental contour (Morse, 1973). However, 4-month-old infants do not distinguish between a sentence spoken with steadily rising *vs.* steadily falling intonational contour, or between a sentence spoken as a statement *vs.* a sentence spoken as a question (Kaplan, 1969). At 8 months of age infants respond differentially only to statement *vs.* question. These differences in findings may be due to the changes in attention and memory span that occur as the infant matures. Older infants may simply be better able to attend to longer sequences (a sentence *vs.* a syllable). On the other hand, the differences found may be due to reorganization of perception. The latter seems to be more accurate, at least insofar as intonational contours are concerned, since even 8-month-old infants did not respond differentially between a sentence spoken with a steadily rising *vs.* a steadily falling contour but only between a statement *vs.* a question even though both types of stimuli were of the same length. A distinct difference may exist between the infant's perception of the structural properties of speech before and after the babbling period. Some further answers to this question might be obtained by reexamining speech sound discrimination in different linguistic contexts besides the CV syllables during the babbling period.

Babbling Period

Suprasegmental Features. During the babbling period itself the data on perception of the structural properties of speech are sparse. The ability to relate a sound stimulus to the existence of a sound-making object does not appear until the 8th to 10th month (Freedman *et al.*, 1969). At 4–5 months the infants showed an orienting response that the experimenters termed reflexive. However, the infants did not attempt to obtain the object. The sound stimulus used in this experiment, however, was a bell and not the human voice. The results of some experiments by Kagan and Lewis (1965) indicate that infants at 6 months of age behave differentially to speech and nonspeech, and that speech, particularly that of a female voice, produces increased vocalization. Infants appear to observe a difference between the features of statements and questions sometime between 5 and 8 months. Earlier, at about 2–4 months, they respond differentially to angry and friendly, familiar and unfamiliar, and male and female voices (Kaplan and Kaplan, 1970). In studies of the behavior of adults in auditory serial recall (Crowder, 1972) a prelinguistic stage in the analysis of the signal which is termed "preliminary acoustic storage" has been found. At this stage in the process of recall the features checked and corrected are pitch, voice quality, location, and loudness. The experimenter suggested that this kind of analysis and storage is the only kind available to the infant. It has also been observed that at about 8–9 months infants will imitate, in their babbled utterances, the intonational patterns produced by their mothers, although they do not imitate the segmental aspects of their utterances (Nakazima, 1962). All these bits and pieces of evidence may indicate that the infant first and primarily observes the suprasegmental aspects of the utterances he hears, rather than their segmental composition, and relates what he hears to speakers and to particular communicative situations. This may be the case despite the fact that the infant at this stage is producing segments in his babblings and that the structure of these segments changes during this period.

Segmental Features. What has been most frequently and carefully observed is that there are structural changes in the utterances produced during the babbling period and during the transition from babbling to words. During the babbling period, utterances increase in frequency and length, and the segmental and syllabic content of these utterances changes (Irwin, 1957; Nakazima, 1962). During the 5- to 6-month period the mean ratio of consonant to vowel frequencies is 0.36. At the 17- to 18-month period it is 0.63 (Irwin, 1946). At the earlier period a large proportion of the consonants being produced contains the features +nasal, +voice, and +grave. At the later period a large proportion of the sounds produced contains the feature +diffuse (Menyuk, 1971, Chap. 3). The frequency of occurrence of syllabic patterns changes over the 13- to 18-month period (Winitz and Irwin, 1958), probably because of the influence of the lexicon being acquired. At the beginning of this period (13th to 14th month) word approximations are observed.

Transition from Babbling to Words

At 13 months, using cardiac rate deceleration as a possible indication of attention, Kagan and Lewis (1965) found that when infants were presented with paragraphs containing familiar words and nonsense syllables read with and without intonation and stress, the greatest deceleration occurred when infants listened to the paragraph containing familiar words read without intonation and stress. Friedlander (1967) in his study of the pattern of selection of varying auditory stimuli by infants aged 11–13 months found that infants in choosing between pairs of auditory signals consistently preferred mother's normal speech and, somewhat later, mother's speech without intonation and stress. It is impossible to produce continuous speech without intonation and stress. Therefore, these passages when read without intonation and stress were probably produced as word lists. If this is the case, these data perhaps indicate that an infant initially pays attention to the suprasegmental features of utterances and then, later, to familiar word length utterances. These data further suggest that another reorganization of the perception of the structural properties of speech takes place during this prelinguistic period. The first may occur in the transition from vocalization to babbling. The second occurs in the transition from babbling to words.

Nakazima (1970) has found that at 6, 7, and 8 months the infant's babbling is repetitive and appears to be largely used for "play" purposes. At 9 months, however, there is a decrease in repetitive babbling and a reorganization of babbling, at what is termed the "level of language," occurs. Simpler sequences are produced and sounds are used as evocation and response to voice stimuli (that is, to call persons and to respond to persons calling) although only meaningless sound sequences are used. By 11 or 12 months he observed that conventional words begin to appear. This is true of infants in both American-English and Japanese linguistic environments. Gruber (1966) also noted a marked shift in the pattern of vocalizations produced by a child. At about 13 months the child always produces utterances of more than one syllable that are quite complicated in structure. As the sequence develops, more and more marked segments are observed in a single utterance. In addition, these utterances are produced frequently. Approximately 1 month later the child produces much simpler and much less frequent sequences of sound, and these later utterances correspond, for the most part, to his native language.

These observations indicate that a little before or a little after the 12th month, a definitive shift in the structure of the utterances produced does occur. Utterances become simpler and less frequent, begin to resemble standard lexical items in their structure, and, according to Nakazima, are no longer simply play performances but are used to signal and to respond. These data taken together with the data on changes in what the infant attends to in the speech signal may indicate an important change in the child's comprehension of the use of speech as well as a change in his perception and production of the structural properties of speech. Changes in the infant's perception of speech, at least as measured by attention and selection, and changes in the child's production of speech seem to occur at approximately the same time. That is, perception and production, in terms of gross performance measures, appear to be closely related at this stage of development.

Integration of Phonological Features and Semantic Properties

The development of the child's perception and production of a word or a small set of words has been examined to determine, among other things, the conditions under which he appears to make the transition from babbling to words and the segmental properties of the words he produces. The process seems to be one of integration of the perception and production of words and the integration of the phonological features and semantic properties of these words. In describing the development of the word "papa" by a child in a Japanese-speaking environment, Nakazima (1970) noted the following sequence of events. When the child was 12 months, the mother taught the child the word with a falling intonation contour. The child reproduced this phonological sequence using [p], [m], [t], [h], and glottal stop for the consonantal segment and reproduced it with a flat, falling, or rising intonation contour on different occasions. At 13 months "papa" was reproduced accurately for the most part, but variations continued to occur. "Papa" was used by the child to refer to mother, father, maid, and other adult males; then to a picture of a male, a dog, a tooth brush, and a toy dog. This sequence was produced when alone as well as when another human was present. Still later the words "pappa" and "momma" were used for both parents and also for the maid. At 17 months the sequence is correctly articulated and used appropriately. A very similar pattern of development of this word was found for a child in an American-English-speaking environment and also for the acquisition of other words by both children. The experimenter concluded that at the early stages of word production, speech perception and production are not yet integrated. Labels and particular objects are also not definitively associated. That is, the concept of label use seems to have been acquired at this stage but not the concept that the label should be used for a particular object. The experimenter emphasizes that active, spontaneous practice (both when objects are present and absent) seems to play an important role in the acquisition both of the phonological properties of words and of their semantic properties.

Greenfield (1969) suggested that a somewhat different sequence in word acquisition takes place. She traced her daughter's learning of the meaning of the word "dada." First, the child spontaneously produced the sequence "dada" during vocal play. Mother or father imposed meaning on this sound sequence by repeating it after the child and indicating by head turning or pointing, as they said the sequence, that this is the name of an object. The child's perception of the segmental features of the phonological sequence used to name "dada" changed over time. At the beginning stages any sequence containing CVCV in which the V is [a] elicited a looking-at-father response from the child.

The role of mothers or caretakers in effecting the integration of speech perception and production and the integration of phonological sequences and semantic properties is not clear in these discussions. Bullowa *et al.* (1964) observed the following stages in the acquisition of the word "shoe." First the mother produces the word "shoe" when the object is present and indicates the association with the word and object. Sometime later the infant attempts to imitate the word and the mother rejects the imitation and produces the correct word. The child's approximate imitation at some later stage is accepted. The child still later produces an approximation to the word when the object is present, and this approximation, although somewhat different from the previous form used, is also accepted by the mother. The child then produces the approximation when the object is absent and receives acknowledgement from the mother. Still later the correct form is produced.

Although this description and the previous descriptions of the sequence in word acquisition shed some light on the conditions under which the transition from babbling to words takes place, it is also clear that different techniques may be used by different infants and mothers during this word acquisition period. Murai (1963–64) has suggested that the sequence of performance that can be observed (for example, imitation then comprehension or comprehension then imitation) is dependent on the technique used by the mother. Some mothers specifically attempt to elicit imitation. Other mothers simply point and name. Probably all mothers do some of both. It may also be the case that differences in the sequence of performance that has been observed (for example, simultaneous use of the word when the object is present and when it is not, or at first only use of the word when the object is present and then later use of the word in both situations) are due to differences in the concepts of the use of language by individual infants (*i.e.,* to name or communicate). Finally, the differences in the sequence of performance that can be observed may be the result of the techniques of observation, that is, the particular samplings of behavior that the experimenter has available to him. The important question concerning the differences in the sequence of performance observed is whether or not these differences have lasting effects on the child's comprehension and use of language. Until we have more careful analyses of the behavioral sequence during this stage of development carried out with a sizable number of children (plus follow-up studies of later development) we will not have an answer to this question. We, of course, also have to be careful of the measures used to assess later development.

Integration of Perception and Production of Segmental Features

Both in the perception and in the production of the segmental properties of words, a sequence of distinctions has been observed. The perceptual differentiation of segmental features by infants aged 11-21 months has been examined in one linguistic environment (Shvachkin, 1966). A developmental sequence in differentiation which closely matches Jakobson's (1968) description of what the sequence should be, in terms of the phonological structure of languages and increasing degree of markedness, seems to occur in the development of perceptual distinctions by the children. However, the design of the experiment, that is, teaching children to differentiate between pictured minimal pair words, causes one to question the generality of the findings. Children from various linguistic backgrounds have been observed to make certain productive distinctions before others. The sequence in which these distinctions are made seems to be similar regardless of the linguistic environment. Further, the sequence of mastery of consonantal segments containing certain features seems to mirror the sequence of proportional usage of consonantal segments containing certain features at an earlier stage of development (Menyuk, 1971, Chap. 3). This process of acquiring productive distinctions continues well beyond the age of 18 months. How closely tied this process is to the development of perceptual distinctions is not clear since at the time when children are producing one-syllable utterances they appear to understand two-syllable utterances. At the time they are observing very general features of the segments of one-syllable utterances in their productions they appear to perceive not only more but different distinctions between these segments. That is, they will use one phonological sequence for a number of words but appear to have no difficulty in identifying particular words within this set (Ervin-Tripp, 1966). Also, one can observe in the productive strategies used by young children, preplanning for the production of the total utterance so that, for example, final sounds appear in initial position ([m k o m] [m k o] for comb) and sequential sounds have an effect across several segments (Smith, 1970). These permutations and effects are not reflected by commensurate perceptual confusions. In addition, the sequence of development of the perception of feature distinctions does not quite match the sequence of development of the production of feature distinctions (Menyuk, 1972).

These findings raise many more questions than they answer since the data on perceptual distinctions during this period of beginning word usage are so sparse. In principle, one could argue that, again, perception of segments exceeds production. One could argue equally well that at this stage the two processes are developing independently and are tied to different kinds of perceptual categorization—words with semantic properties and phonological features for perception, and semantic features and syllabic units for production (Menyuk, 1973a). The process of integration of the perception and production of the speech signal at the segmental level takes place over a long period of time. The evidence for this is not only behavior which indicates that children appear to perceive segmental differences before they can produce them, but also the fact that delayed auditory feedback of the speech produced does not appear to act as a disruption of ongoing speech behavior until about 2 1/2–3 years of age (Yeni-Komshian, Chase, and Mobley, 1967). Before this age infants seem to monitor or listen to the delayed signal, as if it were any speech stimulus rather than a signal related to their own production.

Semantic Properties of Words and Sentence Structure

The child's comprehension of the semantic properties and the phonological features of words and their integration during the period of development from one word to two words has not been examined in any detail. What has been studied are the words produced and the context in which they are produced to determine the meaning (for the child) of the lexical item itself. Children initially use words to name objects as a whole rather than observing the properties of these objects, and to label states, conditions, and activities which vary (for example, gone, down, open, broken) rather than to mark attributes (MacNamara, 1972). In the acquisition of properties of lexical items the following observations have been made: overgeneralization occurs, the same lexical item is used when talking about different things (hot for both hot and cold); no generalization occurs, an item is used only when talking about a specific thing (chair used for a specific chair); nondifferentiation occurs, several lexical items are used when talking about the same thing (horse and dog are used for dog) (Menyuk, 1971, Chap. 6). In addition, there seems to be a sequence in the particular properties that are observed by the child. A basic, perhaps universal set of unmarked properties, closely tied to the human's ability to perceive and categorize spatial then temporal aspects of environmental phenomena, appear to be observed first, and then marked properties in these categories are observed (Clark, 1973; see Clark's chapter in this book for a fuller discussion of these data).

There have been few experimental studies of the child's perceptual categorization of objects and events and the relationship of these categorizations to words during the one-word stage of development. A possible exception is a study by Nelson (1972). The children in the study were aged 18–24 months. Since there was no indication of the structure of the language being produced by these children, it is possible that these children were at the 2- to 3-word stage of sentence generation. The experimenter asked these children to identify, by either naming or pointing, objects that were represented by outline drawings, detailed drawings, or photographs. The objects were either familiar or unfamiliar and ambiguous (*i.e.,* those objects which share the features of other objects or have many members in their class) or unambiguous. Both ambiguous and unambiguous familiar objects were recognized significantly more often in their detailed (both detailed drawing and photographs) than in their outline state. This difference was not observed with less familiar objects. Significantly more names were given to both familiar and ambiguous items. The following developmental sequence was suggested by the experimenter. The earliest concepts are those of definition of action or function of objects. Initially there are a few unique concepts and no perceptual contrasts are observed. Then overspecificity, in terms of criterial attributes, is demanded. Finally, criterial attributes for class membership are complete and well defined and are extended to new members of the class on the basis of shape or form. Clearly the limitation of items in this study to names of objects decreases the generalizations that can be drawn from it. However, it is encouraging in the sense that it suggests that examination of the criterial attributes used for classification of words is possible with very young children.

There have been very few studies of the comprehension of sentence structure at this early stage of development. An exception is a study by Shipley, Smith, and Gleitman (1969). The responses of children aged 15–30 months to varying types of utterances were examined. The utterances were either the noun alone, a verb plus noun, a telegraph utterance of the type "Please, X, noun, verb" or an imperative. The objects named by the nouns were present in the room. The population was divided into two groups: the less advanced (primarily one-word users) and more advanced (primarily two-word users). Relevant responses were categorized as touching, looking, carrying out the task, repetition of the utterance, or a reply to the command. It was found that with the less advanced children (primarily one-word users and, therefore, the subjects of interest in this discussion) relevant responses were obtained most frequently to the noun in isolation and to the word-separated delivery of the telegraph utterance. The presence of a known or familiar item was the primary factor in obtaining a relevant response, and any sentence context at all appeared to make recognition of the known word more difficult. These results indicate that comprehension of structure as well as production of structure is limited to the word for these children and that at this stage comprehension and production are closely matched. In contradiction to these findings are other observations showing that infants not only pay attention to a word in a sentence but appear to interpret differently structured utterances in different ways although they themselves are only producing the topic noun of the sentence. For example, Lewis (1963, p. 59) noted that when an infant is asked "Where are the flowers?" the infant crawls to them or points to them, but when asked to "Smell the pretty flowers" he does not point to them but smells them. These may be practiced ritual actions in particular linguistic and situational contexts and, thus, reflect no real comprehension of the relationships expressed in the sentence. However, the question of what the infant does comprehend in the sentence he hears still remains unanswered. More experimental studies are needed to examine the infant's comprehension of structure at the one-word stage of development. Both utterance structure (for example, sentence type, relationships expressed, prosodic features) and situational structure (for example, presence and absence of topic objects, use of gesture and expression) need to be controlled and varied.

Table 1. Stages in the Perception and Production of Linguistic Properties

	Production	Perception
Stage I	Vocalization	Acoustic differences of syllabic length segments
Stage II	Babbled utterances marked prosodically	Beginning of differentiation of segmental features?
Stage III	Babbling; sequence of proportional usage of features of speech sounds	Differentiation of supra-segmental features
Stage IV	Syllable length utterances	Attention to word length utterances; beginning of integration of phonological and semantic features
Stage V	Words marked prosodically; general features of speech sounds in syllables observed	Observation of semantic properties of words; beginning of integration of perception and production of speech sounds; observation of semantic relations in sentences?

As was indicated earlier, there are clearly more questions than answers in this area of assessment of the perception of the structural properties of language during this developmental period. Table 1 presents a condensed summary of the findings of studies which have examined both the perception and production of linguistic structural properties of speech during this period.

COMPREHENSION OF THE FUNCTION OF ASPECTS OF LANGUAGE

Cry utterances obviously serve a communicative purpose since they initiate responses from the environment. The relationships between the structure of the cry and the differential responses these cries obtain have been speculated about at great length. Spectrographic analyses have indicated that cries do have differing structures and that these differences are tied to different situations (hunger, pain, discomfort, etc.). No careful studies have been carried out to examine the correlations between different cries and different responses from the environment. At any rate, cries do elicit responses from the environment from birth on and obviously continue to do so for many years. The important question is, when does the infant become aware of the communicative function of cry and noncry utterances and cease to vocalize only in response to physiological drives? That is, when are vocalizations used purposively to communicate with caretakers? It should be noted that noncry as well as cry utterances have been observed in the first weeks of life.

Early Communication

In a sampling of mother-infant communicative interaction from age 49 to 105 days, it was found that there were, during this period, particular sequences in which alternations between mother and infant vocalizations occurred non-randomly (Bateson, 1971). During these sequences there was frequent vocalization by both the mother and the infant, there was no crying by the infant, there was sustained eye contact and no caretaking activities were going on. These situations generally occurred after active caretaking periods. The mother and infant were always less than 1 yard apart and the mother was frequently squatting on the baby's level. Communicative interaction in a noncry situation (the experimenter terms it "conversation") appears to go on at a very early age.

Another study examined the communicative interaction of 50 infants aged 12 weeks and their mothers (Lewis and Freedle, 1972). The experimenters found that both infants and mothers actively participated in a chain of activities in which the behavior of each participant, both vocal and nonvocal, was significantly determined by the behavior of the other. These chains were initiated by the infants as well as the mothers. A significant relationship was found between mothers' vocalizations to infants' vocalizations (both cry and noncry), and, in general, the strongest pairing that occurred was vocalization to vocalization. There were, however, "considerable" individual differences and sex and socioeconomic status differences in the vocalization interactions observed. Girls vocalized more to mothers' behaviors than boys. Boys showed less differentiation of who was the object of mothers' vocalizations (self or other), and mothers talked more to girls than boys. Higher socioeconomic status (SES) infants differentiated more in terms of who was the object of mothers' vocalizations, lower SES infants' vocalizations were more frequently sustained by mothers' vocalizations, and lower SES mothers' vocalizations more effectively elicited vocalizations. Higher SES mothers vocalizations tended to inhibit their infants' vocalizations; that is, their infants appeared to listen more to their vocalizations. Higher SES mothers more frequently responded with vocalization than with other behaviors. These findings indicate that communicative interaction of a vocal nature dominates mother-infant chains of interaction at a very early age.

There are individual differences in patterns of vocal interaction at a very early age that are, perhaps, due to individual differences *per se,* sex, and socioeconomic status. In the previous section we stressed the importance of follow-up studies to examine the effect of particular techniques used by mothers to engage their children in the word game and the effect of how their children do, indeed, participate in the game. Lewis and Freedle have follow-up data on a few of the infants in the population described above. At 2 years of age the spontaneous speech of these children was analyzed. Their expression of semantic relations in these utterances (for example, subject-verb and verb-object) and the mean length of their utterances was determined. Their knowledge of prepositions and adjective contrasts and their performance on the Peabody Picture Vocabulary Test was assessed. It was found that at 2 years of age their rank order of language development, as measured in the manner indicated above, matched their rank order at 12 weeks in terms of amount of vocalizations, the amount of quiet play, the amount of maternal play, and the degree to which they differentiated between themselves and others as being the object of mothers' vocalizations. The assumption of the experimenters is that linguistic competency and degree of linguistic competency grows out of the communication matrix that begins at a very early age. However, it is not clear from this study what factors in the communication matrix, as described, lead to linguistic competency much less to differences in linguistic competency at age 2. There may be situational factors which lead to differences in the amount of vocalization, or the degree of differentiation as to whom the mother is addressing in her vocalization, etc., which may play an important role in the development of linguistic competence. But the descriptions provided do not clearly indicate what these factors might be.

Communication interaction takes place between mother and child at a very early age. The pattern of this interaction (especially as described by Bateson, 1971) seems to be one of vocalization, listening, answering, and, particularly on the part of the mother, further vocalization to elicit a response if one is not immediately forthcoming. However, we cannot conclude from these studies that the infant is purposively engaging in primitive conversation, but only that these events take place. Eventually the infant does appear to engage in purposive noncry vocal interaction with his caretakers and with himself. The question is, is he already doing this at 2–3 months of age?

Communication and Suprasegmental Features

As was stated earlier, the infant has been observed to behave differentially to particular patterns of the suprasegmental aspects of the utterances that he hears at a very early age (2–3 months). The development of intonational patterns which match those of adults has been traced by Tonkova-Yampol'skaya (1969). Sound "intonograms," which measured fundamental frequency, time, and intensity, were used to measure utterances. At approximately 2 months "narration" and "assertion" utterances which rise gradually and then fall in intensity and fundamental frequency appear. Requests and emotional requests which have a sharp peak and then rise slightly or markedly at the end of the utterance in both intensity and fundamental frequency appear at about the 7th month. Commands which have a sharply rising and then falling fundamental frequency and intensity pattern appear at about the 10th month. The narration-assertion utterances, and the request and command utterances are about 1/2 the duration of the emotional request utterances. Therefore, although differential patterns of cry (anger, pain, hunger, fretfulness, etc.) presumably occur at the very earliest stages of development, differential patterns in noncry utterances do not appear in the vocalization of infants until about the 6th and 8th month of life. Nakazima (1962) noted that imitation of intonation patterns begins at this age and that at 9 months, calling to persons and response to calling occurs (Nakazima, 1970) although only meaningless sounds, primarily vocalic in nature, are used. This behavior seems to indicate two things. First, it seems unlikely that the noncry use of suprasegmental features grows out of cry vocalizations given the marked difference in the time at which differential cry patterns and differential noncry patterns appear. Second, this behavior may indicate comprehension of the use of differential contours to express the differential meanings of assertion, request, and command. A much more careful analysis of the situations in which these utterances are produced, the structure of the utterances themselves, the responses of caretakers to these utterances, and the responses of infants to the responses of caretakers is needed before one can conclude that differing intonational contours are being purposively used at this stage. Shortly after this period, at about 12 months, the use of conventional words begins.

Differences in Communicative Style

Nelson (1971) has found that some children at this stage of development (from 1 year on) primarily use single words that are clearly articulated while others primarily use phrases that are so phonologically obscure that they are difficult to analyze. Not only is the form of the language primarily used somewhat different for the two groups of children, but the function of the language used appears to be different. The one-word producers appear to use language primarily to name things, and the unanalyzable phrase users appear to use language to direct others and to express needs and feelings. These differences appear to be somewhat related to the content of their mothers' speech when talking to them, and this, in turn, appears to be related to the educational level of the mothers. Another factor might also account for the differences. Eight of the 10 children who use language primarily to name are firstborn, and 5 of the 8 children who use language primarily to express needs and feelings are later children. It seems that there are differences not only in the sequence of performance that can be observed in the use of first words (for example, imitation then comprehension or *vice versa*) but also in the form and function of these first words. How these differences in the earliest production of words can affect the course of later development is not clear. Both groups of children use language for both functions and differ only in proportion of usage. A possibility, however, is that these early differences are early indicators of different conceptualizations about the primary use of language. These conceptualizations could, logically, strongly influence the course of later development especially if they are not altered by later and differing experiences.

An interesting question concerning this study is why the experimenter categorized some utterances as expressions of needs and feelings and others as names. Some clues as to the possible basis for these categorizations come from another study (Dore, 1973). Observations were made of the interaction of 10 infants aged 10 to 14 months with their mothers and a familiar teacher in a nursery school setting. The interactions of four of the children were video-taped. Taping took place periodically when these children were producing one-word utterances until there was some evidence of the beginning of two-word utterances. The data used for analysis were the child's utterances, his nonlinguistic behavior, his mother's response, and the context. The children's utterances were transcribed phonetically, and a system was devised for marking suprasegmental features of the utterances: falling, rising, level, and rising-falling. The experimenter found what appeared to be three different "styles" of interaction. There were some children who primarily produced unconventional phonological sequences (*i.e.,* not words) but marked with different intonational contours. Another group of children primarily used conventional words that were not differentially marked suprasegmentally. A third group of children used both conventional words and differential suprasegmental marking. The report of the experiment contains detailed data on two of the children who represent the extremes in style. One girl produced primarily conventional words without differential marking (*i.e.,* most utterances had the unmarked terminal fall). She seemed to use language most often to codify environmental phenomena rather than to interact with her mother or the teacher. The other child, a boy, produced few conventional words, but almost all of his utterances were marked differentially and were directed toward other people. His suprasegmental marking developed during this period so that more and more differences in marking were observed whereas no additions or changes of suprasegmental marking were observed in the utterances produced by the girl. In total, 67% of the boy's utterances and 23% of the girl's utterances were directed toward other people. The experimenter concluded that there are some children who primarily develop cognitive schema of the structure of language and other children who develop prosodic schema. These differences may be due to innate personality characteristics, sex, or the types of interactions that mothers engage in with their children during this one-word stage of development. Roughly speaking, the girl's mother seemed to manipulate her child (for example, engaging her in naming games) whereas the boy's mother seemed to be manipulated by her child.

A study of the suprasegmental structure of the utterances of a child (aged 18 months) who was primarily producing one-word utterances was carried out using spectrographic analysis of these utterances (Menyuk and Bernholtz, 1969). This child was older than the children observed in the previous study and could be described as belonging to the third group of children found by the experimeter. Most of her one-word utterances were conventional words and appeared to be marked differentially suprasegmentally. The lexical items selected for analysis were those that were found repeatedly in the tape-recorded samples and consisted of names (sometimes marked with possessive), "no," two nouns ("door" and [dadi] for "doggie"), a verb ("touch") and a particle ("up"). None of the utterances selected was an imitation of utterances produced by the mother, but, rather, they were spontaneous productions of the child. Seventy utterances were isolated, rerecorded, and analyzed spectrographically. A randomized tape of these utterances was prepared and presented to two listeners who were asked to categorize them as declaratives, questions, and emphatics. There was 81% agreement between the listeners in categorizing the utterances. Where disagreement occurred between listeners on an utterance, it was found that one listener categorized some of the emphatics as tense or worried statements whereas the other listener categorized them as emphatics. Spectrographic analysis showed a general characteristic of each type of utterance. Declaratives terminated with a falling fundamental frequency contour, questions terminated with a rising fundamental frequency contour, and emphatics had a sharp rise (sometimes a doubling of frequency) and then fell in fundamental frequency contour during the utterance. It was also found that the mother was responding for the most part (some utterances were ignored) in accordance with the word, the suprasegmental aspect of the word, and the context. Most statements were responded to with other statements which agreed or disagreed with what the child had said (for example, "yes, you can," "no, it's not"), questions were responded to with either a repetition of the question and another question or simply another question (for example, "What about it?," "Is that Chrissie's frog?") and emphatics were responded to by emphatics or action (for example,"O.K!","We've got to!," "Yes!," picks her up).

It is clear that the child's purpose in producing these utterances was not simply to codify an object or an event in the environment but to interact with another or to manipulate another concerning the object or event. It is also clear that purposeful effort is needed to generate questions and emphatics, and that this effort was being employed by the child with a range of lexical items. If, indeed, it is the case that infants at a previous stage of development have already abstracted and categorized differences in suprasegmental patterns, then it seems possible that at this stage the suprasegmental features of statements, questions, and emphatics have been abstracted and categorized and are purposively used with words to generate these sentence types. However, as was indicated, the question of whether or not the child has abstracted and categorized different patterns of suprasegmental features at the stage before one-word use and is using these patterns purposively still remains. The responses of children, at the one-word stage of development, to questions, statements, and emphatics need also to be experimentally explored.

Communication with Self and Others in One-Word Utterances

In addition to the question about the purposive expression of various sentence types, there are also questions about the purposive expression of relations in one-word utterances. Greenfield *et al.* (1972, in press) hypothesized that knowledge of the semantic relations of referents in a concrete context could be used by the child to learn how relations are expressed in a child's particular language. They hypothesized further that at the one-word stage the child may be expressing a proposition made up of a specific referent combined with particular situational features and prosodic features and used for specific purposes (to make social contact, to wish, to command, to declare, to question, etc.). For example, the child says "away" after pushing a toy away and is indicating that the toy is away, or the child says "pooh" when referring to the dirtiness of himself and is indicating that the baby is pooh. Later, at the two-word stage, both aspects of the semantic relation are expressed and the child says "toy away" and "baby pooh." The experimenters argue that one need not postulate expression of an underlying syntactic relation even at the two-word stage since word order has no relevance to the question of underlying semantic structure and, indeed, cannot be used to discover relations in two-word utterances. Only the situation can reveal these relationships. The same method of using the situation to discover relationships can be applied to one-word utterances.

To examine these hypotheses, a study was carried out in which diaries were kept of the utterances of two boys, their actions (gestures, looking, pointing), the situations in which the utterances occurred, and the interpretations of the mother and an objective observer. The procedure used for categorizing utterances was as follows: the child produced an utterance, the mother expanded the utterance or stated what the child meant, and the observer indicated agreement or disagreement. One boy's language development was examined from 8 months, 19 days to 21 months, 8 days and the other from 7 months, 22 days to 22 months. An order of emergence of relations as indicated by agreement between mother and observer is described in the report.

The order of emergence is, roughly, as follows. At the earliest stages "pure performatives" (utterances which cannot be expanded any further) such as "hi" and "bye-bye" are observed. Then other performatives, first, naming (of objects seen or heard) and then vocatives (calling the person named) emerge. Objects of demand then appear and are followed by the negative and later the affirmative. The negative is considered a kind of action and it is at this time that action of an agent emerges. The same sequence of use of the negative (first rejection, then nonexistence, then denial) is observed at this stage as has been observed in the 2- and 3-word sentence stage. A process, termed "decentering" by the experimenters, then begins. Action performed by an agent initially always referred to the child himself as agent. Later, other agents are referred to (mommy "gone"). Inanimate objects of action appear and are at first objects of the child's own action and later objects of other humans' actions. States or actions of inanimate objects are then referred to. Changes in state or action are referred to before constant attributes. Possession and habitual location then emerge. Location initially refers to path rather than end point. For example, the terms "up" and "down" appear first in these types of utterances and then later particular place is referred to ("table," "chair," "truck"). Experiencer (person who is recipient of action) and agent of action then appear. The latter indicates contrast between the actions of others and self. Finally, modifications of an event, questions, and conjunction and oppositions appear.

The experimenters offer the following arguments for the validity of their descriptions of the structure of one-word utterances. The same word is used to express different relations. Therefore, the relationships expressed are independent of specific vocabulary. There is an order in the emergence of expressed relations, and, one might add, this order fits in with other descriptions of aspects of perceptual development. Old words are used in different ways at different stages of development. Finally, related semantic functions seem to emerge at the same time. For example, the negation of rejection, which is classified as reaction to action of others, and action of object appear simultaneously.

The question again arises as to whether or not children are purposively using language to express these relations at this stage of development. That is, it is not clear that they have abstracted and categorized the concepts of agent of action, action of object, location and possession of object, etc., and are purposively using these categorizations to express differential meaning. Although contextual information and more careful analysis of the structural properties of the utterances produced do add to our knowledge of the possible content and structure of these one-word utterances, descriptive research, thus far, has not clarified the issue. These observations have led to differing hypotheses about the structure of these one-word utterances. They are considered to be sentences expressing a syntactic relationship or sentences expressing a semantic relationship or words expressing a codification of experience. Some of the arguments are based on differences in definition of terms (what is a sentence?). Some are based on the kind of evidence mustered for the argument to explain the behavior observed (contextual evidence, prosodic as well as segmental features of utterances, interpretations of caretakers, presuppositions about comprehension preceding production). Some arguments address themselves to the question of explanation of further

Table 2. Stages in the Comprehension of Use of Aspects of Language

	Use	Aspect
Stage I	Manipulation of environment	Differential cry
Stage II	Communicative function	Alternation of vocalization with mother
Stage III	Manipulation of environment; communicative function	Babbling marked prosodically
Stage IV	Manipulation of environment; communicative function; categorization of objects and events; categorization of semantic relations in sentences?	Words plus prosody plus situation

development; that is, what precursors to later development can be found in earlier development to explain the structural changes that occur? Table 2 presents a summary of the findings of studies which have attempted to examine the child's comprehension of the function of aspects of the language during this developmental period.

SOME FINAL COMMENTS

In this discussion the child's perception of the structural properties of language and his comprehension of the communicative use of these properties were arbitrarily separated. The findings of studies during this period indicate how interdependent these aspects are. The child "communicates" effectively from birth on by means of his cry vocalizations, and yet noncry vocalization begins at an early age, changes, and develops. These changes and developments seem to be a product of his physiological maturation, his changing communicative needs, and his ability to relate these needs to particular aspects in the language. The last is due to his perceptual development. How these factors interact with one another at various stages of development is not clear, nor is the structure of the child's knowledge of these relationships at various stages of development clear. In addition, the relationships between perceptual development and productive development are also not clear. There are stages at which these two processes seem very closely tied (for example, the transition period from babbling to words) and other stages at which either the data are nonexistent (during the babbling period) or the data are too sparse (during the one-word period) to come to any conclusions about relationships between the processes.

Methods of obtaining and analyzing data have contributed to the arguments concerning the child's perception of the structural properties of the language, his comprehension of the use of aspects of the language, and the relationships between these two competences at various stages of development. That is, in some instances, conclusions are based on reexaminations of previously collected data (old diaries), and in other instances, on the data of studies being carried out by the experimenters themselves. In some instances the data were obtained by audio-recording, either by written transcription or tape recorder, and in other instances by audio-visual recording. The data have been analyzed by phonetic transcription or by spectrographic analysis. In some instances the situation has been observed, and in other instances it has not. The latter observations are either a gross outline of what is occurring or a detailed analysis of situation and interaction (for example, a frame by frame analysis of video-tape records).

At each stage of development both the context of language generation and the structure of the utterances produced (both child and other) need to be more carefully analyzed and methods of data collection standardized. However, this does not resolve the problem of determining whether or not the categorizations of the experimenters are really the categorizations of infants and children. Perhaps experimental studies of the comprehension of the structural aspects of utterances in particular contexts can lead to answers to these questions. A way of doing this is to observe whether or not the child accepts the experimenter's categorization.

As a final comment, group and individual differences in time of onset of new stages of development, differences in amount of vocalization, and differences in the degree to which infants can differentiate who is the object of the mothers' vocalizations have been observed. At a somewhat later stage (the one-word stage) both differences in the form (one-word or jargon) and function (to categorize objects and events or to communicate with or manipulate others) have been found. At a still later stage (at 2 years) differences in the mean length of utterances, in the structure of these utterances, and in the degree of comprehension of the meaning of words and classes of words have been found. The reasons for these differences at any stage of development are not made clear by these studies, nor are the relationships between differences at various stages, although social and sex differences appear to be related to the performances observed. To find these reasons and to determine these relationships are important tasks not, one would hope, for the purpose of modifying the linguistic behavior of children who are developing normally so that all children are alike in the form and function of their language, but to understand what factors initially contribute to differences and what effect these differences have on the course of development.

For the purpose of developing appropriate intervention programs for children who deviate markedly in their language development from children who are developing language normally, the facts and conditions of moving from one stage of language acquisition to another are particularly important to establish. What has been observed with these children is that they appear to spend exceptionally long periods of time at specific stages of semantic, syntactic, and phonological development (Menyuk, 1973b). It is possible that these periods of arrest are due to the fact that reorganization of linguistic data is needed in order to progress further. To develop effective intervention programs it would then be necessary to understand both the linguistic problems involved in reorganization and the cognitive organization and environmental demands upon which this organization depends.

REFERENCES

Bateson, M. C. The interpersonal context of infant vocalization. Quarterly Progress Report, Research Laboratory of Electronics, Massachusetts Institute of Technology, No. 100, 170—176, Jan. 15, 1971.

Bullowa, M., Jones, L. G., and Duckert, A. The acquisition of a word. *Lang. Speech,* 1964, 7, 107—111.

Clark, E. What's in a word? On the child's acquisition of semantics in his first language. In T. E. Moore (Ed.) *Cognitive Development and the Acquisition of Language.* New York: Academic Press, 1973.

Crowder, R. G. Visual and auditory memory. In J. F. Kavanagh and I. G. Mattingly (Eds.), *Language by Ear and by Eye.* Cambridge, Mass.: M.I.T. Press, 1972, pp. 251—275.

Dore, J. The development of speech acts. Unpublished doctoral dissertation, Baruch College, City University of New York, New York, 1973.

Eimas, P. D., Siqueland, E. R., Juscyzk, P., and Vigorito, J. Speech perception in infants. *Science,* 1971, *171,* 303.

Eisenberg, R. Auditory behavior in the human neonate: Functional properties of sound and their ontogenetic implications. *Int. Audiol.* 1969, *8,* 34—45.

Ervin-Tripp, S. Language development. In L. W. Hoffman and M. L. Hoffman (Eds.), *Review of Child Development,* New York: Russell Sage Foundation, 1966, pp. 55—105.

Freedman, D. A., Fox-Kolinda, B. J., Margileth, D. A., and Miller, D. H. The development of the use of sound as a guide to affective and cognitive behavior—a 2 phase process. Child Develop., 1969, *40,* 1099—1105.

Friedlander, B. The effect of speaker identity, inflection, vocabulary and message redundancy on infants' selection of vocal reinforcers. Paper presented at meeting of Society for Research in Child Development, New York, March, 1967.

Greenfield, P. M. Who is "Dada"? Some aspects of the semantic and phonological development of a child's first word. Unpublished paper, Research and Development Center in Early Childhood Education, Syracuse University, Syracuse, 1969.

Greenfield, P. M., Smith, J. H., and Laufer, B. Communication and the beginning of language: The development of semantic structure in one word speech and beyond. Harvard University, Cambridge, Mass., in press.

Gruber, J. S. Playing with distinctive features in the babbling of infants. Quarterly Progress Report, Research Laboratory of Electronics, Mass. Inst. of Tech., No. 81, 181—186, April, 1966.

Irwin, O. C. Phonetical descriptions of speech development in childhood. In *Kaisers Manual of Phonetics,* Chap. 2. Amsterdam: North Holland Publishing Co., 1957.

Irwin, O. C. Infant speech: Equations for consonant-vowel ratios. *J. Speech Disord.*, 1946, *11*, 177–180.

Jakobson, R. *Child Language, Aphasia and Phonological Universals.* The Hague: Mouton, 1968.

Kagan, J. and Lewis, M. Studies of attention. *Merrill-Palmer Quart. Behav. Develop.,* 1965, *4*, 95–127.

Kaplan, E. L. The role of intonation in the acquisition of language. Unpublished doctoral dissertation, Cornell University, Ithaca, 1969.

Kaplan, E. L. and Kaplan, G. A. The prelinguistic child. In J. Eliot (Ed.), *Human Development and Cognitive Processes.* New York: Holt, Rinehart and Winston, 1970, pp. 358–381.

Lewis, M. M. *Language, Thought and Personality.* New York: Basic Books, 1963.

Lewis, M. and Freedke, R. *Mother-Infant Dyad: The Cradle of Meaning.* Princeton, N.J.: Educational Testing Service, 1972.

MacNamara, J. Cognitive basis of language learning in infants. *Psychol. Rev.,* 1972, *79*, 1–13.

Menyuk, P. Clusters as single underlying consonants: Evidence from children's production. In *Proceedings of VIIth International Congress of Phonetic Sciences.* The Hague: Mouton, 1973a, pp. 1163–1166.

Menyuk, P. *The Development of Speech.* Indianapolis: Bobbs-Merrill, 1972.

Menyuk, P. *The Acquisition and Development of Language.* Englewood Cliffs, N.J.: Prentice-Hall, 1971.

Menyuk, P. The developmental implications of deviant language acquisition. In J. I. Nurnberger (Ed.), *Early Development,* Res. Publ. A.R.N.M.D., Vol. 51, 1973b, pp. 210–220.

Menyuk, P. and N. Bernholtz. Prosodic features and children's language production. Quarterly Progress Reports, Research Laboratory of Electronics, M. I. T., No. 93, April, 1969, pp. 216–219.

Morse, P. A. The discrimination of speech and nonspeech stimuli in early infancy. *J. Exp. Child Psychol.,* in press.

Murai, Jun-Ichi. The sounds of infants. *Stud. Phonol.* 1963–64, *3*, 21–24.

Nakazima, S. A comparative study of the speech developments of Japanese and American English in childhood. (Part three) *Stud. Phonol.* 1970, *5*, 20–35.

Nakazima, S. A comparative study of the speech developments of Japanese and American English in childhood. *Stud. Phonol.* 1962, *2*, 27–39.

Nelson, K. The relation of form recognition to concept development. *Child Develop.* 1972, *43*, 67–74.

Nelson, K. Presyntactical strategies for learning to talk. Paper presented at Society for Research in Child Development, Minneapolis, 1971.

Preston, M. and Yeni-Komshian, G. Studies of the development of stop consonants in children. Haskins Laboratories, SR–11, 1967.

Shipley, E. F., Smith, C. S., and Gleitman, L. R. A study in the acquisition of language. *Language,* 1969, *45*, 322–342.

Shvachkin, N. K. H. 1966. Development of phonemic speech perception in early childhood. Izvestia Akad. Pedag. Nank RSFSR, 1948 Vyp. 13 Abstracted by D. I. Slobin in F. Smith and G. A. Miller (Eds.), *Genesis of Language:* Cambridge: M.I.T. Press, 1966, pp. 381–382.

Smith, N. V. The acquisition of phonology. Cambridge University Press, London, 1973.

Tonkova-Yampol'skaya, R. V. Development of speech intonation in infants during the first two years of life. Translated in *Sov. Psychol.* 1969, *7*, 48—54.

Truby, H. M., Bosma, J. F., and Lind, J. Newborn infant cry. *Acta Paediat. Scand.*, Suppl. 163, 1965.

Winitz, H. and Irwin, O. C. Syllabic and phonetic structure of infants' early words. *J. Speech Hear. Res.*, 1958, *1*, 250—256.

Yeni-Komshian, G., Chase, R. A., and Mobley, R. L. Delayed auditory feedback studies in the speech of children between 2 and 3 years. Annual Report, Neurocommunications Laboratory, Johns Hopkins University School of Medicine, Baltimore, 1967, pp. 165—188.

CHAPTER NINE

RECEPTIVE LANGUAGE IN THE MENTALLY RETARDED: PROCESSES AND DIAGNOSTIC DISTINCTIONS

Richard F. Cromer

Medical Research Council, Developmental Psychology Unit, Drayton House, Gordon Street, London, WC1H OAN, England

The process of understanding is complex. Understanding understanding is even more complex. Yet any program of intervention intended to increase the knowledge of a human organism must explore the language comprehension process, because we acquire knowledge primarily through language. Paula Menyuk has reviewed the studies of receptive language. She is concerned mainly with receptive processes in the earliest months of life in normal children. By contrast, this chapter deals more specifically with language comprehension processes in the mentally retarded and across a more extended age range.

As Menyuk has pointed out, there are few experimental studies concerned primarily with comprehension. If this is true for normal children, it is even more true of the retarded. Therefore, in order to talk more meaningfully about the processes underlying deviant language development, it will often be necessary to cite studies which have dealt with productive aspects of language. This is not necessarily a limitation.

Some tests of comprehension tap only one function of language. For example, many studies of understanding have employed methods in which the child's behavior serves as the dependent variable. The independent variable has most often consisted of commands and requests (*e.g.,* "Put the car *on* the cup" *vs.* "Put the car *in* the cup," etc.). But the giving and carrying out of verbal instructions is only one function of language. Other experimenters, however, have employed contrasting pairs of pictures encoding grammatical features (*e.g.,* Berko, 1958; Fraser, Bellugi, and Brown, 1963).

Carroll (1972) has outlined some of the problems in defining language comprehension. In his review, he reminded us of a useful technique for studying comprehension devised by Forsyth and Rubenstein (1966–67). They employed a device in which they could present the subject with a limited portion of a sentence, for example, only the first two or three words. When the subject comprehended these, he pressed a button causing the next segment to appear. One was then able to relate the time taken to comprehend to the particular characteristics of the segment which had been presented. These characteristics could be varied according to the experimenter's purpose, and included length, position in the sentence, grammatical characteristics, and the like. Danks (1969) used a similar technique to study the differential effects of grammatical quality and meaningfulness on comprehension time. I know of no studies using this technique on retarded children.

In any case, it will be possible to learn something about how children acquire language from studies both of production and of comprehension. There are two points to be made in this review which are really interdependent. First, what is important in language acquisition is not so much *what* is comprehended by an individual or a group of individuals, but *how* they come to comprehend it, that is to say, the *processes* involved in language comprehension. The second point is the importance of distinguishing carefully different types of mental retardation when looking at language development. Indeed, it is somewhat inaccurate to talk about "language development in the mentally retarded." Differing diagnostic groups will have differing *processes* which may be responsible for quite different developments during the acquisition of language.

The following is a descriptive review of the literature. The quality of the experimental procedures and interpretations is sometimes questionable, as will be pointed out.

STUDIES GIVING EVIDENCE OF DELAY IN RETARDATE LANGUAGE

It has often been remarked that a characteristic of mental retardation is that the developmental processes are the same as in normal children but that they proceed at a slower rate. Karlin and Strazzulla (1952), for example, studied 50 retarded children living at home. They divided their sample into three IQ range groups: those with an IQ of 15–25; those in the range 26–50; and a group with IQs of 51–70. With increasingly lower IQ they found an increased delay in the appearance of several developmental milestones including the age of first sitting and first walking. General indications of linguistic development also showed delay. The mean age of the first occurrence of babbling, single word utterances, and sentences was increasingly greater with lower IQ.

Lennenberg, Nichols, and Rosenberger (1964) made a 3-year study of 61 Down's syndrome children aged 3–22 years who were living at home. Using the stages "mostly babble," "mostly words," "primitive phrases," and "sentences" on which to rate each child, they found that it was not IQ that best predicted language development, but chronological age and the passing of particular motor milestones. Furthermore, in imitation tests, the Down's syndrome children performed like younger normal children. These findings were interpreted as supporting the notion that language acquisition depends on the development of the central nervous system. Before a certain degree of maturation, the child is unable to make use of particular aspects of language input. A mother's efforts to teach the child to say words before that time will be of no avail. Once the child has reached a certain maturational level, he will learn many different words. In other words, Down's syndrome children are slower in their maturational development and are thus slower in their language acquisition. Lenneberg *et al.* concluded from their study that Down's syndrome children are arrested at primitive but normal stages of language development and that they do not evidence bizarre language behavior.

Normal but developmentally delayed language stages are reported in other retardates as well. Graham and Graham (1971) studied nine retarded children living in a residential facility. This sample was composed of four children diagnosed as encephalopaths, two as cultural-familial retardates, two with congenital cerebral deficit, and one of uncertain classification. These children were 10–15 years old with IQs from 26 to 64. Their mental ages were 3:6–10:0 years. The Grahams collected conversational data and submitted this to a linguistic analysis in which they wrote the underlying strings of the utterances and the elementary transformations (*e.g.,* addition, deletion, substitution) and generalized transformations (those acting on two or more underlying strings to produce a single derived structure) that were used by each child. They found a trend from lower mental age children producing sentences containing base string rules only and few or no transformations, to higher mental aged children using three or more transformations. The Spearman rank-difference correlations between mental age and such factors as percentage of sentences containing no transformations, percentage of sentences containing three or more transformations, and the average number of transformations used, were all in the 0.90's. The average sentence length also steadily increased with mental age (MA) from 3.8 lexical items at MA 3:6 to 8.0 lexical items at MA 10:0. The use of more generalized transformations also increased with mental age. From the linguistic analysis, the Grahams concluded that non-Down's syndrome retardates develop the rules of language at a slower rate but in much the same way as normal children.

Byrne's study (1959) of both athetoid and spastic cerebral palsied children again found delayed but normal development. Although she found that the 74 children in her population were seriously retarded on the accuracy of consonants, they had nevertheless developed earliest those sounds which also appear first in normal children. On other language features, the cerebral palsied children also showed delay. In general, they were about 3 months behind normals in their use of single words, about 1 year behind in their use of two-word sentences, and about 4 years behind in using three-word sentences. These children, then, were delayed, but Byrne found that their language and articulatory skills followed the same sequential pattern as is observed in normal children.

Probably the most linguistically sophisticated study yet carried out on the language behavior of retarded children is that by Lackner (1968). He collected productive language samples from five retarded children, all diagnosed as suffering from congenital or early acquired encephalopathy. These children lived in the MIT clinical research center for 8 weeks and were recorded three times a day. Randomly selecting 1000 sentences for each child, Lackner proceeded to write the transformational phrase structure grammars for these five retarded children. His findings show that sentence length, measured in words, increased with mental age and was the same as for normal children at that mental age. Structurally, there was a regularity in the order of appearance of sentence types as mental age increased. Furthermore, a given sentence type was found only if all sentence types of a lower complexity were also found. Phrase structure rules became more differentiated and specific with increasing mental age. Lackner also noted that none of the structures generated by the rules was incompatible with normal adult usage. Each phrase structure grammar, at each increasing mental age, seemed to be a subset of the grammar at the next level of complexity.

The same children were also given tests of imitation and comprehension. Lackner found that the *number* of transformations which were understood, as well as the number of transformations used, increased with mental age. In addition, the *types* of transformations and their combinations also increased with mental age. These children, like normal children, could imitate and comprehend sentences constructed from their own vocabulary which corresponded to the sentence types used in their own spontaneous speech, but they could not understand or imitate sentences of more advanced types. Lackner concluded that retardation had not resulted in a different form of language behavior. The language of normal and retarded children was not qualitatively different. Both groups followed similar developmental trends. However, severely retarded children may become arrested in their language development and consequently remain at a lower stage of normal development.

There have been a few studies on subnormals which have focused primarily on comprehension. For example, Lovell and Dixon (1967) administered a version of the Fraser, Bellugi, and Brown test of imitation, comprehension, and production (1963) to 80 educationally subnormal (ESN) children—40 subjects each at ages 6 and 7. In Britain, a child is classified as ESN if he is not able to keep up with normal schooling and is about 2 years behind in his school subjects. This usually means an IQ in the range of 50–70. Lovell and Dixon's two age groups had mean IQs of 61–66. In addition, 100 normal children were also tested—20 each at ages 2, 3, 4, 5, and 6. They found, as Fraser, *et al.* had observed in normal children only, that for all their groups, including the retarded children, imitation was always in advance of comprehension, which was always in advance of production for all 10 grammatical types tested. Furthermore, the 6-year-old ESN children performed almost exactly like 3-year-old normal children. Seven-year-old ESN children performed like 4-year-old normals. These findings, then, again support the notion of developmental delay.

Some studies have made use of Berko's test of morphology (Berko, 1958). Newfield and Schlanger (1968) compared normals and subnormals on the acquisition of morphological rules in this manner. They found that the order of acquisition of the allomorphs used in morphological constructions was very similar for the two groups. Children in both groups had mastered the most regular and common allomorphs first. In other words, retarded children learn morphology in a manner comparable to normal children. The learning pace is slower, but the differences are merely quantitative rather than qualitative. Another aspect of their findings was that both groups did better on supplying the morphological inflections to real words than to nonsense words. For example, children found it easier to supply the plural "glasses" for the singular "glass," than to supply "tasses" for the nonsense word "tass." Furthermore, the retarded were less able to generalize from the familiar words to the new (nonsense) words than were the normals. Dever and Gardner (1970) independently obtained the same results. However, they noted that the incorrect responses by the retarded children to the nonsense words often consisted in merely repeating the test word, *e.g.,* they would simply say "wug" instead of "two wugs." But Dever and Gardner also noted that the retarded children could and did produce the morphemes correctly in their spontaneous conversation. Thus, their lack of generalization might have been due to lack of knowledge of what was expected in the test situation or to unknown factors inherent in the use of nonsense words.

Lovell and Bradbury (1967) had also used the Berko test on 160 ESN children in England in groups ranging in age from 8 to 15. The over-all mean IQ of these children was 70. Comparing their results to Berko's results on normal children, they found that the 14- and 15-year-old ESN children performed more poorly than Berko's normal children of about age 6. At that time, Lovell and Bradbury speculated that the ESN children suffered from a relative failure to use a universal rule and to generate the morphological endings to new words, and that they would therefore have to learn more of the specific endings of words than normal children who would more readily apply generalized rules to new words. This interpretation was open to doubt on several grounds. For example, as we will see later on, there is evidence that even severely subnormal children are capable of generalization (O'Connor and Hermelin, 1963), and the ESN children in the Lovell and Bradbury study are only mildly retarded. Furthermore, there is no evidence that linguistic rules are less generalized in the spontaneous speech of these children. Informal observation even suggests that some language errors arise from incorrect overgeneralization of particular rules. In any case, Bradbury and Lunzer (1972) decided to submit the problem to closer analysis.

In the later experiment, 18 ESN children of chronological age 9:0–10:0 and 18 normal children of chronological age 6:0–7:0 were used. Various subgroups had to learn one of three morphological rules (plural, past tense, or possessive) marked by a nonsense particle attached to 10 nonsense words. In some groups, the rule was "universal," meaning (in their terminology) merely that all 10 words were followed by the same nonsense particle to mark the grammatical feature. Another subgroup had to learn a "dichotomous" rule in which 5 of the words were marked with one suffix and 5 were marked with a different suffix. This is analogous, for example, to plurals in written English where one adds either -s or -es to the singular. (Spoken English, of course, has three, not two forms.) Finally, a third subgroup learned an "arbitrary" rule in which all 10 nonsense words had a different suffix to mark the grammatical feature. The results showed that the number of trials required to learn the universally applied rule was significantly less than for the other two types of rules. The other two types were equally difficult to learn. Both required about twice as many trials as the universally applied type. More significant, however, was the fact that these results were identical for both the ESN and the normal groups of children. Bradbury and Lunzer concluded that the earlier hypothesis was wrong. Educationally subnormal children are capable of learning the linguistic rule. However, a transfer task to 30 new items presented only once was also given. Here, the subnormals were less successful than the normals. This is puzzling since the original learning task was itself a kind of transfer task. The experimenters speculated that it may possibly be due to something in the nature of the one-trial method, or perhaps that the subnormal children, when faced with a new task, were less ready to search through and use strategies available to them.

In summary, the most usual finding from the various studies using Berko-type tests is that the acquisition of language features by retarded children is basically the same as that by children of normal intelligence, but at a slower pace. In addition, there has been the suggestion by some experimenters that the retarded do not generalize these rules quite as readily as do normal children, at least when nonreal words or items have been used.

STUDIES GIVING EVIDENCE OF DIFFERENCES IN RETARDATE LANGUAGE

Substandard but Normal Processes

The notion that some processes which are essential in the acquisition of language, though not lacking in retarded children, may nevertheless be far less utilized by them, means that one would expect to find divergences from normal children either in the eventually resulting language or in the use to which language is put. There are many studies on the use of language as a mediating function. For example, in recognition experiments, even when it can be shown that severely subnormal children have the ability to assign verbal labels, they may be relatively handicapped in forming such verbal connections spontaneously when they are paying attention to objects (Bryant, 1965, 1967; also see review by Bryant, 1970). When they were *forced* to verbalize, however, Bryant found that differences between normals and subnormals disappeared. Bryant argued that the severely subnormal suffer from a restriction of attention unless verbal labeling is introduced. Moreover, Morris (1972, in press), in a number of carefully designed experiments, has shown that the benefit of verbalization is due not to mediational properties as such but solely to the increased attention to the stimulus material which results from the enforced verbal labeling. It would be in this sense, then, that normals and subnormals might differ, *i.e.*, in the *use* to which they put language.

Our main concern in this review, however, will be in processes which might lead to differing linguistic outcomes during the child's development. One possible clue to these processes might lie in any differences observed in subnormals and matched mental age normals. Spreen (1965) reviewed a number of studies which led to the conclusion that retardates evidence a small lag in such measures as sentence length, sentence complexity, discrimination of speech sounds, and percentage of nouns used, as compared to matched mental age normals. But the retardates were superior in vocabulary size. Bartel, Bryen, and Keehn (1973), however, did not find this superiority over normals in a group of retarded trainable pupils attending special education classes. There was no difference between these children and matched mental age normals in the use of lexical items. But the retarded group was inferior in the use of grammatical categories.

Other studies have also found that subnormals lag behind their mental age counterparts in their use of particular grammatical features. Semmel, Barritt, and Bennett (1970) administered a Cloze task consisting of various grammatical structures to groups of institutionalized and noninstitutionalized educable mentally retarded (EMR) children and to two groups of normal children—one matched for chronological age and the other matched for mental age with EMR children. There were 20 children in each group. The mean IQ of the EMR children was about 70. In the task, a tone was presented in the place of the missing word. The child had to provide a missing word in order to "make good sense." Both groups of EMR children had significantly lower scores than the two normal groups on the ability to give grammatical, meaningful sentences. These experimenters interpreted their results as showing that the retarded children were not merely suffering from a simple time lag, but that they had a greater difficulty on the Cloze task than would be predicted from their mental age. One can note, however, in these results, that both the EMR and normal children evidenced similar trends on the same grammatical form classes. For example, all children found the noun slots easiest to fill, and all found verbs to be the most difficult. In general, then, the findings would appear to argue merely for an especially greater lag rather than for grammatical differences, although it was noted by the authors that deleted adjectives were particularly difficult for the institutionalized EMR children. There is also some problem in interpreting these results in that the errors made by

EMR children were mainly of a type which was categorized as "nongrammatical and nonmeaningful." They did not make significantly more responses which were called "nongrammatical, meaningful," which might have been expected if the test were truly tapping only grammatical ability.

Carlton and Carlton (1945), in a much earlier study of the oral language of mentally defective adolescents, provided some evidence that there are true grammatical differences to be found. They collected speech samples from 61 institutionalized subnormals (mean IQ 59.6); 80 noninstitutionalized subnormals (mean IQ 67.5); and a group of normal children matched on mental age, sex, and socioeconomic status (mean IQ 101). Although they used a notion of correctness based on a conception of how language ought to be spoken according to prescriptive grammars, one can nevertheless sift from their data those utterances which would be considered errors in the sense currently used by linguists. What is of interest is that Carlton and Carlton found seven errors (of which at least three would be considered errors in the modern sense as well) made by both groups of defectives which were not observed in any normal child. This would appear to support the notion that possible process differences have led to a different end result observable in language differences between adolescent subnormals and their matched mental age peers. However, we do not know from the Carlton and Carlton study whether the errors made by the subnormals and not found in the normal children would in fact be found in normal children of a lower mental age. That is, we cannot be sure whether the grammars of these children were different or whether the subnormal children were merely more greatly retarded in their language development than would be indicated by their mental age.

A similar problem occurs when we try to interpret the interesting results reported by Sinclair (see Sinclair-de-Zwart, 1969) on the comprehension abilities of a group of adolescent severely retarded children (IQ 50 and below). The child's task was to carry out actions which the experimenter described. Sometimes the experimenter used the linguistic patterns used by normal operational stage children (as defined by Piagetian tasks), and sometimes the linguistic patterns of normal nonoperational children were used. When the descriptive terms used by normal nonconserving children were used, e.g., *"Donne beaucoup à la fille, et peu au garcon"* (Give a lot to the girl and a little to the boy), the severely retarded children were able to carry out the action correctly and consistently. However, when the experimenter used the descriptive patterns of normal conserving children, e.g., *"Donne plus à la poupee-fille, moins au garcon"* (Give more to the little girl, less to the boy), the retarded children were incapable of carrying out the actions consistently. The way this result differs from that found with nonretarded children is that normal nonoperational children *could* understand the linguistic patterns of operational children in the comprehension task, with the exception of a few 4-year-olds. It would appear that the nonoperational severely retarded children were more deficient than the nonoperational normal children. However, based solely on the reported data, such a conclusion is not warranted. We are not given the mental ages of the retarded children but are merely told that they had IQs of 50 or below and had chronological ages of 8–15. It was also noted that the youngest normals (the 4-year-olds) also failed in comprehending instructions couched in the terminology of operational children. Therefore, it may be that the subnormal children were not behaving differently from normal children, but merely behaving like the youngest normals. And this may have been because the subnormals were of a similar mental age to those youngest children, or, if they were of a higher mental age than 4:0 years, that they were more greatly retarded than their mental age would indicate.

So far, two major types of findings have been reviewed. First, there were a number of studies which seemed to give evidence that in some instances of subnormality, language development was normal but merely delayed. The second group of studies, however, provided some evidence that the language processes of subnormals may be slightly different from that of nonretarded children, since the resulting language they produce or the language features they are able to comprehend may be excessively retarded beyond what would be expected based on matched mental age samples. Before turning to studies which seem to indicate that major *differences* in language acquisition processes may occur in specific types of subnormality, it will be necessary to take a slight digression into the problem of the influence of *nonlinguistic* cognitive processes on language acquisition.

Cognitive Explanations and Their Limitations

Piagetian theory has emphasized the importance of the developing cognitive abilities of the child (Piaget, 1970a,b; Piaget and Inhelder, 1969). In Piaget's view, language is dependent on and shaped by underlying cognitive structures, and it reflects the thought processes made possible by those structures at different stages of development. It has even been argued that the appearance of language at about the age of 18 months and not sooner is due to its dependence on the cognitive structures achieved during the sensorimotor period. Hermine Sinclair (1971), a linguist working in the Piagetian framework, has argued, for example, that it is only at the end of the sensorimotor period that the child has reached the stage where he is cognitively able to differentiate himself as an active person distinct from the objects he acts upon. This presumably gives rise to the conscious need for communication. In addition, other sensorimotor schemata are said to account for corresponding linguistic abilities observed in language acquisition. For example, Sinclair claimed that the ability to classify actions must be developed before the categorization of linguistic elements into major categories such as noun phrase or verb phrase is possible. The sensorimotor ability to order things both spatially and temporally permits a linguistic counterpart, namely concatenation of these linguistic elements into structured phrases. The newly developed ability to relate objects and actions to one another is the cognitive condition necessary for the development of such functional grammatical relations as "subject of" and "object of." In other words, it is only at the end of the period of sensorimotor development that, to use Sinclair's words, "the child possesses a set of coordinations of action-schemes which can be shown to have certain structural properties which will make it possible for him to start comprehending and producing language" (Sinclair, 1971, p. 127).

If these assertions can be shown to be true, then the implications for language development in the severely retarded are obvious. Unless the child possesses the cognitive structures attained by children of normal intelligence at the end of the sensorimotor period of development, language intervention programs would be of little benefit.

In addition to these earliest processes, later developing cognitive abilities appear to determine what the child can comprehend and produce in language. For example, Slobin (1966) found that the emergence of the conditional in Russian-speaking children was somewhat later than might be expected given the ease with which hypotheticals are linguistically formed in that language. He speculated that the cognitive complexity of the meaning of that linguistic form accounted for its late emergence. Similar results have been found for a number of linguistic features related to complex temporal notions (Cromer, 1968). For example, before the child has the ability to decenter temporally, from one point of view in time to another, he does not use entire categories of both lexical items and grammatical structures. These categories, which include such notions as "timelessness," "hypotheticalness," and "relevance" of one time to another (e.g., as is often expressed by the perfect tenses in English), appear to become operative at about the age of 4½ years. Before this age, the child has some linguistic forms which he uses, however, only in a limited way to express the meanings of which he is capable. On the other hand, after certain cognitive changes have occurred, he uses these old forms to express the newer meanings, and, in addition, he begins to acquire other more advanced forms which code the newer meanings. Slobin (1973) has developed this notion of the cognitive prerequisites for the acquisition of grammar and has provided a good deal of linguistic evidence in support of it, much of it from non-European as well as European languages. Roger Brown (1973) has presented evidence that the first grammatical distinctions the child makes with verbs are those which encode the types of meaning he is credited by adults with expressing with his uninflected verbs just prior to the acquisition of these new linguistic forms. Indeed, a substantial number of studies indicate that many aspects of language acquisition depend on the development of particular cognitive operations which make certain meanings possible. (See Cromer, 1974b, for a review of such studies.) Again, if these hypotheses are correct, one would not expect subnormals with lower mental ages than those at which such cognitive abilities appear in normal children to be able to comprehend or produce linguistic forms which express meanings dependent on those abilities.

The importance of both cognition and meaning in determining language features has been stressed by a number of recent theories. In Fillmore's (1968) case theory of grammar, for example, underlying meanings play a primary role. McCawley (1968) suggested a specifically semantic deep structure as opposed to the grammatical one proposed by Chomsky (1957, 1965). Schlesinger (1971a,b) has put forward a theory taking into account the speaker's intentions, and these are based on cognitive capacities. However, while many studies and the recent theories to which they have given rise point to specific cognitive developments as *necessary* prerequisites for the acquisition of language or of particular grammatical forms, one must also ask whether such cognitive developments are *sufficient* to explain those acquisitions. There is some evidence that they are not.

This point has already been put forward by Brown (1970). He argued that the grammatical relations of language are defined by linguists in purely formal terms. In early child speech, these formal relations may be more or less perfectly coordinated with semantic rules, but the two are not the same. Some striking evidence for this assertion has come only recently from an experiment carried out by Hughes (1972, to appear) in England.

Hughes, under the direction of Dr. Neil O'Connor at the Medical Research Council, was investigating the communication abilities of children who had been diagnosed as receptive aphasics. These children have normal intelligence as measured by nonverbal tests, but they are unable to acquire language in spite of intensive efforts to achieve this in special schools over a period of years. Hughes decided to use materials similar to those used by Premack (1969) to teach chimpanzees to communicate. She constructed a number of magnetic-backed, meaningless shapes to serve as symbols which could be manipulated on magnetic boards. Through the use of gestures coupled with some reinforcement for correct choices, she was able to teach children to use the shapes as signs for particular objects. In addition she was able to teach verbs such as "give" and "point to," and finally she taught them a number of language functions, including direct and indirect objects, negation, modifiers, and questions. Children not only understood the system in a number of generalization tests but were able to manipulate the shapes so as to produce "utterances." These children were able to acquire rapidly the language functions taught in twice-weekly, half-hour sessions over a total period of only 10 weeks. Thus, their ability to understand and even communicate such functions was unimpaired. But they were not able even to comprehend the basic grammatical relations in language. We do not know why aphasic children are unable to acquire language. Probably there are many reasons, and no doubt these vary from one individual to another. But there is also the possibility that at least in some of these children there is some impairment of a specifically linguistic mechanism of the type Chomsky would hold is innate in human individuals.

While cognitive operations of particular types can be shown to be a necessary prerequisite for the acquisition of language in general or for the acquisition of particular grammatical features, there may be something more specifically linguistic which is also necessary for language acquisition to occur. In other words, the possession of a sensorimotor intelligence cannot in itself explain the *expression* of that intelligence in language. When examining some of the impaired processes found in different types of subnormality, it will be of interest to keep this in mind. Some groups may suffer from an impairment of one type of cognitive process or another while other groups of subnormals may lack language altogether because of more specific linguistic handicaps.

Language Impairment due to Different Processes

In order to look at what effects some of the different cognitive processes may have on language acquisition, we can first look at a study not of retarded children, but of adult aphasics. Unlike the developmental aphasics in the Hughes study, however, these were normal speaking adults until brain damage resulted in their aphasia. In adults, the site of damage determines the nature of the aphasia. For example, in Wernicke's aphasia, in which there has been damage to the posterior temporal lobe, the patient often appears to be grammatically fluent, but his words lack semantic relationship. By contrast, the language of aphasics suffering from a frontal lesion in Broca's area is characterized by a loss of grammatical structure. These patients retain meaningful words but no longer mark them grammatically. (Such neurological findings, incidentally, lend credence to a Chomskian type of linguistic analysis which treats grammar and semantics as separate entities.)

Myerson and Goodglass (1972) applied a transformational grammatical analysis to the language of three Broca's aphasics: a 30-year-old college-educated man, a 54-year-old woman factory worker said to have "a seventh grade education," and a 28-year-old man with 2 years of college. These three patients were differentially impaired with the first mentioned, the 30-year-old, being the most severely impaired, and the 28-year-old, the least. The grammatical analysis given by Myerson and Goodglass will be of interest for linguists and psycholinguists since it may give some hints concerning elements to look for and blind alleys to avoid in normal language analysis. For example, they found that the use of intonation was independent of the ability of the individual to use syntax for the expression of ideas. For our purposes, however, I want to focus on one result. This grammatical analysis of patients with differing degrees of impairment revealed that the limitations paralleled the order of acquisition by the child. There was an inverse correlation between the severity of the aphasia and the number of specific types of distinctions that could be made in the base component, as well as in the number and types of rules which were used to generate surface structures. Furthermore, the number of base-generated constituents which could actually be expressed in any utterance decreased with increasing impairment. This number increased over time, however, as a patient improved. This, too, reminds one of similar developmental observations in normal children acquiring language.

Bloom (1970) made a convincing case for a cognitive limitation on production of utterances by the child. The interpretation of children's utterances in conjunction with a situational analysis revealed that children organize linguistic categories in a hierarchical structure such that they can add categories without increasing sentence length. Bloom postulated a "reduction transformation" by which the child is able to delete some categories while adding or expanding others. She gave several examples from her data in which a child made a number of consecutive utterances demonstrating the child's capacity simultaneously to delete some elements during expansion of others so as to remain within his "production limit." For example, whenever the subject of a sentence was expressed, either the verb, the object, the adverbial phrase, or more than one of these was omitted.

Other investigators have found evidence for a cognitive deficit in the processing of language rather than in its production, or more precisely, the deficits of production found in some language-deviant groups may be traceable to impoverished mechanisms responsible for comprehension. This is, of course, in contrast to Bloom's normal children, who were demonstrated to have an understanding of the grammatical relationships but a limitation in production capacity which prevented their fully extended expression. For example, Menyuk (1964, 1969) studied a group of children aged 3:0–5:11 who had been labeled as "infantile" in their use of language. She studied both their spontaneous speech and their responses in a repetition task which had also been administered to young normal speaking children. She found that at any level throughout the age range, the syntactic structures used by the language-deviant group did not match the structures used by normal speaking younger children. These children were using deviant rather than "infantile" (i.e., delayed) language. Furthermore, the repetition task revealed significant differences between the groups. For normal speaking children, structure, not sentence length, determined whether or not a sentence was accurately repeated. Even with sentences of up to nine words in length for children as young as 3 years of age, length was not a factor which determined successful repetition. The correlation between sentence length and its nonrepetition was only 0.04. By contrast, the correlation for the language-deviant group was 0.53. Furthermore, the types of mistakes made in this task revealed that sentence length was an important factor for these children. The omissions they made were almost invariably of the first part of the sentence, whereas the last things heard were the most frequently recalled. The errors by normal speaking children, on the other hand, were mainly modifications of trans-formational structure. Menyuk also noted that the language-deviant children had a poorer auditory memory than normal speakers. Their short term memory for utterances of only three to five morphemes in length was severely limited. Menyuk speculated that if a child could not keep an utterance of more than two or three morphemes in his short term memory, he would be severely limited in being able to carry out a deepening linguistic analysis of the language. This would result in his having impoverished, limited, and in some cases even different hypotheses and rules concerning language.

In England, Graham has been conducting research on educationally sub-normal children using a similar hypothesis about the effects of a short term memory limitation on language (Graham, 1968, in press; Graham and Gulli-ford, 1968). He has found, for example, that both repetition and comprehen-sion scores on sentences increase regularly with short term memory measured by random words and digits. Relating the notion of short term memory to the amount of computation required by sentences of varying syntactic complexity, Graham interpreted the results he obtained as evidence that children are unable to process sentences that make demands on short term memory which are beyond their capacity.

It would appear, then, that among the cognitive factors which affect language acquisition, limitations of a "production span" and of short term memory would be significant. Bloom's evidence supports the notion that younger children are limited in the amount they can produce in a single utterance. Menyuk and Graham have shown the importance of limited short term memory on the comprehension of language and thus also on its produc-tion by younger normal children, language-deviant groups, and educationally subnormal children. But such limitations are not the only ones possible. Graham, for example, in a personal communication, noted that the correla-tion between comprehension and the ability to repeat a sentence was still significant when short term memory effects were partialed out. Lee (1966) made a study of children who were called "language-delayed." She also found that these children were not merely following the natural pattern of develop-ment at a slower rate. She found instead that the language-deviant child fails to make some of the linguistic generalizations upon which syntactic develop-ment depends. For example, normal children use designative and predicative constructions from the two-word level, *e.g.,* "there ducks," "really hungry." But the language-deviant child does not use such constructions, according to Lee. What is important to note is that this difference is claimed to be occurring even at the two-word level, that is, at a level which would be assumed to be within both the short term memory capacity and the "produc-tion span capacity" of the language-deviant child. There are a number of studies of other groups whose language disabilities cannot be due to limita-tions of this type. One such group is severely subnormal autistic children.

Autistic children, of course, show the characteristic from which the condition takes its name, namely, extreme withdrawal and failure to relate to other persons. In addition, these children have a tendency to stereotyped and ritualistic forms of behavior, motor mannerisms, inappropriate responses to sensory stimuli, and language impairment or complete lack of speech. Indeed, the most frequently noted feature of this condition is the severe language impairment. Hermelin and O'Connor (1970) provide the best scientific description of autistic children, along with a number of experiments which examined their mental processes, including studies of their deficiencies in perception, language, coding, seriation, and recall. Although autism can occur at any intelligence level, most reports show a strong link with subnormality, and most autistic children have IQs below 60. Owing to their language impairment, autistic children have sometimes been confused with or compared to developmentally aphasic children. However, Bartak and Rutter (in press) have provided a useful study in which it was shown that the two groups can be reliably differentiated and present entirely different kinds of language impairment. For example, children in the autistic group showed significantly greater I-you pronoun reversal, echolalia, steretoyped utterances, and inappropriate remarks than the aphasic children.

There is recent evidence that autistic children differ even in their cries from normal children and from other subnormal children. Ricks (1972, in press) compared the cries of these groups. The normal children were 8–12 months of age. The autistic children were 3–5 years of age, as were the matched nonautistic subnormal children. First, under controlled conditions, Ricks elicited four types of messages from each child: a frustrated sound, a requesting sound, a greeting sound, and a sound expressing pleased surprise (*e.g.,* the sound made when a novel and exciting event occurred). This was done by setting up real situations which stimulated the child to produce the appropriate "message." The cries thus elicited were tape-recorded. Special tapes were then made by appropriate splicing so that the following experiment could be conducted. Six parents of normal children and six parents of autistic children each listened to the tape-recorded sounds of four babies. Since each child made four sounds, each parent had 16 sounds to identify, but of course, the sounds were presented in random order. Parents of a normal child heard their own baby, two other normal English babies, and one non-English baby. Parents of autistic children heard their own child, two other autistic children, and one nonautistic retarded child of the same age. The parents were given four tasks: 1) they had to identify and label all 16 sounds, 2) they had to identify their own child, 3) the parents of normal children had to identify which child was the non-English child, while the parents of autistic children had to identify the nonautistic subnormal child, 4) the parents heard the request sounds of six babies and had to pick out their own child from among these. The results showed that parents of normal children could easily identify the messages, but to their great surprise they could not pick out their own child. In addition, they correctly identified the messages of the non-English child but could not pick out which child was non-English. By contrast, the parents of autistic children could only identify the messages of their own child and could easily tell which child was their own. They could, in addition, identify the messages of the nonautistic retarded child, but they could not identify the cries of the other autistic children. Two things are noteworthy from these results. First, the retarded, autistic children do not seem to use the vocabulary of intonated signals used by normal children and instead have their own distinctive cries. By contrast, the cries of normal children have a marked similarity and these signals seem to be independent of language background. Second, the nonautistic retarded children evidenced normal cries which could be identified by adults.

At a later age, too, autistic children show differences in processes underlying language, and it is here that we see that a limitation of memory span cannot be the causative factor. It has been demonstrated that the number of units or "bits" of information that can be retained in the span of immediate memory by an individual can be increased by recoding these bits into larger units or "chunks" (Miller, 1956). One method of doing this is to make use of syntactic structure. People are able to retain in their immediate memory many more words than would be indicated by digit span tests if these words form grammatical sentences. Many subnormal autistic children, including those who have some speech, appear to lack this ability to make use of syntactic structure. One study of this deficiency is by Frith (see Aurnhammer-Frith, 1969). She studied 16 autistic children, using only those who had some speech. These children had a mean chronological age of 11:6. A comparison group of 16 normal children (mean chronological age 4:3) was matched to the autistic group on digit span. In addition, the groups were of comparable mental age (4:9 and 3:11) as measured by the Peabody Picture Vocabulary Test. The task in Frith's experiment was to repeat messages of various controlled lengths, some of which were grammatical and meaningful sentences while others consisted of words merely strung together in random order. The results showed that normal children greatly benefited from sentence structure, but the autistic children benefited significantly less. The significant differences on the structured sentences are especially striking when one recalls that the children in the two groups were prematched for digit span capacity.

Other groups of subnormals do not share this inability to profit from sentence structure. Hermelin and O'Connor (1967) directly compared 12 subnormal autistic children and 12 severely subnormal nonautistic children matched on the basis of their immediate memory span for digits and on scores from the Peabody Picture Vocabulary Test. The severely subnormal children were a heterogeneous group but no Down's syndrome children, epileptics, or children with obvious sensorimotor dysfunction were included. The immediate recall task was to repeat words arranged either randomly or in sentences. The results showed that, while severely subnormal nonautistic children did significantly better with sentences than with random sequences, no significant difference was found with the autistic children.

It has also been noted that many autistic children have an immediate memory span equal to that of normal children. This is not true of other subnormal groups, who in general have an extremely short memory span (O'Connor and Frith, 1973). But the nonautistic subnormal children make use of sentence structure to increase the number of "bits" they can retain and are thus able to equal the performance of autistic children with greater memory spans since the autistic children do not increase the number of "bits" they retain under the structured sentences condition. It is apparent that the cognitive processes underlying language differ significantly in severely subnormal autistic children, other subnormal children, and children of normal intelligence. Are there other subgroups of subnormality which show specific deficits in the processes responsible for language?

LANGUAGE PROCESSES IN OTHER DIAGNOSTIC GROUPS

A major problem in studying any process in different subgroups of subnormals is that so small a proportion of mentally subnormal individuals is diagnosable at all. Richards (1970) has recently made a comprehensive compilation of specific conditions which are diagnosable by clinical examination and medical history. His list of 27 identifiable conditions includes such well known entities as cretinism, Down's syndrome, Laurence-Moon-Biedl syndrome, amaurotic family idiocy, and de Lange syndrome, as well as a number of lesser known and more recently differentiated conditions. A second problem is that it is often difficult to collect a large enough sample of some of these groups to make a meaningful study of the impaired processes. The few studies which are available tell us very little about language processes. They usually provide merely a description of the level of language attainment in general terms.

Garstecki, Borton, Stark, and Kennedy (1972) examined the language and speech of three children with Laurence-Moon-Biedl syndrome. One child's language was unintelligible. A second used sentences which were described by these authors merely as structurally and functionally incomplete. The third and oldest case (age 17 years) had some short sentences which were described as structurally incomplete. We are told only that the structural complexity of these sentences was below that of a normal 3-year-old.

Diedrich and Poser (1960) made a case study of two phenylketonuric children. During 3 years on a controlled phenylalanine-low diet, there was marked improvement in language, but again this is unspecified.

It has been speculated that in some groups, the language of subnormals may be superior on some measures to that found in normal children. For example, it has sometimes been reported that children with internal hydrocephaly are rather verbose and evidence fluent, adult-like speech usage, with a precocious vocabulary. To examine this, Fleming (1968) collected speech samples from 11 hydrocephalic children aged 4:0–8:1 with IQs ranging from 73 to 101. With a median IQ of 94, this group was of near normal intelligence. Their speech was compared to a control group of normal children matched for chronological age, IQ, sex, race, socioeconomic status, and school grade placement. The speech samples were all taken from the children's responses to an apperception test. Fleming found no evidence for verbosity in the hydrocephalic children, in either total number of responses, total number of words, or mean length of response. Indeed, the only significant difference which was found was that the hydrocephalic children had more inappropriate responses, such as situational conversation and unrelated responses. Fleming concluded that the hydrocephalic children give a false impression of verbosity because of their verbal spontaneity and social aggressiveness.

It has often been suggested that the language abilities of Down's syndrome children differ from those in other subnormal groups. Lyle (1960) found, for example, that the effects on language of institutionalization were greater on Down's syndrome children than on other retarded groups. Others, however, have disputed the notion that children with Down's syndrome differ in their language ability (Jordan, 1966; Evans and Hampson, 1968). Again, few studies have been directed at the underlying processes. There is, however, some recent experimental work comparing Down's syndrome children and non-Down's syndrome severely subnormal children with children of normal intelligence on the types of phonological rules they use. It is useful first to sketch a background to this recent work.

It is becoming increasingly accepted that the child does not merely imitate sounds. Rather, he produces them according to a systematic set of phonological contrasts. This position was put forward by Jakobson in 1941 (see Jakobson, 1968). Basically, his theory asserts that the infant discriminates features of sounds which are represented by phonological contrasts such as vocalic-nonvocalic, voiced-voiceless, nasal-oral, grave-acute, etc. As he grows older, the infant makes an increasing number of contrasts until he has identified all the sounds in the language on the basis of these distinguishing features. It is further claimed that these contrast rules appear in the child's productions in a constant order across various languages. Details of theories of this type can be found in Chomsky and Halle (1968), Jakobson (1968), Jakobson, Fant, and Halle (1952), and Jakobson and Halle (1956). A good short summary of this position is also available by Palermo in his chapter on language acquisition in Reese and Lipsitt (1970). In addition, it is possible to write sets of cooccurrence rules which describe the production and omission of sounds in particular phonological contexts. Smith (1973) has been making a longitudinal study of phonological acquisition in this light. He has elaborated a set of rules used and their change over time by a normal speaking child. Under his supervision, Dodd (unpublished manuscript) has been comparing the phonological rules of normal and Down's syndrome children (see Smith, in press). In one experiment, she compared 10 normal and 10 Down's syndrome children matched for mental age and social background, on their spontaneous and imitated naming of 50 pictures of familiar objects. The mental age range of these children was 2:3–4:9. She found that 23 phonological rules could be derived from the data of the normal children. These rules account for all "errors" made by the normals; that is, the rules were applied consistently by the normal children both within and across subjects. An example of these rules would be that [s] deletes preconsonantally so that "spoon" becomes "poon" in the child's version. Similarly, [l] and [r] are deleted postconsonantally so that "flower" becomes "fower," and "train" becomes "tain." Dodd found that the children with Down's syndrome used the same 23 rules, but they did so inconsistently, and many of their errors could not be accounted for by any phonological rules. Some of their errors consisted of repetition of one syllable of a word so that, for example, the child would say "denten" for "dentist" or "meta-meta-mato" for "tomato." In other cases there was reduction of words so that only vowels were uttered (*e.g.,* "e-e" for "elephant"). In still other cases there was complete deletion of consonant clusters (*e.g.,* "wi--ers" for "whiskers"). There were also many inconsistent sound substitutions. For example, [p] and [b] might be substituted for by [m], [f], [sh], [n], or [ch], by the same child. More recently, Dodd has tested a group of severely subnormal children matched with the Down's syndrome children and normals on mental age. Her results indicate that the non-Down's syndrome severely subnormals perform like mental age-matched normals. They follow the rules consistently whereas the Down's syndrome children did not. What might account for the differences in children with Down's syndrome?

O'Connor and Hermelin (1963) reviewed evidence from a number of experimental studies that Down's syndrome children differ from other subnormals in that they lack muscle tone. They hypothesized that this hypotonia might conceivably impair kinesthetic feedback. This cannot be the cause of the phonological differences between Down's syndrome children and normals in Dodd's experiment, however, since she also found that children with Down's syndrome made significantly fewer errors in imitation compared to their spontaneous utterances (whereas normals make the same number of errors on spontaneous and imitated trials). In other words, it is not that Down's syndrome children lack the ability to form these sounds. Lenneberg (1967) also found that children with Down's syndrome have the ability to imitate words better than they could produce them spontaneously.

Another possibility is that the Down's syndrome children are deficient in their ability to abstract and/or generalize rules. However, it should be noted that a good deal of the data on the children with Down's syndrome in Dodd's experiment could be accounted for in terms of the same 23 rules that normals used. Subnormals appear to have the ability to formulate language rules. One can recall, for example, the Newfield and Schlanger study (1968), cited earlier, that showed that subnormals learned morphological rules in a manner comparable to normal children, as seen in the Berko test of morphology. Furthermore, there have been a number of studies using reinforcement techniques to train mentally retarded children on various language rules such as the use of the plural morpheme (Guess, Sailor, Rutherford, and Baer, 1968; Guess, 1969; and Baer and Guess, 1971). These studies have included Down's syndrome children in their small samples. Since these children can be trained to give the proper response in the appropriate context, it must be assumed that they can perceive the morphological differences and can abstract the appropriate rule. In addition, these experimenters have demonstrated the ability of the children to generalize the plural rule to new instances. It would appear, then, unlikely that the performance by the Down's syndrome children in Dodd's experiment, *i.e.*, their production of so many utterances not in accordance with any phonological rules, was due to their inability to formulate or generalize such rules.

Yet another possibility is that the Down's syndrome children's performance may be due to a failure of long term motor programs. Crome and Stern (1967) noted that children with Down's syndrome have an abnormally small cerebellum, compared both to normal brains and to other parts of their own brain. Furthermore, the cerebellum is important in motor performance and motor learning. It may be, then, that Down's syndrome youngsters suffer from a deficit in their long term motor programs directly traceable to anatomical abnormalities. Frith and Frith (in press) have recently compared matched groups of children with Down's syndrome, autistic children, and normals on a simple tapping task and on the ability to track motorically on a pursuit rotor. They found that the Down's syndrome children had adequate eye and hand coordination and could initially perform the tracking task. However, unlike the other two groups, the youngsters with Down's syndrome did not improve their performance with rest periods. The Friths hypothesized that Down's syndrome children may be more dependent on visual and kinesthetic feedback, whereas normals are able to depend on more long term motor programs. This is also supported by the fact that children with Down's syndrome were also unable to increase the speed of their tapping. Presumably, increasing tapping speed may disrupt motor feedback. Dodd suggested that the same hypothesis may possibly account for her data. It will be recalled that the performance of Down's syndrome youngsters was superior on imitation to that on spontaneous utterances. Imitation may require only short term motor planning whereas production may require different and more long term plans. A deficit in this planning ability may be responsible for the large number of non-rule-governed phonological responses in the spontaneous naming of objects by the children with Down's syndrome.

These, of course, are hypotheses which attempt to explain the obtained results. For our purposes, what is more important are the results themselves which indicate that processes having some part to play in language acquisition may differ in Down's syndrome children, other subnormal subgroups, and children with unimpaired mental functioning. On the other hand, this review began with some evidence that at least some types of subnormals differ in their language abilities merely in terms of delay. However, if speculation concerning the possibility of a critical period for language acquisition in human beings is true, it may be that delay itself may lead to different processes being used for acquiring language.

DELAY ITSELF AS A FACTOR IN CAUSING DIFFERING PROCESSES

A series of recent experiments (Cromer, 1970, 1972a, b, 1974a) examined the acquisition of a particular linguistic structure as it relates to the language acquisition process. This structure, first studied by Chomsky (1969), is the one usually rendered by linguists as the contrast pair "John is *eager* to please" and "John is *easy* to please." In the first, the adult English speaker knows that "John" is the actor. He does the pleasing. In the second sentence, however, the native speaker knows that "John" serves as the patient; someone else pleases him. Such sentences often serve as examples that the surface features of sentences we hear do not define the basic grammatical relations and are therefore unable to provide the information necessary for adequate comprehension. However, if the listener recovers an abstract representation of the sentence which displays properties which define the basic grammatical relations (the deep structure), appropriate comprehension becomes possible (see, *e.g.,* Bever, Fodor, and Weksel, 1965a, b; McNeill, 1970a, b; Miller and McNeill, 1969; and Wanner, 1968). How this knowledge is acquired has received little experimental attention.

I have been using a series of sentences of this type which encode the actions a child is to carry out with two hand-puppets—one the head of a duck and the other the head of a wolf. In a warm-up session the child is shown that either animal can bite the other, and he carries out these actions with the puppets. He is then given a series of sentences, and he demonstrates his comprehension of these by carrying out the action corresponding to his interpretation. Take, for example, the following sentences:

The duck is *keen* to bite.
The wolf is *tasty* to bite.
The duck is *easy* to bite.
The wolf is *willing* to bite.
The wolf is *hard* to bite.
The duck is *glad* to bite.
The duck is *fun* to bite.

These sentences have an identical ordering of elements. The only clue for the proper interpretation (recovery of correct deep structure) is in the adjective which is used. For ease in discussing this structure, adjectives like "happy," "keen," "willing," and "glad," which when used in the space indicate that the deep structure subject is the same as the surface structure subject and that it is the named animal who does the biting, have been labeled S-adjectives. Adjectives like "tasty," "easy," "hard," and "fun," which indicate that the other or nonnamed animal does the biting, have been called O-adjectives. There are also adjectives like "bad," "nice," and "nasty," which are ambiguous in this structure in that either deep structure interpretation is possible when they are used. They depend for their interpretation on the situational context. The eight sentences just cited use unambiguous S- and O-adjectives, and when adults are asked to perform this task they do so without difficulty (Cromer, 1974a). Children do not acquire adult competence on this structure until rather late—about 10 years of age. There are various stages in their acquisition.

In the earliest stage, or what I have called the "primitive rule" stage, the child always shows the named animal as doing the biting. He thereby gets all S-adjectives correct but consistently misinterprets O-adjectives. At the same time, however, he correctly shows the nonnamed animal to be doing the biting if a passive sentence is used, such as "The wolf was bitten." Thus, it is not the case that the child thinks he must show the named animal as doing the biting. Rather, he is not yet aware that with this particular surface structure, various deep structures are recoverable depending on which adjective is used. By mental age 6:3 as measured on the Peabody Picture Vocabulary Test, the child has entered the intermediate stage. The child has somehow come to the realization that various interpretations are possible, but he has not yet learned which adjectives indicate which deep structure. He therefore makes many errors, sometimes treating an S-adjective as an O-adjective and *vice versa*. Furthermore, he is very inconsistent from one day to the next, getting right some sentences he previously performed incorrectly, but also missing some he had interpreted correctly only 1 day before. Finally, at about chronological age 9 or 10, he seems to reorganize his categorization of English adjectives and he performs all sentences correctly in the adult manner. Educationally subnormal children pass through the same stages. They too no longer use the primitive rule for interpreting all sentences after mental age 6:3. And several years later, at about chronological age 14, 15, and 16 years, these children suddenly become able to comprehend sentences of this type in the normal adult manner.

There are, then, two aspects to the acquisition of this structure. First, there is the realization that various interpretations are possible depending on which word is used in the space. This realization marks the end of the primitive rule stage. Second, the child must now learn the structural properties of each adjective in order to determine which deep structure to recover. I have focused my attention on the second aspect and have conducted a number of experiments to see how the learning of structural properties of these adjectives might occur. I hypothesized that children might learn which were the S-adjectives and which were the O-adjectives by hearing them in related transformations. That is, some transformations allow S-adjectives but do not allow O-adjectives; others allow O-adjectives but exclude S-adjectives. A simple contrast pair illustrates this concretely. Take the S-adjective "glad" and the O-adjective "fun." The former can be used in frames such as "I'm always *glad* to read to you," but the latter cannot. "I'm always *fun* to read to you" is ungrammatical. Conversely, the frame, "Reading to you is _____" allows O-adjectives but excludes S-adjectives: "Reading to you is *fun*" is a grammatical sentence, but "Reading to you is *glad*" is not. In various learning experiments, nonsense words were presented to children in these related transformational frames which structurally differentiated the two types of adjectives. Then, the same nonsense words were used in the test structure, "The wolf is _____ to bite" to see if the child had been able to learn the structural properties from the related transformations. In these experiments, some children performed by using certain response strategies and it is on these strategies that I want to concentrate here. A response strategy was inferred whenever a child answered an entire set of test sentences in an identical fashion, *e.g.*, always showing the named animal, or always showing the nonnamed animal as doing the biting.

In one experiment with normal children (Cromer, 1974a), it was observed that all primitive rule stage children used the primitive rule for their answers to sentences with the nonsense words, that is, they always continued to show the named animal as the actor. Just over half of the intermediate stage children used some kind of set strategy, but only half of these used the primitive strategy; the other half used what can be called an O-strategy, that is, they always showed the nonnamed animal as the actor for all test sentences. Finally in the group of children who were able to treat normal adjectives correctly in the adult manner (the "passers"), a quarter used set strategies for the sentences with nonsense words, but now, almost all of these strategy-using children used the O-strategy; practically none used the primitive strategy. Thus, in normal children, increasingly greater use was made of the O-strategy by children of increasing classification level.

It may appear odd that the more advanced children make increasing use of a strategy of treating all new instances as if a transformation of basic grammatical relationships has occurred. However, such a strategy is possibly explicable in terms of a linguistic universal connected with what is called the marked and unmarked concept (see Greenberg, 1966, for a review of the marked/unmarked concept in linguistics). Marking in linguistics means to add something, some particle or element to the unmarked form. Thus, grammatically, the plural is marked by many languages in contrast to the singular. Furthermore, it has been observed that in many linguistic contrasts, the member which is the marked form is universally the same in all languages where that contrast is made.

Miller and McNeill (1969) reasoned that the unmarked features are the ones produced as a matter of course. They do not require a decision on the part of the speaker. Children first acquire only the unmarked features of language and only later begin to use marked forms. Recently, McNeill, Yukawa, and McNeill (1971) have carried the argument one step further. They have proposed that, when children are acquiring particular structures in their language, they will actually expect to find as overtly marked those forms which correspond to the universal principle of marking. That is, children will actually seek overt marking for the universally marked (or secondary) forms as opposed to unmarked (or primary) ones. For example, they were examining the acquisition of direct objects (a primary form) and indirect objects (a secondary form) by Japanese children. Japanese marks both of these forms overtly with a postposition particle. However, in accordance with the universal principle, children should expect the indirect object to be the marked form. The results of McNeill *et al.* seem to indicate that children did better on some artificially manipulated sentences when only the indirect object was marked with a particle than when both direct and indirect objects were marked as is normally done in adult Japanese. Though they do not say so explicitly, what is really being claimed is that empirically found linguistic universals have a psychological reality in that children acquiring language will actually expect linguistic marking to indicate the same side of a contrast pair as is found in all languages where that contrast is made.

In the structure I have been examining, the primary form would be the one corresponding to "The duck is *glad* to bite," while the secondary form, "the duck is *fun* to bite," indicates that a change in basic grammatical relations has occurred. However, both "glad" and "fun" may be considered to be marked forms in contrast to the set of adjectives which are ambiguous in this structure. As mentioned earlier, when such an adjective (*e.g.*, "nice") is used, one may recover either deep structure; indeed, it is interesting to note that such adjectives are allowed by both types of differentiating frames. We can say both, "I'm always *nice* to read to you" and "Reading to you is *nice.*" In other words, adjectives like "glad" and "fun" can be considered marked forms in contrast to the unmarked ambiguous adjectives just as in Japanese both direct and indirect objects are marked in the adult grammar. But just as Japanese children expect to find the indirect object marked, so analogously might English children expect the secondary form in this structure to be marked. Thus, when they hear words used in these differentiating frames, they treat all "marking" (if these frames can be said to "mark" these forms) as indicating that the surface subject is derived from an *object* in an embedded sentence in the deep structure, rather than treating them as primary forms with untransformed deep structure relationships. This might account for the increasing use of the O-strategy in intermediate and passing children. Furthermore, if this is truly a specifically linguistic process rather than a more general cognitive one, other predictions are possible. One property of linguistic strategies appears to be declining use of them by persons beyond the critical period of language acquisition. It may be that one reason that adults have difficulty in contrast to children in acquiring second languages or in reacquiring their own after organic impairment, is that they are unable, or at least unlikely, to bring such principles to bear in their learning. Experiments on normal adults on this structure using a series of nonsense words to be learned reveal that no adult ever made use of the O-strategy, even though nearly half used a response strategy for their answers. But their response strategies, like those of the youngest children, were always the primitive strategy of showing the named animal as the actor.

It is with educationally subnormal children that the possibility of a critical period of language acquisition may be important. Thirty-one educationally subnormal children were tested on this structure and took part in a learning experiment using nonsense adjectives in the related transformational frames (Cromer, 1972a). Children were again divided into those who were primitive rule users when real adjectives were used, those who were intermediate, and those who were at the adult level. The results revealed that the same percentages of the subnormal children in each of these categories used set response strategies as did normal children. That is, nearly all primitive rule users used that strategy for their answers to the sentences with nonsense words. About 50% of intermediate children used set response strategies on the new words, and about 25% of the passers did so. But unlike normal children, their strategies were always of the primitive rule type. No child ever used the O-strategy (see Table 1). This is in stark contrast to the normal children, who increasingly used the O-strategy at higher classification levels. In other words, these educationally subnormal children performed like nor-

Table 1. Presponse Strategies to New (Nonsense) Words*

Groups	Response types		Total strategy use
	Primitive strategy (S-strategy)	O-strategy	
Normal children	%	%	%
Primitive rule users (N = 10)	100.0	0.0	100.0
Intermediates (N = 17)	29.4	29.4	58.8
Capable of passing (N = 26)	7.7	19.2	26.9
ESN children			
Primitive rule users (N = 12)	91.7	0.0	91.7
Intermediates (N = 8)	50.0	0.0	50.0
Capable of passing (N = 11)	27.3	0.0	27.3
Adults (N = 19)	42.1	0.0	42.1

*Reprinted by kind permission of Butterworths Publishers, London.

mal adults. No one in either group ever made use of the type of strategy which is hypothesized to be related to a linguistic universal which might be connected with language learning. It may be, then, that these educationally subnormal children, who are 14, 15, and 16 years of age, are beyond the critical period for language acquisition. That is, like normal adults, they have passed beyond the period when they are likely to make use of such language-specific abilities. A more extended review of the argument and the specific data can be found in Cromer (in press).

It should be noted that the lack of such a strategy does not prevent the subnormal child from acquiring this structure. These children, with a mean IQ of about 65, come to comprehend this linguistic structure in the adult fashion when real adjectives are used, at about 15 or 16 years of age. The particular strategy hypothesized to show the psychological reality of a linguistic universal has nothing to do with acquiring adult competence on this structure, but it may affect other structures and throw some light on the processes underlying language acquisition. The evidence so far is only suggestive. More direct studies of linguistic universals are needed to determine whether they have any psychological validity. If they do, one will want to know whether they cease to operate with great efficiency after a certain chronological age. If this is the case, then the mere fact of language delay may cause differing processes to be used during the acquisition of language by older subnormal children.

CONCLUSION

Throughout this chapter, I have emphasized two related points. First, one cannot talk about linguistic competence in the mentally retarded. There are differing subgroups who may evidence very different language abilities. Second, there should be a greater emphasis placed on the processes by which language is acquired rather than on merely describing the linguistic level of any group. Of course, such descriptions are necessary, but they should serve as starting points in discovering the processes which may be deficient in a particular group. O'Connor and Hermelin (1963) have listed several possible deficits which have been studied to account for cognitive problems in mentally retarded individuals. These include perceptual impairment, deficits of cue selection and attention, deficits in the ability to transfer learned principles, and encoding and decoding deficits. These and others may also help to account for the language acquisition difficulties in some groups of subnormals.

In this paper, evidence has been reviewed which shows that some subnormals are merely delayed in their language acquisition. Other studies have indicated that some subnormals are more delayed than their mental age would indicate. There has been some evidence, however, that deficits of certain cognitive abilities, e.g., limited short term memory span, may be responsible for the kinds of linguistic structures that can be comprehended and eventually produced. In some groups, as in severely retarded autistic children, very general cognitive abilities not related to short term memory may be impaired. Some of these abilities may be specifically linguistic. Evidence for this was seen in the crying signals of young autistic children. Experiments with nonretarded developmentally aphasic children also point to the strong possibility of specific linguistic impairment in some children. There has also been speculation that deficits in long term motor programming may impair the language acquisition process. Finally, it was hypothesized that language delay in itself may lead to different processes being used for language acquisition after a critical period. These are only some of the possible processes which may affect language acquisition. It is to be hoped that such underlying deficits will be examined in greater depth.

REFERENCES

Aurnhammer-Frith, U. Emphasis and meaning in recall in normal and autistic children. *Lang. Speech,* 1969, *12,* 29–38.

Baer, D. M. and Guess, D. Receptive training of adjectival inflections in mental retardates. *J. Appl. Behav. Anal.,* 1971, *4,* 129–139.

Bartak, L. and Rutter, M. L. Language and cognition in autistic and aphasic subjects. In N. O'Connor (Ed.), *Language, Cognitive Deficits and Retardation.* London: Butterworths, in press.

Bartel, N. R., Bryen, D., and Keehn, S. Language comprehension in the mentally retarded child. *Except. Child.,* 1973, *39,* 375–382.

Berko, J. The child's learning of English morphology. *Word,* 1958, *14,* 150–177.

Bever, T. G., Fodor, J. A., and Weksel, W. Is linguistics empirical? *Psychol. Rev.,* 1965a, *72,* 493–500.

Bever, T. G., Fodor, J. A., and Weksel, W. Theoretical notes on the acquisition of syntax: A critique of "context generalization." *Psychol. Rev.,* 1965b, *72,* 467–482.

Bloom, L. *Language Development: Form and Function in Emerging Grammars.* Cambridge, Mass.: M.I.T. Press, 1970.

Bradbury, B. and Lunzer, E. A. The learning of grammatical inflexions in normal and subnormal children. *J. Child Psychol. Psychiat.,* 1972, *13,* 239–248.

Brown, R. The first sentences of child and chimpanzee. In R. Brown, *Psycholinguistics: Selected Papers by Roger Brown.* New York: The Free Press, 1970, pp. 208–231.

Brown, R. *A First Language.* Cambridge, Mass.: Harvard University Press, 1973.

Bryant, P. E. The effects of verbal labelling on recall and recognition in severely subnormal and normal children. *J. Ment. Defic. Res.,* 1965, *9,* 229–236.

Bryant, P. E. Verbalization and immediate memory of complex stimuli in normal and severely subnormal children. *Brit. J. Soc. Clin. Psychol.,* 1967, *6,* 212–219.

Bryant, P. E. Language and learning in severely subnormal and normal children. In B. W. Richards (Ed.), *Mental Subnormality: Modern Trends in*

Research. London: Pitman Medical and Scientific Publishing Co., 1970, pp. 150–163.

Byrne, M. C. Speech and language development of athetoid and spastic children. *J. Speech Hear. Disord.*, 1959, *24*, 231–240.

Carlton, T. and Carlton, L. E. Errors in the oral language of mentally defective adolescents and normal elementary school children. *J. Genet. Psychol.*, 1945, *66*, 183–220.

Carroll, J. B. Defining language comprehension: Some speculations. In J. B. Carroll and R. O. Freedle (Eds.), *Language Comprehension and the Acquisition of Knowledge.* Washington D.C.: V. H. Winston & Sons, 1972, pp. 1–29.

Chomsky, C. *The Acquisition of Syntax in Children from 5 to 10.* Cambridge, Mass.: M.I.T. Press 1969.

Chomsky, N. *Syntactic Structures.* The Hague: Mouton, 1957.

Chomsky, N. *Aspects of the Theory of Syntax.* Cambridge, Mass.: M.I.T. Press, 1965.

Chomsky, N. and Halle, M. *The Sound Pattern of English.* New York: Harper & Row, 1968.

Crome, L. C. and Stern, J. *The Pathology of Mental Retardation.* London: Churchill, 1967.

Cromer, R. F. The development of temporal reference during the acquisition of language. Unpublished doctoral dissertation, Harvard University, Cambridge, Mass., 1968.

Cromer, R. F. "Children are nice to understand": Surface structure clues for the recovery of a deep structure. *Brit. J. Psychol.*, 1970, *61*, 397–408.

Cromer, R. F. The learning of surface structure clues to deep structure by a puppet show technique. *Quart. J. Exp. Psychol.*, 1972a, *24*, 66–76.

Cromer, R. F. The learning of linguistic surface structure cues to deep structure by educationally subnormal children. *Amer. J. Ment. Defic.*, 1972b, *77*, 346–353.

Cromer, R. F. Child and adult learning of surface structure cues to deep structure using a picture card technique. *J. Psycholing. Res.*, 1974a, *3*, 1–14.

Cromer, R. F. The development of language and cognition: The cognition hypothesis. In B. M. Foss (Ed.), *New Perspectives in Child Development.* Harmondsworth, Middlesex: Penguin Books, 1974b, pp. 184–252.

Cromer, R. F. Are subnormals linguistic adults? In N. O'Connor (Ed.), *Language, Cognitive Deficits and Retardation.* London: Butterworths, in press.

Danks, J. H. Some factors involved in the comprehension of deviant English sentences. (Doctoral dissertation, Princeton University) Ann Arbor: University Microfilms, 1969, No. 69-2735.

Dever, R. B. and Gardner, W. I. Performance of normal and retarded boys on Berko's test of morphology. *Lang. Speech*, 1970, *13*, 162–181.

Diedrich, W. M. and Poser, C. M. Language and mentation of two phenylketonuric children. *J. Speech Hear. Disord.*, 1960, *25*, 124–134.

Evans, D. and Hampson, M. The language of mongols. *Brit. J. Disord. Commun.*, 1968, *3*, 171–181.

Fillmore, C. J. The case for case. In E. Bach and R. T. Harms (Eds.), *Universals in Linguistic Theory.* New York: Holt, Rinehart & Winston, 1968, pp. 1–88.

Fleming, C. P. The verbal behavior of hydrocephalic children. *Develop. Med. Child Neurol.*, 1968 *Suppl. 15*, 74–82.

Forsyth, D. and Rubenstein, H. In Seventh Annual Report, Harvard University: The Center for Cognitive Studies, 1966–1967, pp. 26–27.

Fraser, C., Bellugi, U., and Brown, R. Control of grammar in imitation, comprehension, and production. *J. Verb. Learning Verb. Behav.*, 1963, *2*, 121–135.

Frith, U. and Frith, C. D. Specific motor disabilities in Down's syndrome. *J. Child Psychol. Psychiat.*, in press.

Garstecki, D. C., Borton, T. E., Stark, E. W., and Kennedy, B. T. Speech, language, and hearing problems in the Laurence-Moon-Biedl syndrome. *J. Speech Hear. Disord.*, 1972, *37*, 407–413.

Graham, J. T. and Graham, L. W. Language behavior of the mentally retarded: Syntactic characteristics. *Amer. J. Ment. Defic.*, 1971, *75*, 623–629.

Graham, N. C. Short term memory and syntactic structure in educationally subnormal children. *Lang. Speech*, 1968, *11*, 209–219.

Graham, N. C. Response strategies in the partial comprehension of sentences. *Lang. Speech*, in press.

Graham, N. C. and Gulliford, R. A. A psychological approach to the language deficiencies of educationally subnormal children. *Educ. Rev.*, 1968, *20*, 136–145.

Greenberg, J. H. Language universals. In T. A. Sebeok (Ed.), *Current Trends in Linguistics*, Vol. III. The Hague: Mouton, 1966, pp. 61–112.

Guess, D. A functional analysis of receptive language and productive speech: Acquisition of the plural morpheme. *J. Appl. Behav. Anal.*, 1969, *2*, 55–64.

Guess, D., Sailor, W., Rutherford, G., and Baer, D. M. An experimental analysis of linguistic development: The productive use of the plural morpheme. *J. Appl. Behav. Anal.*, 1968, *1*, 297–306.

Hermelin, B. and O'Connor, N. Remembering of words by psychotic and subnormal children. *Brit. J. Psychol.*, 1967, *58*, 213–218.

Hermelin, B. and O'Connor, N. *Psychological Experiments with Autistic Children.* Oxford: Pergamon Press, 1970.

Hughes, J. Language and communication: Acquisition of a non-vocal "language" by previously languageless children. Unpublished bachelor of technology thesis, Brunel University, 1972.

Hughes, J. Acquisition of a non-vocal "language" by developmentally aphasic children. To appear.

Jakobson, R. *Child language aphasia and phonological universals.* The Hague: Mouton, 1968 (originally published in 1941).

Jakobson, R., Fant, C. G. M., and Halle, M. *Preliminaries to Speech Analysis: The Distinctive Features and Their Correlates.* Cambridge, Mass.: M.I.T. Press, 1952.

Jakobson, R. and Halle, M. *Fundamentals of Language.* The Hague: Mouton, 1956.

Jordan, T. E. *The Mentally Retarded.* Columbus, Ohio: Merrill, 1966.

Karlin, I. W. and Strazzulla, M. Speech and language problems of mentally deficient children. *J. Speech Hear. Disord.*, 1952, *17*, 286–294.

Lackner, J. R. A developmental study of language behavior in retarded children. *Neuropsychologia*, 1968, *6*, 301–320.

Lee, L. L. Developmental sentence types: A method for comparing normal and deviant syntactic development. *J. Speech Hear. Disord.*, 1966, *31*, 311–330.

Lenneberg, E. H. *Biological Foundations of Language.* New York: Wiley, 1967.

Lenneberg, E. H., Nichols, I. A., and Rosenberger, E. F. Primitive stages of language development in mongolism. In D. McK. Rioch and E. A. Weinstein (Eds.), *Disorders of Communication* (Research publications of the Association for Research in Nervous and Mental Disease, Vol. XLII). Baltimore: Williams & Wilkins, 1964, pp. 119–137.

Lovell, K. and Bradbury, B. The learning of English morphology in educationally subnormal special school children. *Amer. J. Ment. Defic.*, 1967, *71*, 609–615.

Lovell, K. and Dixon, E. M. The growth of the control of grammar in imitation, comprehension, and production. *J. Child Psychol. Psychiat.*, 1967, *8*, 31–39.

Lyle, J. G. The effect of an institution environment upon the verbal development of imbecile children. III. The Brooklands residential family unit. *J. Ment. Defic. Res.*, 1960, *4*, 14–22.

McCawley, J. D. The role of semantics in a grammar. In E. Bach and R. T. Harms (Eds.), *Universals in Linguistic Theory*. New York: Holt, Rinehart & Winston, 1968, pp. 124–169.

McNeill, D. *The Acquisition of Language*. New York: Harper & Row, 1970a.

McNeill, D. The development of language. In P. H. Mussen (Ed.), *Carmichael's Manual of Child Psychology*, Vol. I. New York: Wiley, 1970b, pp. 1061–1161.

McNeill, D., Yukawa, R., and McNeill, N. B. The acquisition of direct and indirect objects in Japanese. *Child Develop.*, 1971, *42*, 237–249.

Menyuk, P. Comparison of grammar of children with functionally deviant and normal speech. *J. Speech Hear. Res.*, 1964, *7*, 109–121.

Menyuk, P. *Sentences Children Use*. Cambridge, Mass.: M.I.T. Press, 1969.

Miller, G. A. The magical number seven, plus or minus two: Some limits on our capacity for processing information. *Psychol. Rev.*, 1956, *63*, 81–96.

Miller, G. A. and McNeill, D. Psycholinguistics. In G. Lindzey and E. Aronson, (Eds.), *The Handbook of Social Psychology*, Ed. 2, Vol. 3. Reading, Mass.: Addison-Wesley, 1969, pp. 666–794.

Morris, G. P. Verbalisation and memory in the mentally subnormal. Unpublished doctoral dissertation, University of London, London, 1972.

Morris, G. P. Verbalisation and memory in the severely subnormal. In N. O'Connor (Ed.), *Languages Cognitive Deficits and Retardation*. London: Butterworths, in press.

Myerson, R. and Goodglass, H. Transformational grammars of three agrammatic patients. *Lang. Speech*, 1972, *15*, 40–50.

Newfield, M. U. and Schlanger, B. B. The acquisition of English morphology by normal and educable mentally retarded children. *J. Speech Hear. Res.*, 1968, *11*, 693–706.

O'Connor, N. and Frith, U. Cognitive development and the concept of set. In A. Prangishvili (Ed.), *Psychological Investigations: A Commemorative Volume Dedicated to the 85th Anniversary of the Birth of D. Uznadze*. Tbilisi, U.S.S.R.: Metsniereba, 1973, pp. 296–300.

O'Connor, N. and Hermelin, B. *Speech and Thought in Severe Subnormality*. Oxford: Pergamon Press, 1963.

Piaget, J. *Genetic Epistemology*. New York: Columbia University Press, 1970a.

Piaget, J. Piaget's theory. In P. H. Mussen (Ed.), *Carmichael's Manual of Child Psychology*, Vol. I. New York: Wiley, 1970b, pp. 703–732.

Piaget, J. and Inhelder, B. *The Psychology of the Child.* London: Routledge & Kegan Paul, 1969 (originally published in 1966).

Premack, D. A functional analysis of language. Invited address before the American Psychological Association, Washington D.C., 1969.

Reese, H. W. and Lipsitt, L. P. *Experimental Child Psychology.* New York: Academic Press, 1970.

Richards, B. W. Clinical syndromes. In B. W. Richards (Ed.), *Mental Subnormality: Modern Trends in Research.* London: Pitman Medical & Scientific Publishing Co., 1970, pp. 1–40.

Ricks, D. M. The beginnings of vocal communication in infants and autistic children. Unpublished doctorate of medicine thesis, University of London, London, 1972.

Ricks, D. M. Vocal communication in pre-verbal normal and autistic children. In N. O'Connor (Ed.), *Language, Cognitive Deficits and Retardation.* London: Butterworths, in press.

Schlesinger, I. M. Learning grammar: From pivot to realization rule. In R. Huxley and E. Ingram (Eds.), *Language Acquisition: Models and Methods.* London: Academic Press, 1971a, pp. 79–89.

Schlesinger, I. M. Production of utterances and language acquisition. In D. I. Slobin (Ed.), *The Ontogenesis of Grammar: A Theoretical Symposium.* New York: Academic Press, 1971b, pp. 63–101.

Semmel, M. I., Barritt, L. S., and Bennett, S. W. Performance of EMR and nonretarded children in a modified cloze task. *Amer. J. Ment. Defic.,* 1970, *74,* 681–688.

Sinclair, H. Sensorimotor action patterns as a condition for the acquisition of syntax. In R. Huxley and E. Ingram (Eds.), *Language Acquisition: Models and Methods.* London: Academic Press, 1971, pp. 121–130.

Sinclair-de-Zwart, H. Developmental psycholinguistics. In D. Elkind and J. H. Flavell (Eds.), *Studies in Cognitive Development.* New York: Oxford University Press, 1969, pp. 315–336.

Slobin, D. I. The acquisition of Russian as a native language. In F. Smith and G. A. Miller (Eds.), *The Genesis of Language.* Cambridge, Mass.: M.I.T. Press, 1966, pp. 129–148.

Slobin, D. I. Cognitive prerequisites for the development of grammar. In C. A. Ferguson and D. I. Slobin (Eds.), *Studies of Child Language Development.* New York: Holt, Rinehart & Winston, 1973, pp. 175–208.

Smith, N. V. *The Acquisition of Phonology.* Cambridge, England: Cambridge University Press, 1973.

Smith, N. V. Universal tendencies in the child's acquisition of phonology. In N. O'Connor (Ed.), *Languages Cognitive Deficits and Retardation.* London: Butterworths, in press.

Spreen, O. Language functions in mental retardation: A review. I. Language development, types of retardation, and intelligence level. *Amer. J. Ment. Defic.,* 1965, *69,* 482–494.

Wanner, H. E. On remembering, forgetting, and understanding sentences: A study of the deep structure hypothesis. Unpublished doctoral dissertation, Harvard University, Cambridge, Mass., 1968.

CHAPTER TEN

DISCUSSION SUMMARY–DEVELOPMENT OF RECEPTIVE LANGUAGE[1]

Joseph E. Spradlin

Bureau of Child Research, University of Kansas, Lawrence, Kansas 66044

Both chapters in this section include the term "receptive language" in their titles. The titles are slightly more restrictive than the topics actually covered. Both writers included material on conceptual development and productive language as well as on receptive language. The rather extensive inclusion of materials relating to other aspects of language was probably due to several factors. First, both writers view receptive language as being so closely tied to conceptual and perceptual processes and productive language that discussing receptive language in isolation would be both difficult and artificial. Secondly, the amount of research reported on language reception is so limited that restricting the content solely to this area would have led to very short papers. Thirdly, both writers appear to believe that both productive and receptive language reflects underlying cognitive processes or competencies and thus whatever is important for production would also be important for reception. Regardless of the reasons, both the principal authors and the conference participants ranged far and free in their discussions.

The two reports deal with different aspects of language acquisition. Menyuk's paper reviews the information on normal infant language development and puts forth some hypotheses concerning what is happening as the infant develops language. Cromer reviewed language research which has been conducted with older normal and handicapped children. Because the papers deal with different areas, the discussion summary for each is presented here separately under the headings "Early Language Development" and "Language Process Differences and Diagnostic Groups."

EARLY LANGUAGE DEVELOPMENT

Menyuk divided her discussion on infant language development into the development of structure and the development of language function. Struc-

[1] The preparation of this paper was partially supported by Grants HD 00870-10 and HD 02528-08 from the National Institute of Child Health and Human Development.

ture refers to the infant's acquisition of the phonological, syntactic, and semantic systems. Function refers to the exchanges infants have with other persons in their environment and how infants use language. Menyuk postulated reorganization of language reception and production at various stages of development rather than a smooth gradual developmental transition. The first stage occurs at about 6 months, when infants begin to babble. Although some infants discriminate certain consonantal phonemes very early in their development, they seem to be unable to produce the complete closure necessary for producing these phonemes until about 6 months of age. Until about this time, according to Menyuk, infant productions are primarily vocalic. At about 6 months, infant vocalizations include more sounds involving closure (*e.g.,* consonantal sounds). This production of consonant-vowel sequences marks the beginning of the babbling stage. There is evidence that some infants discriminate their mother from other persons. It was even suggested that infants might be able to discriminate when they were being addressed from when they were not being addressed as early as 3 months of age.

On the function side, some infants engage in long verbal exchanges with their caretakers prior to 3 months of age. There were various interpretations of these early exchanges. Some participants suggested that such exchanges might be a kind of language acquisition universal on which later language development is based. Bowerman noted that her own daughter had engaged in exchanges relatively early, but that these exchanges decreased later. She asked whether such exchanges might not be akin to such early reflexes as the walking reflex, which decreases as infants get older. Menyuk (in this volume) reported that Bateson did not find such a decrease in vocal exchange.

Of particular interest were the changes which apparently take place in a child's vocalizations and response to other's vocalizations between about 8 and 14 months of age. During this time, the infant's production pattern changes from one of babbling and complex intonation patterns to one which consists primarily of short word length utterances. Infants also may show a preference for listening to single words rather than sentences. Preliminary observations suggest that during this period many children are acquiring first words. Menyuk suggested that the period is a second major phase of reorganization and that two major types of integration are occurring. First, production and perception are becoming integrated (the lag between perception and production narrows). Second, the semantic properties and the phonological sequences are becoming integrated. That is, phonological sequences begin to serve as labels for semantic referents. Some participants suggested that the integration of semantics on phonological sequence begins when infants recognize that there are two types of events–1) words or symbols and 2) the events to which they refer. Premack noted during the discussion that he had observed what he thought to be this type of classification in young chimpanzees. Furthermore, he indicated that such a separation was a minimal condi-

tion for early labeling behavior to develop. However, the experimental procedures for demonstrating such a reorganization of classification were not
immediately apparent to the participants.

Menyuk suggested that perhaps children with language problems would
show considerable delay in reorganization at the various stages. If the stages
can be delineated, and if they can be demonstrated to be predictive of later
language disorders, they would have considerable implication for early detection of children with language problems. Moreover, it is also possible that
these stages would be critical points for early intervention. However, the data
which would allow us to predict children's language levels at 4 or 5 years
from their vocalization and auditory perception at age 1 year to 18 months
are not currently available.

Menyuk has developed a series of hypotheses concerning the language
development of infants. These may prove useful both in predicting the course
of language development and in developing language intervention procedures.
However, Menyuk's cautions concerning the inadequacies of the infant language data base should not be overlooked.

The difficulty in conducting research on infant language development is
readily apparent. Perhaps the greatest advances have been made in the study
of infant auditory preception (Eimas, this volume; Morse, this volume;
Butterfield and Cairns, this volume). Researchers have developed methods
for recording objectively and sometimes reliably the responses of infants to
linguistic auditory stimuli. Moreover, there is some indication that gross
results can be replicated across infants. Some of the findings have even been
replicated in different experimental laboratories (Butterfield and Cairns, this
volume).

Conducting research on infant development of productive language presents extreme measurement and recording problems. Much of the exciting
research on the development of infant language has been conducted by
individual researchers observing a limited number of infants over a long
period of time. These researchers analyze and interpret the utterances of
infants in terms of the total context in which they occur. Such research has
been productive in generating exciting hypotheses concerning infants' basic
conceptual systems and how these relate to infants' language structure.
However, this research does present problems. There have been few attempts
to demonstrate that independent observers would classify and record infant
language events in the same way. Secondly, since observational research is
extremely time-consuming, there have been few replications across infants by
different researchers. Finally, the focus on the environmental context to
interpret the child's utterances may yield misleading information concerning
infant's language systems. For example, common opinion is that infants talk
only about events in their immediate environment. Many utterances of
infants are unintelligible to observers, and many of those utterances which are
intelligible are intelligible only because of the supporting environmental

context. Could it be that failure to observe infants talking about events not present in their environment represents an adult listener's failure rather than a behavioral characteristic of infants?

The difficulty in conducting language development research is extreme, but constructing a theory of infant language development is even more difficult. There are no guidelines concerning what are and are not acceptable data on which to generate a theory of infant language acquisition. Even such accepted research requirements as observer reliability are very difficult to obtain in infant language development studies. A demonstration that observers agree on specific infant behaviors would be a minimal requirement prior to accepting data as the foundation on which a theory of infant language acquisition would be developed.

Even if reliable observations are made with one infant, there is no assurance that the same observations can be replicated with other infants. Such replications would be required for a general theory of infant language acquisition.

There is considerable excitement in the area of infant language development. Participants of the conference noted that infant language research and theory suggest points of intervention. However, applied benefits will probably come after there is a body of reliable and replicable data. Such benefits currently appear to be far in the future.

LANGUAGE PROCESS DIFFERENCES AND DIAGNOSTIC GROUPS

Cromer proposed that the language deficiencies of mentally retarded children might result from different language processes than those which occur in normal children and that, furthermore, there might be process differences among the various classes of mentally retarded children. The paper went on to discuss 1) research comparing the language of normal and retarded children; 2) relation of cognition and language; 3) research on the language processes of such language-deficient diagnostic groups as autistic and aphasic children; and 4) research comparing the strategies of normal children, retarded adolescents, and normal adults in dealing with sentences such as "John is easy to please" and "John is eager to please."

Comparisons of the Language of Normal and Retarded Persons

The studies which compared the language of normal and retarded children evoked considerable discussion. Many of the participants had serious reservations concerning the rationale for the classifications on which such studies are based. It is customary to view mental retardation as a classification based on some organic characteristic of children. Such a view is inaccurate. Operationally, mental retardation turns out to be a classification based on social and behavioral factors. According to one participant (Lawrence Turton) a child is most likely to be placed in a class for retarded children if 1) he is from an ethnic or minority group, 2) he is in a school which has a school psychologist, and 3) the school psychologist is capable of giving only a limited number of intelligence tests. Turton further suggested that those studies which showed no language process differences were not surprising since in fact there were probably few differences between the group other than those related to social class. He further added that different results might be obtained with severely retarded children.

Richard Dever pointed out during the conference that even when differences were obtained between normal and retarded children the results were probably not too meaningful since the behavior demonstrated in the test situation is often quite different from behavior exhibited in the child's natural environment. To illustrate this point, he cited his own research finding that scores on the Berko Test had little relationship to children's use of English morphology in the natural environment (Dever, 1972). He also presented an anecdote in which nonverbal children were asked to babysit a "nervous" rabbit. They were told they could calm the rabbit by talking to him. Under these conditions the "nonverbal" children exhibited a greater amount of speech and variety of structures than they did in other school situations.

Since the language comparisons between normal and retarded children are an attempt to investigate the relationship between language tests and intelligence tests, one should give careful attention to the nature of both types of tests. Many of the writers in the field of language treat an intelligence quotient as a unitary construct independent of the test which yields the intelligence quotient. However, a closer look at the common intelligence tests suggests that mental ages or intelligence quotients on the various tests are not equivalent. The Peabody Picture Vocabulary Test is a vocabulary reception test. The Columbia Mental Maturity Scale is a visual concept evaluation test. It requires no auditory reception language for high performance. The Stanford Binet Scales use a variety of both verbal and nonverbal factors in testing. To obtain a high intelligence quotient, the child must both understand spoken language and express himself in spoken language. Each of these tests constitutes a definition of intelligence. The relationship between intelligence and the scores on any given language test depends on which intelligence test is used.

Staats pointed out that on many occasions the same behavior (or lack of behavior) is used to classify a child as having low intelligence as is used to classify a child as having language problems. He suggested that a great deal of the confusion concerning the relation of intelligence to language would be reduced by a careful analysis of the stimuli presented and the responses obtained on language and intelligence tests. At this point one participant pointed out that even when the same measures were correlated, the results of different studies were often different. The participant suggested that perhaps the measures are no good. At this point Donald Baer made a statement which specified a major source of the confusion in the area of language and intelligence measurement. This statement was so clear that it merits direct quotation:

I'd like to make a grammatical point. "Measures," I think, implies the phrase "measures of blank"—a prepositional phrase, as I recall.

I think the issue here is not that measures are no good, but they are not *measures,* because there is no proper "of blank" put behind them. All measures are *behaviors* that are looked at in a variety of situations and a variety of ways.

Behavior is subject to environmental control. There is a well-codified set of laws which describes that; and most of these measures, it seems to me, ignore those laws. What they represent probably are not contradictory testimony about some underlying "of X" which they're supposed to be measures of; but instead, they represent a variety of ways of looking at a variety of behaviors, frequently in ignorance of the conditions that are important to the control of those behaviors.

The anecdote about the rabbit is exactly an anecdote about that. I think we get into a great deal of confusion, consequently, because we think of them as measures *of something,* when in fact, they're simply a variety of responses being looked at under a variety of very important conditions which are largely ignored.

Thus far questions have been raised concerning the validity of the retardate-normal comparative procedures, the independence of items on intelligence and language measures, the representativeness of language and intelligence test results, and the adequacy of control procedures in test situations. Even if all these questions could be answered adequately, it is unlikely that gross group comparisons of normal and retarded could reveal process differences associated with different diagnostic classifications. Since normal-retarded comparative studies include a variety of types of retardates with different language processes, it is unlikely that group studies will show process differences. It is more likely that a variety of the stable individual process differences shown by some subjects may be masked by error variance occurring in the total group. Furthermore, if each language test is given only once, there is simply no way of separating variance associated with stable individual differences from variance associated with the lack of control discussed by Baer.

Relation of Cognition and Language

Cromer, like other participants at the conference, holds that cognitive development may be a necessary prerequisite for language development. An example of a cognitive prerequisite is the contention that an infant must be able to classify actions before such major categories as a noun phrase and a verb phrase are possible. No specific techniques were suggested for determining whether an infant classifies actions; however, procedures can probably be developed for discovering such action classifications independent of either language comprehension or production. One way of defining action classification independent of comprehension is through the study of imitative behavior. If a child imitates several different actions, he then classifies those acts and perhaps has one prerequisite to comprehending the label for action. Recent studies by Striefel (personal communication) suggest that severely retarded children who do not imitate motor acts have considerable difficulty in learning to follow simple verb-object commands. If these preliminary data hold up, it might suggest that comprehension and production training should not be begun until the child has an imitative motor repertoire.

Language Deficits of Aphasic and Autistic Children

Although Cromer considers cognitive development necessary to language development, he does not consider it sufficient. In a report cited by Cromer, Hughes (1972) conducted training research with aphasic children which supported the hypotheses. Using children who used a symbolic system similar to that reported by Premack (1970), Hughes taught nonverbal aphasic children to associate shapes with particular objects and actions and to use such language functions as direct and indirect object, negation, and questions. These children were then able to use the symbols to communicate. Carrier (1973) has reported similar findings with severely retarded children and adult aphasics. The Premack type of symbolic system suggests both research and therapy questions. Are the deficits shown by some of these children limited to the auditory-vocal system, or are there more general deficits involving organization of transitory signals regardless of whether they are auditory, visual, or tactile? If deficits exist for all transitory signals, it would appear to be a problem of short term memory or organizational functions. It is possible that (for some children) failure to learn an auditory language is related solely to auditory processes. For others it relates to more general cognitive deficits.

Therapeutically, there is the possibility that after a child has been taught a visual motor symbolic system he might be able to learn an audio-vocal language system. Preliminary work by Carrier (1973) suggests that this may be true for some severely retarded nonspeaking children.

Autistic children were also presented in Cromer's paper as a group who show specific language process deficits. In a report cited by Cromer in his chapter, Aurnhammer-Frith (1969) indicated that autistic children who were matched with normals on the Peabody Picture Vocabulary Test and a digit repetition task did not profit from grammatic structure in their sentence repetition as did normal children. The failure of autistic children to greatly improve their repetition span when structured sentences are the stimuli has led Hermelin and Frith (1973, see Cromer's chapters) to conduct a series of interesting studies. In their studies, normal, retarded, and autistic children were matched on mental age and were compared for their repetition of both structured and unstructured verbal material. In general, their results indicated that neither word classes nor structure aided the autistic group's recall. Both normal and retarded group's recall were aided by word classes and structure. The autistic groups did not differ from normals and subnormals on visual motor patterns. This finding suggests that, for at least some autistic children, their classification and organization problem is confined to the auditory vocal system. If this is true, then a visual symbol system such as those used by Premack (1970), Hughes (1972, see Cromer's chapters), and Carrier (1973) should be effective in teaching some autistic children a communication system. Hermelin's and Frith's report does not include individual data, and so it is not possible to determine what percentage of children within each group performed in the manner represented by the group mean.

The data by Aurnhammer-Frith (1969) and Hermelin and Frith (1973, see Cromer's chapter) suggest that among children classified as autistic there are children who do not profit in recall from auditory structure. Cromer seems to think that similar process deficits might be found among other traditional groups. At this point it is well to distinguish between types of diagnosis. Although the terms "aphasia," "autism," and "mental deficiency" imply organic conditions, operationally they turn out to be behavioral classifications. Children who engage in many stereotyped movements, have severe temper tantrums, avoid eye contact, withdraw from people, and are echolalic are likely to be classed as autistic. Children who interact socially, handle materials well, show evidence of hearing but who do not exhibit language have a high chance of being labeled aphasic. Children who score low on intelligence tests and show rather general behavioral deficits and who do not have unique language or stereotyped behavior are likely to be called retarded. On the other hand, some of the diagnostic classifications discussed by Cromer are not behavioral classifications. Cretinism, Down's syndrome, Laurence-Moon-Biedel syndrome, and phenylketonuria are not behavioral classes but biological classes. Attempts to relate behavior process deficits to biological diagnostic classes have not proved very fruitful in the past. There are probably several reasons for the failure to find close relationships between behavior and etiological classes. With nearly all biological conditions the organic effects are variable. For example, some Down's syndrome children show congenital heart malformations while some do not. Even when highly similar appearing gross neurological conditions are present, there may be significant differences in the more molecular aspects of neurological morphology and function. And there may be early environmental factors which have considerable effect on both language and nonlanguage behavioral processes of handicapped infants. Language characteristics contribute heavily to the diagnosis of autism and aphasia. The fact that differences between these groups and other groups have been reliably demonstrated suggests a strategy. That strategy is to select children with language deficits and then make careful long range attempts to determine if stable language process differences are found. One could then go on to study the effects or lack of effects of remediation attempts. Such a careful analysis of language processes might aid in predicting and remediating language handicaps of children and also yield important information concerning the processes involved in normal language development.

Linguistic Strategies of Normal Children, Normal Adults, and Retarded Adolescents

Cromer's chapter is based on the thesis that retarded children may exhibit different language acquisition processes than normals. One possibility he suggested is that language delay itself results in different language processes. Cromer's thesis is both highly tentative and complex. However, I will present it as I understand it. First, there are linguistic universals. Second, with linguistic universals involving contrasts (*e.g.*, plural, singular), the same member is marked in all languages if only one contrast member is marked. Third, the unmarked member is the one which is most common or most natural. Fourth, children have a *critical period* during which they are particularly responsive in learning markings involved in language universals. Fifth, after the critical period, adolescents and adults can acquire the language, but they use different acquisition processes. So, if a retarded person is delayed in language learning, he will then use different processes to acquire these linguistic universals. Data for most of the critical aspects of this hypothesis are meager. However, Cromer had conducted a series of studies which he related to the hypothesis. These studies investigated the responses of normal children, normal adults, and retarded adolescents to sentences such as "The wolf is *tasty* to bite" or "The wolf is *eager* to bite." Cromer presented the child two animals such as a wolf and an alligator and determined whether the child had the named animal or the nonnamed animal do the biting. This procedure was carried out with adjectives which describe an actor (happy, willing, and glad), adjectives which describe the recipient of the action (tasty, easy, hard, fun), adjectives which are ambiguous (bad, nice, and tasty), and nonsense words used in an adjectival context. Cromer reported that prior to 6 years, 3 months, normal children typically have the named object do the biting (S strategy) regardless of the type of adjective presented. After 6 years, 3 months they go into an intermediate stage and during this stage some children have the nonnamed object doing the biting (O strategy). At about 10 years of age normal children are able to respond correctly to both subject-modifying and object-modifying adjectives. Cromer reported that normal adults are able to respond correctly to subject-modifying and object-modifying adjectives. Educationally subnormal adolescents acquire this ability by about age 13, 14, or 15 years.

When normal children at the intermediate stage and above were presented nonsense adjectives, some (7 of 43) exhibited a type S strategy and some (10 of 43) exhibited a type O strategy. All normal adults who exhibited a strategy (8 of 19) and all retarded adolescents who exhibited a strategy (7 of 19) exhibited a type S strategy (7 of 19).

Cromer interpreted these data as indicating that children during a critical period are very sensitive to secondary forms and that adults and retarded adolescents have passed through this critical period for the easy acquisition of linguistic universals.

The results of the experiments and these interpretations yielded a lively discussion at the conference. The issue of the reality and the utility of linguistic universals brought many diverse views to the surface. Several participants pointed out that a few years ago the notion of any kind of unlearned aspect of language functioning was dismissed as nonsense. However, recent theory and data suggest that certain phonological patterns may be universal and that certain acoustic distinctions are present soon after birth. Currently, it is respectable to talk of innate acoustic feature detectors. This group of participants found it very likely that humans may be uniquely wired to detect certain more complex language universals.

Other members of the group were highly skeptical concerning the existence of linguistic universals. Part of the disagreement concerning the existence or nonexistence of linguistic universals stemmed from the definition. Schlesinger suggested that there were at least two uses of the term "linguistic universal." One use is strictly tautological. Language is defined in terms of certain characteristics. If a system does not have those characteristics, then it is not a language. Thus, by definition there are certain linguistic universals. A second type of universal is an empirical universal. Language is defined and then languages are studied to determine if they have certain characteristics common to all languages which are not necessitated by the definition. Schlesinger went on to suggest that if one language could be found that did not have a specific characteristic, then that characteristic could not be considered as a linguistic universal. Moreover, Schlesinger stated that there is little evidence for such universals.

Cromer said that Schlesinger's definition was too stringent and that a linguistic universal was simply a marking or characteristic which a number of languages shared and which had psychological reality. Nevertheless, Cromer agreed that the evidence for linguistic universals is not overwhelming.

The issue of critical periods has also raised some questions. The fact that some normal children exhibited a strategy not exhibited by any normal adults or retarded adolescents may indicate a critical period which has been passed by adults and adolescents. It might also simply be the result of a variety of other factors differentially affecting adults, adolescents, and children. For example, normal adults are not usually in elementary classrooms with a high emphasis on language arts, and retarded adolescents may be in a very different language environment than normal elementary age children.

There is really no reason for a subject to use any particular strategy. One might speculate that very minor manipulation would bring about an adult who used an O strategy. What would happen if five nonsense adjectives were introduced and given O-type meanings and then the normal adult was presented a new nonsense adjective according to Cromer's procedure. It would be surprising if the adult did not exhibit an O-type strategy for those new nonsense adjectives. The same might also be true for ESN adolescents. If such gentle training procedures could result in O-type strategies, what would be the implications for the critical period hypothesis?

During the final part of the discussion, attempts were made to explore possibilities for designing an experiment for evaluating the psychological reality of linguistic universals. There was some agreement that if a linguistic universal had psychological reality, children should learn to mark the secondary form more readily than to mark the primary form and leave the secondary form unmarked. Since most languages mark the plural form of a noun and leave the singular form of the noun unmarked, plural markings were viewed as a likely candidate for study. Children should be able to learn a system which marks the plural noun and leaves the singular unmarked more rapidly than they could learn a system which marks the singular form and leaves the plural unmarked. A study by Guess, Sailor, Rutherford, and Baer (1968) was put forth as an example of a study which suggested that the marked plural was more easily learned than the marked singular. Guess *et al.* first taught a severely retarded child to label two objects with the plural label and a single object with the singular label. Then they revised training and taught the child to name single objects with the plural label and plural objects with the singular label. The reversal took more trials to reach criterion than did original learning.

The Guess *et al.* (1968) study was deemed by Baer as simply being inadequate to test the notion of the psychological reality of the linguistic universal. Baer implied that, had the subject first been trained to label the single object with plural label and then trained to label two objects with the plural label, the reversal once again might have taken longer than initial training. The group concluded that a group design or perhaps a design involving repeated reversals would be required to answer the question of whether it is easier for children to learn to mark the plural form or the singular form of the noun.

Closely related to the issue of psychological reality of linguistic universals is the notion of developmental sequences during language acquisition. Menyuk asked whether any language structures might be trained in any order. Most of the participants said no, that some language behaviors were prerequisite to other language behaviors and thus it was necessary in training to follow specified orders of training. There was a much smaller group at the conference that believed that perhaps almost any language could be taught in any order and that if this extreme statement was not true, then the orders and sequences were less fixed than many at the conference were assuming. For example, many at the conference seemed to be suggesting a kind of linear A→B→C programming. Others were suggesting that, perhaps something needed to be trained before C but the sequence might be A→B→C, A→D→C, or A→N→C. That is, while the sequence might not be totally unrestricted, there are alternatives for teaching sequences. A colleague of mine has stated that the issue of what can be trained in what order is not the critical question. He suggests that the critical issue for training is "whether it is more efficient to teach certain language structures prior to others?" His implied answer is that some sequences of training must be better than others. Perhaps the determination of such sequences is a fruitful direction for language training research (Kenneth Ruder, personal communication).

SUMMARY

The two preceding chapters resulted in a variety of interesting hypotheses concerning language development and language intervention. Menyuk hypothesized that language acquisition in infants takes place as a series of reorganizations of receptive and expressive processes. The phases of reorganization are thought to be blocked or prolonged in retarded children. Moreover, these phases of reorganization are suggested as important times for introducing language intervention techniques. If such periods of reorganization exist, then perhaps careful observation during these periods would predict later language acquisition. Such a prediction would be a major breakthrough in early language acquisition because predictions of later language acquisition from early acquisition are currently quite risky. However, the hypotheses Menyuk put forward are highly tentative and must be supported by reliable and replicable infant language acquisition data before they can have practical implications for intervention programs.

Cromer hypothesized that there are a variety of retarded children and that different groups of retarded children may present different cognitive and language acquisition processes. This hypothesis suggests not only that researchers look very closely at the gross language deficiencies of large groups of children labeled as retarded, but that researchers look very carefully at language process differences among handicapped children. Such a careful look at processes will require both an insightful set of hypotheses concerning basic language processes and a high level of skill in behavior control and evaluation. The requirements suggest collaborative research among language experts and behavioral scientists. The Chula Vista Conference has promoted such collaborative efforts.

REFERENCES

Aurnhammer-Frith, U. Emphasis and meaning in recall in normal and autistic children. *Lang. Speech*, 1969, 12, 29—38.
Carrier, J. K., Jr. Application of functional analysis and a non-speech re-

sponse mode to teaching language. Kansas Center for Research in Mental Retardation and Human Development: Parsons, Kans., Parsons Research Center Report 70, 1973.

Dever, R. B. A comparison of the results of a revised version of Berko's Test of Morphology with the free speech of mentally, retarded children, *J. Speech Hear. Res.,* 1972, *15,* 169–178.

Guess, D., Sailor, W., Rutherford, G., and Baer, D. M. An experimental analysis of linguistic development: The productive use of the plural morpheme. *J. Appl. Behav. Anal.* 1968, *4,* 297–306.

Hermelin, B. and Frith, U. Psychological studies of childhood autism: Can autistic children make sense of what they see and hear? *J. Spec. Educ.,* 1971, *5,* 107–117.

Premack, D. A. A functional analysis of language. *J. Exp. Anal. Behav.,* 1970, *14,* 107–125.

IV DEVELOPMENTAL RELATIONSHIP BETWEEN RECEPTIVE AND EXPRESSIVE LANGUAGE

CHAPTER ELEVEN

TALKING, UNDERSTANDING, AND THINKING

Lois Bloom

Departments of Psychology and Speech Pathology, Teachers College, Columbia University, New York, New York 10027

The relationship between understanding and speaking has barely been touched on in language development theory and research. Children's early speech has clearly received the lion's share of attention. In contrast, what children understand of what they hear has been virtually ignored, largely because of the difficulties involved in measuring comprehension, not because of a lack of interest. A major problem in evaluating comprehension is that children's responses are multidetermined—what the child does depends on many things in addition to what he hears. In contrast, child speech can be written down or otherwise recorded and, if nothing else, simply reported or described. However, there has also been an unfortunate tendency to take comprehension for granted, in the light of what little anecdotal and experimental evidence has been reported. The result is that the prevailing view of the developmental relationship between the two is, quite simply, that comprehension necessarily precedes production at every step along the way. However, as awareness about the processes involved in speech development has increased, there has been a growing interest in comprehension development, and deeper questions than whether the one precedes the other have begun to emerge. In particular, one would like to know more about the factors that contribute to understanding messages, how such factors relate to producing messages, and the relation of both to linguistic and cognitive development.

Understanding and speaking do not develop separately, with children learning different "rules" for each. Inasmuch as communication depends upon the extent to which the semantic intention of the speaker matches the semantic interpretation of the listener, the knowledge that each has could not be independent. An intuitively likely hypothesis about the developmental relation between the two is that both speaking and understanding depend upon the same underlying information (or competence), but each manifests a

1 The preparation of this paper was supported in part by Research Grant HD 03828 from the National Institutes of Health. The opinions and ideas presented here have benefited from discussions and collaborations with Janellen Huttenlocher, whose studies of comprehension have been particularly enlightening.

different performance mode. The theory of generative transformational grammar has described the linguistic knowledge of adult speaker-hearers as a grammar that can be influenced by different kinds of performance variables. In this view, understanding and speaking would involve learning the same words and linguistic structures, with different performance capabilities emerging at different times. Inasmuch as it is necessary to process words and semantic-syntactic structures in order to learn them, the production of speech might appear to be dependent upon the prior development of comprehension. But, while it is most probably not the case that speaking and understanding are altogether separate developments, it is by no means clear that the emergence of speech and understanding shadow each other.

Another hypothesis that will be proposed here is that the two represent mutually dependent, but different underlying processes, with a resulting shifting of influence between them in the course of language development. In short, it will be suggested that the developmental gap between comprehension and speaking probably varies among different children and at different times and may often be more apparent than real.

Before attempting to deal with the questions of the nature of speech and comprehension and the relation between them in development, it will be helpful to review how their interaction has been described in diaries or case histories of development and in recent psycholinguistic studies of young children. As will be seen, there is most often a strong assumption of a necessary temporal priority in the relation between comprehension and speech development. For example, according to McNeill, "children probably add new information to their linguistic competence mainly by comprehending speech" (1970, p. 102). Observations of small children, by both experimenters and parents, have almost always produced the strong impression that children somehow respond to much more language than they can actually say themselves. However, it also happens that there has always been a certain amount of skepticism in the early diaries about the nature of children's comprehension and exactly what it is in speech events that children are responding to when they appear to understand what is said. More recently, there has been growing skepticism about linguistic comprehension in the psycholinguistic literature as well.

THE COMPREHENSION-PRODUCTION GAP

Several studies have recently demonstrated that infants as young as 2 months of age perceive acoustic differences between sounds (Eimas et al., 1971; and Moffit, 1971) and between different intonation contours at 8 months (Kaplan, 1970). This ability to hear the difference between two sounds (such as [b] and [p]) involves a different set of capacities than is involved in the ability to associate an acoustic event (a word) with some aspect of the environment. However, the one is embedded in the other inasmuch as the child who recognizes a relationship between a word and an object must necessarily discriminate the word from among other acoustic events that he also hears. Thus, the child must have developed a primitive ability to segment acoustic units within the larger acoustic event of heard speech (which, in turn, has had to be differentiated from nonspeech acoustic events).

First Words

Certain repeated acoustic events begin to stand out in the stream of speech that the child hears towards the end of his 1st year. A number of investigators (for example, Guillaume, 1927; Leopold, 1939; and Lewis, 1951) have emphasized intonation and stress variations as major factors influencing this primitive segmentation. According to Lewis (1951) children respond to intonation before they respond to phonetic form and will respond similarly to adult utterances with different phonetic form if the intonation contour is the same. To explain the child's transition from response on the basis of intonation to response on the basis of phonetic form, Lewis suggested that

> the child responds affectively both to the intonational pattern of what he hears and to the situation in which he hears it. And at this very same time he hears a phonetic pattern, inextricably intertwined with the intonational pattern and—in many cases—linked expressively or onomatopoetically with the situation. Then his affective response fashions a new whole out of these experiences, this new whole including the intonational pattern, the situation, and the phonetic pattern. When at last the phonetic pattern acquires dominance so that irrespective of the intonational pattern it evokes the appropriate response from the child, we say that he has understood the conventional word (p. 122).

> [Thus], in the earlier entries [in Lewis' diary account] the child's response to a word is largely affective and conational—consisting of the initiation or inhibition of an act as the result of the affective state aroused by the word; while in the later entries his response is increasingly directed to and concerned with one particular element in his experience—an "object" (p. 146).

Lewis has described the beginning of comprehension in terms of the affective coalescence of intonation contour, phonetic form, and situation into "a new whole," which is, presumably, the primitive mental representation of semantic information linking acoustic linguistic events (intonation and phonetic patterns) with visually perceptual, nonlinguistic (situational) events.

With respect to the relation between comprehension and emerging speech, Lewis noted a 1-month lapse between understanding reference to objects and, not until 17 months, the clear use of words for objective reference, for example "ba" (bath), "ba" (button), "ha" (honey):

> It is clear that the changes in the child's responses to words parallel the changes in behavior accompanying his own speech, the latter development following, stage for stage, some months after the former. Along both lines we see a progressive increase in the reference to specific objects within the situation, and ultimately reference even to objects which are not actually present (p. 147).

Lewis did not, however, relate the early influence of intonation for emerging comprehension to the use of intonation in early speech.

Spitz (1957) has described the early development of awareness of prohibitive "no" as the child's first semantic notion. His explanation of its emergence is based upon the exaggerated and often abrupt change in emphasis and affect in mothers' speech that accompanies the stern "no" and head shake as the child starts to crawl about and investigate. Spitz described the beginning of comprehension in the association between a word, "no," and a set of events or *behaviors* that have been defined for the child by his mother as "prohibited." In this case, the child needs to associate the acoustic event with events that transcend the perceptual properties of different objects. Thus, plants, electric wires, knives, and matches share common reference, even though they *look* quite different, because they have been associated with "no" and the accompanying prohibiting behavior from an adult. Although prohibitive "no" is often reported in the diary studies to be responded to by children in their 1st year, there have been no reports of prohibitive "no" in children's earliest speech. Indeed, the use of prohibitive "no" develops *after* the use of "no" to signal the other semantic notions of nonexistence, disappearance, rejection and denial (Bloom, 1970, 1973).

Leopold (1939) reported that the beginning of his daughter Hildegard's comprehension was at 8 months, and was, at first, limited to:

> her own name ... [which] usually induced her to turn her head expectantly toward the speaker. There was no doubt that she referred these sounds in some way to herself. ... In the second half of the ninth month she took a decisive step forward: both speaking and understanding began [although] it was speaking in a very rudimentary sense (p. 21).

Subsequently the word "Daddy" and prohibitive "no, no!" ... "made her pay attention, stop crying, and look around." Leopold reported that understanding increased rapidly thereafter while progress in speaking was slight. However, the earliest words that were understood: her name, "Daddy," and "no, no!" were not among the first words in Hildegard's subsequent speech.

Some time toward the end of their 1st year, then, children may indicate recognition of an association between an acoustic event and an object by a shift of gaze toward the object, or an arrest of attention. Usually such objects and events are among the most familiar to the child. My daughter, Allison, first recognized the word "birds" in association with the mobile above her dressing table and then, shortly after, the word "music" in association with the record player in her room, before her 1st birthday. Unfortunately, the information that exists about emerging comprehension as children begin to associate sounds and referents is anecdotal in just this way.[2] The diary studies (Lewis, 1951; Leopold, 1939; Guillaume, 1927; etc.) reported first instances

---

[2] Janellen Huttenlocher is currently investigating children's ability to recognize and discriminate linguistic stimuli in the first 2 years.

of such behavior but did not report whether or not such responses persisted after they were first observed. For example, Allison's original responses to "birds" and "music" were arrest of attention and shift of gaze toward the objects, but it was not clear if she responded consistently to these words thereafter. She did not recognize the words "birds" and "music" in any situations other than her mobile and her record player for many months. Moreover, neither of the words "birds" or "music" were among the first words that she said, when she began to say words 3 months later. Although speech recognition preceded speech production by 3 months, there was not a one-to-one correspondence between early recognized words and later spoken words.

There have been reports of overinclusion of reference for the first words that children say, where a word is used in situations which seem to share a common element for the child, but not necessarily for the adult (Bloom, 1973; Clark, 1973). For example, Werner (1948) described a child's use of "afta" to designate a drinking glass, a pane of glass, a window, and also the contents of a glass. The child did not understand the word used in each situation before using it himself because there is little likelihood that he heard the word in the same situations, but that did not keep him from using it. It appears that, for comprehension, the child needs to experience a word in each instance in order to understand it. But in speech, as in saying "afta," for instance, the child may not previously have heard the word used in the same context. Thus, it is not the case that production depends on prior comprehension for each instance in which a word is used. Although the child needs to have heard the word in order to say it in the first place, he may well learn to understand the word by learning how to use it—that is, by generalizing or associating properties of the situation in which he first heard the word to new situations.

Even though the first words that the child says are not necessarily the same words that are first understood, there seem to be other kinds of similarities between early production and early comprehension. For one, children respond initially to names of particular objects or persons, and first words also make reference to particular objects or persons (such as "birds" in reference only to birds in a mobile and "music" in reference only to a particular record player). For another, among the earliest words that children say are words like "more" to specify another instance or recurrence of an object or event, or "gone" to comment on the disappearance or nonexistence of objects—that is, children also recognize behaviors which different objects can share. There are different objects that can go "up" or be "up," and different things can be prohibited, etc. The use of the words "afta," "more," "up," and "gone" are similar in reference to the child's early comprehension of prohibitive "no," because the same word is ascribed to referents with different figurative properties. Thus children seem to learn words in reference to particular objects, such as "Mommy," "bottle," and "blanket," and in reference across perceptually different objects, such as "no," "more," and "gone" for both comprehension and production. More important than any temporal continuum in development between understanding and talking is the fact that both result from the interaction of mutually influential underlying processes.

From Single Words to Sentences

Once children are well into the use of single word utterances in the 2nd year, the question of related development in comprehension assumes a different form. The question in the 2nd year of development is whether or not children process the syntax of sentences that they hear in order to understand sentences, even though they themselves say only one word at a time. The prevailing assumption has been that children do understand a great deal more than they are actually able to say in this period of time, and such presumed understanding is often used as an argument for the claim that single word utterances are holophrastic or "one-word sentences."

As pointed out by Bloom (1973), children between 1 and 2 years of age do appear to understand a great deal that is said to them and often seem to respond appropriately to complex statements and directions. But the directions and statements they respond to so readily refer to their immediate environment more often than not. Utterances in the speech of mothers addressed to children are frequently redundant in relation to context and behavior, and language learning no doubt depends upon the relationship between the speech the child hears and what he sees and does. There are, as yet, no reports of studies that attempt to evaluate whether or not children using single word utterances understand sentences in nonredundant contexts as well as they understand what is said to them about what they can see or hear, or what they do, aside from often repeated and familiar phrases. For example, the statement, "Will is going down the slide," spoken to a child who has been playing with Will on the playground, would be likely to cause her to look for Will or look toward the slide. If children do not understand sentences that refer to relations among objects and events that are not immediately available, then the extent to which they analyze the semantic-syntactic structure for understanding is certainly questionable. Thus, the same statement "Will is going down the slide" or the question "Is Will going down the slide?" would most probably draw a blank if the child hears it at the dinner table or while taking a bath.

Leopold (1939) pointed out that comprehension during the period when speech is limited to single words depends primarily on the child being able to recognize the highly stressed and salient words in an utterance. Adults speaking to children help them understand by repeating key words and exaggerating stress. Guillaume (1927) vividly described the elaborations through gesture, emphasis, and repetition that are used to help very young children understand what is said to them. For example, "Give Grandma a kiss. Grandma. Give her a *kiss.* Give *Grandma* a kiss" with pointing and pursing the lips, and maybe even turning the child's head toward Grandma would most probably produce the desired result. While such a description may seem somewhat extreme, such cues as repetition, exaggeration, pointing, and gesture come to be automatic for the adult, and children no doubt come to look for such cues and use them for getting meaning from the stream of speech that they hear. Several recent studies of mothers' speech to children have demonstrated that their sentences are shorter, simpler, and more redundant than speech to adults (Broen, 1972; Snow, 1972).

The important issue in relating development in comprehension to development in speaking is the relation between the child's mental schemas for processing such linguistic and nonlinguistic cues, on the one hand, and the mental processes which result in utterances, on the other hand. The cues of repetition, exaggeration, pointing, and gesture are also present in the child's own behavior in the 2nd year, but it is not at all clear how such behaviors relate to the child's perception of such cues produced by others. Children's gestures have frequently aroused interest (for example, McCarthy, 1954), but there have been no studies of the development of kinesic movement in relation to the development of speech. An important issue that remains to be resolved is how children's developing gestures relate to the systematic and conventional system of gestures and "body language" used by adults.[3] But, further, one would like to know how the child's movements augment his speech, and whether the interaction between expressive movements and speech relate to the child's perception of combined gestural and auditory cues from adults.

One investigation that attempted to tap children's understanding during the single word utterance period was reported by Shipley, Smith, and Gleitman (1969) using data from two groups of children: one group used only single word utterances, the second group used telegraphic two- and three-word sentences. Children were presented with commands that directed them to act on an object in their immediate presence. The commands were varied as 1) single words, *e.g.,* "ball;" 2) telegraphic, *e.g.,* "throw ball;" or 3) well formed "throw me the ball." The first finding that was reported was that children who used only single word utterances themselves, responded most often to single word commands, providing no support for the idea that comprehension exceeds production in this period of development. Moreover, the tasks did not evaluate whether or not the children analyzed the structure

[3] Bambi Schieffelen, at Teachers College, Columbia University, is currently involved in just such an investigation, using the video-taped material in Bloom (1973).

of the sentences, inasmuch as merely touching the ball or picking up the ball was accepted as a positive response.

The second finding reported by Shipley, Smith, and Gleitman (1969) was that the older children who were using two- and three-word utterances preferred to respond to well formed commands rather than to telegraphic or single word commands. However, this second result cannot be taken as evidence that comprehension exceeds production if the well formed commands manifested the same syntactic structure represented in the children's own telegraphic, that is, *reduced,* utterances. It has been pointed out that early two- and three-word utterances are often reductions of more complete underlying structure (Bloom, 1970). For example, the actual utterances "read book" and "Mommy book" would have the fuller underlying structure *Mommy read book* given 1) the relevant nonlinguistic state of affairs (Mommy reading, or about to, or supposed to read a book) and 2) evidence elsewhere in a large enough corpus of utterances that the child understands the linguistic relations between agent (of an action) and object (affected by the action).

There seems to be an asymmetry between the child's understanding words and understanding relations between words in the transition from using single word utterances to using longer, structured speech toward the end of the 2nd year. On the one hand, the child needs to understand something of the semantics of a word in order to respond to the word when he hears it spoken by someone else. For example, in order to recognize the association between the acoustic event "milk" and the substance *milk* that is available and offered to him with regularity in his daily routine, he must have perceived and mentally represented, however primitively, the acoustic configuration of the word. On the other hand, the child does not need to know or to understand the semantic-syntactic relations between words, that is, the *structure* of sentences, in order to respond when someone talks about the actual relations between *Mommy* and *book,* or between *Baby* and *milk,* or between *ball* and *floor,* when 1) he already understands the words separately, and 2) such objects and relations occur along with the utterances that make reference to them.

Knowledge of semantic constraints and knowledge of syntax are necessary for understanding linguistic messages that do not refer to the contexts in which they occur. In such utterances, the "meaning" is in the linguistic message alone. But when a sentence is redundant with respect to the context in which it occurs, then the amount of information which the child needs to get from the linguistic message is probably minimal. There is, then, another asymmetry between understanding and speaking multiword utterances in that children do not have to process syntax to understand reference to relations among immediate events, but children do need to learn something about the syntax of the language and semantic constraints in order to talk about such relations in any coherent way. Thus, knowing a word and knowing a grammar, and understanding structured speech and using structured speech, apparently represent different mental capacities. It may be misleading to consider that such capacities develop in linear temporal relation. Such differences between the manifestations of underlying knowledge about aspects of language have not, as yet, been touched on in language development research. They will be explored further, after first considering how the interaction between speaking and understanding has been described in recent psycholinguistic experiments with somewhat older children.

PSYCHOLINGUISTIC TASKS TO COMPARE COMPREHENSION AND PRODUCTION

Several different experimental attempts have been made to investigate the relationship between understanding and speaking in the course of development. Three procedures that will be considered here are: 1) the Imitation-Comprehension-Production (ICP) tasks devised by Fraser, Bellugi, and Brown (1963); 2) training tasks; and 3) the use of elicited imitation.

In the Fraser, Bellugi, and Brown ICP tasks, 3-year-old children were presented with pairs of pictures that portrayed 10 different grammatical relationships such as between subject and direct object. Each pair of pictures presented two contrasting representations of a relation, for example, a *girl* pushing a *boy,* and a *boy* pushing a *girl.* The investigator presented each pair to the child, saying, "Here are two pictures, one of a boy pushing a girl, and the other of a girl pushing a boy." In the imitation task the children were asked to repeat one or the other sentence "The boy is pushing the girl" or "The girl is pushing the boy." In the comprehension task the children were asked to point to the picture that goes with one of the sentences: for example, "Show me the picture of the girl pushing the boy." In the production task, the children were asked to say a sentence for one of the pictures. The results of the experiment were that imitation was easiest and production was most difficult, leading Fraser, Bellugi, and Brown to conclude that imitation precedes comprehension and comprehension precedes production in the course of language development. Subsequently, Lovell and Dixon (1967) repeated the ICP tasks with 2-year-old children, with the same results and apparent confirmation of the conclusion that children are able to imitate and then understand certain linguistic structures before they use them.

There are several problems in accepting the results of the ICP test. For one, in the production task, the children have already heard the sentence in the introduction to the instructions "Here are two pictures, one of a boy pushing a girl, and the other of a girl pushing a boy," which gave some support to the child for making up his own sentence. Imitation was the easiest task, but it was also the case that the length of the sentences presented for imitation was always within the children's auditory memory span. Children have difficulty repeating sentences that exceed memory span even when they themselves are able to produce the same sentences spontaneously at a different time, as will be seen subsequently in the discussion of elicited imitation.

Fernald (1972) has recently challenged both the methodology and the conclusions of the ICP test. He pointed out that the response possibilities were not equated for the comprehension and production tasks and, in part, favored higher scores for comprehension. In pointing to a picture in the comprehension task, the child could be either right or wrong, depending on which picture he chose, and no other responses or behaviors from the child were considered. However, in the production task, Fraser, Bellugi, and Brown had counted irrelevant responses as errors. Fernald repeated the experiment but equated the response possibilities for both comprehension and production, and when looking at only the correct or incorrect responses in both tasks, comprehension and production were essentially the same. Baird (1972) also questioned the procedures of the ICP tasks. Other research reports have contradicted the evidence of the comprehension-production gap in language development.

Keeney and Wolfe (1972) tested the production, imitation, and comprehension of subject-verb agreement for number in English sentences by 46 3- and 4-year-old children. Production of subject-verb agreement was evaluated in the children's spontaneous speech; 94% of 906 utterances were correct for number agreement; and there were no errors in sentences with the copula "be." More than one-half of the sentences had pronouns rather than nouns as subjects. The authors concluded from this sample that the children reliably inflected verbs for number agreement with subject nouns in their spontaneous speech. In the imitation task, sentence stimuli were either grammatical or ungrammatical (for subject-verb agreement) and did not exceed memory span, for example "The bird is singing." Verbatim responses were scored; 83% of the grammatical sentences were repeated verbatim while only 51% of the ungrammatical sentences were repeated verbatim. However, in 93% of the ungrammatical sentences not repeated verbatim, the children corrected the noun and verb inflection, again demonstrating that they knew the rule for producing subject-verb agreement in sentences.

The results of three comprehension tests in the Keeney and Wolfe experiments were not so clear cut. In one of the comprehension tests, the verbal test, children were presented with either a spoken singular or plural verb and asked to say a subject-noun that agreed in number; results of this test indicated that the children were responding to the verb number inflection in that they most often produced subject-nouns in agreement. In the second and third tests, the children were asked to point to one of a pair of pictures that represented a bird or birds, acting out either a full spoken sentence, in one test, or only the spoken verb of a sentence, in the other (verbal) test. In responding to the full sentences, the children were most often right (apparently responding to the noun number), but in responding to the verb alone they were not. Based on the results of this experiment, Keeney and Wolfe concluded that the children did not understand the relation between verb inflections for number and the meaning of singular or plural, even though they could produce subject-verb agreement for number in their speech: "in reference to the verb number inflection, then, production does indeed precede comprehension."

There are a number of questions that can be asked of the Keeney and Wolfe results—some of which were raised by the authors themselves. They pointed out, for example, that numerosity is a cognitive notion with respect to objects and is effectively signalled by the singular-plural inflection of nouns. The verb inflection is essentially redundant, and moreover, contradicts the noun inflection in form. Thus, a singular noun has no inflection, but plural nouns add [-s]; whereas the agreeing verb adds [-s] for singular nouns and nothing for the plural: "the bird sings" and "the birds sing." The result is that "sings" and "bird" are singular; "sing" and "birds" are plural.

One might indeed question whether the verb inflection actually means singular *vs* plural apart from the noun (or pronoun) number. Expecting children to recognize its quasi-semantic function may be a metalinguistic task that is beyond their capabilities at 3 and 4 years. The fact that the inflection was fully productive in their spontaneous speech was evidence that they had learned a syntactic rule which they could not identify. Such learning may reflect a certain integrity of the linguistic system as the child is learning it. That is, learning one aspect of the system necessarily entails knowing related aspects, so that knowing plural rules for nouns and speaking sentences will predict the use of verb agreement. In this case, as with lexical items, using a linguistic form may be a means of learning it.

In a recent study by Lahey (in press) there is support for the idea that children may incorporate surface features of the language into their speech before they fully understand the underlying meaning distinctions that such forms represent. Lahey compared 4- and 5-year-old children's comprehension of coordinate, center-embedded relative clause, and right-branching relative clause sentences under four conditions of presentation: 1) with both prosody and syntactic markers, 2) with markers but without prosody, 3) with prosody but without markers, and 4) with neither prosody nor markers. The children were asked to act out such sentences as "the cow hit the pig that chased the deer" with toy animals, and the number of semantic-syntactic relationships that were acted out was scored.

Lahey reported that coordinate sentences were easiest to understand and right-branching sentences were the most difficult, which was in contrast to the report by Menyuk (1969) that nursery school children *produced* more right-branching sentences than center-embedded sentences. Further, scores for center-embedded sentences were significantly lower when prosody was eliminated, but syntactic markers were present. Lahey concluded that word order was the major linguistic cue that the children used to process the sentences presented to them, even though they were at the age when children produce many syntactic markers in their spontaneous speech. Some of the children in the study spontaneously reproduced the sentences as they acted them out and either repeated the marker or supplied it when it was missing but, nevertheless, did not demonstrate the relationship that was marked by the relative pronoun.

Two studies have compared the ability of younger children to respond to word order variations in comprehension tasks with their ability to use word order in their own speech. Wetstone and Friedlander (1973) reported that children who used two- and three-word utterances with consistent word order responded equally as well to both normal word order and varied word order in questions and directions presented to them. Chapman and Miller (1973) used object manipulation to compare children's comprehension and production of subject-object order in semantically reversible sentences with animate and inanimate subjects and objects. They reported that children used appropriate subject-object order in speaking significantly more often than in responding to subject-object cues in a comprehension task.

Of particular interest in the Chapman and Miller study was the result that the two younger groups of children (with mean length of utterance less than 2.5 morphemes) responded correctly at less than chance level to sentences with an inanimate subject and an animate object, indicating that they were responding to the animacy of the nouns more often than they responded to word order to determine the relationship of each noun to the verb. Although Chapman and Miller did not report the corresponding information for production, that is, the extent to which the children used animate or inanimate nouns as sentence subjects, their comprehension result is consistent with other reports that animate nouns predominate as sentence subjects in children's early sentences (Bloom, 1970; Brown, Cazden, and Bellugi, 1969). It appears that semantic-syntactic knowledge of verbs influences comprehension and production similarly in early development. The semantics of verbs determines the selectional restrictions on nouns as subjects and objects, and the verbs that predominate in early grammar are those verbs that allow reference to people doing things and inanimate objects being acted upon. Eventually, children need to learn 1) that the semantic-syntactic restrictions with such verbs as "hit, chase, bump, push, pull, and carry" (the verbs used in the Chapman and Miller tasks) can be relaxed to specify inanimate agents and effect on animate objects and 2) that word order can override certain selectional restrictions of verbs as a stronger linguistic device. Again, as with lexical items and grammatical morphemes, using word order may be a means of learning more about its grammatical function, as the child actively applies his knowledge to new situations and thereby expands on it.

Training Tasks

In a study by Guess (1969) two severely retarded boys, each 13 years old and with reported mental age of 4.5 years, were trained for the acquisition of the plural morpheme. When trained to understand the forms, the subjects did not generalize to expressive use at the same time. Subsequently, after being trained to use the plural forms correctly, successful reversed receptive training did not generalize to reversed expressive use. Guess concluded that the subjects' ability to learn to understand the plural morpheme was independent of their ability to learn to use it.

In a follow-up study, Guess and Baer (1973) trained four retarded subjects concurrently in both comprehension and production of different allomorphs, either [-s] or [-z], of the plural morpheme. Subjects were trained to understand one plural form and to produce a different plural form. The findings indicated that even when trained concurrently to both understand and use the plural morpheme so that new, untrained stimuli were responded to correctly, three of the four retarded subjects exhibited partial or no generalization of performance from comprehension to production or *vice versa* with the same plural allomorph. As Guess and Baer pointed out, other studies have used a learning paradigm and have demonstrated the effectiveness of training in one modality (production or comprehension) for facilitating performance in the other, for example, studies of articulation (Winitz and Preisler, 1965; and Mann and Baer, 1971).

The most relevant issue with respect to the relative importance of understanding and using a speech form in the process of learning it has to do with the many variables that interact to affect each. On the one hand, one might well question how it is possible for an individual to use a linguistic structure or form without knowing something about it. However, the important fact is that both understanding and the use of a linguistic form—whether a particular word, a grammatical morpheme, or a syntactic structure—depend on a great many variables, both linguistic and nonlinguistic. The studies by Guess and Guess and Baer compared the effects of specific training for auditory discrimination and expression of a grammatical form, and their results indicated that there was little mutual influence between the two kinds of performance within the contingencies of the reinforcement paradigm. In the experimental situation, the contingencies of reward might be strong enough to preclude any behavior that is not directly reinforced. Even though subjects included new instances within the response category (when they supplied the learned morphemes to novel words), the variables that defined the response behavior were necessarily constrained. It is not clear what the subjects knew that led them to say or respond to the plural morpheme.

In a naturalistic situation, a child might respond to the form when he hears it, but what he understands of the form might be heavily dependent on the situation in which he hears it or on the state of affairs to which it refers. By the same token, a child's use of a particular form cannot be taken as unequivocal evidence that he knows the form so that he can understand and use it in unlimited reference and in any situation. As will be seen, this fact becomes quite important when one considers children's performance in elicited imitation tasks.

Elicited Imitation

An important limitation in studies of speech output has to do with the constraints of topic and context as influences on the grammatical structures or words that children use. That is, what a child says depends on what he is talking about. One needs to obtain large samples of speech in order to be assured of some degree of representation of the child's linguistic knowledge. But the time involved in collecting and processing large speech samples has limited the number of children that can be studied in this way, so that other techniques for tapping children's knowledge are necessary. One such technique that has received some attention is having children repeat phrases and sentences. It is possible to prepare sentences that present specific structures one might want to test for in different groups of children. The underlying rationale for presenting such sentences to children to imitate has been that the child will process sentences that exceed auditory memory span according to what he knows about grammar. As a result, it has been argued, one can tell how much he understood of the original sentence by looking at how much of the meaning of the original sentence is preserved in his own repetition of it, and his repetition will provide evidence of his own coding abilities for production. The underlying premise in elicited imitation tasks, then, is that if a sentence is too long for the child to hold in memory he will process the meaning of the sentence, and his imitation of it, although shorter and inexact, will provide some evidence of 1) the extent to which he understood it and 2) what he knows about speaking such sentences.

The technique has been used with different research questions in mind. Menyuk (1963) had children imitate well formed (by adult standards) sentences and utterances produced by children that did not conform to the model language. Others have compared imitations of standard English and black English sentences by black speakers (for example, Labov, 1968) or by black and white speakers (for example, Baratz, 1969). Rodd and Braine (1971) attempted to assess the ability of 2-year-old children to repeat a variety of phrase structures.

In order to further explore the relation between spontaneous speaking and elicited imitation, one of the children studied longitudinally by Bloom and her associates, Peter, was asked to play a repetition game. Peter had been identified as an imitator in natural speech inasmuch as an average of one-third of his different utterances consisted of repetitions of something spoken by someone else (Bloom, Hood, and Lightbown, 1974). Thus, Peter imitated easily in naturalistic situations, and he played the game when presented with sentences to elicit imitation. The following exchanges took place between an adult investigator and Peter, age 32 months, 2 weeks, as they played "Simple Simon says."[4]

Simple Simon says:	Peter:
1. This is a big balloon.	This a big balloon.
2. This is broken.	What's broken?
3. This is broken.	That's broken.
4. I'm trying to get this cow in there.	Cow in here.
5. I'm gonna get the cow to drink milk.	Get the cow to drink milk.
6. You made him stand up over there.	Stand up there.

These sentences were among a list of 14 sentences presented to Peter. He readily attempted to repeat all but two: "That is not bigger" and "What's that on your leg?"

Looking at his responses to the sentences 1—6 above, one might conclude a) that Peter probably understands but cannot produce the copula "is," as in examples 1—3; and b) Peter may or may not understand, but he cannot produce causal connectives such as "gonna," "trying," and "made" in examples 4—6. However, all of the 14 sentences presented to Peter for imitation had actually been produced by Peter spontaneously the preceding day, as follows:

Speech event:	Peter:
2 and 3. (Peter showing airplane with broken tail to investigator)	This is broken.
4. (Peter trying to get a colt's feet to fit into a barrel)	I'm trying to get *this* cow in there.
5. (Peter, holding the cow, going to the toy bag to get barrels)	I'm gonna get the cow to drink some milk.
(Peter returning with the barrels)	I'm gonna get the cow to drink some milk.
6. (Peter trying to get investigator to spread an animal's legs, so that it will stand in a spot he had cleared for it)	You made him stand up over there.

It appears, then, that given the support of contextual events and his own behavior, Peter's spontaneous speaking ability exceeded his ability to imitate

---

[4] From data collected in collaboration with Patsy Lightbown and Lois Hood. The numbered utterances on the left were presented by an adult investigator for Peter to repeat.

sentences presented to him for imitation. When asked to reproduce sentences that did not relate to immediate context and behavior, he could not produce the very same utterances he himself had produced with such support. In pointing out that their subject also could not reproduce the same sentence she herself had said earlier, Slobin and Welsh (1973) suggested that intention, in addition to context, contributed to the support for the production of messages.

Intention to speak and contextual support from the actual existence of a referent for the utterance are two factors contributing to production performance that are missing in elicited imitation performance and in comprehension tasks. Thus, a child's saying a sentence originates with 1) an internal state of knowing, needing, or intending; plus 2) a referent in context and behavior; plus 3) linguistic knowledge about structure and semantic constraints. In responding to a sentence that he hears in the certain absence of 1), and the possible absence of 2), the child can depend only on 3). Talking and understanding are clearly different behaviors and seem to involve something more than simply a temporal relation in the course of their development.

BETWEEN UNDERSTANDING AND SPEAKING

A disparity between perception and production has been presumed for a long time in speech and psychology as well as in art, and various attempts have been made to understand and explain it (see, for example, Olson and Pagliuso, 1968). Among the most often quoted examples of the difference between perception and production is the fact that children are able to recognize geometric shapes long before they can reproduce them. Adults can recognize and appreciate a work of art but few, indeed, can reproduce one. Some small children can hear the difference between "*l*ight" and "*w*hite" and yet cannot say the words differently themselves, saying "white wight;" and individuals learning a second language often understand more than they can say.

Among the explanations of the disparity that have been offered, there is reference to memory factors affecting recognition and recall (Mandler, 1967); the knowledge of extra details or attributes that is needed for reproduction as opposed to recognition (Maccoby and Bee, 1965); and the intervening mental reconstruction of an image as the basis for reproduction (Piaget and Inhelder, 1970). Such explanations have not been explicitly extended to young children learning language, but they may contribute to an exploration of the developmental relationship among understanding, talking, and thinking. The memory load for saying a sentence is presumably greater than for understanding, inasmuch as the individual needs to recall the necessary words and their connections to say them, but these linguistic facts are immediately available to him when he hears them spoken by someone else. The child can experience a sentence as more or less independent of its parts, but saying sentences involves bringing together the elements to form a whole. In recognizing a word or a sentence, a child relates what he hears to existing perceptual schemas, but saying the word or sentence involves reconstructing an intervening representation in the form of a "symbolic image" (Piaget and Inhelder, 1971). In Piaget and Inhelder's view, the latter is more difficult.

It is not clear how representational images relate to either the acoustic signals that the child hears or the speech that he himself produces. Both seem to involve the reconstruction of existing schemas, but, perhaps, at different levels of complexity. It is worth considering that the mental representation that gives rise to an utterance is cognitively less complex than the search for an "existing" perceptual schema that is triggered by hearing speech.

One might consider that in the course of development, both linguistic events (A) and nonlinguistic events (B) provide input that is perceived and organized at (C) in Figure 1. What the child knows of language—that is, that information that allows him to both understand and produce messages— is represented by (C) and depends upon the mental organization and integration of (A) and (B). Whether one speaks of images, concepts, or schemas, there is necessarily some form of mental representation of events. There is not a one-to-one relation between (A) and (B), that is, between linguistic facts, on the one hand, and items and events in the real world, on the other. Rather, there is a necessary internal mental representation of experience, and language is a means for coding or mapping experience.

What are some of the factors that may be involved in producing and understanding messages, in the course of language development, given the basic premise represented by (C) above: that language does not code reality,

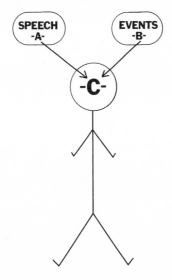

Fig. 1.

but, rather, language codes the individual's intervening mental representation or his experience of reality? The question is an enormously complicated one, and there does not appear to be existing evidence as yet that will lead directly to an answer. At best, what is offered here is a highly tentative and partial account that might lead to the formulation of testable hypotheses for obtaining such evidence.

With respect to producing messages, it has been observed repeatedly (for example, Leopold, 1939; Brown and Bellugi, 1964; Bloom, 1970) that children typically talk about what they are doing or what they can see in the immediate "here and now" in which their utterances occur. Thus, a child might climb on a tricycle and announce "ride trike," or fit a peg into a hole and comment "this fit" or "no fit" (if it doesn't). Child utterances are redundant with respect to the context in which they occur, and to which they also refer, more often than not. Adults, in marked contrast, do not ordinarily talk about what they see or what they are doing when the listener is there to see for himself. In adult discourse, an utterance that bears no relation to the perceivable situation can elicit an appropriate response that also does not relate to what the speakers see or hear or do at the same time.

Egocentricity is often invoked to account for the fact that children seem not to take into account the information that is already available to the listener—or, indeed, to take the listener into account at all. A second point that can be made is that mother's speech to children is probably no less redundant, and indeed, language learning probably depends on the fact that mothers will not typically discuss finances or an argument with a friend when they talk to their children. Rather, when the young child comes into a room with a ball, the typical comment might be "You've got a ball" or "That's your red ball," or "Do you have a ball?" Thus, it might be argued, that children talk in the "here and now" because their parents talk in the "here and now" (to them). However, both the fact that the child is centered on his own actions and perceptions when he produces messages, that is, his egocentricity, and the fact that mothers' speech to children is also redundant with respect to context may well be related to another cause: that young children are strongly dependent on the support of nonlinguistic context for both producing and understanding messages.

It is important to emphasize that it is not the immediate context *per se* that supports the child's message or that enables him to decode messages, but, rather, it is the child's mental representation of the circumstances and events in nonlinguistic context. Thus, in Figure 1, the nature of the child's mental representation at (C) will determine the extent of his success at producing and understanding messages. Consider Figure 2, in which a linguistic signal (A) encodes an event (B).[5] It is proposed that, in early development, the

---

[5] The following diagrams are presented here with full awareness that they are incomplete. They hypothetically schematize some of the observations about the relation

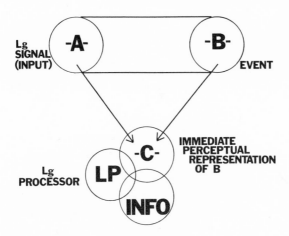

Fig. 2.

success of the child's understanding the message in (A) would be dependent upon the extent to which the child understands the relations in (B), with the immediate perceptual representation of the event as the source of the child's information at (C). The linguistic signal may function simply to call attention or focus the child on the event, and extent of understanding would be relatively independent of the complexity of the signal, with limited linguistic processing at LP.

Similarly, in Figure 3, the child is again presented with an event (B), but it is the child who produces the linguistic signal (A) relative to event (B), as output. Here, the success of the child's producing the message depends, again, on the immediate perceptual representation of the event (B) but also on his ability to use a linguistic processor for coding the information in (C). Given the states of affairs represented in Figures 2 and 3, comprehension may well exceed or at least be equal to production depending on the need for and use of a linguistic processing mechanism. In both, the same information about event (B) is available at (C), but linguistic processing appears to be necessary for producing messages about event relationships (multiword utterances), but not necessary for understanding such messages, when these relate to immediately perceived events. But if understanding is greater than talking, it is important to recognize that understanding can be largely nonlinguistic— which, at least at this early stage of development, would seem to close the comprehension-production gap.

This appears to be a plausible account of at least part of the relation between understanding and speaking in the period when children say only

between understanding and speaking in language development that have been discussed. They are offered, tentatively, for the purposes of discussion and, hopefully, further elaboration after relevant empirical study.

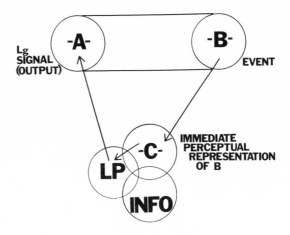

Fig. 3.

one word at a time—given the information referred to earlier and other accounts as well (Bloom, 1973). That is, children in the single word utterance period say only one word at a time because they do not yet know a linguistic code for representing information through semantic-syntactic relations between words. The fact that children are limited to single word utterances is evidence that they do not know enough about semantic-syntactic structure to say sentences; how much they know of semantic-syntactic structure for understanding sentences remains to be determined.

What of the relation between understanding and speaking when children are using multiword utterances? The conditions in Figures 2 and 3 continue to prevail; that is, there is still the perceptual representation of immediate events at (C) to support both encoding and decoding. It can now be assumed that the linguistic mechanism is more complex and functions to provide information from the linguistic signal that the child receives, in addition to coding the information that the child puts into messages. Here the relation between comprehension and production is less clear cut and needs to be tested by careful comparative research. The temporal lag at this point in development, if it exists, appears to assume that production itself is evidence of comprehension, but that assumption remains to ,be verified as well. The results reported by Chapman and Miller (1973) suggested that comprehension during early development of grammar depends upon lexical decoding, with semantic relations between words cued by the relations between objects in event contexts *at the same time* that children are using knowledge of syntax (word order) to say sentences.

It seems that the major task for the child in the course of language development is the ability to speak and understand messages that are independent of external situations or internal affectual and need states. Language emerges as truly creative in the sense described by Chomsky (1966)—the ability to speak and understand indefinitely many sentences, never spoken or heard before—only through a very gradual process that no doubt continues well into the school years. Thus, language development probably culminates when the child becomes capable of the logical operations described by Piaget (1956), and language becomes for the child truly a means of knowing, at about age 12. But while the achievement of the ability to use a linguistic code relatively independent of context may be the major task of language development in the school years, it certainly has its beginnings in the early preschool years and, further, may never be completely achieved in the adult years, as will be discussed subsequently.

With respect to understanding that is independent of the situation in which it occurs, consider Figure 4. Here, the linguistic signal must be processed at LP, the linguistic processor, first. As the signal is processed, there is no support in the immediate perceptual representation for representing the information in the message. The linguistic signal is the only external source of information about the message. Therefore, information from the LP must be compared with what the child already knows (INFO in cognitive memory) in order to obtain a mental representation of the message at (C) and thereby understand it.

Speaking that is independent of the situation in which it occurs would be schematized as in Figure 5. Here, it is the mental representation at (C) that precipitates the linguistic signal, but the representation originates internally, from the information in the child's cognitive memory (INFO). Thus, the utterance codes what the child already knows. The LP receives the information for linguistically representing the content of the message, in the form of a mental representation, image, or schema at (C).

Comparing speech in Figure 5, where there is no external event (B), with

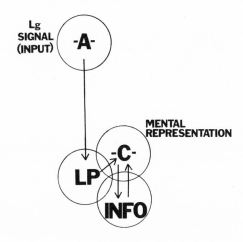

Fig. 4.

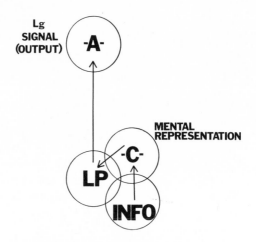

Fig. 5.

speech in Figure 3, where there is an external event (B), one can see that where there is an external event to be talked about, message content is more immediately accessible at (C) to the LP for linguistic processing for output. Although there is necessary interaction between (C) and stored INFO in order for the child to know what he sees in (B), the mental representation for the content of the utterance is in the immediate perception. Similarly, one can compare understanding in Figure 4 where there is no event (B), with understanding in Figure 2, where there is an external event (B) that interacts with the message (A).

In this account, one can see how young children's speech occurs most often in relation to immediately perceived events, and children apparently understand speech in relation to immediately perceived events. The diagrams (Figs. 2 and 3) do not explain speech and understanding in the "here and now"; they offer no new information but simply schematize speech and understanding in the "here and now" so that it is possible to see how it is characteristic of early development.

Comparing speaking and understanding, it is not difficult to understand why comprehension in Figure 2, where there is an external event (B), would occur more readily than where there is not an external event, as in comprehension in Figure 4 and speaking in Figure 5. However, the comparison that may be more pertinent to the language development evidence that was discussed earlier is between understanding and speaking in the absence of an external event (B), the comparison between events in Figures 4 and 5. Here, it is possible that understanding may well be less than or equal to speaking, because, in understanding, the mental representation of the content of the message originates with the linguistic signal (A), and the information for mental representation available at (C) is limited, first, to information from the linguistic processor. However, producing an utterance originates with the mental representation at (C) which provides information to the linguistic processor for semantic representation.

Piaget and Inhelder (1971) argued that the need for constructing the mental image or schema makes production difficult. It would certainly make production in the absence of an event (B) more difficult than production given an external event to talk about. But it also appears that creating the mental representation as input to linguistic encoding may be cognitively less complex than deriving a mental representation as a result of linguistic decoding. In this regard, one can compare children's utterances that occur in discourse, in response to what someone else says, with utterances that originate spontaneously. In current research in progress (Bloom, Higgins, and Hood, forthcoming), data from four children consist of records of discourse between child and others (investigators and mothers) from the age of approximately 19 months to 3 years. The children produced far fewer utterances in response to what someone else said than they produced spontaneously. Communicative effectiveness was greater for utterances that were not responses to adult utterances, that is utterances that originated with what the child was thinking about, or did, or saw. Further, communicative effectiveness increased developmentally for utterances that were contingent on preceding utterances from an adult. The argument is, essentially, that what an individual knows about an event will determine his ability to both speak and understand messages that code that event and, further, either the event in actual context or the mentally represented event will always be a richer source of information about messages than a linguistic signal alone.

Several experimental studies have demonstrated that what a child knows about an event will influence how he interprets a message about the event. Given the same linguistic message, the child will have greater or lesser difficulty interpreting it depending upon what he already knows about the state of affairs encoded in the message. In a series of experiments, Huttenlocher (1968a, b; 1971) has demonstrated that messages such as "The red truck pushes the green truck" will be responded to with varying delay depending on whether one or the other or neither of the objects is already placed in a three-space track or ladder. Thus, the child's ability to determine the relationship between two nouns in a sentence is determined in part by how the corresponding objects appear to him in the situation in which the sentence occurs.

Earlier it was said that the major achievement in language development is the ability to use a linguistic code independently of the situational contexts in which utterances occur. In attempting to explain the development away from dependence on context, it is necessary to recognize the continual development of increasingly more complex systems of mental representation of both linguistic and nonlinguistic information. Also, it is clear that even in adults, context continues to be important. Recent research by Johnson, Bransford, and Solomon (in press) and Bransford and Johnson (1972) has demonstrated how the availability of context and prior knowledge can influence comprehension and recall of linguistic messages by adults.

Bransford and Johnson pointed out that understanding a sentence is "a joint function of input information and prior knowledge." They presented five groups of subjects with a prose passage read to them under the following conditions: 1) no context (simply hearing the passage); 2) context before (seeing an appropriate pictured context before hearing the passage); 3) context after (seeing the picture after hearing the passage); 4) partial context (seeing a pictured context with the relevant items rearranged); and 5) no context, but two presentations of the passage. Subjects then rated the passage on a 7-point scale of comprehension difficulty and then were asked to recall (in writing) the passage as accurately as possible, or at least write down as many ideas as they could. Subjects who received the pictured context before hearing the passage recalled twice as much or more than subjects in any of the other conditions. Their mean comprehension rating was 6.1 (where 7 was the highest rating), while other ratings ranged from 2.3 to 3.7. According to Bransford and Johnson's results, adults understand more from hearing a prose passage when provided with an overt context. Moreover, their subjects reported that they attempted to mentally create situational context when they only heard the prose passage.

It appears that the mental representation of linguistic features of meaning continues to be influenced through adulthood by the interaction of informational, contextual, and pragmatic constraints. The above schematic diagrams are obviously very gross in their representation of the enormously complex interactions that take place with speaking and understanding. The components themselves need to be described and explained, and such explanation should result in considerable refinement of the network of their interaction. However, they do make it possible to see some of the sources of variability in speaking and understanding performance that have been observed. The performance of a particular child will differ to the extent to which learning and maturation have influenced development in any of the component systems: the mechanism for linguistic processing, cognitive memory, and capacities for mental representation of experience.

In summary, the only conclusion that seems appropriate to what has been presented here is that there is not enough information at the present time to explain the relationship between speaking and understanding in language development. At best, the research that has been done is contradictory and inconclusive. However, it is important to emphasize that the relationship is probably never a static one but, rather, shifts and varies according to the experience of the individual child and his developing linguistic and cognitive capacities.

REFERENCES

Baird, R. On the role of change in imitation, comprehension and production. Test results. *J. Verb. Learning Verb. Behav.*, 1972, *11*, 474–477.

Baratz, J. A bidialectal task for determining language proficiency in economically disadvantaged Negro children. *Child Develop.*, 1969, *40*, 889–901.

Bloom, L. *Language Development: Form and Function in Emerging Grammars.* Cambridge, Mass.: M.I.T. Press, 1970.

Bloom, L. *One Word at a Time: The Use of Single Word Utterances before Syntax.* The Hague: Mouton, 1973.

Bloom, L. Language development. In F. Horowitz, E. Hetherington, S. Scarr-Salapatek, and G. Siegel (Eds.), *Review of Child Development Research*, Vol. 4. Chicago: University of Chicago Press, in press.

Bloom, L., Higgins, L., and Hood, L. The development of child-adult discourse. Forthcoming.

Bloom, L., Hood, L., and Lightbown, P. Imitation in language development: If, when and why. *Cognitive Psychology*, 1974, 6.

Bransford, J. and Johnson, M. Contextual prerequisites for understanding: Some investigations of comprehension and recall. *J. Verb. Learning Verb. Behav.*, 1972, *11*, 717–726.

Broen, P. The verbal environment of the language learning child. *ASHA Monogr.*, 1972, *17*.

Brown, R. and Bellugi, U. Three processes in the child's acquisition of syntax. *Harvard Educ. Rev.*, 1964, *34*, 133–151.

Brown, R., Cazden, C., and Bellugi, U. The child's grammar from I to III. In J. P. Hill (Ed.), *Minnesota Symposium on Child Language*, Vol. 2. Minneapolis: University of Minnesota Press, 1969.

Chapman, R. S. and Miller, J. F. Early two and three word utterances: Does production precede comprehension? Paper presented at the Fifth Annual Child Language Research Forum, Stanford University, Stanford, April, 1973.

Chomsky, N. *Cartesian Linguistics.* New York: Harper & Row, 1966.

Clark, E. What's in a word? On the child's acquisition of semantics in his first language. In T. Moore (Ed.), *Cognitive Development and the Acquisition of Language.* New York: Academic Press, 1973, pp. 65–110.

Eimas, P., Sigueland, E., Jusczyk, P., and Vigorito, J. Speech perception in infants. *Science*, 1971, *171*, 303–306.

Fernald, C. Control of grammar in imitation, comprehension, and production: Problems of replication. *J. Verb. Learning Verb. Behav.*, 1972, *11*, 606–613.

Fraser, C., Bellugi, U., and Brown, R. Control of grammar in imitation, comprehension and production. *J. Verb. Learning Verb. Behav.*, 1963, *2*, 121–135.

Guess, D. A functional analysis of receptive language and productive speech: Acquisition of the plural morpheme. *J. Appl. Behav. Anal.*, 1969, *2*, 55–64.

Guess, D. and Baer, D. An analysis of individual differences in generalization between receptive and productive language in retarded children. *J. Appl. Behav. Anal.*, 1973, *6*, 311–329.

Guillaume, P. Les debuts de la phrase dans le language de l'enfant. *J. Psychol.*, 1927, *24*, 1–25.

Huttenlocher, J., Eisenberg, K., and Strauss, S. Comprehension: Relation between perceived actor and logical subject. *J. Verb. Learning Verb. Behav.*, 1968a, *7*, 527–530.

Huttenlocher, J. and Strauss, S. Comprehension and a statement's relation to the situation it describes. *J Verb. Learning Verb. Behav.*, 1968b, *7*, 300–304.

Huttenlocher, J. and Weiner, S. Comprehension of instructions in varying contexts. *Cognitive Psychol.*, 1971, *2*, 369–385.

Johnson, M., Bransford, J., and Solomon, S. Memory for tacit implications of sentences. *J. Exp. Psychol.*, in press.

Kaplan, E. Intonation and language acquisition. *Papers and Reports on Child Language Development.* Stanford: Committee on Linguistics, Stanford University, 1970.

Keeney, T. and Wolfe, J. The acquisition of agreement in English. *J. Verb. Learning Verb. Behav.*, 1972, *11*, 698–705.

Labov, W., Cohen, P., Robbins, D., and Lewis, J. A study of nonstandard English of Negro and Puerto Rican speakers in New York City. Vols. I and II, Final Report, Cooperative Research Project, Office of Education, 1968.

Lahey, M. The use of prosody and syntactic markers in children's comprehension of spoken sentences. *J. Sp. Hear. Res.*, in press.

Leopold, W. *Speech Development of a Bilingual Child.* Evanston, Ill.: Northwestern University Press, 1939–49.

Lewis, M. *Infant Speech, a Study of the Beginnings of Language.* New York: Humanities Press, 1951.

Lovell, K. and Dixon, E. The growth of the control of grammar in imitation, comprehension, and production. *J. Child Psychol. Psychiat.*, 1967, *8*, 31–39.

Maccoby, E. and Bee, H. Some speculations concerning the lag between perceiving and performing. *Child Develop.*, 1965, *36*, 367–377.

Mandler, G. Verbal learning. In T. Newcomb (Ed.), *New Directions in Psychology*, Vol. 3. New York: Holt, Rinehart & Winston, 1967.

Mann, R. and Baer, D. The effects of receptive language training on articulation. *J. Appl. Behav. Anal.*, 1971, *4*, 291–298.

McCarthy, D. Language development. In L. Carmichael (Ed.), *Manual of Child Psychology.* New York: Wiley, 1954.

McNeill, D. *The Acquisition of Language: The Study of Developmental Psycholinguistics.* New York: Harper & Row, 1970.

Menyuk, P. A preliminary evaluation of grammatical capacity in children. *J. Verb. Learning Verb. Behav.*, 1963, *2*, 429–439.

Menyuk, P. *Sentences Children Use.* Cambridge, Mass.: M.I.T. Press, 1969.

Moffitt, A. Consonant cue perception by twenty- to twenty-four-week old infants. *Child Develop.*, 1971, *42*, 717–731.

Olson, D. and Pagliuso, S. (Eds.) From perceiving to performing: An aspect of cognitive growth. *Ontario J. Educ. Res.*, 1968, *10*, No. 3.

Piaget, J. *The Psychology of Intelligence.* Patterson, N.J.: Littlefield, Adams, 1960.

Piaget, J. and Inhelder, B. *Mental Imagery in the Child.* New York: Basic Books, 1971.

Rodd, L. and Braine, M. Children's imitations of syntactic constructions as a measure of linguistic competence. *J. Verb. Learning Verb. Behav.*, 1971, *10*, 430–443.

Shipley, E., Smith, C., and Gleitman, L. A study in the acquisition of language: Free responses to commands. *Language*, 1969, *45*, 322–342.

Slobin, D. I. and Welsh, C. A. Elicited imitation as a research tool in developmental psycholinguistics. In C. A. Ferguson and D. I. Slobin (Eds.), *Readings in Child Language Acquisition.* New York: Holt, Rinehart & Winston, 1973.

Snow, C. Mothers' speech to children learning language. *Child Develop.*, 1972, *43*, 549–565.

Spitz, R. *No and Yes.* New York: International Universities Press, 1957.

Werner, H. *Comparative Psychology of Mental Development.* New York: Science Editions, 1948.

Wetstone, H. and Friedlander, G. The effect of word order on young children's responses to simple questions and commands. Paper presented to the Society for Research in Child Development, 1973.

Winitz, H. and Preisler, L. Discrimination pretraining and sound learning. *Percept. Mot. Skills*, 1965, *20*, 905–916.

CHAPTER TWELVE

THE RELATIONSHIP BETWEEN COMPREHENSION AND PRODUCTION

David Ingram

Department of Linguistics, University of British Columbia, Vancouver 8, British Columbia, Canada

Several years ago, it was quite fashionable to assume that comprehension precedes production. This position is evident in McCarthy's famous review in 1954: "Most writers agree that the child understands the language of others before he actually uses language himself" (p. 520). McCarthy went on from there to discuss the issue of the gap between comprehension and production. Some recent experiments also support the claim of comprehension ahead of production, in particular Fraser, Bellugi, and Brown (1963) and Shipley, Smith, and Gleitman (1969). In the last 2 years, however, this position has undergone a radical shift. There is a certain skepticism in the air about this previously accepted position. The skepticism has ranged from claiming that the relationship between them is one of mutual dependence (Bloom, 1973b) to asserting that production actually precedes comprehension (Chapman and Miller, 1973). In fact, it is now fashionable to deny the previous assumption.

This chapter holds that comprehension does precede production, and that it could never be any other way. That is, it is proposed that *comprehension ahead of production is a linguistic universal of acquisition,* and that the empirical issues involved here are not this claim but rather the nature of comprehension and production and the gap between them. We shall attempt to show what is meant by the claim and to clarify some misunderstandings that have led to alternate positions. Much of the problem results from the fact that it is unusual to find anyone actually explaining what is meant by saying that one precedes the other. We hope to show that current findings to the contrary are actually supportive of the traditional position.

POSSIBLE RELATIONSHIPS BETWEEN COMPREHENSION AND PRODUCTION

In its most literal sense, the quotation from McCarthy could be taken to mean that the child has complete understanding of language before uttering a word. This is given in I as the strongest possible claim in favor of comprehension preceding production.

I. All comprehension of language is complete before any production begins.

Anyone who has observed a child developing language in a normal manner knows that this is not the case. Rather, it appears that very little of language is comprehended when the first words appear. Even so, there is an interesting related claim that is relevant to the issue.

Ia. All or much of comprehension of language may be complete before any production begins, and the converse situation is never found.

Evidence for Ia comes from those cases where there is deviation from what is otherwise normal.

The classic case is that described by Lenneberg (1962) of a child who showed extensive comprehension of English yet could not produce any speech. The subject was an 8-year-old boy suffering from anarthria, a congenital inability to acquire motor speech skills. The child was tested for comprehension by being asked to respond to a series of questions and commands. He was able to do so appropriately, even when the contextual influences were reduced by such procedures as absence of the mother, transmission of instructions through earphones, and requiring active responses beyond nodding simply yes or no. Also, the stimulus items were sufficiently complex that it appeared unlikely that the child was picking out key words rather than following English syntax. From these tests, Lenneberg concluded that the child had normal understanding of English.

An example of a child who achieved partial comprehension of language without speech is that of the wild boy of Aveyron as reported in Itard (1932) and discussed in Brown (1958). The child was found living alone in the Caune Woods in France and upon capture showed no signs of knowing language. It was estimated that he was 12 years of age and had been living in isolation for at least 5 years. For the next 5 years Itard worked with the child and was able to establish understanding of several words and phrases. During this time, there was no productive speech except for two exclamations "Oh, Dieu!" and "lait!" Even though there were apparent limits on the extent of the child's understanding, it was obviously ahead of speech production which was virtually nonexistent.

Examples such as these point up the study of language function through dysfunction. In each case there is evidence that comprehension *may,* under unusual circumstances, develop with virtually no similar development of production. The converse situation, however, of extensive development of production but no comprehension, has never been recorded. This was discussed by Lenneberg (1962):

> However, there is no clear evidence that speaking is ever present in the absence of understanding. . . . An empirical test of speaking without understanding might be as follows: a child acquires nothing but words

that have no meaning to him (by blind imitation) and learns the formal principles governing the generation of sentences. He will now utter sentences out of context and irrelevant to situations by established common sense standards; he would also have to be demonstrably incapable ever to respond appropriately to commands formulated in natural language. My assertion is that such a condition has never been described as a congenital, developmental problem (p. 232).

He then went on to conclude the traditional view of this relationship: "It is thus likely that the vocal production of language is dependent upon the understanding of language but not vice versa (p. 232)."

Another source of potential support for Ia comes from bilingual speakers who have been inactive from one of the languages for a number of years. Although an empirical example, the only evidence we have at this point is anecdotal. In every case, the speaker typically claims retention of some or all comprehension, but a loss of production. This is also the case when children acquire the language of their country and are exposed to, but are never required to speak, a second language occasionally used in the home. Conversely, there is no known report of a person maintaining good productive knowledge of a language but having lost comprehension. A claim of this sort would be something like: "I speak it beautifully, but I don't know what I'm saying!" Empirical research into this area should yield valuable information about the relation between these two aspects of language and should provide evidence supporting the traditional position.

While Ia provides a situation that may occur, the question still remains concerning what relationship holds in the normal language acquisition setting. Few would deny that improvement of over-all comprehension and production normally occur simultaneously, unlike the possible but uncommon situation in Ia. (There is a possible exception here in regards to phonological development.) In the normal case, the argument comes down to the comprehension and production of specific grammatical phenomena. One possible relationship is that expressed in II.

II. Complete comprehension of a specific grammatical form or construction is complete before it is ever produced.

It is my impression that in some cases II has been interpreted as the traditional view.

It is not difficult to prove that II is untenable. The most current and obvious counterevidence comes from the use of children's early words and their extensions to other objects. The child will first apply a word according to a very general feature, *e.g.*, [± animate] and then use the word to apply to every real word object that meets that feature, even though the child may have never heard the object referred to by that word. Examples are Pollock's (1878) child's use of "baba" and Lewis' (1963) example of "tee," both applied to animate objects. Discussions of the direction of semantic differentiation that takes place can be found in the works of Ingram (1971), Menyuk (1971, pp. 172–174), and especially Clark (1973).

The rejection of II, however, does not necessarily mean the rejection of the traditional view that comprehension precedes production. The observations above about overgeneralizations, for example, are not recent findings about language acquisition. They were being made as early as 1878, as Pollock's diary attests. They were typical of most of the early diary studies at the beginning of this century. It is apparent from these observations that the previous investigators were aware of the fact that children did not show complete comprehension before production. In light of this, the traditional position is actually that one stated as IIa.

IIa. *Some* **comprehension of a specific grammatical form or construction occurs before it is produced.**

This position is being defended in this study. Also, as will become evident, it is held that the traditional notion claims no more than this. The implication that this position claims more than is stated in IIa has resulted in problems in interpreting the view that comprehension precedes production. These will be discussed more fully in the following section.

COMPREHENSION PRECEDES PRODUCTION

A number of factors provide counterevidence to the position of IIa. These concern the occurrence of overgeneralizations, the discrepancy between order of appearance of grammatical forms and constructions in comprehension and production, the observation that comprehension in some cases is the same as production, the use of forms with no apparent understanding, and the results of experimental studies. Upon closer examination, however, each one can be seen to provide either evidence in favor of the traditional view or else no evidence either way.

Overgeneralizations

The data from children's overgeneralizations of words is counterevidence to II but not to IIa. The use of overgeneralizations by children shows that the structure of their lexical items differs from that of the adult versions. This fact, however, needs to be kept distinct from another question that can be asked about these data. Does the child's overgeneralization, in every case, reflect the child's comprehension? That is, does the child who, for example, uses "button" to refer to all round objects, actually understand the word to mean "round object?

In some cases it is apparent that the comprehension is reduced. This is seen in experimental studies, *e.g.,* Donaldson and Wales (1970), Clark (1971), and interview situations where the child discusses his understanding, Piaget

(1928). However, there are other cases where the limited productive use does not necessarily reflect a similar comprehension.

One kind of example comes from early lexical items such as the early use of "papa" or an equivalent form for the adult word "father." It is very common to find that this word at some early point comes to be used by the child to mean "man." This has been interpreted by some people to mean that "papa" means something like "man," *i.e.,* that the child understands the word in the same way that he uses it. However, there is cognitive evidence that the child knows his father by this point. In cases like this, children still understand the adult's use of "papa" to refer to this specific individual. The child's comprehension of "papa" contains more information than the child's productive lexical item.

A second example comes from the use of grammatical forms, this specific case being a comparison of children's comprehension and production of personal pronouns. In Webster and Ingram (1972), there were several cases of children who showed perfect understanding of the gender distinctions between "he, she, him, her" but did not reflect this in their spontaneous speech. One child, for example, used "he" for both "he" and "she" and "him" for both "him" and "her." Going solely on the production of pronouns by this child, one might say that he did not understand the gender distinction. The perfect results on the comprehension testing showed that this was not true.

In these examples, it is evident that there is often a distinction between those features needed to describe a child's understanding of a word and those needed to represent his production. This difference can be reflected in the difference between what linguists refer to as semantic and syntactic features. When a child acquires language, he has to learn both of these for the lexical items of the particular language. Gender, for example, is both a semantic and syntactic feature in some languages. In German, the word for "child" is "Kind" which is syntactically neuter even though semantically it is either masculine or feminine. Using the practice suggested in Ingram (1970) of enclosing semantic features in square brackets [ ] and syntactic features within angles < >, we can hypothesize entries for the pronouns "he" and "she," for the child mentioned above.

"he"	"she"
[+ Animate]	[+ Animate]
[+ Human]	[+ Human]
[+ Masculine]	[+ Feminine]
<+ Pronoun >	<+ Pronoun >
<+ Masculine >	<+ Masculine >

The semantic features of gender have been acquired, as is evidenced by the understanding, whereas the syntactic feature in current use is <+masculine>. It appears that children will acquire several semantic features for a word and then use one of these as the syntactic feature, *i.e.,* a feature to mark the way that words are encoded. In regards to the discussion of "papa," the word in this example will have the following structure:

"papa"
[+ Animate]
[+ Human]
[+ Masculine]
[+ Specific]
< + Masculine >

The children have the semantic feature [+ specific] used here simply to represent the fact that the term refers to a specific person, even though syntactically the feature is <+ masculine > which allows the word to be used in reference to all males. It is not yet limited to a specific person.

Overgeneralizations of the kind discussed since the earliest diary studies do not constitute evidence against comprehension ahead of production, but rather evidence for the way children acquire features. Some features are first comprehended, and one or more of these are picked up by the child in his own productive utterances. Studies such as those reviewed by Clark (1973) show that only the most basic features may be acquired before production begins. Also, this may be a natural result of the child's own cognitive limitations. The issue is the nature of comprehension and production, not that the former does not precede the latter. The traditional view of IIa predicts that the direction of generalization will always be the same, *i.e.*, that the child's productive speech will rely on some feature of the child's comprehension, and never the opposite. In the Webster and Ingram study, none of the 30 subjects showed appropriate use of the four pronouns but defective understanding.

Appearance of Words in Comprehension and Production

It has been discussed by Bloom (1973b) that the first words that the child produces are not always the first words that the child understood. For example, her daughter Allison first recognized the words "birds" and "music" even though they were not among the first words subsequently produced by her. Although not proposed by Bloom as such, this could be taken as evidence against comprehension preceding production since there is an apparent discrepancy in the operation of the two.

Upon close examination, this observation is not counterevidence at all. The position stated in IIa makes no claims that the first words understood must be the first produced. The only claim it does make is that the first words produced must have also been noticed or understood to some extent. A variety of factors may contribute to this discrepancy. Obvious ones include attention, memory, and frequency of exposure. Leopold's daughter Hildegard was cited by Bloom as another example of a child whose first words produced were different from the first understood. Interestingly enough, Hildegard also had a number of words in her early speech that dropped out at a later time. This could also happen in comprehension where words understood at one point might drop out for periods of time. There is no guarantee that words will either appear or be maintained in either comprehension or production in any systematic fashion. The point is that observations such as this do not provide counterevidence to the claim that comprehension precedes production. If they are claimed to, they are based on a misunderstanding of the position. As stated, this claim argues no more than is stated in IIa. The issue involved in examples such as Bloom's is that of the gap between comprehension and production.

Comprehension Equals Production

Thus far, I have discussed the traditional view in terms of individual lexical or grammatical forms rather than syntax. In terms of the latter, IIa also claims that some understanding occurs before production occurs. Arguments against the traditional view often take the form that a) there are cases where the two are equal, and b) there are cases where the production of a grammatical feature is different from its comprehension.

A common claim from traditional child language research is that children understand more syntax than they produce. This is exemplified by claims that this can be demonstrated for children in the early stages of language development through both comprehension and production data. Two early periods have specifically come under discussion. The first of these is the holophrastic or one-word utterance stage, that time between approximately 1:0 and 1:6 during which children's utterances consist of one word at a time. At least two studies have observed utterances and postulated during this period underlying semantic structures of more than a single unit (Greenfield, Smith, and Laufer 1973; Ingram, 1971). (The latter study is less direct on this point since it dealt with word utterances in general, many of which occurred after the outset of two-word utterances.) An example would be that an utterance such as "up" might be either agent-act or object-state dependent on what the child was attempting to say. While neither study claims any syntactic knowledge on the part of the child at this point, the postulation of these semantic relations in children's grammar implies that there is understanding of them in adult speech.

Shipley, Smith, and Gleitman (1969) have studied the comprehension of four holophrastic children through giving them commands to follow. The commands were divided into adult forms, *e.g.*, "Throw me the ball" and child forms, the latter subdivided into verb + noun (V-N) commands, *e.g.*, "Throw ball" and noun (N) commands, *e.g.*, "ball!" The holophrastic children preferred child commands to adult commands, as judged by the child's touching the object mentioned. Among the children, two preferred V-N to N commands, one responded more or less equally to both, and one preferred single word commands. The authors concluded from this: "Those who appear to be at the single-word, or holophrastic, stage in production prefer to respond to speech at or just above their own productive limit (the V-N and N commands)" (Shipley, Smith, and Gkitman, p. 331).

The second group to be studied is that one often referred to as at the telegraphic stage, *i.e.*, those children beginning to combine words into sentences of two or more words per utterance. At the onset of telegraphic speech, children will use sentences that reflect an underlying subject-verb-object structure even though no sentences with all three will occur. Bloom (1970) has shown that this period will be marked by N-V, V-N, and N-N constructions which lead to postulating an underlying N-V-N. Here there is syntactic evidence implying competence with the more complex structure even though it is never completely found in their own speech. Shipley, Smith, and Gleitman included in their study a group of seven telegraphic children. All responded significantly better to the adult commands than to child commands, showing their comprehension to be ahead of their production. They concluded: "just those utterance types they themselves did not use were more effective as commands: the telegraphic children responded most readily to the well-formed sentences" (p. 331).

Bloom (1973) has recently criticized the basis for claiming comprehension ahead of production for both of the above groups. In each case, however, it appears that the arguments put forth are not really against the traditional view in IIa, but rather against the assumption that the gap between the two is always uniform and sufficiently long. The traditional view defended in this paper makes no claims about the length and predictability of the gap between comprehension and production. This was pointed out in the section above on the order of appearance of items in the two. Likewise, arguments that comprehension and production may be *closer* together than originally supposed for certain constructions does not deny the precedence of comprehension.

In terms of holophrastic children, Bloom (1973a) questioned the findings that there are complex semantic relations underlying children's early one-word utterances. Although this conflicts with results of studies done by Greenfield, Smith, and Laufer (1973) and Ingram (1971) and deserves further discussion and resolution, the relevant issue here is that her position does not contradict IIa. There is no claim, for example, that children utter meaningful utterances at the holophrastic stage and yet have no understanding of adult speech. Results such as these violate the traditional view. Concerning the possibility that the comprehension of syntax by holophrastic children may be much closer or equal to their own production, the results of Shipley, Smith, and Gleitman still remain to be explained. Two out of the four children showed a marked preference for the more complex commands.

Concerning the telegraphic children, Bloom (1973b) suggested that the operation of reduction transformations results in creating the impression that comprehension is greater than production. The child who uses N+V, V+N, and N+N constructions, for example, is proposed to have an underlying N+V+N structure where one of the constituents is deleted by a reduction transformation. Therefore, the claim that the child understands N+V+N constructions actually means that the comprehension is equal to production since reduction rules distort the fact that the child has an underlying N-V-N. She concluded from this that comprehension equals production in these cases.

As pointed out by Wall (1972), there appears to be a specious use of "transformation" involved with this argument, the result of confusing the different roles of competence and performance. As defined by Chomsky (1965), the term "competence" refers to the abstract rule system of language while "performance" concerns the use of this rule system through speaking and listening. Transformations are rules of linguistic competence, constrained by innate limitations on what can be a possible rule of grammar. The reductions discussed by Bloom, however, concern linguistic performance in speaking. That is, while the child's competence may have a structure of the form N+V+N, there is a performance limitation that only two of these may appear in any one utterance. Wall discussed this at some length:

> If facts such as these indicate anything at all, it seems to me that they point to deletion in performance rather than by transformational rules. Any transformation that deletes one of three constituents without regards to its identity or its serial or hierarchical position in the tree is formally very different from any other transformational rule that has even been seriously proposed . . . it seems more plausible that the source of the deletion is in performance rather than in competence (p. 25).

If reductions such as these are interpreted as limitations on production, not competence, and the child's understanding is taken to be one of the underlying N+V+N structure, then the child's understanding here is ahead of the child's production.

Two further points can be made concerning limitations of this kind. One is that one of the reductions in the Shipley, Smith, and Gleitman study would be that of the indirect object in sentences like "throw me the ball." This is different from the deletions in Bloom (1970) which discussed primarily subject, verb, and object deletions. The development of sentences such as the above and its transformationally related form "Throw the ball to me" still await comprehensive study in both comprehension and production. It may be premature to generalize the observations from the other constructions to them. Second, the issue of reduction as a performance or competence phenomenon still does not contradict IIa, which makes no claims concerning the length of the gap between comprehension and production. Contrary data would need to show that children are comprehending less than they are actually producing.

The second kind of evidence that can be brought up concerns cases where the child appears to have different production and comprehension of a grammatical form or structure. This, however, is not because of a violation of IIa; it is the result of the child's *organization* of the data he is constantly hearing. The child is not simply in a position of receiving and then producing linguistic structures but is also organizing that input and making hypotheses about it based on what limitations there are on the structure of grammar. The end results of hypotheses such as these may occasionally be structures that appear different from the child's comprehending abilities. The first existence of some comprehension, however, is necessary for this to occur.

An example of this is the use of personal pronouns by some children in acquiring English. There are two children in the literature who have been observed to use English personal pronouns in a manner remarkably different from that of the adult language. The first of these is Mackie, a child observed by Gruber (1967). In acquiring the English subject and object pronouns, Mackie used the object ones as topics of his sentences, in either initial or final positions. Examples are "him bear" to mean "he is a bear" and "catch me" to mean "I can catch it," the latter showing the variation in word order. The subject pronouns, on the other hand, only occurred as subjects of sentences and were analyzed by Gruber as being part of the verb phrase in the child's grammar, based on the over-all analysis of topicalization. The object pronouns operate as noun substitutes but the subject ones do not, appearing instead to be used much like an affix on the verb. The sentences "her go way" *vs.* "she go way" would differ in structure as shown below. The trees are altered from the way Gruber would present them to leave the pronouns as the only distinction from how these would be ordinarily shown in adult English.)

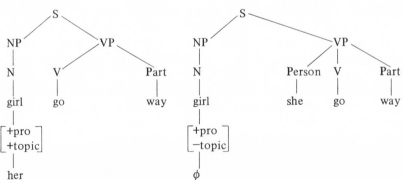

Here the "her" form is used as a pro-noun, *i.e.,* a substitute for a noun. When the subject is not topicalized, the zero (ϕ) form occurs. "She," meanwhile, is not used as a pro-noun, but rather as a person affix on the verb.

While at first glance this analysis may appear unusual, it turns out that there is at least one other case from the limited data available on children's use of pronouns that show the same strategy. Brown and Bellugi (1964) commented on the use of personal pronouns by Adam, one of the three children in their longitudinal study. In this case, Adam used both nouns and pronouns in his sentences simultaneously. Examples are "Mommy get it ladder," "I miss it cowboy boat," and "I Adam drive." Here it may also be that the pronouns in question have been analyzed by the child as person affixes on the verb, rather than pronouns. If this is true, Adam would have said Mackie's sentence shown in the second tree above as "Girl she go way," including the noun in the sentence.

The question arises as to how the child arrives at productive speech of this sort, where the child's utterances are different from what he is hearing and, in some ways, show more sophisticated structure than that of his comprehension. The answer is that the child has understood the function and role of person and pronouns in English and has made a hypothesis about the underlying structure of the sentences that contain pronouns. This hypothesis is based on what the child knows about what is a possible personal pronoun system in language. In Ingram (1970), we observed that languages split into two types concerning person pronouns. The first type is like English where all person pronouns are noun substitutes and occur as part of noun phrases. The second type, which I refer to as person-copying languages, has noun substitutes as English and also has person affixes on the verbs, much like the second diagram above. If these two types are universal alternatives, then every child acquiring a language will have to decide which type his own language belongs to. Mackie and Adam appear to have made a wrong guess about English, analyzing the structure as one where person copying occurs. This analysis, however, depends on *some* prior understanding of the kind of data the child is dealing with. This is in keeping with the traditional view. Also worth noting is the fact that IIa does not claim that the child will always understand correctly. Those times when the child does not, in fact, provide some of the most interesting and revealing data on acquisition.

Use of Meaningless Forms

There are occasional observations that children will use some forms in their speech without apparent understanding of their meaning. One such case is a reference by Lenneberg (1967) to a personal communication from Roger Brown. "There were instances in his sample in which plural inflections were used productively at a time when experiments on the child's semantic progress indicated that he did not yet know what this particular suffix signals" (p. 285). Since this has not to date been reported on in detail, it is difficult to refute or accept this as evidence against the traditional view. One important aspect that would need to be known is what is meant by productive use. Also, the extent of phonological influence would need to be investigated in suffixes such as the plural. Velten's child (1943), for example, has final substitutes of [č → ts] and [st → ts], along with words like [zats] "socks" and [wuts] "weeds" where there was rare occurrence of a singular. These under superficial analysis could be taken as plural markers rather than part of the lexical item.

If cases such as the above are possible, it is interesting to speculate on how weakly IIa needs to be stated. Slobin (1971) discussed a weak version of IIa:

> Constraints on production and comprehension are intimately related—especially in child speech, where the forms the child uses in his own speech must be those he has been able to perceive in the speech of others (pp. 345–346).

That is, one could conceivably alter IIa to IIb.

IIb. Some perception of a specific grammatical form or construction occurs before it is produced.

One would then say that in the Brown data the child has perceived the plural endings and is placing them on words without having yet understood them.

IIb, however, is untenable. First of all, all the evidence discussed before this section is in support of IIa, *i.e.,* that there is some understanding of forms before their use. Second, even the Brown example supports IIa rather than IIb. There are two ways a child might productively use plurals without comprehension. The first is to use them whenever a numeral is involved, *e.g.,* "ball" but "two balls." The second way is to randomly generate plurals on nouns. In each one, there is evidence of some understanding of the form. In each, the child has categorized the ending as one which *only* appears on nouns. Also, in the first case, the occurrence with numerals reveals the relationship to numerosity. A true example of IIb would be where the child picks up the -s ending and puts it on all of his words in some random fashion, including all parts of speech. Even then, the phonological influence of perceptual schema would need to be kept in mind, *i.e.,* Waterson (1971).

A second apparent example of meaningless usage that I have seen is a child who was using the pronouns "he" and "she," although there was no apparent understanding of the gender distinction. While the Webster and Ingram (1972) data revealed this as an unusual situation, its occurrence showed some understanding of the nature and function of "she" as an anaphoric element of the language. It was never used indiscriminately in any other context than that as a substitute for "he." Just as in the data from overgeneralizations, the child was at least aware of the general syntactic features of the word, *i.e.,* < +pronoun, −first mention, +definite >. There is some understanding of its use before its production.

Besides showing IIb incorrect because of some understanding of the grammatical usage of apparent counterexamples, IIb can also be shown wrong from the existence of word creations in children's speech. Word creations are cases where the child makes up his own word to name objects or actions. Here the child has never perceived the form in question, in the sense of hearing the particular word used in the context that he himself has selected to use it in. At the same time, word creations do not affect IIa since it does not claim that the child needs to name things with the same phonological entries as the adult. Thus, the child may understand "tree" to refer to "objects with open leaves," and create his own form, based on his phonological system, to refer to such objects. Such a form is not one based on the child's perception.

Word creations have been discussed most often by the earliest studies in language acquisition, *e.g.*, Lukens (1896), Chamberlain and Chamberlain (1904). One problem is that some so-called word creations are explainable as reductions of adult forms. Velten, for example, claimed that his daughter's form of [bap] for *lamb* was an invented form. Stampe (1972), however, has shown that it can be derived from the adult form by general phonological processes. Also, many such creations are actually the result of vocal play, *e.g.*, Chamberlain's child, and are not recurrent forms of the child's lexicon. If word creations can be shown to exist apart from these two considerations, however, they constitute counterevidence to IIb.

Results from Experimental Studies

The classic psycholinguistic study cited as evidence of comprehension ahead of production is that of Fraser, Bellugi, and Brown (1963), in which 12 3-year-old children were given tasks for the comprehension and production of 10 grammatical contrasts. The results indicated that the comprehension of the items was ahead of the production. Lovell and Dixon (1967) replicated the study on 2-year-old children with the same results. Recently, Fernald (1972) has criticized the scoring done in these studies, claiming that their decision to count irrelevant responses on the production task as error biased the results in favor of comprehension. Using a more equal method of scoring, he was able to show in his replication of this study that comprehension and production were very close together, with no significant difference between them.

Two points are relevant here for studies such as these and the traditional view of comprehension ahead of production. The first is that the results of Fernald do not necessarily contradict the position stated in IIa. To show that these two dimensions of language processing are closer than may have been assumed to date does not contradict that the one still precedes the other. To do this, one would need fairly consistent results showing production to be ahead. Second is the question of whether or not it is justifiable to compare comprehension and production tasks in the first place, particularly when the tasks cross a number of different grammatical contrasts. One can argue *ad nauseam* about how one task might be in some way easier than another, or that the relationship between comprehension and production will differ from one grammatical contrast to another, especially if the same kind of task is involved. Awareness of this problem is apparent in studies such as those by Clark (1971), where there is virtually no attempt to compare the comprehension and production in terms of one being better than the other. The best candidates for questions such as this one appear to be those that deal with a single grammatical feature and use more or less spontaneous speech as the production task, although there are even problems with this approach.

Besides showing comprehension and production to be possibly very close together, some experimental research now is attempting to show that production exceeds comprehension. The first study to do this is that of Keeney and Wolfe (1972). Looking at subject-verb agreement in English, the authors studied 46 3- and 4-year-old children on its production in spontaneous speech and imitation, and its comprehension as tested on three comprehension tasks. Use was close to perfect in the spontaneous utterances and on two of the three comprehension tasks there was a significant tendency to respond to the number marking of the verb. On the other task, however, there was no significant response to the verb number. This task, referred to as the pictorial test, required hearing a verb alone and then pointing to one of two pictures showing the action of the verb, one showing one bird doing the action and the other showing two birds involved in the same action. Pointing to the former picture would be correct for an inflected verb and the latter picture for an uninflected one, e.g., "hops" vs. "hop." From the poor performance on this task, the authors concluded production ahead of comprehension.

There are at least two points that need to be kept in mind in interpreting results like these. The first is the methodological questions involved in testing subject-verb agreement by giving a single verb form, particularly when uninflected, and then requiring a response from the observation of visual forms. As mentioned by the authors, the child may look at one of the two birds on the plural picture and process it as the singular. More seriously, there is the question whether or not the task is a possible one for children of this age. As pointed out in Bloom (1973b), the nature of the task may have been beyond the capacity of the children. Also, there was no testing of adult speakers to verify the validity of the kinds of responses they assumed the task would elicit from native English speakers.

The second point concerns the interpretation of the results, even if we assume for sake of argument that the methodological problems were resolved. Throughout the article, it is apparent that they consider number agreement on the verb as reflecting a combined semantic-syntactic process. Their conclusion is that the child has only acquired part of it, i.e., the syntactic part, but not the semantic side. "The correct inflection is produced by a purely syntactic rule" (p. 705). This, however, ignores the facts that there is a distinction between syntax and semantics and that subject-verb agreement is a syntactic rule, not a semantic one. First of all, the distinction between the verb [-s] inflection and the zero is not strictly one of number since the unmarked form, e.g., "hop," can also be used for singular form "I" and "you." The syntactic feature involved is really something like $<$ ±3rd person singular > where the zero form is < -3rd person singular >. Second, the numerosity involved in this process is in the noun which has both semantic and syntactic features of number. The semantic and syntactic features may be the same, *e.g.,* "dogs," or different, *e.g.,* "scissors," the latter always taking a syntactic feature < -3rd person singular > regardless of the semantic number of the noun. Once the syntactic feature for number is determined on the subject, a purely syntactic rule operates to copy this feature onto the verb.

Since the authors consider subject-verb agreement to be a semantic-syntactic process, they assume that they can test for sentence number by contrasting inflected and uninflected verbs. In an earlier study, Keeney and Smith (1971) used nonsense noun subjects in pairs such as "The snup jumps" *vs.* "The snups jump" and found no understanding of number in 4-year-old children.

> Thus, with regular verb inflection as the only reliable cue for sentential number, the children responded at chance level on the comprehension test, indicating that they did not understand the meaning of the verb inflection (quoted from Keeney and Wolfe, p. 699).

Keeney and Smith took this to mean that production may be ahead of comprehension, and Keeney studied this further in the study under discussion. The point here, however, is that subject-verb agreement is not a semantic-syntactic rule, but rather a syntactic rule. Consequently, this inflection has no "meaning" in the sense that it is not a semantic feature. As a syntactic feature, its processing in sentences with only verb marking is suggested to be the following. The speaker can ascertain the syntactic feature of the noun, based on the number of the verb. Once the syntactic feature of the noun is determined, one can establish the semantic number of nouns, *based on what one knows about the word classes of English.* Take the following sentences:

a.   The sheep are jumping.
b.   The sheep is jumping.

From the number of the verb, the English speaker can determine the syntactic number of the noun subjects. Then, we know that the noun "sheep" in English belongs to a class of words whose semantic number is the same as its syntactic number, and therefore can determine the semantic number of the subject. Compare those, however, with these sentences.

c.   The scissors are falling.
d.   The scissors is falling.

Here, we can determine the syntactic number of the noun from the syntactic number of the verb. "Scissors," however, belongs to a class of nouns in English whose semantic number is not determinable from its syntactic number. Rather, it always takes a syntactic number of < -3rd person singular >.

Since verb agreement is only a syntactic rule, what we learn about these sentences is not their semantic numerosity, but rather their syntactic numerosity. In this case, we learn that sentence d is ungrammatical.

This distinction between semantic and syntactic number can be used to place into perspective the results of both Keeney and Smith (1971) and Keeney and Wolfe (1972). In Keeney and Smith, pairs such as the following were used, with nonsense forms as subjects.

    e. The snups jump over the box.
    f. The snup jumps over the box.

Since agreement is a syntactic process, the only thing that can be determined in these sentences is the syntactic features of the nonsense nouns. Since the children do not know these words as English words, they have no prior knowledge about what class they belong to. That is, they do not know whether their semantic number is supposed to be the same as the syntactic number or not. Similar results were found in Berko's study (1958) where plural inflection for "glass"-"glasses" was high (91% correct), whereas the use of the plural for the nonsense forms of similar structure were low, *e.g.,* "tass"-"tasses" (36%). Children at these ages (4–7) appear to establish word classes for certain less general processes of language, and only later establish a rule for them. The English adult who responds to sentences e and f by establishing semantic numerosity is hypothesizing a rule that all nouns entering English that are uninflected for plural will undergo the same rule as "sheep," "fish," etc., *i.e.,* that semantic number equals syntactic number. The establishment of minor rules such as these appear to be late occurrences in language acquisition.

Concerning the results of Keeney and Wolfe, it is apparent that one needs to distinguish between comprehension and production of semantics, and the comprehension and production of syntax. Since subject-verb agreement is a syntactic process, the issue of comprehension ahead of production cannot deal with semantic issues, but rather syntactic ones. It is apparent from the verbal and sentential tests in Keeney and Wolfe that children do have syntactic understanding of how agreement operates. Thus, their findings do not contradict IIa. They cannot make any conclusions about semantic comprehension since it is not directly a semantic rule.

Another experiment that casts doubt on the position in IIa is that of Guess (1969), in which comprehension and production are shown to be potentially different in dealing with the same grammatical feature. Guess was able to train two mentally retarded boys to use plural inflections productively and at the same time understand them in a different manner, by interpreting inflected forms as singular and uninflected ones as plural. The results show a certain independence of comprehension and production. Evidence of this sort from spontaneous utterances has already been discussed above. There it was claimed that apparent differences result from children's reorganizing the data according to hypotheses they have made about the structure of language. In some way, the above experimental condition is one which forces alternate hypotheses on the child. The interesting aspect was that there appeared to be no subsequent influence of one on the other.

It is hard to see the implications of a study like this for the traditional view of comprehension ahead of production. For one thing, the language of the children was more or less confined to the experimental setting. For example, there was no preliminary testing of either child to see if they showed any understanding of the singular-plural distinction. The only pretesting was to make sure they did not produce it. Second, there was no collection of spontaneous speech after the productive training of the plural to see if the two children would use plural outside of the experimental situation. Also, there is the question of how long such a situation could be maintained in a natural language, *i.e.*, of having comprehension and production proceed in opposite ways, before one would begin to influence the other. Lastly, and most relevant to IIa, is the question of how much of the production task was also a comprehension test. The child must label appropriately either a single object or a group of objects. To do this, the child would need to come to some understanding of the use of plural. Here the normal process of understanding by hearing plural nouns used with groups of objects is replaced by a training task showing the production of plural coincides with numerosity. This is grossly analogous to the situation where someone teaches himself a language from a textbook and consequently learns to produce it without hearing it. Thus, when first confronted with a speaker of the language, this person's production will exceed his comprehension. This deals with two different uses of comprehension, however, as separated above in IIa and IIb. The use of comprehension by Guess is as in IIb, in the sense of perceiving, whereas the experimental situation is creating a productive ability involving a cognitive understanding beyond perception. The results in this way can be taken as showing that understanding can be learned independent of auditory perception. The fact that deaf children can learn language shows that understanding needs to go beyond perception. Thus, while Guess' results contradict IIb, they are not so clear in the case of IIa.

SUMMARY

Upon closer examination, a number of cases of proposed counterevidence to the claim that comprehension precedes production can be challenged once the traditional position is clarified. Proposed counterevidence is based in many cases on misunderstandings of what the traditional position asserts. These misunderstandings include:

1. The gap between comprehension and production is systematically long and predictable.

2. Complete comprehension precedes production.
3. Comprehension involves auditory perception in all cases.

Related to the last one is the fact the term "production" in the traditional view has been misunderstood. Production means the use of a grammatical form or construction with no apparent understanding. Once these points become clarified, it is apparent that the empirical issues are really the nature of comprehension and production, and of the gap between them, rather than whether comprehension precedes production.

THE RELATIONSHIP TO PHONOLOGICAL DEVELOPMENT

We have discussed the relationship between comprehension and production in terms of syntactic and semantic acquisition, arguing that some comprehension inevitably precedes production. The question then arises whether or not the same relation holds when children acquire the phonological system of any language. The relationship in this area is usually referred to as perception *vs.* production.

Thus far, the assumption that perception precedes production has more or less existed without challenge. Rather, the research has dealt with the nature of both, and the gap between them. In terms of these, there are two controversies of particular interest. One has to do with the influence of perception on production in the development of the child's phonological system. The second concerns the implications of recent results in infant perception on linguistic development.

Regarding the first controversy, some linguists have maintained that the child's perception of adult utterances is quite advanced and that the development of phonology primarily concerns the development of production. Stampe (1969), for example, discussed acquisition as a series of substitutions for adult forms that are assumed to be appropriately perceived. Also, Smith (1970) has argued for advanced perception, arguing that the development of phonology is primarily overcoming a set of "incompetence rules" which interfere with the production of accurately perceived forms. This position, however, is in conflict with experimental data. Schvachkin (1948/1973) studied phonemic perception in young children through the comparison of labeled objects whose names consisted of nonsense words differing by a single sound. By doing this, he was able to show that the development of perception was a gradual process with a consistent sequence of discriminations. This study was replicated for English by Garnica (1971), who also resolved a number of the methodological problems of the earlier study. The latter study also showed that discriminatory ability is not complete by the onset of speech and that it develops along with productive abilities. Arguments have also been presented on the basis of children's productive speech by Waterson (1971) to show that perception is not as far ahead of production as was originally believed. Waterson presented evidence that children structure utterances based on perceptual schemas, the latter reflecting the more salient perceptual features of the words the child is attempting to discriminate. This position was also defended by Ingram (1973).

It is interesting to compare the nature of this controversy with the one discussed earlier for syntax and semantics. Here, there is recent evidence which suggests less of a gap between the two than originally supposed. Likewise, as reinterpreted above, much of the research on comprehension and production in syntax shows that the two may be closer than expected. Research in both phonology and grammar, then, can be seen as revealing a common finding of proximity between understanding and producing.

The results of studies done by Schvachkin and Garnica appear to conflict with recent results in the area of early infant perception. Eimas *et al.* (1971) have shown that children as young as 1 year and 4 months can discriminate between the stop consonants [p] and [b]. Schvachkin and Garnica both found the voice-voiceless distinction to be a late one, acquired as late as the 3rd year. How does one reconcile results like these? Elsewhere (Ingram, 1973) we have suggested that it is necessary to distinguish between *acoustic* and *linguistic* perception. The studies with infants are dealing with the former, which is an ability to discriminate perceptually without any recourse to language. Language, on the other hand, consists of sound-meaning correspondences. Linguistic perception adds the requirement of categorizing the signal perceptually into representations of meaningful elements. This abstraction process results in reducing radically the otherwise effective ability of acoustic perception. By having their stimulus items name real word objects, Schvachkin and Garnica have introduced meaning into their studies, which are subsequently studies of linguistic perception.

From current results, it appears that the earlier position of IIa can be extended to apply to the situation found in phonological development. Maintaining the distinction between linguistic and acoustic perception, IIa can be stated for phonology as:

III. Some linguistic perception of a word occurs before it is produced.

The word "some" is important here, as it was for IIa. It reflects the fact that this perception can be and often is incomplete at the time of production. Again, the crucial issue concerns the gap between them.

FINAL REMARKS

We have tried to clarify the traditional position that comprehension precedes production. In doing so, we have examined a number of observations that could be taken as counterevidence to show they do not contradict the traditional position and that they are based on a misunderstanding of what it means to say that the one precedes the other. Lastly, we have also tried briefly to relate this topic to phonological acquisition and point out the similarities in research findings. These findings combine to reflect a general trend toward considering receptive and productive language as closer than expected.

Throughout, we have noted that the real issue is the gap between the two. This concerns both the over-all gap and variations on specific grammatical features. Also, it is especially important to determine individual variations that are involved. Some children appear to say everything they know, others much less so. In the latter case, the child's comprehension appears far ahead of production. This is often true of children with language disorders. It is with this question of gap between comprehension and production that the most fruitful research will take place.

REFERENCES

Berko, J. The child's learning of English morphology. *Word*, 1958, *14*, 150–177.

Bloom, L. *Language Development: Form and Function in Emerging Grammars.* Cambridge, Mass.: M.I.T. Press, 1970.

Bloom, L. *One Word at a Time: The Use of Single Word Utterances before Syntax.* The Hague: Mouton, 1973a.

Bloom, L. Talking, understanding, and thinking. 1973b. This volume.

Brown, R. *Words and Things.* New York: The Free Press, 1958.

Brown, R. and Bellugi, U. Three processes in the child's acquisition of syntax. *Harvard Educ. Rev.*, 1964, *34*, 133–151.

Chamberlain, A. F. and Chamberlain, I. C. Studies of a child. *Pedagog. Seminary*, 1904, *11*, 264–291.

Chapman, R. and Miller, J. Word order in early two and three word utterances: Does production precede comprehension? Paper presented to Stanford Child Language Research Forum, 1973.

Chomsky, N. *Aspects of the Theory of Syntax.* Cambridge, Mass.: M.I.T. Press, 1965.

Clark, E. V. On the acquisition of the meaning of *before* and *after*. *J. Verb. Learning Verb. Behav.*, 1971, *10*, 266–275.

Clark, E. V. What's in a word? On the child's acquisition of semantics in his first language. In T. E. Moore (Eds.), *Cognitive Development and the Acquisition of Language.* New York: Academic Press, 1973.

Donaldson, M. and Wales, R. J. On the acquisition of some relational terms. In Hayes, J. R. (Ed.), *Cognition and the Development of Language.* New York: Wiley, 1970, pp. 235–268.

Eimas, P. C., Siqueland, E. R., Jusczyk, P., and Vigorito, J. Speech perception in infants. *Science*, 1971, *171*, 303–306.

Fernald, C. Control of grammar in imitation, comprehension, and production: Problems of replication. *J. Verb. Learning Verb. Behav.*, 1972, *11*, 606–613.

Fraser, C., Bellugi, U., and Brown, R. Control of grammar in imitation, comprehension, and production. *J. Verb. Learning Verb. Behav.*, 1963, *2*, 121–135.

Garnica, O. K. The development of the perception of phonemic differences in initial consonants by English-speaking children: A pilot study. *Pap. Rep. Child Lang. Develop.*, 1971, *3*, 1–30.

Greenfield, P., Smith, J., and Laufer, B. *Communication and the Beginning of Language: The Development of Semantic Structure in One Word Speech and Beyond.* New York: Academic Press, 1973.

Gruber, J. Topicalization in child language. *Found. Lang.*, 1967, *3*, 37–65.

Guess, D. A functional analysis of receptive language and productive speech: Acquisition of the plural morpheme. *J. Appl. Behav. Anal.*, 1969, *2*, 55–64.

Ingram, D. On the role of person deixis in underlying semantics. Doctoral dissertation, Stanford University, Stanford, 1970.

Ingram, D. Transitivity in child language. *Language*, 1971, *47*, 888–910.

Ingram, D. Phonological analysis of a child. Unpublished paper, 1973.

Itard, J. M. G. *The Wild Boy of Aveyron* (Translated by G. and M. Humphrey). New York: Century, 1932.

Keeney, T. J. and Smith, N. D. Young children's imitation and comprehension of sentential imitation and comprehension of sentential singularity and plurality. *Lang. Speech*, 1971, *14*, 372–383.

Keeney, T. J. and Wolfe, J. The acquisition of agreement in English. *J. Verb. Learning Verb. Behav.*, 1972, *11*, 698–705.

Lenneberg, E. H. Understanding language without ability to speak: A case report. *J. Abnorm. Soc. Psychol.*, 1962, *65*, 419–425.

Lenneberg, E. H. *Biological Foundations of Language.* New York: Wiley, 1967.

Lewis, M. M. *Language, Thought, and Personality in Infant and Childhood.* New York: Basic Books, 1963.

Lovell, K. and Dixon, E. The growth of the control of grammar in imitation, comprehension, and production. *J. Child Psychol. Psychiat.*, 1967, *8*, 31–39.

Lukens, H. Preliminary report on the learning of language. *Pedagog. Seminary*, 1896, *3*, 424–460.

McCarthy, D. Language development in children. In L. Carmichael (Ed.), *A Manual of Child Psychology.* New York: Wiley, 1954, pp. 492–630.

Menyuk, P. *The Acquisition and Development of Language.* Englewood Cliffs, N.J.: Prentice-Hall, 1971.

Piaget, J. *Judgement and Reasoning in the Child.* London: Routledge and Kegan Paul, 1928.

Pollock, F. An infant's progress in language. *Mind*, 1878, *3*, 392–401.

Schvachkin, N. V. Development of phonemic speech perception in early childhood (In Russian). *Izv. Akad. Pedag. Nauk RSFSR*, 1948, *13*, 101–132. Translated into English in C. Ferguson and D. Slobin (Eds.), *Studies of Child Language Development.* New York: Holt, Rinehart, and Winston, 1973.

Shipley, E., Smith, C., and Gleitman, L. A study in the acquisition of language: Free responses to commands. *Language*, 1969, *45*, 322–342.

Slobin, D. Developmental psycholinguistics. In O. Dingwall (Ed.), *Survey of Linguistic Science.* University of Maryland: Department of Linguistics, 1971.

Smith, N. The acquisition of phonology. Unpublished paper, 1970.

Stampe, D. The acquisition of phonetic representation. Papers from the 5th Regional Meeting, Chicago Linguistic Society, 1969, pp. 433–444.

Stampe, D. A dissertation on natural phonology. Doctoral dissertation, University of Chicago, Chicago, 1972.

Velten, H. The growth of phonemic and lexical patterns in infant language. *Language*, 1943, *19*, 281–292.

Wall, R. Review of L. Bloom, *Language Development: Form and Function in Emerging Grammars. Lang. Sci.*, 1972, *19*, 21–27.

Waterson, N. Child phonology: A prosodic view. *J. Ling.*, 1971, *7*, 179–211.

Webster, B. and Ingram, D. The comprehension and production of the anaphonic pronouns *he, she, him, her* in normal and linguistically deviant children. *Pap. Rep. Child Lang. Develop.*, 1972, *4*, 55–78.

CHAPTER THIRTEEN

DISCUSSION SUMMARY–DEVELOPMENTAL RELATIONSHIP BETWEEN RECEPTIVE AND EXPRESSIVE LANGUAGE

Robin S. Chapman

Department of Communicative Disorders, University of Wisconsin, Madison, Wisconsin 53706

In the preceding two chapters, Lois Bloom and David Ingram discussed the developmental relationship between receptive and expressive language. Bloom concluded that the relationship is one of developmentally shifting influence between two mutually dependent, but different, underlying processes. Ingram argued that the relationship, as it has traditionally been understood, is a unidirectional one in which some comprehension of a specific grammatical form or construction must occur before (or at the same time as) it is produced.

During the conference, this topic evoked a lively and difficult debate over the issues of what constituted comprehension and production, what developmental relationship could be said to hold between the two processes, how the comparison could be made, and why these particular relationships might hold. That the debate would be lively could have been predicted from the issues. That it would be difficult was not unexpected, but the difficulty was compounded by the fact that Bloom was unable to attend the conference in person.

The actual discussion took that erratic form typical when participants with multiple concerns speak to multiple issues in a single order. The intent of this summary is to sort out the different threads of concern and enlarge upon some of them rather than to preserve the fabric of the original interchange. Something of its design can be conveyed, however, by noting that during the course of the session participants argued that the relationship between comprehension and production was obviously, and variously, all of the following: analytic, an object of empirical study, or untestable; necessary, only to be expected, or fortuitous in the context of the natural language learning situation; unchanging with production equal to comprehension, unidirectional with comprehension preceding production, unidirectional with production preceding comprehension (of syntax), or not unidirectional at all; and uniformly or variously "gapped" with respect to specific constructions.

An important source of such disarray among the conferees was definitional. It is to this topic—of what was variously meant by "comprehension" and "production" and the consequences of each view—that we first turn here. Methodological issues in comparing the two processes and explanations of putative developmental relationships will be taken up in ensuing sections.

WHAT WAS MEANT BY "COMPREHENSION" AND "PRODUCTION"

"Comprehension" and "production" were most often used to refer to the processes by which listeners obtain meaning from utterances and speakers encode meaning into utterances. These definitions, which have seemed sufficiently precise for everyday use among psycholinguists, proved distressingly imprecise in the discussion of their developmental interaction.

As Bloom pointed out in her chapter, multiple cues are available for comprehension and production. This recognition proved to be crucial to the disentanglement of conflicting statements about the developmental interaction of the two processes. To speak to the issue of developmental interaction, it becomes necessary to specify the scope of one's claim by stating which forms (X) and which cues (Y) are meant. In particular, failure to make X and Y explicit in the following phrases led to apparently contradictory claims which the additional information would have reconciled: comprehension of X on the basis of Y; production of X on the basis of Y. For instance, following Bloom's analysis and points made during the discussion, the speaker's intended meaning could be grasped by the listener on the basis of any one of the following mediating events: the syntactic-semantic analysis assigned to the sentence; the observed relations among objects and events in the immediate environment; the relations among objects and events previously mentioned in the conversation; or the usual relations among the mentioned objects and events in the listener's past experience. Similarly, Bloom pointed out that nonlinguistic context as well as intention to send a particular message may play crucial roles in the use of grammatical forms and structures in production, citing apparently reduced command of structures in children's later elicited imitations of their own utterances (see Bloom's footnote 4).

There was general recognition among conference participants that the contextual cues offered alternate routes to the encoding and decoding of meaning. When the uses of the terms "comprehension" and "production" during the discussion are further specified according to linguistic or contextual cues, however, four versions of a claimed relationship can be identified.

1. **Comprehension of an utterance containing a grammatical form or structure, on the basis of at least some linguistic or contextual cue, precedes the production of that form or structure on the basis of at least some linguistic or contextual cue.**

In this version, the basis for comprehension need not be the grammatical form or structure in question. Indeed, the utterance itself may play a very secondary role to the situation in leading the listener to its meaning. Further, the cues used in comprehension are *not* asserted to be identical to the cues used in production. That is, a statement of the form "comprehension of an utterance with X structure on the basis of Y cues precedes production of an utterance containing X structure on the basis of Z cues" is an instance of this position. The frequency with which this view appeared in discussion suggests that it is this version which is ordinarily understood when someone asserts that comprehension precedes production.

One consequence of this view is that it makes certain questions difficult to ask. For instance, it becomes difficult to state what evidence would be necessary to conclude whether or not the same underlying syntactic, semantic, or conceptual knowledge is playing a role in both comprehension and production, for the elliptical mode of expression implies that the knowledge used in achieving the underlying representation of meaning will be the same in both processes.

A second consequence of this view is that it allows one to argue, as Ingram appeared to do, that only a case of *meaningless* production of a form or structure constitutes a counterexample to the claimed relationship, because one may otherwise assume that the speaker comprehends at least the utterances he produces and hence that comprehension and production are, at least, equivalent. Few discussants adopted the latter position, in which only meaningless productions of forms (*e.g.,* Adam's "Why—why not?" questions) could serve as counterinstances, but a large number understood and used the terms to mean *comprehension, however accomplished,* and *production, however accomplished.* Thus the demonstration that Adam, Eve, and Sarah produced the plural morpheme correctly 90% of the time at the same time that they indicated no comprehension of the plural morpheme in a controlled test (Brown, 1973) would be countered by the objection that the comprehension test situation—but not the production test situation—omitted the situational context which would serve as a cue in ordinary discourse.

Discussants adopting these uses of the terms argued that the important questions have to do with the extent of the gap between comprehension and production for a given structure or form, the way in which the gap may change with time, the degree to which the gaps for different structures differ, and an explanation of why gaps exist at all. These questions can also be asked in the other versions of the relationship to be considered, but they assume a secondary status. Ingram's chapter suggests that, given the view in version 1, the weight of the evidence overwhelmingly supports the conclusion that comprehension precedes (or is equal to) production. The direction of the relationship, then, does not come into question. In the two versions to follow, however, it is the direction of the relationship which is precisely the critical question.

**2 and 3. Comprehension of an utterance containing a grammatical form
or structure, on the basis of just that form or structure as cue,**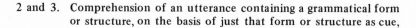

(2. precedes/ 3. follows) the control of that form or structure in production on the basis of at least some linguistic or contextual cue.

These were a second, relatively common, and third, relatively infrequent conference view of the relation between comprehension and production of a grammatical form or structure. In these versions, *comprehension of X* is understood to mean that *X* itself can be used as the cue to meaning. The meaningful presence of *X* in the child's production is taken as the operationalization of production.

These two versions hew more closely to Bloom's dissection of comprehension as a multiply cued process, but they are relatively uncritical in establishing the criteria for control of *X* in production, given Bloom's demonstration that production will vary with the contextual support available. With respect to comprehension, however, these versions allow the questions to be raised of what specific comprehension strategies (using linguistic or nonlinguistic information) first lead to the understanding of grammatical structures and forms and how these comprehension strategies change prior to the ability to use the form or construction itself as the sole cue.

Whether that ability to use the linguistic cue as the clue to meaning is achieved before or after the ability to produce a particular grammatical structure is a nontrivial question. The little direct evidence available indicates that, for at least some structures (*e.g.*, word order signaling subject and object; noun plural), the structure or form is controlled in production before it serves as a cue in comprehension (*e.g.*, Chapman and Miller, 1973; Brown, 1973). For other structures, version 2 may be correct: no difference or comprehension preceding production (*e.g.*, Ingram's report of pronoun usage in this volume; Fernald, 1972).

Finally, a fourth version of the relationship can be identified which would state production as well as comprehension cues specifically. This view is a logical extension of the positions taken by conferees during the discussion session and would seem to be the view set forth by Bloom in her chapter. It is, in fact, not a single statement but a series of statements of possible relationships holding between comprehension of *X* on the basis of *Y* cues and production of *X* on the basis of *Z* cues where *X, Y,* and *Z* are all specified in a given claim. One of the more important instances of this series of statements would be the following.

4. (For instance:) Comprehension of an utterance containing a grammatical structure or form, on the basis of just that form or structure as cue (precedes/follows) the control of that form or structure in production on the basis of *Z* cues from immediate context.

This is an inelegant attempt to cast Bloom's recognition of multiple cuing in production as well as comprehension into a form parallel to the more frequently used conference versions. At this point the search for a single relationship necessarily ends and a far more detailed search for the development of successive strategies for talking and understanding takes place. The question of when the child can be credited with a grammar—and whether that grammar is initially used in both modalities—assumes new importance.

This version 4 formulation of the issues leads one to look for possible production strategies linking aspects of context and experience to production prior to the full emergence of a production grammar. Several possible relations between specific cognitive attainments and specific achievements in production were proposed by discussants. David Premack suggested that for the case in which one first trained in production, the gap between production and comprehension would be greater when the subject's production was a description than when it was a demand or an imperative, since the latter (but not the former) might require the sort of internal representation of the act which could mediate transfer between the two modalities.

Donald Morehead argued that the achievement of representational thought would be a necessary precursor to the child's ability to learn to comprehend a sentence lacking immediate context. Dale remarked that the relation between the achievement of object permanence and related achievements in the linguistic domain was probably of that necessary-but-not-sufficient nature discussed in Cromer's chapter, citing as an example his own impression that children's use of discourse remote in time and place to the event emerges only about 6 months after the age at which object permanence is achieved.

Similarly important in the version 4, or Bloomian, view are the questions about comprehension strategies that were raised by proponents of versions 2 and 3: what are the comprehension strategies for sentences in context, prior to the use of grammatical cues? Are there also comprehension strategies for sentences lacking context? Chapman and Miller's (1973) report that their subjects understood sentences with animate subjects and inanimate objects even though situational context cues were not present suggests the existence of the latter sort of comprehension strategy. An examination of those production data, such as Bloom suggests, does not indicate that children are more often correct in producing sentences describing animate subject-action-inanimate object events than in describing other events; nor did they more frequently give the sentence subject in describing these events in contrast to other events. The relation of the apparent comprehension strategy to production, then, is at present unclear.

It is just this sort of question, however, which Bloom's analyses of the two processes brings into focus. The question of the relationship between receptive and productive language becomes the issue of how strategies for comprehension and production relate to one another at any point in developmental time, for given structures and given cues to their meaning. Whether these specific comparisons can be made will depend in part on whether the methodological issues raised in the next section can be satisfactorily resolved.

METHODOLOGICAL ISSUES IN COMPARING COMPREHENSION AND PRODUCTION

The few experimental studies directly comparing comprehension and production have taken comprehension to mean comprehension on the basis of the lexical item or grammatical structure alone as cue. Not the least of the assessment problems is the identification of just what contrasts in stimuli will permit this conclusion. The production tasks coupled with these comprehension tasks have asked the child to describe a picture or event, thus providing context for the encoding task. Some experiments have also provided alternate models of the sentence. That is, the comparisons roughly embody versions 2 and 3 of the conference's definitional uses. Whether the production situations used in these tasks closely approximate the natural settings of language use, in which the child intends to send a particular message, and whether they *should* provide the full panoply of input available to the child in spontaneous speech are matters not directly debated, although reflection upon the discussion and Bloom's chapter suggests that they should be.

Dale's suggestion that we find ways to test comprehension, production, elicited imitation, and spontaneous imitation with and without context speaks to this same issue. That it cannot be solved as neatly as the factorial language suggests becomes apparent when one considers what task should be used to operationalize production without context.

The foregoing problems of how best to operationalize comprehension and production were noted only in passing during the conference discussion, since differential definitional use provided potent distraction from this topic. Not noted at all, but important to remember, is the way that "developmentally precedes" has been operationalized. In the experimental and training studies discussed during the session, this relationship was inferred from comparative task difficulty rather than longitudinal data demonstrating order of emergence. There is, of course, no logically *necessary* connection between ease of task and developmental ordering of the two processes, for a given structure and set of cues. If longitudinal data are used to determine order of emergence, the problems of establishing criteria for acquisition in each mode and the comparability of the criteria across modes emerge. The development of criteria for acquisition of underlying structures and forms in production was discussed at length by Bloom (1970) and Brown (1973).

When ease of task is the variable from which developmental priority is inferred, participants noted that the direct comparison of ease of comprehension and production has been recently shown to present methodological problems sufficiently nontrivial to dissolve or reverse reported significant differences upon their solution (Baird, 1972; Fernald, 1973). One such problem noted in the discussion is that of scoring the production data for control of just that form or structure that is also being tested in comprehension. A second problem commented upon is that production tasks, but not comprehension tasks, typically provide a third response category of unscorable and missing responses. The existence of this category of response in production but not comprehension leads to incommensurate guessing probabilities in the two tasks and hence incomparable data (Baird, 1972). The problem is not a negligible one since missing and unscorable production responses occur frequently (*e.g.,* 20–80% of the time) with 2- to 3-year-old children.

Fernald (1972) made changes in scoring and eliminated the third response possibility in his replication of Fraser, Bellugi, and Brown (1963), showing no over-all significant difference. Which of these changes contributed more importantly to the outcome of Fernald's study was one of the questions that discussants raised. It is worth noting that Fernald's solution of the incommensurate guessing probabilities by assigning responses in the third category for production to right and wrong categories on a 50-50 basis makes the tasks comparable only at the cost of assuming that these responses indicate an internal state of inability to produce the structure or form in question correctly. Fraser, Bellugi, and Brown (1963) had similarly viewed failure to produce a response as a wrong response. This assumption can stand some scrutiny, however, when the subjects are as notoriously inattentive and innocently uncooperative as the 2- and 3-year old. One technique, only partially implemented in a current study (Chapman and Miller, 1973), is to test on the entire set of items repeatedly in each mode, so that the conditional probabilities of giving correct and incorrect responses on a trial, given previously correct, incorrect, or unscorable responses, can be estimated. This approach still requires the assumption that contrasting pairs of stimuli within the comprehension and production tasks are equally often unscorable (Martin, 1973), an assumption that should be empirically confirmed.

Finally, in comprehension tasks where incorrect responses are being analyzed for evidence of comprehension strategies, it should be observed that David Premack's point in session II is relevant: it is necessary to show that the child's response patterns indeed vary lawfully in some way with the stimuli, rather than as a simple product of response preference given a "don't know" state of the organism. Should cross-modal comparisons still prove possible, as well as interesting, conference participants advanced a number of candidate theories to account for obtained relationships. These are summarized in the next section.

EXPLANATIONS FOR DEVELOPMENTAL RELATIONSHIPS BETWEEN COMPREHENSION AND PRODUCTION

The explanations offered by conferees for why a particular relationship between comprehension and production might hold were at least as various as the different versions of that relationship. Most explanations were rooted in the language acquisition history of the child. Within that framework, four types of explanation could be identified: those based on mechanisms of acquisition, those based on performance history, those based on reinforcement history, and those based on what was learned. It should be noted that the original predictions of difference made by Fraser, Bellugi, and Brown (1963) were based on the additional task demands placed on the subject responding in each mode.

Explanations Based on Acquisition Mechanisms

Some argued that prior comprehension of certain words or structures is the necessary input to the language learning device eventually reproducing those structures, so that the relation between comprehension and production is a necessary consequence of the nature of the language learning mechanism. This use of terms would appear to correspond to version 1 of the conference definitions; similar arguments could be constructed for the other version.

Menyuk suggested an opposite view in raising the query of whether Bloom intended to make the argument that the production of the structure was in some way useful in achieving comprehension. Donald Morehead earlier had observed that repetition of sentences prior to the attainment of Piaget's sensorimotor stage 6, when mental representation is possible, might serve in place of the mental representation of the sentence for purposes of comprehension. (Comprehension in the absence of production, prior to the stage of mental representation, should not occur, he argued.) The end of the discussion period closed off elaboration of this provocative line of argument.

Explanations Based on Performance History

Several participants proposed that sheer amount of practice in the two process modes would be sufficiently different to account for better performance in one modality than the other. Participants did not agree, however, on which modality the child had more practice in, comprehension (in context) or production (in context). The need for data was recognized.

Schiefelbusch pointed out that the mother-child dyad in which communicative interchange first takes place is the natural laboratory in which to investigate relations between comprehension and production as well as other questions about acquisition mechanisms (*e.g.*, Lewis and Freedle, 1972; Broen, 1972; Snow, 1972). He observed, however, that the nature of this interaction would appear to provide the infant with practice in both roles, that of initiator and responder, equally.

Explanations Based on Reinforcement History

Baer, on the basis of work with the retardate (Guess and Baer, 1973), argued that any empirically determined gap between production and comprehension would simply reflect the differential reinforcement contingencies in the natural environment. He noted that in the laboratory training can produce an initial gap in the direction of comprehension or production simultaneously for different allomorphs of the same morpheme. He further argued that the eventual generalization across modality observed in one subject was also a product of reinforcement history, since altering reinforcement contingencies could persuade the nongeneralizers to generalize to the other mode and the generalizer to stop generalizing. (Donald Morehead disputed the possibility of replicating this task with infants by arguing that comprehension alone could not be trained until the child has achieved the Piagetian level of mental representation.)

Explanations Based on What is Learned

David Premack focused on the need to explain the emergence of complete transfer between modalities rather than initially differing performance levels; the latter, he argued, were only to be expected since the organism, initially, would be learning different things. He reported eventual transfer across modalities in his chimp without explicit experimental intervention—as also occurs in the child, he argued. (Whether reinforcement for generalization existed implicitly was a point of contention with Baer.) The crucial question to ask, he stressed, would be "what is the system that emerges and makes transfer possible?"; that is, what learning or maturation or what occurs to transform the nontransferring chimp or child to one who shows complete transfer?

AN AFTERWORD

The view that comprehension precedes production has been widely accepted among students of child language, but, as some participants observed prior to the conference, little of a theoretically interesting nature has seemed to follow from that fact. The two preceding chapters mark an end to this era in child language research. Ingram, in his careful review of the diary studies, showed what the statement has traditionally meant; Bloom, in her innovative and insightful reconsideration of the problem, has transformed it utterly.

The discussion of these two chapters summarized here should make it plain that it will take us some time to understand and absorb that transformation and its consequences fully. A major stumbling block will be learning to state our hypotheses about comprehension and production with more care for the multiple cues which may play a role in each of those processes. More care, too, will be required for methodological issues. If the points raised during the discussion are any indication, however, that care will be repaid by the emergence of a number of theoretically interesting and specific questions about the relation of the child's cognitive and linguistic attainments to speaking and understanding in the natural language learning situation. In particular, the discussion of these issues at the conference marked a watershed, for many of us, in turning from models of *what* the child knows to models of *how* the child knows.

REFERENCES

Baird, R. On the role of chance in imitation, comprehension, and production test results. *J. Verb. Learning Verb. Behav.* 1972, *11*, 474–477.

Bloom, L. *Language Development: Form and Function in Emerging Grammars.* Cambridge, Mass.: M.I.T. Press, 1970.

Bloom, L. *One Word at a Time.* The Hague: Mouton, 1973.

Broen, P. Ann. The verbal environment of the language-learning child. *ASHA Monograph 17,* Washington, D.C.: ASHA, December, 1972.

Brown, R. *A First Language.* Cambridge, Mass.: Harvard University Press, 1973.

Chapman, R. and Miller, J. Word order in early two and three word utterances: Does production precede comprehension? Paper presented to the Fifth Annual Child Language Research Forum, Stanford University, April 7, 1973.

Fernald, C. Control of grammar in imitation, comprehension, and production: Problems of replication. *J. Verb. Learning Verb. Behav.*, 1972, *11*, 606–613.

Fraser, C., Bellugi, U., and Brown, R. Control of grammar in imitation, production, and comprehension. *J. Verb. Learning Verb. Behav.*, 1963, *2*, 121–135.

Guess, D. and Baer, D. An analysis of individual differences in generalization between receptive and productive language in retarded children. *J. Appl. Behav. Anal.*, 1973, *6*, 311–329.

Lewis, M. and Freedle, R. *Mother-Infant Dyad: The Cradle of Meaning.* Research Bulletin. Princeton, N.J.: Educational Testing Service, 1972.

Martin, E. Personal communication to R. S. Chapman, June 1, 1973.

Snow, C. Mother's speech to children learning language. *Child Develop.*, 1972, *43*, 549–565.

V NONSPEECH COMMUNICATION

CHAPTER FOURTEEN

TEACHING VISUAL LANGUAGE TO APES AND LANGUAGE-DEFICIENT PERSONS[1]

David Premack and Ann James Premack

Department of Psychology, University of California, Santa Barbara, California 93106

LANGUAGE-FREE TESTS

Measurement of Perceptual Echolalia

In 1965, Metz and Premack worked with a group of institutionalized children, all of whom had some degree of language deficiency. Some were able to communicate verbally. Others never communicated but repeated what had been said to them a moment earlier (echolalia), or hours, or even weeks earlier (delayed echolalia). Such a child when asked, "What is your name?" would reply, "What is your name?" If not spoken to directly, the child was likely to repeat long instructions heard at an earlier time, such as, "Don't go in there now. I don't want to see you in here now, Mary. Wash your hands." Although it was not possible to reconstruct the model for every speech episode, it is reasonable to suppose that one must have existed, for there was no independent evidence of productive speech.

Verbal Echolalia. The first test presented to the children was mainly an effort to understand echolalia. Why did these children repeat what was said to them? Were they imitative in speech only? Social behavior is acquired mainly by modeling or imitation, yet social behavior is conspicuously absent in these children. If we wanted to consider that the echolalic might be imitative in nonverbal behavior, it was necessary to devise a test that could demonstrate this possibility. We also considered that the echolalic child might be no more imitative than a normal child, but that he lacked the normal child's access to nonimitative alternatives. An echolalic child, when questioned by an adult, is pressured to respond. If the child were permitted *not* to respond, the child would not be imitative, but silent instead. This type of child is not allowed the option of silence, however, for the adult insists on some kind of dialogue. Failing to understand the adult question, but obliged, nevertheless, to speak, the child can either repeat what is said to him or generate speech at random.

[1] The research reported here was supported by United States Public Health Service Grant MH-15616. We are indebted to Richard Metz, a co-investigator on the project with echolalic children, and to Mary Morgan, Debby Barone, and Amy Samuels who were the principal trainers of the chimpanzees and the autistic child.

Demonstration of Perceptual Echolalia. To obtain answers to some of the above questions, we designed a test to determine if perceptual responses could be classified as imitative or nonimitative. The tests utilized a number of familiar objects and proceeded as follows. The experimenter placed an object before the child, asked "What goes with this?" and waited for the child to pick one of a variety of objects that were arranged in front of him. If the experimenter offered, say, a doll from his set of alternatives, and the child selected a doll from his set of alternatives as well, the child's response was considered imitative. If the child picked some object other than a doll, the choice was classed as nonimitative. But nonimitative responses can be defined in a more illuminating way. They can be seen as constituting a positive category which can serve to assess the several kinds of *perceptual* nonimitation that are possible. We considered at least three classes of such responses, which differed on *a priori* grounds in the degree of association or dependence between the two items that were involved in each response.

1. The first class, labeled perceptual halves (PH), was defined by the use of dismembered objects, mainly bisected asymmetrical ones. A typical instance consisted of the experimenter placing a doll's body before the child, and the child responding with the choice of a doll's head. If the subject responded by selecting another doll's body, the response would be imitative. In selecting the head, the subject completed rather than duplicated the stimulus. The highest degree of association (between stimulus and response objects) was considered to be found in this class. Some of the objects used in this series included: blossom and stem, cup and handle, doll body and doll head.

2. The second class, labeled perceptual associates (PA), consisted of objects that had two separable parts, but which were normally found together as a single functioning unit. Examples included: jar and lid, lamp and bulb, shoe and lace.

3. The third class, labeled functional associates (FA), consisted of two separate objects that are normally used together, but each of which is an intact item as such and can be used alone. Examples included: cup and saucer, mirror and hairbrush, hammer and nail.

4. The last class, called null associates (NA), were essentially objects paired at random. In this test, it consisted of objects that were not duplicates of each other and did not fulfill any of the above associative conditions. Examples included: wagon and tub, lamp and shoe, hammer and lace.

We divided a group of institutionalized children (ages 4–12) into nonoverlapping subgroups of four children each, in terms of the amount of echolalia they showed on a speech test. In the experimental group, 15–80% of the subjects' responses to the examiner's questions were echolalic. In the age-matched control group only 0–8% of the subjects' responses were echolalic. Members of the two groups were tested individually, in counterbalanced order, on three different procedures.

In the first procedure, the children were trained to make all three kinds of nonimitative or associative responses, *i.e.*, to identify and put together perceptual halves, perceptual associates, and functional associates. They were then given two transfer tests identical to the first tests except that entirely new objects were used. In the first transfer test, imitative responding was possible since the subject's array of objects always included an object that was identical to the experimenter's test object. In the second transfer test such an object was not included and imitative responses were not possible.

Three different arrays of objects were used in the first step, each consisting of eight objects. One array consisted of a toy banana, washcloth, railroad car, medical cup, spoon, car rear, comb, and green block; this was used to teach both perceptual parts and functional associates. A car rear and front served as an instance of perceptual parts, while a washcloth and soap instanced functional associates. Each array was used to teach two different types of nominitative response. The other two arrays were used to teach perceptual associates and perceptual parts in the one case, and in the other, perceptual associates and functional associates. There were comparable sets of eight objects included in these arrays.

Each child was trained in the following manner. The experimenter placed a test object immediately before the subject in a small box, and asked, "What goes with this?" The subject was taught to select one object from the array before him and place it in the box. If the child failed to respond within 3 sec, passive guidance was used. Whether the subject responded correctly or not, the order of the array was rearranged and the subject was advanced to the next trial. On correct responses, the subject was told "good" and given a piece of food. The food reward was gradually reduced to every third or fourth correct response over the course of training. When the subject performed incorrectly, the subject was told "no" and given nothing.

The two kinds of trials given on each array, for example, functional associates and perceptual parts, were arranged according to a Gellerman (1933) series with a restriction of a maximum of two successive trials of the same kind. The child was trained to a criterion of 9 out of 10 correct responses on each problem. When he met this criterion on both problems in the array, he was advanced to the next array. The order in which the arrays were given was randomized over subjects and was the same in both groups. The main dependent variable was the number of trials required to reach criterion on each of the three arrays.

All children reached criterion and were advanced to the next procedure. Five new arrays were used, all of which contained objects that were not used in training. For example, one of the five arrays consisted of the following objects: cup, shoe, cup handle, hairbrush, wagon, lace, mirror, and tub. The cup and handle represented the class of perceptual parts; shoe and lace the class of perceptual associates; brush and mirror the class of functional associates; and tub and wagon the class of null associates. Each array contained eight problems, two for each level of association including null association. In addition, the subject's array always included an object identical to the test object, so that an imitative response was possible on every trial. Each object in the array was presented to the subject only once, along with the question, "What goes with this?" From his array of objects, the child could select an item that was: a duplicate of the test object, a perceptual part, a perceptual associate, a functional associate, or a null associate. If the subject's choice belonged to the class of perceptual parts, perceptual associates, or functional associates, he was told "good" and given a snack. He was told "no" and given nothing for any other class of choices. The order of objects in each array was random and was the same for all subjects. Problems were presented in the same random order for all subjects.

The third procedure was exactly like the second one except that imitative responding was not possible. The five arrays were reconstituted, using the same objects as in the second test, but the subject's array never contained an item identical to the test item. As before, each array contained eight problems, two for each of the four associative levels, and each object was presented only once. The child could respond with the choice of object that was a perceptual part, perceptual associate, functional associate, or null associate. Correct and incorrect responses were handled as they had been in the second procedure. Forty responses were made by each subject on both the second and third procedures, eight responses for each of the five arrays. The test results were as follows.

1. The experimental group took an average of almost 39 trials to reach criterion on the first step, compared to only about 9 for the control group, $p < 0.05$, Mann-Whitney U-test (two-tailed). Neither group showed a significant difference over the three associative levels (Friedman two-way analysis of variance), though the numerical differences tended to be in the predicted direction, especially in the control group; for example, 1.25, 3, and 4.25 average trials to criterion for perceptual parts, perceptual associates, and functional associates (14, 4, and 23, figures for the experimental group).

2. On the first transfer test, in spite of the pretraining on associative responding, imitation was the dominant response for both groups. The experimental group made only 17 associative responses out of a possible 160 responses; the corresponding figure for the control groups was 54 responses. Although the control group made three times as many associative responses as the experimental group, the difference was not significant. Nor was the difference in associative levels significant, though numerical differences were in the predicted direction for both groups, *e.g.,* 8, 7, 2, and 22, 17, 15, total correct responses for PH, PA, FA, for the control and experimental groups, respectively.

3. On the third test, with imitative responding not possible, the two groups differed significantly in the number of associative responses. The experimental group made an average of 20 associative responses compared to an

average of 28 for the control group, $p < 0.05$, Mann-Whitney U-test (two-tailed). For both groups the number of correct responses varied in the predicted direction with associative level. For PH, PA, and FA, total correct responses were 37, 27, and 16 for the experimental group and 40, 37, and 35 for the control. The levels difference was significant for the experimental group, $p < 0.05$, Friedman two-way analysis of variance, but not for the control group.

How much correct responding was masked by imitation? How did this vary with the associative level of the problem? The total number of correct responses that were given to items previously eliciting an imitative response, was about the same for both groups, 59 and 56 for the experimental and control groups, respectively. However, this difference is confounded by the fact that the experimental group had more opportunities for correction (since they made three times as many imitative responses on the second procedure). An unconfounded comparison is given by the percentage of imitative responses that were corrected. This was 90% for the control group and only 66% for the experimental group, significant at $p < 0.05$ by Mann-Whitney U-test (two-tailed). The number of corrections made varied in the predicted direction with associative level in both groups; for PH, PA, and FA, 28, 18, 13 and 21, 18, 17 for experimental and control groups, respectively. The difference was significant for the experimental group at $p < 0.04$ Friedman two-way analysis of variance, but not for the control group. Thus the children who were more imitative in speech were also more imitative in visually mediated nonverbal responding. These results are the first of several which show parallels between verbal and nonverbal behavior.

The ability of the echolalic child to make appropriate associative responses when imitation was precluded is a prognostically sanguine sign. It suggests that these children may actually possess appropriate response modes which are masked in the usual situation by a dominant imitative response. At a given developmental stage, imitation may be the dominant response mode in all children, but in the normal child it is subsequently supplanted by other response modes. The present results suggest that with echolalic children the training program should eliminate imitation as a possibility and strengthen alternative responses. Then, conceivably, even when imitation is readmitted as a possibility, the appropriate response alternatives will be able to compete successfully with it. Notice that this objective can be easily realized with the present language training procedure. Since the experimenter makes the words, he can eliminate the imitative alternatives. Later he can readmit them and test the success of his training.

Assessment of Language Comprehension

Although nearly all the children in the hospital had some degree of language deficiency, the ward staff persisted in attempting to control all children by verbal instruction. The possibility that some of the children might not understand language did not seem to arise. What, in actuality, was the level of language comprehension in these children?

We tested language comprehension in the same eight children in whom we measured perceptual echolalia. First, we established a word recognition vocabulary for each child, by teaching the child to point to the one item in a set of four (objects, photos, or pictures) that correspond to the spoken word. The names of objects were assessed, along with those of some properties and actions. Property names were also tested for extension: if the child could apply "broken" to a bottle, could he extend the application to a door that was off its hinge, or to a motor that did not work? Most of the children were able to match 90 and 180 degree rotated objects to the standard and to match objects to pictures. All children proved to have some recognition vocabulary, including not only the names of objects, but also those of properties and actions. Vocabularies were substantially larger in the nonecholalic children; they also had less difficulty with the perceptual transformation.

Plurals, Negatives, Passives. With the already established word recognition vocabularies, a number of simple tests were made for various morphological and grammatical distinctions. Included in these were tests for: plural, negation, passive, multiple subjects, adjectival modification, and other forms of word combinations. Sentence comprehension received extensive testing, mainly because both parents and ward staff tended to overestimate comprehension in the children, mistakenly assuming sentence comprehension existed when no more than word recognition was involved. For instance, when a child is told, "Let's go for a ride," and the child heads for the car, the adult takes this activity as evidence of sentence comprehension. No test is made of the child's response to the alternative sentences, "Let's not go for a ride," We took a nice ride yesterday," "Children in Arabia ride camels." In these cases, too, the child may head for the car, in which case all one could conclude is that the child is able to extract the key word "ride" from a variety of contexts.

In all the tests presented, two or more alternatives were placed before the subject. One was baited, and the child was given an instruction that permitted him to identify the baited object. The alternatives were typically objects or pictures. These were familiar enough to be in the subject's word recognition vocabulary, except on those series of tests where unnamed, unfamiliar, and/or nonsense objects were deliberately used. On the tests for pluralization, for example, the alternatives consisted of a chair and two chairs. The child was told to "Take chair" on some trials, and "Take chairs" on others, always with heavy emphasis on the terminal sibilance. On some versions of this test, the child was required to repeat the instructions before choosing; or sometimes a stronger albeit artificial inflection was tried, *e.g.,* "spoon *vs.* spoonda," "chair *vs.* chairda."

Tests of Sentence Comprehension. Sentence comprehension tests progressed from the simple instruction to "Take X" in the presence of one object, to the complicated instructions that named all of the several objects present, but stated that only one of them was correct. The position of the key word in the sentence was varied systematically over the course of the tests, as were the complexity of the sentences and the devices used to inform the child which object was correct. Some tests for negation and the passive were embedded in this series. For instance, on some trials, the subject was told "Don't take X," "X is wrong," "X is not the one," "No, not X," etc. "Don't, no, not" were the main negatives tested.

Tests involving word combinations such as noun-noun pairs, adjective-noun pairs, or noun-verb pairs employed four alternatives. For instance, for the instruction "Take red chair," the alternatives were pictures of a red chair, red bed, green chair, and green bed. The noun-verb pairs also used pictures as alternatives, while the noun-noun pairs mainly used objects.

The echolalic children, in addition to having smaller vocabularies, gave virtually no evidence of comprehension of either syntactic or morphological distinctions. When sentences were given that named both of the two alternatives present, all of the echolalic children failed the test. That is, if a dog and cat toy were present, and the child was told, "The dog gave it to the cat," "The cat took it from the dog," etc., the nonecholalic child responded correctly most of the time, but the echolalic child responded at chance. The failure to comprehend sentences confirmed the earlier suspicion that success on day-to-day verbal instruction from ward personnel was based on the child's responding at the word level. To an instruction that contained a key word, the child carried out what he had learned to be the appropriate motor act. The ability to do so was probably facilitated by the limited set of response alternatives that ward life required of them, such as heading in a given direction, following the attendant, interrupting an activity, but little else.

Language Comprehension Compared with Language Production

The child with echolalia failed the test for pluralization and the negative as well. Not surprisingly, he also failed the test on the passive, a test which stymied most of the control children as well, though it was the only test that the control children failed. Some of the echolalic children could process pairs of words of all three varieties, noun-noun, adjective-noun, and noun-verb. One rather curious finding involved a nonverbal match-to-sample version of the test which was conducted with only one echolalic child. The child was unable to carry out object-object matching when the alternatives were placed on the horizontal but was successful when the objects were arranged on the vertical.

Interestingly enough, both pluralization and negation, which were failed in the comprehension mode by all echolalic children, were clearly marked in the spontaneous speech of all the children. Extensive speech records on these children, collected over a period of 2 years, showed clear evidence of the use of plurals and negatives. Thus, Mary, as an example, employed all forms of negation in her spontaneous speech with sentences such as "You're not going for a ride today. . . . Don't go in there now. . . . No, you can't. . . ." but showed no comprehension of any negative form. The spontaneous speech of these children is grammatical, well articulated, and, depending on the age of the child, apt to contain all of the morphological markers. But it is not true productive speech, if we mean, minimally, speech that the child can understand when it is used by a second party.

These tests suggested that the simple criterion, degree of echolalia, could divide the children into groups capable of profoundly different kinds of language function. One group clearly understood language, while the other group just as clearly did not. The whole group of children represented a heterogeneous collection of individuals loosely connected by such labels as "emotionally disturbed, . . . institutionalized, . . . and psychotic. . . ." This assessment of such a diverse group of children by so simple a criterion was a surprise. Even more so was the inclusion of the subgroup of children who had virtually no sentence level comprehension at all. Since the time when these tests were conducted, we have dealt with some retarded children who, unlike the group of echolalic children, did not even have word recognition vocabularies. In a very real sense, the child who has progressed to words, but not beyond, is a greater mystery than one who has neither words nor sentences. Why would a child acquire words but be unable to acquire either inflections or word combinations?

The acquisition of distinctions based on word order and inflection probably requires attention to features that are more subtle than those involved in simple word-object associations. Yet these children do have both word-property and word-action associates, though admittedly in limited number and with a somewhat curtailed range of applicability. Their failure to acquire the plural inflection is the more puzzling given Slobin's finding (1973) that in normal children the terminal part of the word is acquired more rapidly. There is a conspicuous absence of social responsiveness in these children, encouraging one to guess that the over-all basis of the deficiency may be the child's invulnerability to social reinforcement. Although not necessary for learning, reinforcement is vital for performance. By determining where the child directs his attention, it may be an indirect though strong determiner of precisely what is learned. Tests of this hypothesis can be derived from astute remedial programs. If with programmed instruction these children acquire what the ecology failed to teach them, the hypothesis could be given some credence.

VISUAL LANGUAGE MAPS COGNITIVE DISTINCTIONS

Language can be viewed as the mapping of existing distinctions. Once language is acquired, it can be used to teach new distinctions, new object classes, for example, and even new logical operations. But if certain perceptual and conceptual abilities are not present, language cannot be acquired at all. In making an assessment of the linguistic potential of both infrahuman and pathological human populations, it is vital to keep these two levels in mind. For instance, the echolalic child who lacks pluralization and who responds incorrectly to "Take X" vs. "Take X's," may do so for several reasons. 1) He may be unable to discriminate X from XX. 2) He may be capable of 1) but be unable to generalize, that is, to recognize that the distinction between Y and YY is the same as that between X and XX. 3) He may be capable of both 1) and 2) but lack only the linguistic marker. The deficiencies involve different levels of processing, the former being deeper than the latter, and in all likelihood they are not equally remedial. Certainly the child who lacks only the linguistic marker has a happier prognosis than the one who is incapable of generalizing the X vs. XX distinction. In fact, all of the echolalic children proved to suffer only from 3), that is, to lack the linguistic marker. They were all subsequently taught either simultaneous discriminations or match-to-sample based on X vs. XX, and they successfully generalized these discriminations. In addition, the one child to whom we subsequently gave explicit training on the plural not only acquired it for the training material, but was able to transfer the distinction to nontraining items.

Concepts that Underlie "Giving"

The true extent of the conceptual structure underlying language is only poorly suggested by our laboratory tests. An inventory of the concepts of a species would clarify the issue; however, we have not gone beyond simple cases, as, for instance, the use of match-to-sample to determine whether or not the subject can match on the basis of object similarity (or color, size, shape, numerosity); whether or not he can match pictures to objects; whether or not he can match one picture to another picture (Premack, 1971). This hardly scratches the surface of the conceptual structure of a species, however.

   The social behavior of a species is a rich source of its conceptual structure, but here, too, the analysis is preliminary. Consider the perceptual prerequisites for a simple and representative verb such as "give." The action named by this verb involves a relation between three terms: a donor, a recipient, and the object of the action. A prototypic case involves the passage of an object from one agent to another. This passage includes not only the object, but the prerogatives of ownership as well. However, ownership does not confer unbounded prerogatives. Legitimate actions can probably be defined for every object, so that these acts, and only these, are permitted the new owner-recipient. Should a recipient act illegitimately, e.g., smash the apple rather than eat it, he is less likely to be made a recipient again. Knowledge of this kind must be within the capacity of the subject if he is to be taught the verb "give."

The subject must also be able to recognize agents on the individual level. In the normal use of the verb, we distinguish "Mary give John X" from "John give Mary X," a usage clearly demanding recognition at the individual level. By the same token, the distinction "You give me X" and "I give you X" would not be possible for a species that did not have a concept of self, as apparently the monkey does not, according to inferences based on its mirror behavior (Gallup, 1970). It is difficult to picture teaching the predicate "give" (in anything like the human sense) to a species that does not itself engage in giving. Stated concisely, for this verb to take its normal arguments, the species must distinguish objects from agents, one individual from another, and himself from others.

How many species besides man fulfill these conditions? Chimps appear to engage in full-fledged acts of giving, both in the field and in the laboratory. Goodall (1965) and others have observed wild chimps to engage in food sharing. Sarah (a 10-year-old language-trained chimpanzee) can be induced to ransack her cage for an item with which she can consummate giving. Consider that giving does not take place until the potential recipient retains what the potential donor has handed over. When, for the sake of experiment, the trainer immediately abandoned whatever Sarah handed him, she would try one object after another until her potential recipient finally retained what she handed him.

Perhaps lesser species (some of the carnivores and even the insects) engage in giving and could be taught names for both the action and the members that engage in the action. But a closer look at the potential examples of "giving" in these nonprimates shows clearly that in primates the predicate has broader applications. The lioness who "gives" meat, for instance, appears to limit the action to one class of objects (meat) and one class of recipients (nuclear family). Training might broaden the conditions of giving, but the "untrained" lion engages in a limited version of giving. This is not so for human giving, nor for chimp giving. The possible objects, donors, and recipients of giving in man seem unlimited, a fact which is reflected in the lack of restrictions on the words that can occur in conjunction with the verb. This is very evident in the literal use of the verb, as when we give apples and doughnuts; but even more clearly in the metaphorical use, as when we "give" a piece of our mind, goodwill, virginity, or our hearts. Because the chimp engages in giving on a very broad level, that is, the objects and recipients are highly varied, it seemed a reasonable transaction to map with language. In fact, it was the first simple transaction that was mapped with language, and it was with "give," specifically, that Sarah's first simple sentences made perceptual contact (Premack, 1971).

Sarah's Language

Sarah's first simple sentence was taught by mapping vocabulary elements to all the perceptual distinctions in the give transaction. Sarah (an African-born female chimpanzee, *ca.* 5 years old at the time of training) and her trainer sat facing each other over a table. The trainer placed a piece of fruit on the table, and Sarah picked it up and ate it. When the procedure became routine, the trainer introduced a plastic word along with the piece of fruit, only the piece of fruit was now less available than was the plastic word. Sarah was shaped to place her plastic word on the magnetized board which was attached to the wall by the side of the table. When she did so, she received a slice of fruit. At first Sarah was always given the correct word along with the piece of fruit. She was given the name for apple, which she placed on the board in order to receive an apple; and she was given the name for banana, which she too placed on the board in order to receive a slice of banana.

Following this training, Sarah was offered two words, only one piece of fruit. If she "named" it correctly by placing its correct name on the board, she received the fruit. Donors in the transaction were Sarah's trainers. For easy identification, each donor wore a necklace from which hung her/his plastic name. (Sarah wore a similar name on *her* necklace, but she was more often a recipient than a donor.) When Mary worked with Sarah, she gave Sarah a plastic name that matched the one on her own necklace to place on the board along with the fruit name. Randy followed the same procedure with her name. Then Sarah was given a choice of proper names. Now Sarah was required to identify both donor and fruit. In addition, her two-word sentences had to meet an order requirement:

Mary	Mary	Randy	Randy
apple	banana	banana	apple

Both the donor and the object classes were relatively straightforward, but the action and recipient classes were not. In all of the transactions, Sarah was always the recipient. It was necessary for her to note the perceptual distinctions possible in this class as well. In mapping recipients, Sarah was given the name 'Gussie" (Sarah's companion), which she placed on the board as required, only to find that her fruit had been given to her friend Gussie. Sarah shrieked, pouted, and stomped. It was clear that the recipient class would consist of one member only unless a new tactic was devised. Sarah was finally cajoled into placing Gussie's name on the board for apple or banana, and when she did so, though Gussie did receive the fruit, Sarah herself was the recipient of her favorite, M and M's. The action of "giving" was contrasted with other actions, in the final step. Sarah was shown that fruits could be *cut*, *inserted* into a container, and *washed*. After the perceptual activities were demonstrated, Sarah was taught the names of the actions, which too, were ordered in the sentence. At the end of this portion of training, Sarah was able to produce several simple sentences such as:

Mary	Randy	Mary	Sarah	Mary
insert	give	give	insert	wash
apple	banana	apple	banana	apple
	Sarah	Gussie		

A Visual Language System

The words in this system consisted of varicolored pieces of plastic of various shapes. There was no relationship between the shapes of the plastic and that of the objects that they referred to. In other words, the shapes did not have an iconic relationship to objects; rather, the relationship between language items and real objects was a completely arbitrary one. The plastic words for colors (such as green, red, etc.) bore no similarity to one another in color. The backs of each plastic form contained portions of metal that were glued on securely, and these adhered to a magnetized board located in Sarah's cage. Sarah's sentences proceeded on the vertical, the columns moving from right to left as sentences increased in complexity. When Sarah's training ended, she had achieved a vocabulary of some 130 words, in the following categories: proper noun, nouns, verbs, adjectives (including colors, shapes, and sizes), particles, quantifiers, prepositions, and logical connectives. More importantly, she was able to produce and comprehend a variety of simple sentences and several types of questions and to process one example of a compound sentence and, surprisingly enough, an example of a complex sentence as well.

Simple Interrogatives, Compound and Complex Sentences

Sarah's language "comments" on the early transactions were all examples of simple sentences, of course. We wondered if it would be possible to teach her the question, since it could serve many purposes in further language training. The procedure once again started at the perceptual level. Sarah was given a set of three objects, two of which matched, and she was required to place that particular pair together. When she was able to match like items reliably on a number of sets of three objects, she was then taught to place her word "same" between the like objects, the word "different" between the unlike objects. The interrogative particle was introduced next. In this series, because Sarah did not have the vocabulary for all the objects presented to her, she did not work on the magnetized board, but on her table. The sentences were "written" out with a combination of plastic words and objects in what we called hybrid sentences. The simple format looked like this:

```
key      ?        key
key      ?        cork
```

or, What is the relationship between a key and a key, between a key and a cork? Sarah's "same/different" were available, and Sarah learned to remove the ? and replace it with the correct word

```
key      "same"      key
key      "different"  cork
```

In the next set of questions, Sarah was given two real objects, a key and a clothespin, which she used to replace the interrogative markers in:

?	"same"	key
?	"different"	cork

Paraphrased, the sentences ask, What is the same as a key, and what is different from a cork?

The use of the concepts of same and different made it possible to arrange questions that could take "yes" and "no" answers as well. Earlier, Sarah had been taught "no" in a situation that banned her from taking certain foods; but she had not yet been taught the affirmative. She was given errorless trials on "yes," using the format:

?	clothespin	"same"	clothespin

or, is a clothespin the same as a clothespin, to which Sarah placed her only word "yes" as a substitute for the interrogative marker. Asked the question:

?	penny	"same"	scissors

she replaced the ? with her only choice, the word "no." After several trials on the above questions, Sarah was given both "yes" and "no" as responses to them. She did as well on the "yes/no" questions as she had on the original "same/different" group.

Sarah was able to proceed very adequately on simple sentences, though some of the concepts taught in this mode were quite difficult. She learned explicitly, for instance, that objects had names, for she was taught, in her own language system, that "fig name of" a real fig, and could thereafter identify it by name. She learned a few colors, shapes, and sizes, writing "red color of apple," "round shape of cracker," "small size of grape," etc. in concise sentences. But a somewhat more complicated problem arose in attempting to teach Sarah a compound sentence. In joining two sentences together using the simple conjunction "and," we can eliminate one set of subjects and verbs, *i.e.,* (John ate a cookie, John ate a grape. John ate a cookie and a grape.) Though we are not confused by the fact that in the conjoined sentence, "a grape" does not have its own subject and predicate, there was no reason to suppose that Sarah would not be confused. There was no particular reason to believe, at the time, that she comprehended the sentence as little more than a string of associations.

In this situation, Sarah was seated before her table, on which was placed an ordinary dish as well as a colorful sand pail and two fruits, an apple and a banana. When she was presented with a simple sentence, such as:

Sarah insert banana pail
Sarah insert apple pail

Sarah insert banana dish
Sarah insert apple dish

she was to follow the instruction of the sentence, *each* of which was given as a separate instruction. Sarah placed the banana or the apple in either the pail or the dish, depending on the written instruction. When Sarah showed that she was adept at reading and correctly interpreting these simple sentences, she was presented with a pair of sentences, an instructional situation she had previously experienced in the learning of the negative.

Sarah   Sarah
insert   insert
apple   banana
pail   dish

The sentences were presented in this fashion so that Sarah would learn that she had two sets of instructions to read and carry out. Next, she was given a variety of sentences that started as two complete simple sentences, but were later reduced to a single compound sentence.

Sarah
insert
banana
pail

Sarah
insert
apple
dish

Sarah followed the above instructions, and

Sarah
insert
banana
pail
insert
apple
dish

were also carried out correctly, even though one "Sarah" was omitted in the instruction. Finally, the omission of the second insert,

Sara
insert
banana

pail
apple
dish

did not disrupt Sarah's performance. In transfer tests, which included verbs other than "insert," and nouns other than those used in the training of this problem, Sarah performed at the same level of accuracy.

The perceptual experience for mapping the conditional was that of contingency or reinforcement training. In terms of experience, Sarah had previously been exposed to a number of simple sentences that contained a variety of proper names, verbs, object names, and the negative. All of the sentence terms followed the instructional rule of introducing only one un-known at a time. In many ways, Sarah's language training resembled the requirements for the production of a sentence: only one term is rewritten at a time. In Sarah's training, only one semantic possibility was, so to speak, rewritten at a time. The procedure reduced the possibility of causing Sarah unnecessary confusion. The rule requiring a single rewrite at a time helps the generative grammarian in the same way. Since Sarah was well instructed in simple sentences of various kinds, the only unknown she needed to be taught on a perceptual level was the conditional "if ... then," which has discontinuous elements in English. To avoid this awkward arrangement, Sarah was taught to use the single element ⊃ which is found in symbolic logic. The training began with:

| Sarah take apple | ? | Mary give Sarah chocolate |

Sarah replaced the interrogative particle with her only alternative, the conditional particle. On the completion of the sentence:

| Sarah take apple | if then | Mary give Sarah chocolate |

Sarah was offered a slice of apple, which she took, followed by a piece of chocolate which she also took. Next, she was presented with the sentence:

| Sarah take banana | ? | Mary not give Sarah chocolate |

which translates: what is the relationship between Mary not giving Sarah chocolate and Sarah taking the banana. Once again, Sarah replaced the interrogative with "if then." Now Sarah was given a piece of banana, but that was all. She received five trials on each of the two sentences, and was then moved along to the next step.

| Sarah take apple | if then | Mary give Sarah chocolate |
| Sarah take banana | if then | Mary not give Sarah chocolate |

| Sarah take banana | if then | Mary give Sarah chocolate |
| Sarah take apple | if then | Mary not give Sarah chocolate |

In this step, Sarah was seated at the table. Before her, there was a slice of apple and a slice of banana, while on the board the trainer arranged one set or the other of the above instructions. Since Sarah was extremely fond of chocolate, she was considered to have understood the instructions correctly if she chose the fruit that promised the chocolate. But this step turned into a fiasco. Sarah made many errors, shrieked her frustration, but continued, nevertheless, to choose the apple at every test. Unfortunately, her early experience with contingency training had always reinforced the apple, not the banana. Faced now with a difficult lesson, she reverted to an early learning pattern. Sarah soon changed her strategy to making alternate choices, and she finally attended carefully to the sentences on her board and performed without error. Once Sarah understood the relationship, she handled her transfer tests with customary accuracy. For instance, both the antecedent and the consequent sentences were changed in her transfer tests:

| Mary take red | if then | Sarah take apple |
| Mary take green | if then | Sarah take banana |

Sarah was required to watch Mary's activity. If Mary took a green card, Sarah was to take the banana, and if Mary took the red card, Sarah was to take the apple. Not only did Sarah have to observe Mary's action, she had also to read the language description of the action, read her consequent instruction, then perform her designated action. Another transfer test involved:

| Red on green | if then | Sarah take apple |
| Green on red | if then | Sarah take banana, |

in which two of her previously learned prepositional sentences were reviewed in the context of the conditional. Here again Sarah performed at her customary level of accuracy, about 80% (Premack, 1971).

The conditional sentence is a complex one and is a very advanced sentence for a chimpanzee to learn. It is not possible to appreciate fully Sarah's ability to process this type of sentence without some review of the learning history that made it possible. In the early stages of language training Sarah was taught that there were relationships between and among a variety of nonlanguage objects, such as between two cups and two spoons, between people, between people and actions, and between actions and objects. Later, when she began to construct sentences on her board, she learned that there were relationships between the words themselves. When Sarah was taught the conditional, she was given the opportunity to learn something far more complicated than that of the relationship between objects, or between words. She learned, now, that there was such a thing as a relationship between sentences, a relationship between two very different kinds of sentences. Sarah was able to use simple sentences and learned to respond correctly to the compound sentence. Sarah began with such sentences as "Sarah insert apple pail, Sarah insert banana dish," and could then perform "Sarah insert apple pail banana dish," and other sentences of this type. But the conditional sentence is neither simple nor compound. It is a complex sentence that connects two simple sentences, in which no deletion of subject or verb is possible since the sentences do not match. "Sarah take apple, Mary give Sarah chocolate," refer to different subjects and different verbs. Since there are no overlapping terms, no simplification of the sentence can occur. Instead, Sarah must learn that what she does at one point in time will affect what will happen at a later point in time. With a slim vocabulary of 130 words, Sarah learned to name persons, objects, verbs, etc. She progressed to a series of simple sentences in which she learned properties, classes, quantifiers, plurals, the copula, and so on. And she comprehended compound sentences, reaching, finally the complex sentence. The training was accomplished by simply mapping language elements to an already existing perceptual structure.

SOME PROBLEMS WITH THE CONCEPTUAL POSITION

To test the thesis that language maps existing distinctions, we use language-free tests to determine if the perceptual or conceptual distinctions are present. If the assessment is positive, words can be instilled through an effective language training program. And, conversely, if the assessment is negative, the language training will fail. That is, given an effective training procedure, a positive assessment should be both a necessary and a sufficient condition for the acquisition of language. This position is troubled on two grounds. First, there are cases in which the assessment appears to be positive, and yet the subject fails to acquire the words. Second, there are cases in which the thesis cannot be tested at all. Certain distinctions seem to be purely verbal, seem to have no preverbal foundation, making it impossible to design a prelanguage test. If it is the case that the subject fails to acquire words in the face of a positive assessment, then a positive assessment is only a sufficient, and not a necessary condition for language mapping. If there are cases in which the thesis is not applicable, we are faced with the possibility that it cannot be applied exhaustively. Examination of examples of both problems can indicate whether or not they are serious.

Problems in Learning "Same-Different"

In order to determine whether or not the subject can be taught to label, say two apples "same," and an apple and a banana "different," we first test the subject's ability to learn generalized match-to-sample. That is, we first determine whether the subject can match two apples and then demonstrate that he can match not only those items but an indefinite set of items as well. Some of the objects used are items that are easily contrasted, such as spoons, cups, pieces of hardware, and so on. After having been trained on 3–10 similar items, all the chimpanzees, Sarah and two new 3- to 4-year-old African-born females, Peony and Elizabeth, were able to show transfer, performing as accurately on the new items as on the training ones. Chimps as young as 3 years of age have no difficulty with the test and could conceivably learn the problem at a still earlier age.

Once the subjects pass the transfer test, we attempt to teach them the words "same" and "different," initially with the same items that are used in match-to-sample. Though Peony and Elizabeth have both learned approximately 30 words, including the names of objects, agents, and actions, they have not yet learned "same" and "different."[2] A similar difficulty has been

---

[2] Both Peony and Elizabeth have since learned "same" and "different." Indeed, Peony responded impressively to an invitation to use these words in a manner different from the one that was taught her. During training she had received these words in a fixed format: the alternative objects A and B on a line, the sample A centered and in front of them, and the word "same" or "different" placed in between the sample and the

reported by Deich and Hodges (personal communication) in their application of the present method to a group of retarded children. Of six children in the group, only one so far has learned "same-different," though all (except one) have learned names for objects and most have learned names for actions and agents as well. Sarah had no difficulty learning "same-different"; neither did the autistic child, whose data will be reported later; nor did the global aphasics trained with the same method (Velletri, Gazzaniga, and Premack, 1973). Nevertheless, a number of other subjects, chimps, and children failed to learn these words. Are the words "same-different" unique, and do they differ from other words? Is the prelanguage test given to the subjects an appropriate assessment procedure?

The "same-different" training consists of placing say, two cups, and a plastic word between the two cups, to produce: Cup "same" cup. Next, a cup and a spoon are set before the subject, along with the plastic word "different," and the subject is required to produce: Cup "different" spoon. These trials are errorless, since only one word is present on each trial. After three to five such trials on both words, the subject is given a choice test, to measure the effectiveness of the errorless trials. If he passes the choice test, he is advanced to the next pair of items, until his performance indicates that he is ready for a transfer test. But if the subject shows no learning when given the opportunity to choose between the two words, he is returned for repeated training on the original items, using errorless training. In the case of the adamant failures, Peony and Elizabeth, the subjects were advanced to new items simply to counteract the boredom that can undermine the total learning situation. Peony and Elizabeth failed to pass the choice test of "same" and "different" in spite of a large number of trials. How are we to reconcile this failure in the face of their ability to do generalized match-to-sample on the very same items?

There are differences between match-to-sample and the "same-different" training which suggest that the former may not be an appropriate assessment of the latter. The physical arrangement of the stimuli differ in the two cases. Three objects are present in match-to-sample and only two in the training of "same-different." The responses required of the subject also differ. In match-to-sample, the subject is required to select an object; in language training to select a word and place it between two objects. These differences are trivial from a normal adult's point of view, but apparently not from that of the young or infrahuman subject.

---

alternatives (see diagram in text). Was Peony's ability to use the words "same" and "different" dependent upon the configuration that had been used consistently in training? To answer this question, we presented the same stimulus material in random arrays. Peony's typical response to the random array was as follows: she put one like object on top of the other, i.e., A on A, and put the word "same" on top of them; then she put the word "different" on top of B, the odd object. Thus Peony's ability to use "same" and "different" was decidedly not dependent upon a fixed stimulus array but showed that kind of generalism or flexibility which we associate with human knowledge.

A second difference between the prelanguage and language task is that the former requires a positive judgment only, while the latter requires both the positive and negative judgments (same-different). The inconsistency can be corrected by teaching *oddity* as well as *matching* to the subjects. Consider the format:

The letters represent objects of different kinds, and the words in each box, the plastic forms that are intended to mean "same" and "different," respectively. In the presence of the word "same" the subject is required to place the alternative A near the sample A; in the presence of "different," to place the object Y near the sample X. This case differs less from match-to-sample than does the original "same-different" training. The subject, in this format, operates upon the objects (not the words) as he does in the case of match-to-sample, and the geometry of the two procedures is very similar.

The original training corresponds to production, while the revised training parallels that of comprehension. Also, the original training requires the subject to produce a sequence that is more an assertion than a request. Production itself has not been difficult for any of the subjects, but all of the production has been confined to requests, *e.g.*, "Debby give apple Elizabeth," and so on. They have not yet produced propositional-like strings. However, "A same A" and "A different B," the sentences that map the original "same-different" training, seem to be assertions rather than requests. Perhaps this contributes to the difficulty in the training as well.

Chimpanzees and retarded children are not the only ones to have difficulty with "same-different." Many normal children from 2 to 5 years of age fail to learn these words in the usual number of trials it takes them to learn most other words. The reasons for the failure can sometimes be identified. Peony and Elizabeth responded to the problem at chance, often showing either a simple position habit or stimulus preference. Many of the younger children also responded in this primitive manner. In fact, all of the 2- and 3-year olds did so. But the 5-year olds tended to adopt a different strategy; they memorized individual cases, rather than induce the rule that was basic to all of the given cases. So, the older children learned each training case to a high criterion and responded at chance only when new stimuli were introduced. Thus, they failed all transfer tests. Curiously, they often showed one-trial learning on the transfer tests. For instance, if the child mistakenly used the word "different" when the new stimulus pair "dog"-dog was introduced as a transfer test, on the next trial, he shifted to "same" and retained this response. With one-trial learning and relatively few transfer trials per training trial, rote memory could be a favorable strategy. Only by increasing the rate at which new pairs were presented would it become unfavorable, and this is something we have not yet done. Still, it is interesting to note, first, that no child adopted a memorization strategy on the simple match-to-sample and, second, that all children, including the 2-year olds, were able to learn that problem. Does the "same-different" situation require that we abandon the thesis that prelanguage comprehension plus a generally successful training procedure add up to a necessary and sufficient condition for instilling its language counterpart? It was the one concept that was difficult to map, no doubt because the prelanguage and language tasks were dissimilar. We prefer to retain the thesis, thus recommending that prelanguage and language tasks be as alike as possible in order for language to map the prelanguage.

Problems Arising from the Absence of the Perceptual Counterparts for Language

Besides the difficulty of the case of "same-different," there is another difficulty that the thesis confronts. This one concerns those cases for which it is not possible to specify a prelanguage test. It is a different kind of difficulty, but probably a more serious one. Earlier we asked if a visual representation could be found for every verbal distinction. If one could be, then one would not encounter any problems, but if linguistic distinctions existed, and no visual representation did, then the thesis could not apply to some cases, possibly very important ones.

For example, it is not clear how we are to represent the logical connectives on a visual basis. The possibilities that we can invent are pale, *e.g.*, wife and daughter, wife or daughter (exclusive or), and if wife then daughter, might be depicted visually by an appropriate series in which: wife and daughter, wife or daughter (exclusive or), and if wife then daughter, are shown alongside pictures of the husband or father. An example is shown below where F, W, and D, stand for pictures of the appropriate parties.

and		*or* (exclusive)		*if-then*	
F_1	$W_1 D_1$	F_1	W_1	F_1	$W_1 D_1$
F_2	$D_2 W_2$	F_2	D_2	F_2	$W_2 D_2$
F_3	$D_3 W_3$	F_3	W_3	F_3	$W_3 D_3$
..	..	..	..	..	..
..	..	..	..	..	..
F_N	$W_N D_N$	F_N	W_N	F_N	$W_N D_N$

Notice that in these displays, the conjunction and conditional differ only in this respect: the conditional involves an order requirement (if W then D $\neq$ if D then W) which the conjunction does not (W and D=D and W). The test would require that the subject be able to repeat the three patterns indefinitely with new items. But does the ability to detect and mimic these patterns or others like them demonstrate comprehension of the logical connectives? It may show only that the subject can distinguish among certain visual patterns. One might try scenarios, rather than designs, action sequences in which: 1) the child smiled and the mother gave him a cookie, 2) either the child smiled or the mother gave him a cookie, and 3) if the child smiled the mother gave him a cookie. After viewing these scenes, the subjects would be shown additional films and be required to match them to the initial scenes. Doing so might show only an ability to abstract a pattern and to mimic it, yet that pattern might be a critical part of the connectives.

It is probably not possible to represent class membership wholly on a visual basis. Physical models can be used here, such as a jar and marbles, but it is not clear what operations the subject must be able to carry out on the model in order that the concept of class membership be realized. More important, it is not clear how to characterize the general set of cases for which visual representation may not be possible. The logical connectives suggest that if the arguments of the predicates are themselves linguistic entities—atomic sentences in the case of the connectives—then visual representation will not be possible. But linguistic arguments may not be the only cases that resist visual representation; class membership is resistant as well.

Makeshift tests can be substituted for formal visual representations in some cases. For example, to test Sarah's capacity for (one of the aspects of) conjunction, we invited her to behave in a so-to-speak conjunctive fashion. We gave her trials on which pieces of fruit were offered in contrast to all of her previous training on which only one piece was offered. For eight trials, despite the presence of more than one piece of fruit, she requested the individual pieces with individual sentences. For example, "Mary give apple Sarah," "Mary give banana Sarah," etc. But on the ninth trial she wrote "Mary give apple banana Sarah" and continued to do the same on subsequent trials, incorporating a third fruit into the sentence when it was offered. We took this as evidence of her ability to conjunct. In adding one (appropriate) word to another, she eliminated redundant elements that would have been present if the same request had been made with separate sentences. The argument is admittedly tenuous and the test suggestive rather than formal.

With if-then or the conditional relation, we were again stymied for a prelanguage test and substituted a prelanguage experience that could be described with the use of the conditional. Sarah was taught that in a choice between apple and banana, apple led to chocolate but banana did not. Her experience could be described with sentences that were highly familiar to her, e.g., "Sarah take apple," "Mary give Sarah chocolate," "Sarah take banana," "Mary no give Sarah chocolate." It remained only to connect these sentences in a way to introduce the conditional particle. Sarah was successful in learning this particle, on a productive basis as well. That is, she could apply the particle to atomic sentences that varied from the ones used in training. Unfortunately, the ability to be influenced by such experience (if apple then chocolate; if banana then no chocolate) merely demonstrates a susceptibility to differential reinforcement and is not a sufficient basis for assuming that the subject can learn to label the conditional relation.

EVIDENCE THAT LANGUAGE MAPS CONCEPTUAL STRUCTURE

Three kinds of evidence support the proposition that language acquisition is a mapping of an already existing conceptual structure. First, there is the fact that the extension of a word is coterminous with that of the perceptual judgment underlying the word. Second, there is the evidence for transfer in several domains. Third, the evidence for productivity takes a most interesting form.

Coterminous Relation between Perception and Language

When Sarah was first taught to request those foods that were placed before her, she was offered only pieces of fruit. The fruit was not prepared in her presence. When she requested fruit, then, she referred to a wedge of apple, a slice of banana, a segment of orange, and so on. Never did she receive an intact fruit. Even peanuts were shelled beforehand and given to Sarah in edible portions.

After Sarah had learned a few fruit names, we began to wonder what the food words meant to her. Could she match the word "apple" with an intact apple, the word "orange" to an intact orange, considering that she had never been given this experience? On one series of matching tests, Sarah was given the word "apple" as the sample, while the intact fruits, apple and banana were offered as choices. On the other series, the relation was reversed, the intact banana was the sample, and the words "banana" and "apple" were the choices. Sarah failed the tests. There was only one pairing on which she performed above chance, and that was "orange"-orange, or its reverse. Evidently the segment of orange retained enough of the properties of the intact fruit, with color perhaps a dominant cue, so that Sarah was able to apply the word "orange" to the slice of orange as well as the intact fruit.

We pitied ourselves for the outcome. If Sarah could not learn relations as simple as these, if she could not apply the word "apple" to a whole fruit, but only some fraction of one, then how could we hope to teach her the considerable intricacies of language that were yet to be instilled? But at the next step, Sarah absolved herself from blame and rescued us from despair. She indicated that her failure to associate the name of the fruit with its intact form was probably not a linguistic problem *per se*. In fact, that the problem was in no way linguistic was shown by removing the words from the match-to-sample procedure and conducting the same set of tests using fruit only, eliminating the names. Now Sarah was required to match either an intact fruit to a portion of the same fruit, or the reverse. She failed these tests in quite the same degree as she had the earlier series. She could not match a piece of fruit to the whole fruit, nor the whole fruit to a piece of it, except for the orange, for which she could do both with some accuracy. She performed as well here as she had with "orange"-orange and its reverse. In other words, there was a perfect agreement between the extension of her perceptual judgment on one side, and the use of the corresponding words on the other. At a later time, given no more explicit training than the opportunity to observe the preparation of the fruit, Sarah learned the part-whole relations. She then passed both the nonlinguistic and the linguistic version of the match-to-sample tests.

Transfer of "Name of" and of the Quantifiers

An example of transfer was seen in the word "name of," which was taught Sarah as the relation between the familiar word "apple" and the object apple, the familiar word "banana" and the object banana. Included in the training were also the standard two negative exemplars: "apple not name of" banana and "banana not name of" apple. The word "apple" had been used with considerable frequency in several different sentences which secured an apple for her: "Mary (or Randy or Debby or Jim, etc.) give apple," and in all these situations, Sarah received the apple. Also, when a trainer wrote "Sarah take apple" and Sarah chose the piece of apple from among the several pieces of fruit, she was allowed to take and keep the apple. The same was true in the more complex instruction, "Sarah insert apple (in) dish." If she put the apple, rather than one of the other fruits in the dish (and not the pail), she was praised and given a tidbit she preferred. Thus, the word "apple" and all other fruit names were used in both the production and the comprehension of sentences. In some cases the apple was obtained in hand, and in other cases, an activity was performed upon apple which yielded something besides apple. Word-object pairs on which Sarah received the above training included "apricot"-apricot, "raisin"-raisin, and so on. She had no difficulty transferring the term "name of" to new cases. For instance, though never trained specifically on "name of" with respect to apricot or raisin, Sarah answered correctly that "apricot name of" apricot, but that "apricot not name of" raisin.

Verbs present the technical problem of having referents that are transient, and we did not attempt to test her extension of "name of" to other grammatical classes. It is possible (though not likely) that "name of" was reserved for members of a particular grammatical class. In any case, Sarah did not confine transfer of "name of" to fruit names; she extended the term to "dish" and "pail" by naming these objects as well.

The quantifiers "all, none, one, and some" were taught Sarah with a narrower inductive base than we used with other words. For instance, a set of crackers, all of which were round, served to teach the word "all" ("All" crackers are round). A set in which one cracker was round, and all others square, taught the word "One" ("One" cracker is round). The words "some" and "none" were taught in a comparable manner. "All, one, none," etc. each referred to an object or objects that differed from the other objects in the set only on the basis of shape. In other words, quantification was restricted to shape variations. Nevertheless, Sarah was able to transfer the quantifiers, not only to new items, but also to items that differed on the basis of color or on the basis of size. For instance, in the presence of a set consisting of three green and two pieces of red apple, she was asked "? apple are green" (What or how many apples are green?). She answered correctly by replacing the interrogative marker with "several," thereby forming the sentence "Several apples are green." She was correct in 9 out of the first 10 trials in this series of transfer tests (Premack, 1971). If she had failed this test, we might have sought to devise training procedures for cross-dimensional transfer. But she succeeded. And she did so in a program that made a minimal contribution to such transfer. The success was Sarah's. In fact, if an organism were deficient in the ability to transfer, it is not clear how the deficiency would be overcome.

Productivity

Productivity is the third kind of evidence that we rely on for defending the thesis that language maps the conceptual structure that antedates language training. Productivity is the process in which a word is used to generate new instances of itself. There is a superficial resemblance between transfer and productivity, but transfer refers to actual or existing words, while productivity refers to possible words. In transfer, a word is applied successfully to instances that are new, only in the weak sense that they were not used in the training of the word. For instance, the word "name of," after having been taught as the relation between "apple" and the object apple, was successfully transferred to the relation between "apricot" and apricot, and "raisin" and raisin. The words "apricot" and "raisin" were not actually used in the training of "name of," but they were well established words in Sarah's repertoire.

Productivity goes a step further by using a word to generate a new word. For instance, we used the word "color of," and the word "chocolate" to generate the new color name "brown." Sarah was given the instruction "brown color of chocolate." In this sentence, "color of" and "chocolate" were repertoire words, but "brown" was an entirely new word. The fact that "brown" was simply a new instance of the concept color, was shown by Sarah's ability to reply correctly in substitution questions, such as: "? color of chocolate," "Brown color of ?," etc. Much more interesting than that, her knowledge of "brown" was shown by the fact that when she was presented with four colored disks (only one of which was brown), and instructed, "Sarah take brown," she responded correctly (Premack, 1971).

Contrast between Transfer and Productivity

Productivity differs from transfer on the basis of class membership: productivity refers to possible members, transfer to actual members. A possible class is one in which maroon belongs as a color, or shape belongs as a property. But, though the classes are named, the actual instances of the class have not yet been named. In productivity, the members of the class are given names. When a subject is learning concepts, instances of the concept are sometimes not named (but can be named later), other instances are named and are active in the subject's repertoire, others are named and used in the specific training of the concept. In performing transfer, the subject, though trained on specific instances of a concept, is able to recognize other instances of the concept from his repertoire. In carrying out productivity, the subject uses a concept in such a way as to name instances of the concept that have never before been named (never existed in his repertoire). Both of these capacities serve to show the knowledge that the subject had before language training began. Concepts have numerous possible instances, and the important consideration is not whether they are or are not named. What is important is the fact that the subject can identify these exemplars as substitution instances in the class. The coterminous relations among perception and language, transfer, and productivity all provide strong evidence of the conceptual basis of language.

RECENT TRAINING OF TWO CHIMPS, ONE AUTISTIC CHILD

In 1970 an autism project at the University of California made available a large population of autistic children. We tested a number of them for language comprehension, in the manner described, and selected the most deficient child in the group. Billy (not his real name) was mute and showed no language comprehension beyond word recognition. He was about 8 years old, suffered impaired vision along with his other defects, and was diagnosed "retarded nonremedial." A year later we obtained two African-born (*ca.* 3 years old) female chimps to replace Sarah, whose strength had begun to outstrip her syntax. The same language training procedure was applied to the child and to the apes, modified in small ways to suit the species.

The chimps sat on a table next to a magnetized writing board. They were taught to place metal-backed pieces of plastic on the board, each of which had a wordlike function. Sentences were written on the vertical. The child sat next to the table, used the same pieces of plastic, and was taught to form sentences on the horizontal in the English style.

Although the initial lexicon might serve to differentiate the subjects—"M & M" and "Frito" in one case, "apple" and "banana" in the other—the target activity, eating, was the same in both cases. So was the social transaction—

giving—in which the target activity was embedded. Thus the first sentences taught were "Amy give M & M Billy," and "Amy give apple Elizabeth (or Peony)." This was made possible by some basic overlap in the social behavior of the two species. Giving, or being given to, is engaged in by all the subjects. This activity was decomposed into its four perceptual classes—objects, recipients, donors, and the act itself—and words were taught for members of all four classes.

The use of permanent visual symbols, rather than gestures or sounds, circumvents the short term memory problem, makes possible the use of errorless training along with the introduction of one unknown at a time, and does not depend upon elaborate motor learning (causing a particle to adhere to a board is something primates do readily). When each new word is taught by arranging it so that its introduction at a marked location in a string of known words has the effect of completing the sentence, three primary sources of difficulty are eliminated: 1) only one new word will be present, so the subject cannot err in choice of words, 2) the blank location in the (potential) sentence is marked (with the interrogative marker) so the subject cannot err as to where in the sentence to put the word, 3) the completing operation always consists of addition, rather than addition plus the possibility of deletion and/or rearrangement.

Transfer from Production to Comprehension

Both Sarah and the autistic child reached a point at which they showed excellent transfer from production to comprehension and *vice versa*. The young chimps have not yet reached this point. An example of their failure is given by the following. The verb "give" was taught them in the production mode with a particular set of object names. Later the verb "take" was taught them in the comprehension mode, with a different set of object names. The transfer test involved applying "take" to the object names that had been learned in the production mode. On the production of two-word (*e.g.*, "give apple"), three-word (*e.g.*, "give apple Peony"), and four-word (*e.g.*, "Debby give apple Peony") sentences, Peony was correct 77, 89, and 80% of the time. Given the same object names on the comprehension test, her performance fell to 58%. Data for Elizabeth were highly comparable: 70, 97, and 75% on the production of two-, three-, and four-word sentences, compared to 57% correct on comprehension tests involving the same object names.

Our first attempt to transfer Peony from production to comprehension was both amusing and informative. She had received hundreds of production trials in which one food was placed before her along with several words. She was required to place the correct word on the board in order to receive the food. In the switch to comprehension, the trainer put one word on the board and then put several pieces of food before her. Peony was to take the food corresponding to the word on the board. Instead she picked up one of the pieces of fruit, smeared it on the writing board, and then ate it. What production had apparently taught her was, roughly speaking, put something on the board, for that you will get something. Moreover, she apparently did not regard something being on the board, the something having been put there by the trainer, as equivalent to the act of putting it there herself. Interestingly, this conflicts with the view that it is invariably the consequence of an act, rather than the act itself, that counts.

First Words

One way in which chimps differ markedly from children, both normal and autistic, and from global aphasics as well, is in the extremely slow acquisition of the first words. It is difficult to state numbers for Sarah since, being unprepared for her long initial failure, we jumped from one procedure to another. After she learned several words, succeeding ones were learned in ever fewer trials. Ultimately she acquired new words in one trial, and trials of a highly informal nature. An unused piece of plastic, thus a potential word, was simply held up alongside a so-far unnamed object, her attention was called to the pair, and henceforth the piece of plastic served as the object's name.

The young chimpanzees had no less difficulty than Sarah in learning their first words. Being prepared for the difficulty in their case, we did not abandon a procedure simply because it was unsuccessful but gave them, mercilessly, hundreds of standard trials until finally the first words were learned. Standard trials consisted of errorless production trials on each of two pieces of fruit, followed by choice trials on the same pair. For instance, a piece of banana was placed before the subject along with the word "banana" and the subject was required to place the word on the board before being given the banana. Comparable trials were given on apple. The subject quickly learned the mechanics on these errorless trials, putting the words on the board and receiving the fruit. Choice trials on which both the words "banana" and "apple" were given in the presence of either apple or banana then revealed that the subject had learned nothing, nothing, that is, of the word-referent pairing. To forestall boredom, a new pair of words was introduced, treated in the same way as the first pair, and sometimes a third and fourth pair as well. Each pair was given errorless trials on individual members, followed by choice trials on the pair. Some idea of the slow acquisition of first words is suggested by Elizabeth's data. She required 1699 trials—423 errorless and 1276 choice trials—before learning her first word. No human subject—normal, autistic, or global aphasic—has required 1/10th that number of trials.

The outstanding difference between the chimps and all members of the human population we have tested so far is that only the chimps are being taught first words; the latter already know words. One might suppose that the global aphasics could be described as wordless, but the relative ease with which they acquired their first (plastic) words suggests that it is more likely that they are not. The alternative interpretation that man forms associations faster than chimps is less tenable. After acquiring a sufficient number of words, the chimp acquires new words in one trial.

The hundreds of initial trials which appear to teach the chimp nothing in fact teach it a great deal, but not specifically with respect to word-referent association (Premack, 1973). Word-referent associations are learned later. Apparently they are not learned until the subject has first learned: 1) the class character of a word, 2) the class character of a referent, and 3) the general rule, any word will go with any referent. The last rule is incorrect, of course, since each word is to be associated with only one referent, yet it is one way of describing the superordinate association between the two classes, word and referent, which the subject appears to learn before going on to acquire specific associations between individual members of the two classes.

On one occasion Sarah used monkey pellets to obtain sips of coffee. No words were available to her at the time and coffee was a novel and desired item. This has all the appearance of an astute instance of transfer. But it is difficult to interpret in that light because Sarah did not yet know a single word. Thus the pellet-coffee association could not be considered transfer since there was no word-referent association from which to derive its transfer. The pellet-coffee association could be understood, however, if we consider that what Sarah had learned to that point was a superordinate association, loosely speaking a rule to the effect that any less valued thing can be exchanged for any more valued thing.

A blunt test of this hypothesis could be made simply by presenting the subject with a mixture of words and pieces of fruit. The subject who has not learned even one specific word-referent association may nonetheless have learned the superordinate association, *viz.*, any word can be used to get any fruit. Such a subject should give the trainer a word each time before taking a piece of fruit and should show no consistent relation between the words it gives and the fruits it takes. We made such a test with Walnut, a 4-year-old, African-born male, who regrettably has not yet learned a word. Loosely speaking, Walnut passed the test. Confronted with a scramble of words and pieces of fruit, he gave the trainer one word and then took four or five pieces of fruit, another word and another handful of fruit, etc. He made four or five such one-to-many pairings before we terminated the test. Either Walnut did not know the one-to-one character of the rule, or greed overcame knowledge. Nevertheless, he was consistent in giving only words for fruit; he never gave words for words, fruit for fruit, or fruit for words.

TRANSFER FROM PLASTIC LANGUAGE TO NATURAL LANGUAGE

The plastic language is a laboratory device of no value in the real world. In teaching it to a human subject, we do so on the premise either that the subject will be indefinitely confined to an artificial environment, or, more hopefully, that the plastic language is a crutch which will help the subject acquire natural language and can be discarded later. We have one piece of data that provides modest support for the hopeful option.

Since the autistic child proved not to know pluralization in natural language (either on the original pretraining assessment or on subsequent assessments made during the course of training), we taught him pluralization in the plastic language. In keeping with the rest of the system we did not use inflection but marked the plural with a separate particle. Training sentences included, "Billy take cookie" *vs.* "Billy take cookie pl," where "cookie" plus "pl" equals "cookies." The plural is an easy distinction and was learned readily.

Having taught him pluralization in the plastic language, we reassessed his comprehension of pluralization in natural language, hoping that perhaps no more than calling his attention to the distinction would prove to be necessary. That was an unfounded hope. Given sentences in natural language equivalent to those given in plastic language, *e.g.,* "take cookie," and "take cookies," he performed at chance. The failure was not surprising for we had done nothing to establish an equivalence between the plural markers in the two systems, between the plastic "pl" particle, on the one hand, and the terminal sibilance of "cookies" on the other.

In the next step we established an equivalence between the two systems in perhaps the most direct manner possible. We laid out a number of plastic words and instructed him in natural language to take certain of them. For example, plastic words for M & M and cookie were displayed and the child was told in natural language "take M & M," "take cookie," etc. The child had no difficulty taking the correct plastic word since all of the plastic words used were names of objects for which he also knew the natural language name.

Next, the plural particle "pl" was placed before the child and he was told in natural language, "take plural." After several errorless instructions of this kind, other plastic words were added to the "pl" particle, and the same instruction was repeated, "take plural." He readily passed the choice test, correctly picking up the "pl" particle when told to "take plural."

Was the above procedure successful in establishing an equivalence between the two systems? We answered the question by retesting the child on natural language. A cookie and a pair of cookies were placed before him and he was told "take cookie" on some trials, "take cookie plural" on others. (To make the systems more comparable we discarded the terminal inflection used in English and brought in a separate particle there too. Thus, to pluralize in laboratory English, one said "dog *vs.* dog plural," "cat *vs.* cat plural," etc.) He made only two errors in 20 trials and performed equally well on transfer tests involving objects not used in teaching the plastic plural marker. The plastic visual system is clearly preferable to no language at all, and it may also prove helpful in speeding the acquisition of natural language.

REFERENCES

Gallup, G. G., Jr. Chimpanzees: Self-recognition. *Science,* 1970, *167,* 86–87.

Gellerman, L. W. Chance orders of alternating stimuli in visual discrimination. *J. Genetic Psychology,* 1933, *42,* 207–208.

Goodall, J. Chimpanzees of the Gombe Stream Research, in I. De Vore (Ed.), *Primate Behavior.* New York: Holt, Rinehart & Winston, 1965, pp. 425–473.

Lieberman, P. *The Speech of Primates.* The Hague and Paris: Mouton, 1972.

Premack, D. Language in Chimpanzee? *Science,* 1971, *172,* 808–822.

Premack, D. Cognitive principles? In J. McGuigan and Lumsden (Eds.), *Contemporary Approaches to Conditioning and Learning.* Washington, D.C.: V. H. Winston & Sons, 1973, pp. 287–308.

Slobin, D. I. Cognitive prerequisites for the development of grammar. In C. A. Ferguson and D. I. Slobin (Eds.), *Studies of Child Language Development.* New York: Holt, Rinehart & Winston, 1973, pp. 175–208.

Velletri, G. A., Gazzaniga, M. S., and Premack, D. Artificial language training in global aphasics. *Neuropsychologia,* 1973, *11,* 95–103.

CHAPTER FIFTEEN

NONVOCAL SYSTEMS OF VERBAL BEHAVIOR[1]

Donald F. Moores

Research, Development and Demonstration Center in Education
of Handicapped Children, University of Minnesota, Minneapolis,
Minnesota 55455

This chapter provides a background for the consideration of linguistic systems which apparently meet all of the criteria traditionally considered necessary for true languages with one exception—they involve the visual-motor channel as the primary means of communication rather than the auditory-vocal. Manual sign languages employed by deaf individuals do indeed constitute legitimate language systems. The nature and use of sign languages will be discussed, and an overview of structural and functional characteristics of what is known as American Sign Language (ASL) will be treated. Suggestions will be made for the educational use of manual communication, and an attempt will be made to dispel some common misunderstandings. Although the major portion of this chapter deals with American Sign Language, related work in Europe is incorporated.

Although some variation of American Sign Language is probably used by a majority of deaf adults in the United States and Canada, American Sign Language remains an exotic language. It is subject to less scientific analysis than many dialects spoken by isolated tribes in the most primitive, inaccessible areas of the world. There are a number of explanations for such neglect. Of primary importance has been the tendency of many educators of the deaf to treat any form of manual communication as behavior that must be repressed. During the 20th century, until the decade of the 1960's all programs for the deaf in the United States professed to follow an oral-only philosophy of education, at least until age 11. After this age, some programs would allow their "oral failures" to be exposed to signs in the classroom. Children were considered failures because they did not meet the one criterion for success—to speak well enough to become part of the hearing world. Because the goal of education was "normalcy," *i.e.,* speaking, a prejudice developed against signs as alinguistic, concrete, and inflexible. Signs were

[1] The preparation of this paper was supported by a grant from the Bureau of Education for the Handicapped, United States Office of Education, Department of Health, Education, and Welfare.

confused with "natural" gestures, reflecting an ignorance of the arbitrary, learned nature of a true language of signs.

A second factor which inhibited the study of manual communication systems was the tendency of many linguists, especially those heavily influenced by Bloomfield (1933), to assume that all languages were primarily spoken and that other forms of communication, *e.g.,* written, were imperfect outgrowths of a basic spoken system. This position was first challenged by the pioneering work of Stokoe (1958). Stokoe has brought the tools of linguistic analysis to bear on American Sign Language and demonstrated that it is a linguistic system with all of the important characteristics of a spoken language: phrase structure, transformational rules, a systematic distinctive feature set for expression, etc.

In addition to the work of Stokoe, other recent developments have increased interest in the function and structure of sign language systems. The input of theoreticians and researchers concerned with the biological bases of language has been considerable. Lenneberg (1967) has advocated the use of graphics, under which he includes signs, with very young deaf children. Bellugi-Klima and her associates at the Salk Institute are conducting a series on the development and use of American Sign Language by deaf children and adults. In a presentation at the University of Minnesota in February, 1972, Chomsky described as "barbaric" the educational practices in the State of Massachusetts which proscribed the use of signs with deaf children.

Another source of interest is generated by ethologists and researchers interested in investigating the growth of communication systems in animals. The work of the Gardners (1969) in teaching signs to the chimp Washoe is well known. Although the theoretical orientations and research objectives of individuals such as Lenneberg and the Gardners are dissimilar, and even in opposition, it is apparent that, as emphasis has shifted from learning to built-in propensities for language, more attention is being paid by various researchers to human nonvocal communication and to animal communication.

A final liberalizing influence, which should not be underestimated, is the growing societal awareness and acceptance of cultural pluralism and the increasing willingness to accept differences. There is less of a press toward conformity to a standard, whether it be the white standard, the Anglo standard, or the hearing standard. In this context, deaf people can be judged as human beings and not on the basis of the extent to which they have mastered articulation skills.

THE AMERICAN SIGN LANGUAGE

The difficulties of dealing with any language are complex. For example, anyone attempting to develop a comprehensive definition of the English language would have to come to terms with the wide variety of dialects spoken in England, the United States, South Africa, and Australia. He would have to decide at which point two dialects of a language differ so much that they become two separate languages. Pushing further, he would find differences in English usage not only between countries but also between regions of the same country. To complicate matters even more, there are observable class differences in the use of English that cut across regional and national lines. The final compounding factor is the fact that individuals themselves easily move from one dialect to another depending upon the circumstances. The style and vocabulary a professor uses in teaching a class or preparing a paper need not approximate in any way the manner in which he expresses himself when his role changes to that of a spectator at a hockey match or a father on a canoe trip with his son.

Historically, the problem of definition might have been solved by reference to a standard dialect. For example, for a number of reasons, mostly political, the English spoken around London assumed a dominant status. Questions of correctness of usage were decided by the prescriptions of the King's English. Most of the early English-speaking settlers of the American colonies, however, came from the midlands and the north of England and spoke different, therefore "inferior," dialects.

There is a present tendency to treat dialects as equals. There is no reason to perceive London English as more correct than any other dialect. Its ascendency reflects political-economic, not linguistic, supremacy in much the same way as the French around Paris and Castilian Spanish became standards.

By making dialects respectable, the problem of definition obviously becomes much more difficult and ambiguous. The English language must be redefined to encompass enormous diversity, an almost impossible task. Most people would eventually be satisfied to conclude that, although they cannot define and describe English, they do have the ability to recognize it when encountered and to understand and use it when the circumstances require.

The difficulties inherent in dealing with the term "sign language," or even American Sign Language, are still more complex. There are deaf children and adults across the United States and Canada using a variety of visual-motor communications systems. At the lowest level a system might consist of home-made gestures invented and understood perhaps by only one class of six or seven students in a classroom excluding parents, teachers, and even other deaf students in the same program. At the other end of the continuum would be an arbitrary, abstract, somewhat standardized system capable of expressing all of the levels and nuances of spoken English. The complicating factor is the fact that signs usually have not been passed down from parent to child; rather they are repressed by most of the adults the child comes into contact with. Young deaf children usually are not allowed more than minimal contact with deaf adults. Typically the children develop a sign system surreptitiously against the wishes of the adults in their environment. At a conference on communication, Falberg (1971) suggested that sign language, in its broadest sense, is the only extant language which has been passed down from child to child.

At one time it was believed that there was a standard of correctness, which was the relatively formal system used in classroom instruction at Gallaudet College, the world's only college for the deaf. Gallaudet Sign was, and is, to the American Sign Language as London English was, and is, to the English Language. As a graduate student with normal hearing at Gallaudet the author learned formal "sign language" in a classroom situation. However, attempts to use the newly learned skills in informal situations quickly demonstrated that there are differences between how some concepts "should" be signed and how they actually were signed. An example would be the formal sign for *animal* which illustrates a beating heart and movement on four feet. Although the deaf students recognized the sign in formal use, they seldom, if ever, used it themselves. Other examples might be the formal and informal signs for *father* and *mother*.

Recently American Sign Language has attracted investigators from a number of disciplines. As representatives of areas such as linguistics, anthropology, developmental psycholinguistics, and psychology have brought their specialized skills, and esoteric dialects, to bear on the phenomenon of manual communication, they have generated, along with some fascinating results, a plethora of terms which are confusing to the layman. A quick survey of recent literature would turn up such examples as Sign, Sign Language, Manual English, Linguistics of Visible English (LVE), High Sign, Low Sign, SEE 1 (Seeing Essential English), SEE 2 (Signing Exact English) and Amerslan. Working definitions of the most commonly used of these terms will be presented below.

DEFINITION OF TERMS

The roots of the American Sign Language do not lie in the English language but can be traced back to a variant of the French Sign Language developed by de l'Epee to reflect French syntax. The French Sign Language was brought to the United States by Laurent Clerc who became the first teacher at the American School for the Deaf in 1817. Although a competent user of English can sign and spell in grammatical English patterns, many of the basic signs remain cognates with the original French ones.

Popular folklore to the contrary, there is no universal sign language. A sign language, as any other language, has many arbitrary characteristics that must be learned. For example, Stokoe (1972) reported that after 6 years he had acquired enough competence to find no difficulty conversing with deaf signers in Paris, though he had no command of spoken French and most of them had no knowledge of English. In England, however, because of the relative lack of mutual intelligibility of signs between regions, he reported that signs learned in Canterbury were of little use in communicating with deaf persons in other parts of Britain. However, in Dublin communication was easier because the manual alphabet was similar and because Irish Sign Language, which also stems from French Sign Language, has many cognates with American signs. Stokoe (1972) also reported that at the 1968 World Federation of the Deaf meeting in Paris as many as six manual interpreters were used at one time to translate speeches into various sign languages. Obviously then, there is no one language of signs. The potential number of sign languages, like spoken languages, is clearly unlimited.

Manual communication encompasses gestural systems from primitive, small group, even idiosyncratic, subsystems limited to the here and now up to highly complex forms which in every way may be considered legitimate language systems. For purposes of convenience, we shall refer to the American Sign Language (ASL) as including those systems in use throughout the United States and Canada which have a high degree of mutual intelligibility, although regional and class variations may exist. Within ASL, as with other languages, there exist different types of linguistic codes which we shall consider either formal or standard[2] variants. In this context the standard system may be thought of as a linguistic system possessing its own rules which do not necessarily follow the same constraints as the formal English system. The more a system accommodates itself to English, by this definition, the more it moves toward being in the formal category. At the extreme might be complete reliance on the manual alphabet without resorting to any signs to provide a one-to-one correspondence to the printed word.

Note that the above is merely one way of classifying manual communication systems. It could be argued that what one called "standard" and "formal" here are, in reality, two languages and that a deaf child of deaf parents might first learn ASL and later in school learn English as a second language. In essence this is the position taken by Cicourel and Boese (1972).

Using manual communication, it is possible to present a word in two different ways. One involves the use of fingerspelling, that is, spelling the word letter by letter using the manual alphabet, which consists of 26 letters with a one-to-one correspondence with traditional orthography. In spelling, the hand is held in front of the chest and letters are represented by different hand configurations. The rate of presentation is equivalent to a comfortable, somewhat slow, rate of speech somewhat faster than the rate of an accomplished typist. Figure 1 illustrates the American alphabet. For contrast Figures 2 to 5 present some of the alphabets used in various parts of the Soviet Union, where fingerspelling is a component of all preschool and primary programs for the deaf.

---

[2] In a linguistic sense, one could refer to high (H) and low (L) variants rather than formal and standard, respectively. The author did this in a previous work (Moores, 1972). Because the terms, "high" and "low" may be interpreted as prejudicial, they are not used in this chapter.

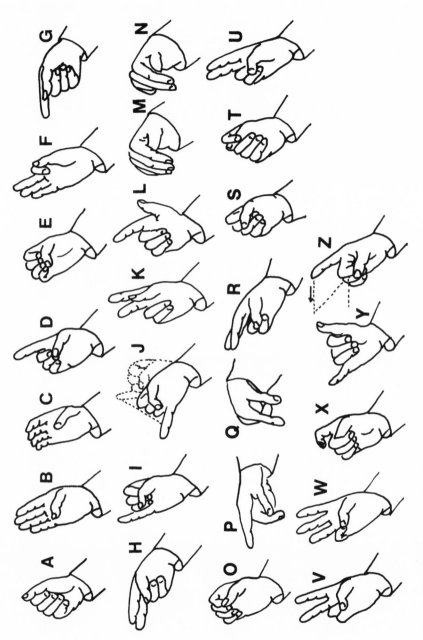

Fig. 1. The American manual alphabet.

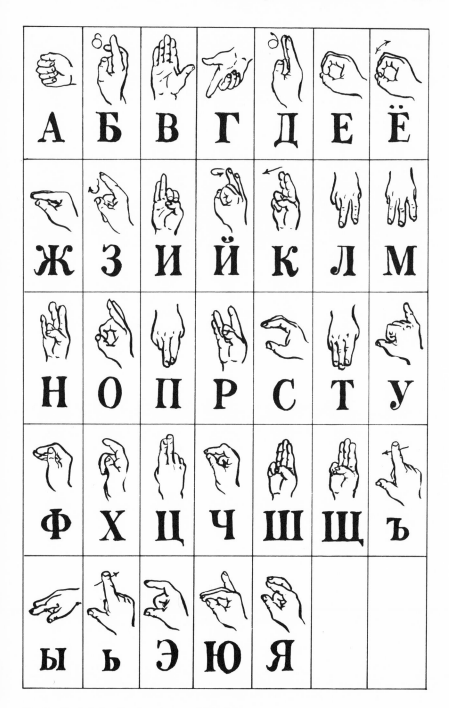

Fig. 2. The Russian Sign Language alphabet. From Gerankina, 1972.

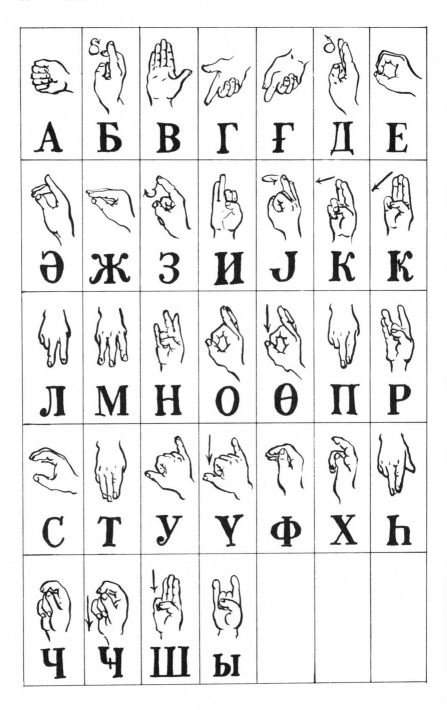

Fig. 3. The Azerbaijan Sign Language alphabet. From Gerankina, 1972.

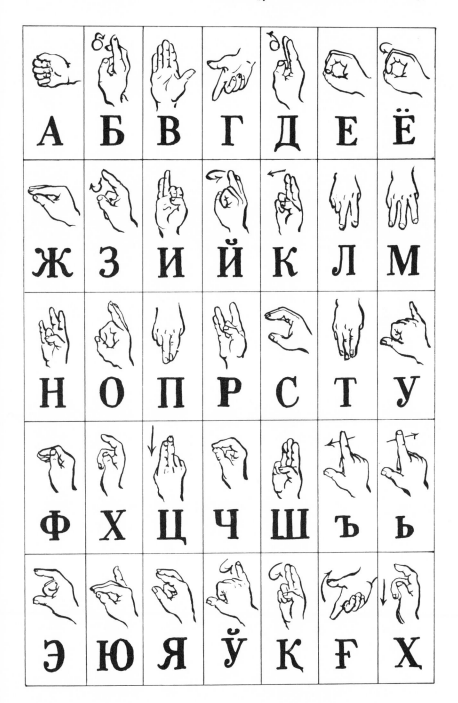

Fig. 4. The Uzbek Sign Language alphabet. From Gerankina, 1972.

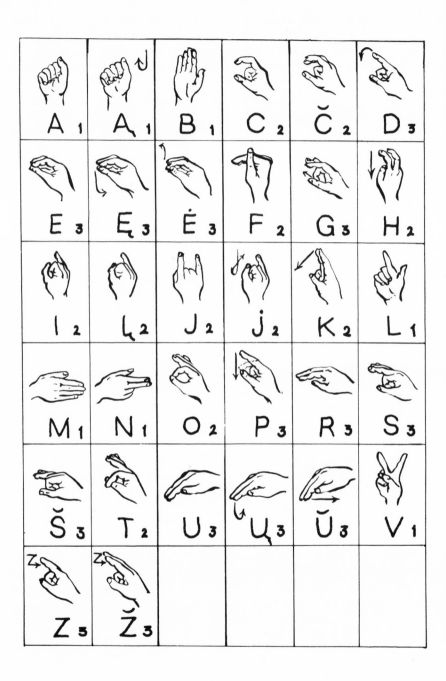

Fig. 5. The Lithuanian Sign Language alphabet. From Gerankina, 1972.

A second way of presenting a word or concept is through a sign which represents a complete idea. Each sign has three elements: 1) the position of the hands; 2) the configuration of the hands; and 3) movement of the hands to different positions. As an illustration the concept *good* is signed in the following way: the left hand, in the "B"' configuration, is held palm up before the chest. The right hand, in the "B" configuration touches the lips. The right hand is then brought down to rest on the left hand. A more complete description of the components of signs will be presented in a following section.

Proficient practitioners of manual communication, then, have a variety of options open to them. They may communicate completely with signs using no spelling or they may communicate completely through fingerspelling. Most individuals tend to use both signs and fingerspelling in their conversations. As a rule of thumb, the more informal a situation, the more signs tend to dominate. As a situation becomes more formal and "English-like" there is a tendency to use spelling to a greater extent.

Opponents of the use of signs have been critical because "the sign language has no copula" or "the sign language has no sign for 'the.' " As we have established, there is no such thing as "the sign language." It should be stressed that anything that can be expressed by speech can also be expressed by the hands. Formal systems force the use of just such elements. If there are elements that cannot be signed, they can be spelled. In passing, one might observe that Russian lacks a copula and Latin lacks a word for *the*. No one has ever suggested on this basis that Russian and Latin do not qualify as legitimate languages.

Refering to Table 1, Native Sign Language, or Amerslan, represents systems in which a minimum of spelling is employed, the copula is omitted, and word order does not necessarily follow English. Much information is presented through context, facial expression, and body posture. This is "the sign language" that has been criticized so frequently. It appears to be related to the public codes identified by Bernstein (1960, 1964, 1972) and will be classified here as a standard form of ASL. Signed English, a formal variant, expresses all aspects of English, including the copula, bound morphemes, and English word order. Notice, Native Sign Language and Signed English are not

Table 1. Major Systems of Manual Communication Presently in Use in the United States

Standard	Formal	Pedagogical (prescriptive)
Native Sign Language	Signed English	SEE 1
Amerslan	Manual English	SEE 2
		Linguistics of Visible English
		Cued Speech

dichotomous, in the author's opinion, but represent two ends of a continuum.

Independent of Signed English, which uses a mixture of signs and fingerspelling, would be Manual English which is pure spelled English without the benefit of any signs.

A number of systems have been developed recently for pedagogical purposes. The best known are Seeing Exact English, Signing Essential English, and Linguistics of Visible English. They will be discussed in a separate section.

LINGUISTIC ANALYSIS OF AMERICAN SIGN LANGUAGE

If ASL is to be considered a true language, it must be demonstrably accessible to linguistic analysis; the visual system would have to possess elements similar to phonemes, the smallest units of sounds in a language. Although it is relatively simple to show equivalence between a sign and a morpheme, little attention has been paid to isolating the distinctive building blocks from which signs are developed in much the same way that spoken morphemes are seen as clusters of consonants and vowels.

Stokoe (1958) developed the concept of a chereme [KERIYM] as a motor analogue to a phoneme. Cheremes constitute the visible distinct elemental units of a sign language much as phonemes constitute the auditory distinctive units of a spoken language.

There are three classes of cheremes, identified as tab (tabulator), dez (designator), and sig (signation). Briefly, the three are defined (Stokoe, 1958) as follows:

tab: Tabulator; the position-marking aspect of sign language activity; specifically, the position in which a significant configuration (dez) makes a significant movement (sig).

dez: Designator; that configuration of the hand or hands which makes a significant motion (sig) in a significant position (tab).

sig: Signation; the motion component or aspect of sign language activity; specifically, motion of a significant configuration (dez) in a significant position (tab).

The three aspects of any sign therefore are 1) the place(s) where it is made, 2) the distinctive configuration(s) of the hand or hands making it, and 3) the action(s) of the hand or hands. Tables 2, 3, and 4 present the cheremes of American Sign Language. A sign may possess one or more of each of the three classes of cheremes. Any sign, then, is a unique combination of 3 or more of the 55 cheremes of American Sign Language. The order of writing the symbols follows a tab, dez, sig sequence.

A Dictionary of American Sign Language has been developed (Stokoe, Croneberg, and Casterline, 1965) using the tab, dez, sig cheremic system. In

Table 2. Tab Symbols for Writing the Signs of American Sign Language*

1.	∅	Zero, the neutral place where the hands move, in contrast with all places below.
2.	◡	Face or whole head
3.	◠	Forehead or brow, upper face
4.	⊔	Midface, the eye or nose region
5.	◡	Chin, lower face
6.	⊒	Cheek, temple, ear, side-face
7.	π	Neck
8.	⊏⊐	Trunk, body from shoulder to hips
9.	⁊	Upper arm
10.	⋏	Elbow, forearm
11.	⍺	Wrist, arm in supine position (on its back)
12.	ꝺ	Wrist, arm in prone position (face down)

*From Stokoe, Croneberg, and Casterline, 1965.

Table 3. Dez Symbols for Writing the Signs of American Sign Language*

1.	A	Compact hand, fist; may be like "a," "s," or "t" of manual alphabet
2.	B	Flat hand
3.	5	Spread hand; fingers and thumb spread like "5" of manual numeration
4.	C	Curved hand; may be like "c" or more open
5.	E	Contracted hand; like "e" or more clawlike
6.	F	"Three-ring" hand; from spread hand, thumb and index finger touch or cross
7.	G	Index hand, like "g" or sometimes like "d"; index finger points from fist
8.	H	Index and second finger, side by side, extended
9.	I	"Pinkie" hand; little finger extended from compact hand
10.	K	Like except that thumb touches middle phalanx of second finger; like "k" and "p" of manual alphabet
11.	L	Angle hand; thumb, index finger in right angle, other fingers usually bent into palm

*From Stokoe, Croneberg, and Casterline, 1965.

(continued)

Table 3. (continued)

12.	ろ	"Cock" hand; thumb and first two fingers spread, like "3" of manual numeration
13.	O	Tapered hand; fingers curved and squeezed together over thumb; may be like "o" of manual alphabet
14.	R	"Warding off" hand; second finger crossed over index finger, like "r" of manual alphabet
15.	V	"Victory" hand; index and second fingers extended and spread apart
16.	W	Three-finger hand; thumb and little finger touch, others extended spread
17.	X	Hook hand; index finger bent in hook from fist, thumb tip may touch fingertip
18.	Y	"Horns" hand; thumb and little finger spread out extended from fist; or index finger and little finger extended, parallel
19.	४	(Allocheric variant of Y); second finger bent in from spread hand, thumb may touch fingertip

Table 4. Sig Symbols for Writing the Signs of American Sign Language*

1.	⌒	Upward movement
2.	⌣	Downward movement
3.	⌁	Up-and-down movement
4.	>	Rightward movement
5.	<	Leftward movement
6.	Z	Side-to-side movement
7.	T	Movement toward signer
8.	⊥	Movement away from signer
9.	I	To-and-fro movement
10.	a	Supinating rotation (palm up)
11.	b	Pronating rotation (palm down)
12.	ω	Twisting movement
13.	b	Nodding or bending action
14.	□	Opening action (final dez configuration shown in brackets)
15.	#	Closing action (final dez configuration shown in brackets)
16.	⅃	Wiggling action of fingers
17.	ə	Circular action
18.	)(	Convergent action, approach
19.	×	Contactual action, touch
20.	ɪ	Linking action, grasp
21.	⧧	Crossing action, grasp
22.	⊙	Entering action
23.	÷	Divergent action, separate
24.	()	Interchanging action

*From Stokoe, Croneberg, and Casterline, 1965.

this system, the previously described sign for *good* would be written in the following way:

• ⌒ $B_T{}^X$: : $\Big\}$ $B_T{}^X$ $\Big\}$ $B_T{}^{txt}$

SOCIOLINGUISTIC CONSIDERATIONS

The work of Bernstein (1960, 1964) in England at the intersection of sociology, psychology, and linguistics has provided new insights into the relationships between social class membership and the function of linguistic codes. From his research Bernstein has posited the existence of two different types of language codes, which he labeled "restricted (or public)" and "elaborate (or formal)" codes.

A restricted code is typified by repeated, redundant utterances with a limited variety of modifiers. It is "now" coded and tends to be concrete and rigid and possess a simple structure. Analysis of communication by means of such a code would unearth characteristics such as 1) short, simple, unfinished sentences; 2) "poor" syntax in relation to a standard; 3) limited use of adjectives and adverbs; 4) infrequent use of subordinate clauses; and 5) minimal reliance on impersonal pronouns. An elaborate code would possess more complex structure and syntax and would be less redundant or predictable. Such a code facilitates abstraction and consideration of hypotheses. The social network and social requirements of advanced civilizations necessitate the development of large classes of people capable of using elaborate codes.

In Bernstein's schema, which was concerned with class differences, the middle class individual learns both an elaborate code and one or more restricted codes. He can move back and forth between codes at will. The lower class child is limited to a restricted code, with serious implications for school advancement and later success. Other forms of language might not be directly comprehended but may have to be mediated through the child's own system. In the classroom the child must translate the code of his teacher through his own structures to make it personally meaningful.

One must be cautious in applying Bernstein's conclusions from work in England to systems of language usage in the United States. Bernstein himself (1972) has decried the misinterpretation of his work, especially in the United States, to the detriment of politically disadvantaged populations. There has been justifiable criticism of attempts, for example, to treat Black English as a restricted, and therefore inferior, dialect which must be eliminated. Recent evidence suggests it is a legitimate complex variant of the English language providing its user with tools of communication as well as any other dialect (Baratz, 1968, 1969a, 1969b; Labov, 1966). It should be noted that a user of Black English can make some distinctions not easily made in standard English. For example, the distinction between "He workin' " and "He be workin' " is a difficult one to make in the standard dialect.

In discussing the role of standard and nonstandard dialects, Baratz (1968) concluded:

He must be able to maintain his non-standard language because it is necessary for him for the majority of his experiences which occur outside the middle class culture. To devalue his language, or to presume standard English is a "better system" is to devalue the child and his culture and to reveal a shocking naivete towards language. Our job then is to teach the child a second language system (dialect if you wish) without denying the legitimacy of his own system (p. 145).

The goal, then, is not to stamp out Black English, Native Sign Language, or Spanish dialects of the Southwest. It is to give the child the skills by which he can move from one system to another, from standard to a formal, when the situation requires it. This is desirable not because the formal system, the relatively formal, prestigious middle class American English, is inherently better but because it is the system shared by a majority of Americans and therefore provides a meeting ground of commonality for communication and participation in the broader culture.

The analogy between the deaf child and the black or Spanish-speaking child should not be pushed too far. True, all may be subject to the scorn of their teachers who may denigrate their methods of communication, but, at least on the outside, the black child or Spanish-speaking child has access to an already developed language system used by parents and peers alike. Deaf children, except for the relatively few with deaf parents, usually do not even have a shared linguistic system with their parents and are subject to repression at home as well as in school. The deaf child is even denied the support and identification that another linguistically different child finds at home and in the neighborhood.

THE LEARNING OF ESOTERIC MANUAL COMMUNICATION SYSTEMS

When a child with normal hearing sets out to learn the language of the adult community, the basic process is a rapid one and is usually completed without observable difficulty prior to his entrance into the educational stream (Brown and Bellugi, 1964; Lenneberg, 1967; McNeill, 1966). The beginning of the deaf child's education, on the other hand, involves an attempt to teach a language system to an essentially alinguistic child (Moores, 1970a). Spurred by a need to communicate and lacking mastery over the auditory-based system, the child will develop small group gesture systems to help him communicate in some basic way (Tervoort, 1961). The existence of these gesture systems is a fact of life and may be observed even in programs which adhere to the so-called "pure" oral method (Kohl, 1966; Lenneberg, 1967; Stafford, 1965; Moores and McIntyre, 1971).

It is worthy of note that these systems are usually constructed by the child. This is in no way analogous to the situation of a child who is constantly exposed to spoken English (or Signed English) and who moves steadily toward the acquisition of adult linguistic proficiency. We are talking about children with almost *no* linguistic input or feedback who are developing methods of communication on their own in the face of a frequently hostile world. These children are in a sense rediscovering, or reconstructing, the wheel.

A primary concern must be the effect that such a system has on the later learning of American English, whether in a spoken, written, or signed form. Tervoort (Tervoort and Verbeck, 1967; Moores, 1970b) studied intensively the development of communication structure patterns in deaf children over a period of years in the United States, the Netherlands, and Belgium in order to assess the relationships between the in-group systems, which he termed "esoteric," and the outgroup, "exoteric" systems of adult Dutch and American English. Although the term "exoteric" may be equated with our previous use of the term "formal, or high," the "esoteric" systems would not be considered standard, or low, variants because of the lack of mutual intelligibility between groups.

In his study, Tervoort reported that children of all ages tended to use signs as the preferred means of communication in their private conversations. There was a consistent growth of grammatically correct usage as a function of age until age 14. After this age, American students continued to improve (show closer approximation to adult English patterns) while the European students leveled off. Tervoort attributed the superiority of the American students, in part, to the positive influence of the educated adult deaf with whom they came in contact. Tervoort stated

> . . . the sign language of the American adult deaf is a source from above, strongly influencing the interchange of the deaf teenager, on campus too, and on the contrary the fact that no such source from above is available for their mates across the ocean with whom they are matched. Once the esotericity of at least part of the subjects' private communication is established as a fact (whether this is a fact that should have been prevented, should be corrected, or even denied, is not the issue here), it is evident that normal need for communication finds a better outlet in an adult arbitrary system, than in uncontrolled and half-grown symbolic behavior not fed from above in educational terms:—it seems clear that the choice has to be: either well controlled, monitored signing tending towards an adult level, semantically and syntactically, or no signing whatsoever; but no signing that is uncontrolled and left to find its own ways (p. 148).

The impact of the continued restriction of students to an esoteric system is dramatically illustrated by the fact that only 2% of the utterances of American children consisted of completely esoteric imitative gestures as compared to 10% of the European total. Some educators of the deaf believe that the English usage of deaf people is poor because of the influence of sign language, which is "ungrammatical." Tervoort's results show that such a position is naive and a causative role cannot be attributed to gestures or signs. It is more logical to conclude that many deaf individuals have difficulty expressing themselves in spoken, written, or signed English because of the imposition of an early linguistically deprived environment.

If such a thing as nonstandard deaf English does exist, its existence may be attributed not to signs but to the influence of inadequate instruction in standard English. In many cases the restrictive factors are provided by the gesture systems unconsciously employed by "oral-only" teachers. An example of this may be provided by the experiences of a deaf graduate student at the University of Minnesota who began instructing deaf junior high students in Minneapolis in the use of Signed English in a program that previously had been "pure" oral. She found that the students had developed habituated signs which were difficult to modify. The most ingrained one happened to be a gesture which covered the use of all interrogative forms. It consisted of holding both upper arms tightly against the body with hands face up, and away from the body, at chest level about 18 inches apart. Tracing back her own school experiences she realized, of course, that this was the common body stance of teachers of the deaf when asking questions of their students. She was struck by the irony of teachers, who have slapped the hands of students for gesturing, unconsciously providing a model of limiting, restrictive gestures. As a result, rather than having at their disposal the means of expressing how, who, what, why, etc., the children are forced to lump them all together into one undifferentiated mass.

From his observations of deaf children in "pure" oral programs in Massachusetts, Lenneberg (1964) reported the following occurrence:

Recently, I had occasion to visit for half a year a public school for the congenitally deaf. At this school the children were not taught sign language on the theory that they must learn to make an adjustment to a speaking world and that absence of a sign language would encourage the practice of lip reading and attempts at vocalization. It was interesting to see that all children, without exception, communicated behind the teacher's back by means of "self-made" signs. I had the privilege of witnessing the admission of a new student, eight years old, who had been *discovered* by a social worker who was doing relief work in a slum area. The boy had never had any training and had, as far as I know, never met with other deaf children. This newcomer began to "talk" sign language with his contemporaries almost immediately upon arrival. The existence of an innate impulse for symbolic communication can hardly be questioned (p. 589).

Perhaps, in establishing evidence for the existence of an innate impulse for symbolic communication, Lenneberg overstated the case in his reference to the child immediately beginning to "talk" sign language. It would seem as logical to have him almost immediately begin to talk Spanish or Hebrew. The American Sign Language possesses many of the properties of spoken languages, including a structure and a relatively abstract, arbitrary referential vocabulary. No one learns to use it almost immediately.

It is also questionable whether a child could pick up "self-made" signs so rapidly. In building communication systems, as Tervoort (1961) noted, groups of deaf children develop esoteric manual "languages" which are unintelligible not only to deaf children in other schools but also frequently to deaf children of other age groups in the same school.

A more parsimonious explanation of the interaction observed might be to assume that, in the course of his 8 years of family interaction, the child learned a limited number of "transparent" easily interpreted gestures which served as the basis for his initial contact with other deaf children.

STRUCTURAL AND FUNCTIONAL CHARACTERISTICS OF SIGN SYSTEMS

Although the study of use of sign languages in adults and the development of sign language proficiency in the child is still in beginning stages, there is enough evidence to make some tentative statements concerning the similarities and differences between auditory and visual systems. As previously mentioned, Bellugi and associates at the Salk Institute are probably devoting greater attention to this area than any other group.

Three characteristics of manual communication systems, at least those used in the United States, which are of potential pedagogical importance are 1) the ikonic nature of many common signs; 2) the motoric, or enactive nature of many signs; and 3) the use of spatial dimensions. Because of the transparent, or easily interpreted, nature of such signs, it is possible that many children are able to receive and express some information at a younger age than children who rely primarily on the auditory-vocal channel. For example, the commonly used signs for *eat, sleep, drink, drive, cry, fight, hug* and *wash* clearly represent the respective actions. Not only are they relatively easy for the child to understand, but he can also make the appropriate signs at an age when most children probably cannot articulate the appropriate words. The advantage is not limited to "verbs" or action words. Signs such as those for *milk* (the motion for milking a cow), water (touching the lips with the "w" configuration), and table (an ikonic representation of the top of a table) are easily understood and presented. Work in progress by Moores and associates suggests that the first word appears in deaf children of deaf parents at an earlier age than it does with normally hearing children. This "ikonicity" and transparency of some aspects of sign languages were probably what led Lenneberg (1967) to his previously cited report on the deaf boy who began using sign language upon his first contact with other deaf children.

Within this context, it is logical to conclude that there may be more understandability across signed languages than across spoken languages, at some levels. For many of the earliest learned signs, *e.g., eat, sleep,* etc., there are probably a limited number of powerful salient characteristics to choose from and we might expect similar signs to develop in different communities. However, a distinction should be made between primitive gestural communication and true sign language communication involving arbitrary learned systems. Even the most ikonic signs illustrate only aspects of objects or actions and are arbitrary even when readily understood. It is also possible that the older a sign system is, the higher the proportion of opaque signs; "opaque" is used here to refer to an unclear connection between a sign and referent. For example, in ASL the sign for *female* is made by running the right hand in an A configuration along the jaw-bone to the front of the chin, apparently referring to strings on the bonnets females wore in bygone days. Similarly, *coffee* is signed by imitation of the motion of grinding coffee beans in a coffee grinder. Over the years the signs have remained constant while the connections to referents have become obscured.

Along the same lines, the proportion of opaque signs probably increases as a sign language is utilized for H as well as L functions. The sign for *psychology* is represented by forming a semblance of the Greek letter ψ with two hands. Religion is signed by touching the right shoulder with the right hand in the R configuration and then pointing straight ahead, keeping the same configuration.

The use of space also provides different dimensions to a sign system and may enable an individual to communicate complex linguistic relationships in a relatively simple way. In other words, if we assume the primacy of cognition over language, a signed language can convey concepts which in spoken American English would be only acquired at a relatively late age. As an illustration, the strings
"I give you"
and
"You give me"

may be differentiated simply by changing the direction of the sign. In the first case the sign *give* moves from the signer to another individual. In the second it moves toward the signer. The same relationships can be expressed for other actions such as *help, hit, tease,* etc. and for nominal and pronominal designations. One project investigator has remarked, not altogether facetiously, that it is a shame that formal English possesses no such power and efficiency.

American Sign Language also shows some relationships that spoken English does not. Signs for polar pairs such as good-bad, open-close, and same-different are made in such a way as to indicate that they are related but differ along some dimension. For example, the sign for *bad* is made in the same way as for good except that as the right hand comes away from the face it is turned palm down before touching the left hand.

Results of investigations by Bellugi (Bellugi, 1972; Bellugi and Fisher, unpublished manuscript) on hearing adults who had deaf parents and were proficient in ASL as well as spoken English indicated that different rates of speech are employed when using speech alone, signs alone, and speech and signs simultaneously to tell stories. Under the three conditions, approximately the same amount of time was required to tell the stories and the amounts of information conveyed were equal. The total number of signs was reported to be less than the total number of words. This finding indubitably may be explained at least in part by their definition of what a sign is. For example, the previously mentioned string *I give you* is coded as one sign and three words. Of primary importance is the fact that the one sign conveys a complete subject-verb-object relationship as clearly as three words.

CHANGING USES OF SIGNS

At the present time the lexicon of signs in ASL is limited. For example, the Stokoe *et al.* (1965) dictionary has approximately 3,000 entries. As signs are used in a variety of settings, the number of signs in use tend to increase. In many cases varieties around a basic sign will develop. As an illustration, although the verb *to be* is infrequently used in informal conversation, it may be expressed by touching the lips with the forefinger and moving the hand straight out. This sign may also be used to express the concepts *true, real, sure.* When individuals wanted to differentiate between different parts of the verb *to be* they would rely on fingerspelling. Now there is a growing tendency to differentiate by using signs. *Be, am,* and *are* are signed in the same manner as the generic *to be* and differ only in their initial configurations, which are *B, A,* and *R,* respectively. *Was* and *were* are differentiated only by their final configurations, *S* and *R.* An even more powerful example of how a family of signs may develop is given by the fact that, except for hand configurations, the following words are all signed in the same manner: *association, class, department, family, group, organization, society, team, union, workshop.*

The proliferation of new signs and the development of variations around commonly used signs are reflections of the growing acceptance of manual communication and its increasingly important role in educational settings. No longer are signs being passed on only from child to child. They probably are now being used educationally with at least some children in a majority of programs serving deaf children. As the demands on and for manual communication have increased, there has been a corresponding growth in the development of pedagogical systems closely related to H variants of English. The two most widely known of these developing programs are Seeing Essential English (SEE 1), developed by Anthony (Anthony, 1971; Washburn, 1971), and Signing Exact English (SEE 2), developed by Gustason, Pfetzinger, and

Zawolkow (1972). The reader is referred to the original sources for complete descriptions of the systems.

Essentially, both systems have a number of characteristics in common. They are being developed for use by normally hearing parents of deaf children as well as for teachers. Conscious attempts have been made to generate new signs for elements which in the past would have been finger-spelled. Thus, signs have been developed for pronouns (he, she, it, etc.), affixes (-ly, -ness, -ment), verb tenses, and articles (an, the) which previously were fingerspelled or omitted.

Both systems use existing signs as a base. However, there are differences. Gustason et al. (1972) especially emphasized that signing should be by word rather than by concept. They offered the example (p. 4) of the word "run" having a variety of meanings, as in to run for office, run up the flag, running water, etc. If signing by concept, each of these meanings for run would be signed in a different way. Gustason et al. recommended one sign for all meanings, arguing that this approach is more compatible with the English spoken by native speakers and, therefore, easier to learn. Because both systems are relatively new, there is no indication at present to the effective-ness of SEE 1 and SEE 2 relative to each other and to the more commonly used Signed English.

Another system which briefly attracted interest was the Cued Speech Method developed by Cornett (1967) in which the manual component is incomplete and not understandable by itself. This is similar to the hand-mouth systems in use in Europe during the 19th Century. Because the child must simultaneously speechread in order to decode the complete message, Cornett advanced his method as a compromise between "oralists" and "man-ualists." Moores (1969a,b) pointed out that Cued Speech represented only one of numerous such compromises and enumerated both theoretical and practical shortcomings of the system. Moores concluded that Cornett had treated the terms "speech" and "language" as equivalent and suggested that the system might be beneficial to the development of articulatory skills but not necessarily prove to be of benefit in language development.

PEDAGOGICAL USES OF MANUAL COMMUNICATION

To refer to the present bloodletting over methodology in education of the deaf as the oral-manual controversy is a distortion of the facts. No present day educator of the deaf advocates a "pure" or "rigid" manual position. All educators of the hearing-impaired in the United States profess to be con-cerned with developing the child's ability to speak and understand the spoken word to the highest degree possible. The difference is between oral-alone educators, who argue that all children must be educated by purely oral methods, and the oral-plus educators who argue that at least some children would progress more satisfactorily with simultaneous or combined oral-manual presentation. In a paper presented to the International Conference on Oral Education of the Deaf, Lenneberg (1967) stressed that the primary goal of education must be language, not its subsidiary skills. Lenneberg went on to criticize educators of the deaf for not distinguishing between speech and language. Stressing that the key is to get as many examples of English into the child as possible, he developed the argument that the establishment of language is not inseparably bound to phonics and urged that graphics be introduced in addition to oral methods at the earliest possible time. Lenneberg included fingerspelling and signs within his definition of graphics. Lenneberg's theoretical position is consistent with Tervoort's (Tervoort and Verbeck, 1967) finding that manual communication had no deleterious effects on speech. It should be emphasized that both Lenneberg and Tervoort recognized the primary importance of oral communication in our society. They advocated balanced, as opposed to rigid manual or rigid oral, communication. At present, although variations exist, four basic methods of instruction may be identified in the United States: The Oral Method; the Auditory Method; the Rochester Method; and the Simultaneous Method.

Oral Method. In this method, also called the Oral-Aural, Oral-Only and Pure Oral method, the child receives input through speechreading (lipreading) and amplification of sound, and he expresses himself through speech. Gestures and signs are prohibited. In its purest form, reading and writing are discouraged in the early years as potential inhibitors of the development of oral skills.

Auditory Method. This method, as opposed to the Oral, is basically unisensory. It concentrates on developing listening skills in the child who is expected to rely primarily on his hearing. Reading and writing are usually discouraged in the child as is a dependence on speech reading. Although developed for children with moderate losses, some attempts have been made to use it with profoundly impaired children. When used with very young children, this approach has been referred to as the acoupedic method.

Rochester Method. This is a combination of the Oral Method plus fingerspelling. The child receives information through speechreading, amplification, and fingerspelling, and he expresses himself through speech and fingerspelling. Reading and writing are usually given great emphasis. When practiced correctly, the teacher spells in the manual alphabet every letter of every word in coordination with speech. A proficient teacher can present at the rate of approximately 100 words per minute. This approach is quite similar to the system of Neo-oralism developed in the Soviet Union (Moores, 1970b).

Simultaneous Method. This is a combination of the Oral Method plus signs and fingerspelling. The child receives input through speechreading, amplification signs, and fingerspelling. He expresses himself in speech, signs, and fingerspelling. Signs are differentiated from fingerspelling in that they represent complete words or ideas. A proficient teacher will sign in coordination with the spoken word, using spelling to illustrate elements of language for which no signs exist, *e.g.,* some function words such as "of, and, the," and indication of some verb tenses.

The term "Total Communication" is being used with increasing frequency. Some people view it as the Simultaneous Method extended downward to very young children while others see it a flexible system encompassing all methodologies. Unfortunately, where methodology is concerned, there is a dearth of functional definitions. Thus, we find a leading oral-only proponent (Miller, 1970) declaring that oralism is not a philosophy but a way of life while a spokesman for oral-plus education (Denton, 1972) defines Total Communication in terms of the rights of children to utilize all forms and avenues of communication.

Recent Trends

Until quite recently, the Oral Method has been predominant. Its ascendency may be traced as far back as the International Congress on Deafness in Milan, Italy in 1880 in which a resolution was passed stating the use of manual communication of any kind would restrict or prevent the growth of speech and language skills in deaf children.

Almost without exception programs for the deaf have followed a completely oral approach with young children. This includes even the so-called "manual" schools in which simultaneous methods of instruction, and deaf teachers, typically have not been introduced into the classroom below the age of 12. In view of this it might be argued that the history of failure of education of the deaf is a history of failure of the completely oral method, that it is more appropriate for children with moderate to severe losses than for those with severe to profound losses. A spate of articles (Karlin, 1969; Bruce, 1970; Miller, 1970) appearing in the *Volta Review,* an American journal dedicated to the advancement of oral methods, has reacted vigorously to such an interpretation.

In view of the frequent bitterness involved over manual communication, it is somewhat surprising to find that until 1965 objective research was almost nonexistent. Most of the available literature still primarily consists of position papers in favor of one or another of the various methodologies. A situation worthy of note is the fact that while most educators of the hearing-impaired have preferred straight oral methods, many psychologists, psychiatrists, and "outside" educators who, for one reason or another, have become interested in the problems of limited hearing have argued for some form of manual communication (Moores, 1970).

Studies of Deaf Children of Deaf Parents Receiving Early Manual Communication[3]

Because there have been no educational programs involving the use of manual communication with young children until recently, many investigators have turned to the study of deaf children with deaf parents who use manual communication in the home. If the use of manual communication is harmful, then deaf children of deaf parents would be expected to be inferior in academic achievement, psychosocial adjustment, and all aspects of communication, including speech, speechreading, reading, and writing. Table 5 summarizes completed studies of deaf children of deaf parents compared to deaf children of hearing parents. Stevenson (1964) examined the protocols of pupils of deaf parents enrolled at the California School for the Deaf at Berkeley from 1914 to 1961 and matched them to deaf children of hearing parents. He reported that 38% of those with deaf parents went to college as compared to 9% of those with hearing parents, and that of the 134 paired comparisons students with deaf parents had attained a higher educational level in 90% of the cases.

Stuckless and Birch (1966) matched 38 deaf students of deaf parents to 38 deaf students of hearing parents at five residential schools for the deaf on the basis of age, sex, age of school entrance, extent of hearing loss, and intelligence test scores. Children with deaf parents were superior in reading, speechreading, and written language. No differences were found in speech or psycho-social development.

Meadow (1966) compared 59 children of deaf parents to a carefully matched-paired group of children with hearing parents. She reported that children with deaf parents ranked higher in self-image tests and in academic achievement and showed an average superiority to their matched pairs of 1.25 years in arithmetic, 2.1 years in reading, and 1.28 years in over-all achievement. The gap in over-all achievement increased with age, reaching 2.2 years in senior high school. Ratings by teachers and counselors favored children with deaf parents on a) maturity, responsibility, independence; b) sociability and popularity; c) appropriate sex role behavior; d) responds to situations with appropriate reactions. In communicative functioning, the group with deaf parents was rated superior in written language, use of fingerspelling, use of signs, absence of communicative frustration, and willingness to communicate with strangers. No differences were reported for speech or lipreading ability.

Commenting on the child's reaction to deafness, Meadow claimed (p. 306) that children with hearing parents viewed their deprivation in terms of

[3] This and the following section are reprinted from Moores, D. *Recent Research on Manual Communication.* Occasional Paper 7, April, 1971, Research, Development, and Demonstration Center in Education of Handicapped Children, University of Minnesota.

Table 5. Studies of Deaf Children of Deaf Parents Receiving Manual Communication*

Investigator	Comparison	Programs	Results
Stevenson (1964)	134 deaf students of deaf parents to 134 deaf students of hearing parents	California School for Deaf, Berkeley	Those with deaf parents were educationally superior in 90% of pair matchings. 38% of students with deaf parents went to college, 9% of those with hearing parents.
Stuckless & Birch (1966)	38 deaf students of deaf parents matched to 38 deaf students of hearing parents	American School for Deaf, Pennsylvania School for Deaf, West. Pa. School for Deaf, Martin School for Deaf, Indiana School for Deaf	Children with deaf parents superior in reading, speech-reading and written language. No differences in speech or psychosocial development.
Meadow (1966)	59 deaf students of deaf parents matched to 59 deaf students of hearing parents	California School for Deaf, Berkeley	Children with deaf parents ahead 1.25 years in arithmetic, 2.1 years in reading, 1.28 years in achievement. Superior in written language, fingerspelling, signs, willingness to communicate with strangers. More mature, responsible, sociable. No differences in speech or speechreading.

Quigley & Frisina (1961)	16 deaf students with deaf parents out of a population of 120 deaf students	Kansas School for Deaf, Michigan School for Deaf, Pennsylvania School for Deaf, Texas School for Deaf, Rochester School for Deaf, California School for Deaf, Riverside	Children with deaf parents superior in fingerspelling and vocabulary. No differences in speechreading and achievement. Children with hearing parents superior in speech.
Vernon & Koh (1970)	32 deaf students with deaf parents matched with 32 recessively deaf students with hearing parents	California School for Deaf, Riverside	Children with deaf parents—an average of 1.44 years superior on academic achievement and superior in reading vocabulary and written language. No differences in speech and speechreading.

*From Moores, 1971.

inability to *speak* rather than an inability to hear. Children of hearing parents tend to ask questions regarding their deafness at a later age than children of deaf parents.

Vernon and Koh (1970) matched 32 pairs of genetically deaf children for sex, age, and intelligence. One group, consisting of recessively deaf children, had hearing parents and had no early exposure to manual communication. On a standardized achievement test the early manual group's general achievement was higher on the average by 1.44 years. They were also superior in reading, vocabulary, and written language. No differences were found in speech, speechreading, or psychosocial adjustment.

In an unplanned ramification of an investigation of the effects of institutionalization, Quigley and Frisina (1961) studied 16 deaf students of deaf parents from a population of 120 deaf day students. They reported that the group with deaf parents was higher in fingerspelling and vocabulary with no differences in educational achievement and speechreading. The group with hearing parents had better speech.

In the only study directly comparing children with deaf parents to children of hearing parents who had completed an intensive oral preschool program, Vernon and Koh (1972) reported that the children with deaf parents exhibited a superiority of approximately one full grade in all areas over the Tracy Clinic oral preschoolers. Children with deaf parents were rated superior in reading with no differences in speech and speechreading.

In the studies presented above it must be emphasized that the children of hearing parents in no way represent multiply handicapped, disadvantaged, or "nonoral" children. Average IQ's for the control groups were reported as 109 by Meadow, 104 by Stuckless and Birch, and 114 by Vernon and Koh. In each case, the socioeconomic status of those with hearing parents was higher; *e.g.*, Meadow had to equate deaf fathers who were skilled craftsmen with professional, managerial, and sales workers among the hearing fathers.

The results reported by Stevenson, Quigley and Frisina, Stuckless and Birch, Meadow, and Vernon and Koh, interesting in themselves, must be evaluated in relation to the richer environment to which children of hearing parents theoretically should be exposed. The socioeconomic status of children with hearing parents is superior. The language and speech limitations of deaf adults have been substantiated extensively. In addition, deaf children of hearing parents are far more likely to receive preschool training and individual tutoring. Meadow reported that 60% of the children with deaf parents received no preschool training as compared with only 18% of those with hearing parents. Half of the group with hearing parents not only attended preschool but had additional experience either at home or at a speech clinic. Almost 90% of the hearing families interviewed had had some involvement with the Tracy Clinic correspondence course, but none of the deaf families had sent for it.

Vernon and Koh emphasized that their sample from the Tracy Clinic represents a select group: An IQ of 114 places a person in the upper 20% of the population; the children received intensive oral instruction and auditory training in a 3-year preschool program; and their parents received professional group counseling and, in some cases, private psychotherapy to help them adjust to deafness in their children.

Given the higher socioeconomic levels, more adequate linguistic and speech skills, and higher academic attainments to be found in the hearing families, in addition to preschool educational and speech training for children with hearing parents, the educational, social and communicative superiority of deaf children with deaf parents takes on added significance. One can only speculate on the attainments of deaf children of hearing parents if, in addition to familial, social, educational, and economic advantages, they had benefited from some form of early systematic communication with their parents.

Preliminary findings in a series of studies being conducted at the University of Minnesota on the language development of deaf children of deaf parents by Moores and associates suggested that deaf children go through the same stages as hearing children in the acquisition of linguistic abilities. The types of linguistic structures produced vary across children, apparently largely dependent in part on whether the mother uses signs in both H and L contexts. Of the three mothers studied most closely, two use both the H and L variants and their children have been observed using different signs for different forms of the verb *to be* and employing bound morphemes such as *-ing*, *-s*, and *-ment*. As such signs are used more and more with young children, it will be interesting to observe the extent to which they stay in informal conversations.

At this point, perhaps it is appropriate to mention the role of deaf teachers in the education of deaf children. Traditionally, deaf teachers have been excluded from day programs for the deaf. Although they have taught in many residential schools, they usually are limited to teaching either older or retarded children. The restrictions are usually related to the belief that deaf children will not develop good speech and language skills if exposed to deaf adults. Based on the evidence gathered indicating the superiority of deaf children of deaf parents in language functioning, academic achievement, and psychosocial adjustment, there is no reason to accept such a position. Newman (1971) has suggested that in many situations a deaf teacher might indeed be superior to a hearing one. Not only has discrimination against deaf teachers been harmful to deaf adults, but their absence might also have adversely affected the educational and psychological development of a large number of deaf children. There is no evidence to support a policy which refuses deaf adults the opportunity to teach deaf children across all ages and levels of intellectual ability.

DIRECT METHODOLOGICAL COMPARISONS IN ACADEMIC SETTINGS

Examination of Table 6 indicates that very few comparative studies have been conducted. Because of the predominance of oral-only methods of instruction in the classroom, especially with younger children, there were almost no comparative data in the various methodologies in the United States prior to 1960. The only exception would be a survey of 43 day and residential programs conducted in 1924-25 (Day, Fusfeld, and Pintner, 1928) which reported that students at the Rochester School for the Deaf enjoyed the highest academic achievement, relative to their ability, of all programs assessed.

For the most part manual communication has not been considered appropriate for "normal" deaf children. In a study of the education of deaf children (Lewis, 1968) in Great Britain, some schools (p. 34) volunteered the following circumstances in which teachers used manual media in class:

Children not developing well orally, from one cause or another.
With dull children.
With children with brain damage or severe language disorders.
With children with cerebral palsy.
With maladjusted children.
With dually handicapped children.
With children of deaf parents.
With immigrant children.
With children transferred from other schools.
To impart information quickly.
To satisfy children's needs for expression.
Experimental use of fingerspelling to help young children to speak.

The predominantly negative connotations toward manual communication held by many teachers of the deaf are clearly revealed in this list. It is almost as if the good, "normal" deaf child must be protected from contamination so that his oral-aural skills will not be affected. Within this context it is interesting to turn to a study conducted in England titled "Survey of Children born in 1947 who were in schools for the deaf in 1962-63." Of 270 deaf children tested only 11.6% had clear intelligible speech and good lipreading ability making it relatively easy for the interviewer to communicate with them by speech (*The Education of Young Deaf Children*, 1967, pp. 11–12).

The pioneering work in development and evaluation of combined methods of instruction in this century can be traced to the efforts of Russian educators over a 15-year period beginning roughly in 1950. As early as 1938 Russians had decided that the Pure Oral Method was a dismal failure. According to Zukov (Moores, 1971), the majority of children by 8th grade could not communicate effectively in any way, whether by speech, speech-reading, reading, or writing. They had deficiencies in every aspect of expressive

Table 6. Direct Methodological Comparisons

Investigator	Comparison	Programs	Results
Morozova (1954)	Oral-only programs *vs.* Neo-Oralism (Rochester Method)	Schools in Soviet Union	Children with fingerspelling master in two years material requiring three years under oral-only method.
Quigley (1969)	Oral-only preschool *vs.* Rochester Method Preschool	American School for Deaf, Indiana School for Deaf	Rochester Method students superior in: a) fingerspelling b) speechreading c) 5 of 7 measures of reading d) 3 of 5 measures of written language. Oral-only students superior in: a) 1 of 5 measures of written language
Quigley (1969)	Rochester Method Elementary and Secondary Programs *vs.* Simultaneous Method Programs	Rochester School for Deaf, New Mexico School for Deaf, California School for Deaf, Riverside, White Plains (N.Y.) School for Deaf, Colorado School for Deaf, Oregon School for Deaf	Rochester Method students superior in: a) all subtests of Stanford Achievement Test b) fingerspelling No differences in speech or speechreading

and receptive language, with inadequacies found in the use of prepositions, pronouns, tense, gender, number, and noun declensions. They confused morphological rules and produced the equivalents of "donuted" for "donuts," "dragonflied" for "dragonflies," and "interests" for "interesting." In other words, they exhibited linguistic weaknesses almost identical to those of deaf students in American programs. Zukov argued that the rigid pure oral method itself was the major factor in the production of children who were unable to speak or speechread. The restriction of language to articulation made the entire education process too inefficient.

To provide the child with tools of communication, especially expressive communication, at an early age, the Russians began experimenting with the combined use of fingerspelling and oral communication, a system they labeled "Neo-oralism." Morozova (1954) reported that 3- and 4-year-old children using fingerspelling could acquire in 2 years that which previously required 3 years to learn under the pure oral method. Martsinovskaya (1961) and Titova (1960) found that fingerspelling facilitated the separation of words into their phonetic composition and significantly accelerated vocabulary growth. It did not hinder articulation or formulation of syllabic structure. Addressing himself to teachers' reservations that children might depend on fingerspelling and not attempt speech, Shif (1969) conducted electrophysiological research which showed close simultaneous coordination of hand and tongue muscles, suggesting that fingerspelling can be part of a coordinated integrated system forming in the speech impellent analyzer.

Of greatest surprise to many American educators is the claim that children educated under Neo-oralism end up more oral than those under the traditional pure oral method because they have a language base and a vehicle of communication from a very early age. This is in direct opposition to the American system where only older children have been exposed to combined oral-manual instruction. In this regard Morkovin (1968) noted:

> The author (Morkovin) spoke with a group of profoundly deaf children who were graduates of the new type of kindergarten at Malokhovka, near Moscow. The children were eight years old and in the second grade of elementary school. They were able to express themselves orally and to ask questions about life in America (p. 197).

Programs for the deaf in the Soviet Union were also visited by officers of the British Department of Education and Science who were charged with investigating the possible place of signs and fingerspelling in the education of the deaf in Great Britain. Following are their reactions (Lewis, 1968).

> The children of four, five and six years old who we saw in class certainly understood their teacher well, and mostly spoke freely and often with good voice, although they were regarded as being profoundly deaf and were unselected groups. We could not judge the intelligibility of the speech, but our interpreter (who had never previously seen a deaf child) said that she could understand some of them. The children were

also very lively and spontaneous, and did not appear to be oppressed by methods used, which might strike someone accustomed to English methods as unsuitable for young children.

It appeared to us, from what we were shown, that the Russians are more successful than we are in the development of language, vocabulary and speech in deaf children once they enter the educational system. This seemed to us a strong point in favor of their method (use of fingerspelling from the very start as an instrument for the development of language, communication and speech), the investigation of which was the main object of our visit (pp. 44–55).

Quigley (1969) attempted to assess the effects of the Rochester Method on achievement and communication in two studies. In the first he compared two preschool programs for the deaf in the United States, one using the Rochester Method and one a traditional oral. After 4 years of instruction the Rochester Method students were superior in fingerspelling, in one of two measures of speechreading, in five of seven measures of reading, and in three of five measures of written language. The control group was superior in one of five measures of written language.

The second study involved a comparison over 5 years of students in three residential schools receiving instruction in the Rochester Method matched with three control groups in contiguous states being taught primarily through the simultaneous use of signs, fingerspelling, and oral means. In all of the schools, the students had been taught by oral-only means when younger. The experimental groups scored higher on all subtests of the Stanford Achievement Test at the end of 5 years. There were no differences at the beginning of the experiment. Applications of Moores' Cloze procedures (Moores and Quigley, 1967) revealed the experimental group to be superior in form class or grammatical functioning with no differences in vocabulary. The experimental group was superior in fingerspelling with no differences in speech and speechreading. Quigley reported that the Rochester Method was not introduced in two of the schools until the children reached age 12. The school which used the method at a younger age was the one which enjoyed the greatest advantage relative to its control (p. 77).

Quigley drew the following implications from the two studies:

1. The use of fingerspelling in combination with speech as practiced in the Rochester Method can lead to improved achievement in deaf students particularly on those variables where meaningful language is involved.

2. When good oral techniques are used in conjunction with fingerspelling there need be no detrimental effects on the acquisition of oral skills.

3. Fingerspelling is likely to produce greater benefits when used with younger rather than older children. It was used successfully in the experimental study with children as young as three and a half years of age.

4. Fingerspelling is a useful tool for instructing deaf children, but it is not a panacea (p. 89).

Beginning in 1969, a growing number of programs for young deaf children have initiated the use of simultaneous oral-manual communication. For the first time researchers are able to investigate the relationship between manual communication and oral language development. Moores and his associates (Moores, 1970b; Moores and McIntyre, 1971; Moores, McIntyre, and Weiss, 1972, 1973) have been conducting a longitudinal evaluation of seven preschool programs for the deaf in the United States which differ along a number of dimensions including methodology, extent of integration of deaf and hearing children, amount of parent involvement, and emphasis on early academic skills.

Among other things, the project is designed to investigate two questions concerning the receptive communication of young deaf children (Moores, Weiss, and Goodwin, 1973):

1. What is the relative efficiency of combined oral-manual compared to oral-only presentation?
2. What is the correlation, either positive or negative, between oral-only receptive abilities and oral-manual receptive abilities?

Table 7 presents information on the programs and subjects involved. A receptive communication test was developed to assess five different but not mutually exclusive modes of communication: 1) sound alone, 2) the printed

Table 7. Program and Subject Characteristics

Program	Mode of instruction	No. of subjects	Chronological age	Hearing level (1969 ANSI)	
				Mean	Range
			months	dB	
A	Oral-only	18	60.17	91.44	71−105
B	Oral-only	15	61.47	93.27	75−110
C	In transition from oral-only to total communication	11	61.82	95.33	88−100
D	Rochester Method	11	64.55	99.45	85−110
E	Total communication	6	61.00	99.33	80−110
F	Total communication	7	64.86	103.00	78−110
G	Variable	6	61.67	93.33	75−105

word, 3) sound plus speechreading, 4) sound and speechreading plus finger-spelling, and 5) sound and speechreading plus signs.

Using vocabulary lists provided by teachers in the seven programs, 20 items representing four levels of difficulty were tested. Three additional multiple choice foils were developed for each item. Alternate choices were balanced in matrix form so that children would have to process an entire phrase rather than part of it in order to make a correct response.

The 20 finished stimuli were randomly assigned to one of five groups, each of which contained one item from every level of difficulty. A sample card was constructed to assist and/or train the child before each new mode of communication was introduced. Programs A and B requested that neither written signs nor fingerspelling be used in testing. Program D requested that signs not be used. These requests were honored.

Examination of Table 8 indicates that the percentages of correct answers increase as dimensions are added. Scores improve from sound alone (34%), to printed word (38%), to sound plus speechreading (56%), to sound and speechreading plus fingerspelling (61%), to sound and speechreading plus signs (72%); t score comparisons between modes (Table 9) indicate the simultaneous presentation of speech and signs was significantly superior to sound alone, the printed word and sound plus speechreading. Sound and speechreading plus fingerspelling was superior to the printed word and sound alone. Sound and speechreading was superior to sound alone and the printed word.

It should be pointed out that the two programs with highest ratings on sound plus speechreading (programs E and G) have exposed children to signs at an early age. It cannot be said that the signs interfere with the children's ability to process spoken communication when signs are absent. If anything,

Table 8. Percentage Correct on Receptive Communication by Programs and Modes of Communication

Program	N	Sound alone	Printed word	Sound + speech-reading	Sound + SR + finger-spelling	Sound + SR + signs	Total % correct
		%	%	%	%	%	%
A	18	32	37	52			45
B	15	40	32	63			52
C	11	25	32	50	48	61	43
D	11	34	36	48	51		44
E	6	33	42	67	71	75	57
F	7	39	54	57	79	75	59
G	6	37	45	75	75	87	60
Totals N	(74)	(74)	(74)	(74)	(41)	(30)	(74)
$\bar{X}$		34	38	56	61	72	50
σ		25	28	29	30	30	20

Table 9. *t* Score Comparisons Between Modes

		1	2	3	4	5
Sound alone	1					
Printed word	2	$t = 0.92$				
Sound plus speech-reading	3	$t = 4.94**$	$t = 3.84**$			
Sound and speech reading plus finger-spelling	4	$t = 5.20**$	$t = 4.14**$	$t = 0.871$		
Sound and speech-reading plus signs	5	$t = 6.62**$	$t = 5.45**$	$t = 2.53*$	$t = 1.51$	

$*p < 0.02.$
$**p < 0.01.$

these children are superior. They do not "take the easy way" and rely on manual communication completely.

In addition, there is no evidence that manual communication inhibits efficient utilization of residual hearing. Two of the three top scoring programs on reception of sound alone (programs F and G) utilize signs from the beginning. To investigate the relationships between modes, Pearson product-moment correlation coefficients between all modes were computed (Table 10). Sound and speech plus fingerspelling correlated with the printed word ($p < 0.01$), speech plus speechreading ($p < 0.05$), and speech and speechreading

Table 10. Correlation Matrix

		1	2	3	4	5
Sound alone	1	1.00				
Printed word	2	0.0598	1.00			
Sound plus speech-reading	3	0.2088	0.1995	1.00		
Sound and speech-reading plus fingerspelling	4	0.1778	0.4702**	0.3326*	1.00	
Sound and speech-reading plus signs	5	0.2474	0.2250	0.2908	0.3773*	1.00

$*p < 0.05.$
$**p < 0.01.$

plus signs ($p < 0.05$). There were no other statistically significant correlations.

Moores, Weiss, and Goodwin (1973) interpreted the findings as indicating that the simultaneous use of residual hearing, speechreading, and signs comprises the most efficient means of receiving information for young deaf children. This finding is in opposition to the untested assumption of Kates (1972, p. 50) that the "American Sign Language" constitutes a different language which detracts from concentration on English. The data suggest that signs, in coordination with oral communication, may facilitate the reception of English.

If manual communication were detrimental to the development of oral receptive skills, we would expect negative correlations between these tests which utilized, in part, manual communication and those tests which did not. On the contrary, low positive correlations were found between all tests. The fact that the sound alone test produced no significant correlations with any other test, although all correlations were positive, suggests that utilization of residual hearing by deaf children is relatively unaffected by manual communication and is dependent upon other factors operating in an educational program.

THE USE OF MANUAL COMMUNICATION WITH OTHER POPULATIONS

Because my observations of the use of manual communication have been restricted to deaf and deaf-blind individuals, comments on the potential usefulness of nonvocal systems with other populations will remain brief, tentative, and speculative. The subject is dealt with in other sections by authors having direct experience with retarded individuals. The interested reader is also referred to reports of Berger (1972), Carrier (1973), and Hollis and Carrier (1973).

It would appear that manual communication might be employed in a variety of ways with retarded children and adults. Depending on the individual it might be used as an aid in the development of speech production and speech perception, as a system for the initiation and maintenance of oral communication, or as the major vehicle of everyday communication.

In a personal conversation with Rynders of the University of Minnesota Research, Development, and Demonstration Center in Education of Handicapped Children, I learned that many Down's syndrome children may have anatomical features which prevent the development of understandable articulatory skills in children who may be capable of understanding spoken communication relatively well. If such proves to be the case, the use of manual communication would provide these children with an effective means of communication with their environment. By extension, it is logical to assume that manual communication would be beneficial for all individuals, retarded or otherwise, who do not or cannot develop adequate spoken language skills.

Limited systems of manual communication might enable severely re-tarded individuals to understand and express basic needs and wants. Hoff-meister and Farmer (1972) introduced a basic set of signs to institutionalized retarded adults with a wide range of hearing losses who had not developed even rudimentary oral communication skills. After a short training period the subjects had developed functional sign vocabularies which enabled them to cope more effectively with their environments.

Another possible use, which has not been recognized even in work with the deaf, is the utilization of the manual alphabet to enhance the develop-ment of oral skills, both receptive and expressive. The approach can be quite effective when used by an efficient speech clinician. The most obvious technique is the use of fingerspelled contrasts, both by the clinician and client, to differentiate between phonemes which differ only in regard to one distinctive feature, such as [p] and [b] or [t] and [n].

SUMMARY

The manual communication systems employed by deaf individuals have thrived for centuries in the face of prejudice, hostility, and attempts by the dominant hearing community at repression. It was argued 200 years ago that the teaching of speech and lipreading (now more commonly referred to as speechreading) would spell the doom of signs, that the system would fade away and die an unmourned death as children acquired oral skills. Since that time periodic waves of enthusiasm have developed for panaceas in the guise of auditory training, integration, early intervention, and parent training. For some reason each of these, worthy in itself, has been viewed as obviating any need for manual communication.

On the basis of experience with deaf children and adults, my view is somewhat different. Manual communication systems have shown a great resilience and ability to endure. This suggests that the systems are meeting an unmet need. I am particularly impressed by the numbers of highly educated deaf adults with excellent receptive and expressive oral skills who also use manual communication in their everyday activities. So long as it retains its power of expression and its utility, manual communication will continue to survive its detractors. In all probability its increasing public exposure on television, in public school systems, and in the theater will probably serve to extend its use to populations other than the deaf.

REFERENCES

Anthony, D. *Seeing Essential English*. Anaheim, Calif.: Anaheim School District, 1971.
Baratz, J. Language in the economically disadvantaged child: A perspective. *ASHA*, 1968, *10*, 143–145.

Baratz, J. Language and cognitive assessments of Negro children. *ASHA,* 1969a, *11,* 87–91.

Baratz, J. and Shuey, R. Teaching black children to read. Center for Applied Linguistics, Washington, D. C., 1969b.

Bellugi, U. Studies in sign language. *Amer. Ann. Deaf,* 1972, pp. 68–84.

Bellugi, U. and Fischer, S. Comparison of the rate of sign language and spoken language. The Salk Institute for Background Studies (Manuscript), La Jolla, Calif.

Berger, S. A clinical program for developing multimedia responses with atypical deaf children. In J. McLean, D. Yoder, and R. Schiefelbusch (Eds.), *Language Intervention with the Retarded.* Baltimore: University Park Press, 1972.

Berger, S. L. Systematic development of communication modes: Establishment of a multiple-response repertoire for non-communicating deaf children. In *Proceedings of the Forty-Fifth Meeting of the Convention of American Instructors of the Deaf,* Little Rock, Ark., 1971.

Bernstein, B. Language and social class. *Brit. J. Sociol.,* 1960, *11,* 271–276.

Bernstein, B. Aspects of language and learning in the genesis of the social process. In D. Hymes (Ed.), *Language in Culture and Society.* New York: Harper and Row, 1964, pp. 251–263.

Bernstein, B. A critique of the concept of compensatory education. In C. Cazden, V. John, and D. Hymes (Eds.), *Functions of Language in the Classroom.* New York: Teachers College Press, 1972, pp. 135–151.

Bloomfield, L. *Language.* New York: Holt, 1933.

Brown, R. and Bellugi, U. Three processes in the child's acquisition of syntax. *Harvard Educ. Rev.,* 1964, *34,* 133–154.

Bruce, W. Assignment of the seventies. *Volta Rev.,* 1970, *72,* 78–80.

Carrier, J. K. Application of functional analysis and non-speech response mode to teaching language. Report No. 7, Kansas Center for Research in Mental Retardation and Human Development, Parsons, 1973.

Cicourel, A. and Boese, R. Sign language and the teaching of deaf children. In D. Hymes, D. Cazden, and V. John (Eds.), *The Functions of Language in the Classroom.* New York: Teachers College Press, 1972, pp. 32–62.

Cornett, O. Cued speech. *Amer. Ann. Deaf,* 1967, *112,* 3–13.

Cornett, O. In answer to Dr. Moores. *Amer. Ann. Deaf,* 1969, *114,* 27–29.

Day, H., Fusfeld, I., and Pintner, R. *A Survey of American Schools for the Deaf.* Washington, D. C.: National Research Council, 1928.

Denton, D. A rationale for total communication. *Amer. Ann. Deaf,* 1972, pp. 53–61.

Falberg, R. National Association of the Deaf Communicative Skills Program Advisory Board Meeting, Tucson, Ariz., February, 1971.

Gardner, R. and Gardner, B. Teaching sign language to a chimpanzee. *Science,* 1969, *165,* 664–672.

Gerankina, A. *Practical Work in Sign Language.* Moscow: Moscow Institute of Defectology, 1972.

Gustason, G., Pfetzing, D., and Zawolkow, E. *Signing Exact English.* Rossmoor, Calif.: Modern Signs Press, 1972.

Hoffmeister, R. and Farmer, A. The development of manual communication in mentally retarded deaf individuals. *J. Rehab. Deaf,* 1972, *6,* 19–26.

Hollis, J. H. and Carrier, J. K. *Prosthesis of Communication Deficiencies: Implications for Training the Retarded and the Deaf.* Parsons: Kansas

416   Moores

Center for Research in Mental Retardation and Human Development, Working Paper 298, July, 1973.
Karlin, S. Et tu oralist? *Volta Rev.*, 1969, *71*, 478e–478g.
Kates, S. *Language Development in Deaf and Hearing Adolescents.* Northampton, Mass.: Clarke School for the Deaf, 1972.
Kohl, H. *Language and Education of the Deaf.* New York: The Center for Urban Education, 1966.
Labov, W. *The Social Stratification of English in New York City.* Washington, D. C.: Center for Applied Linguistics, 1966.
Lenneberg, E. *Biological Foundations of Language.* New York: Wiley, 1967.
Lenneberg, E. The capacity for language acquisition. In J. Fodor and J. Katz (Eds.), *The Structure of Language.* Englewood Cliffs, N. J.: Prentice-Hall, 1964, pp. 579–603.
Lewis, M. *The Education of Deaf Children.* London: Her Majesty's Stationery Office, 1968.
Martsinovskaya, E. N. The influence of fingerspelling on the reproduction of the sound-syllabic structure of a word by deaf children. *Spetsial Shkala,* 1961, *102*, 22–28.
McNeill, D. Developmental psycholinguistics. In F. Smith and G. Miller (Eds.), *The Genesis of Language.* Cambridge, Mass.: M.I.T. Press, 1966, pp. 65–84.
Meadow, K. The effect of early manual communication and family climate on the deaf child's development. Unpublished doctoral dissertation, University of California, Berkeley, 1966.
Miller, J. Oralism. *Volta Rev.,* 1970, *72*, 211–217.
Montgomery, G. The relationship of oral skills to manual communication in profoundly deaf adolescents. *Amer. Ann. Deaf,* 1966, *111*, 557–565.
Moores, D. Cued speech: Some practical and theoretical considerations. *Amer. Ann. Deaf,* 1969a, *114*, 23–27.
Moores, D. A question of accuracy and sufficiency. *Amer. Ann. Deaf,* 1969b, 114, 29–32.
Moores, D. Psycholinguistics and deafness. *Amer. Ann. Deaf,* 1970a, *115*, 37–48.
Moores, D. Evaluation of preschool programs: An interaction analysis model. In *Proceedings of the International Congress in Education of the Deaf,* Stockholm: 1970b, Vol. 1, pp. 164–168.
Moores, D. Review of B. Tervoort and Verbeck, Analysis of communicative structure patterns in deaf children. *Amer. Ann. Deaf,* 1970c, *115*, 12–17.
Moores, D. *Recent Research on Manual Communication.* University of Minnesota Research and Development Center: Occasional Paper No. 7, April, 1971.
Moores, D. Communication - Some unanswered questions and some unquestioned answers. *Amer. Ann. Deaf,* 1972a, pp. 1–10.
Moores, D. Neo-Oralism and education of the deaf in the Soviet Union. *Except. Child.,* 1972b, *38*, 377–384.
Moores, D. and McIntyre, C. *Evaluation of Programs for Hearing Impaired Children: Report of 1970–71.* Minneapolis: University of Minnesota, Research, Development and Demonstration Center in Education of Handicapped Children, Research Report No. 27, 1971.
Moores, D., McIntyre, C., and Weiss, K. *Evaluation of Programs for Hearing Impaired Children: Report of 1971–72.* Minneapolis: University of Minnesota, Research, Development and Demonstration Center in Education of Handicapped Children, Research Report No. 39, 1972.

Moores, D., McIntyre, C., and Weiss, K. An analysis of signs, language and speech in the communication of young deaf children. *Sign Lang. Stud.*, 1973, *2*, 9–28.

Moores, D. and Quigley, S. Cloze procedures in assessment of language skills of deaf persons. In *Proceedings of International Conference on Oral Education of the Deaf.* New York: 1967, pp. 1363–1382.

Moores, D., Weiss, K., and Goodwin, M. Receptive abilities of deaf children across five modes of communication. *Except. Child.*, 1973, *39*, 22–28.

Morkovin, B. Language in the general development of the deaf child. *ASHA*, 1968, *10*, 195–199.

Morozova, N. G. *Development of the Theory of Pre-school Education of the Deaf and Dumb.* Moscow: Institute of Defectology, Academy of Pedagogical Sciences, 1954.

Newman, L. As a deaf teacher sees it. *Deaf Amer.*, 1971, *23*, 11–12.

Quigley, S. *The Influence of Fingerspelling on the Development of Language, Communication, and Educational Achievement in Deaf Children.* Urbana: University of Illinois, 1969.

Quigley, S. and Frisina, R. *Institutionalization and Psychoeducational Development in Deaf Children.* Washington, D. C.: Council for Exceptional Children, 1961.

Shif, Z. *Language Learning and Deaf Children's Thought Development.* Moscow: Institute of Defectology, 1969.

Stafford, C. Fingerspelling in the oral classroom. *Amer. Ann. Deaf*, 1965, *110*, 483–485.

Stevenson, E. A study of the educational achievement of deaf children of deaf parents. *Calif. News*, 1964, *80*, 143.

Stokoe, W. Sign language structure. In *Studies in Linguistics.* Buffalo: University of Buffalo, Occasional Paper No. 8. 1958.

Stokoe, W. *Semiotics and Human Sign Languages.* The Hague: Mouton, 1972.

Stokoe, W., Croneberg, C., and Casterline, D. *A Dictionary of American Sign Language.* Washington, D. C.: Gallaudet College, 1965.

Stuckless, E. and Birch, J. The influence of early manual communication on the linguistic development of deaf children. *Amer. Ann. Deaf*, 1966, *111*, 452–460, 499–504.

Tervoort, B. Esoteric symbolism in the communicative behavior of young children. *Amer. Ann. Deaf*, 1961, *106*, 436–480.

Tervoort, B. and Verbeck, A. *Analysis of Communicative Structure Patterns in Deaf Children.* Groningen, The Netherlands: V.R.A. Project RO-467-64-65 (Z.W.O. Onderzoek, N.R.: 583-15), 1967.

Titova, M. Peculiarities in mastering pronunciation amongst deaf children who are beginning to learn speech through dactylic language. *Spetsial Shkala*, 1960, *97*, 20–28.

Vernon, M. and Koh, S. Effects of manual communication on deaf children's educational achievement, linguistic competence, oral skills and psychological development. *Amer. Ann. Deaf*, 1970, *115*, 527–536.

Vernon, M. and Koh, S. Effects of preschool compared to manual communication on education and communication in deaf children. In E. Mindel and M. Vernon (Eds.), *They Grow in Silence.* Silver Spring, Md.: National Association of the Deaf, 1972.

Washburn, A. *Seeing Essential English.* Denver: Community College of Denver, 1971 (Manuscript).

CHAPTER SIXTEEN

DISCUSSION SUMMARY–NONSPEECH COMMUNICATION

Richard B. Dever

Department of Special Education, Indiana University, Blooming-ton, Indiana 47401

The two papers in this section took two different tacks. The Premacks' paper dealt primarily with ways of looking at language, while Moores' paper dealt primarily with nonspeech methods currently employed by deaf people. For this reason the two papers were discussed separately during the conference and will also be discussed separately here.

David Premack, in his opening remarks, stated that the aim of his enterprise was to arrive at some of the dispositions that are critical to language development and to devise tests to discover if these dispositions are present or not present in a specific organism. Behind this statement was his contention that an animal cannot be expected to develop a linguistic representation for a concept if it cannot grasp it abstractly first. Therefore, a way must be found to discover whether or not the concept is present before any attempt at language training can be made. Then, if the concepts are found to be testable, effective training based on the results of that testing can proceed. Because of this, the Premacks' see their work as having many implications for the training of children who have not learned their language. To a question asking for the necessary cognitive prerequisites for language, Premack stated 1) that a two-term verb-relation competency was required for the development of linguistic representations of entities such as "name of," "color of," "same-different," and the conditional particle, and 2) that clear evidence has been obtained in a number of animals that discriminative use of such concepts must be present before the linguistic representation of them can be developed.

This triggered discussion centered on two questions. The first question was: Is the verb actually a relational term or simply a label for an action in much the same way that many nouns are labels for objects? No real answer developed, but it was pointed out that others have attempted to respond to the same kind of question, (e.g., how it might be possible to infer the presence of constituent structure and the relations between items in child language learning). In working with adults, it has been possible to rely on intuition in trying to find the answer, but in working with children this has not been the case. As stated above, no real answer to the question developed during the discussion, and Premack thought that the question simply might be too strong for the tools at hand.

The second central question was: Do children initially learn two-term relations? This question seemed to revolve around the Premacks' notion of "two-term." In their system it is a functional classification, referring, for example, to the relationship between the "subject" and "direct object." The "verb" that relates these functions is seen as a "two-term" relator. Because the Premacks' plastic language is, in effect, a language foreign to American English, it was difficult for some of the participants to relate the "two-term relator" concept to the problems faced by retarded children who must learn English. For example, the Premacks' two-term relation includes functions expressed by both transitive verbs and the equative verb "be" in English. It also appears to exclude the entire concept of intransitive verbs. Moreover, ideas expressed in English by "be" are expressed in the plastic language by a number of different "verbs." For example, the plastic sentence, "Red-color of apple," and "Square-shape of-cracker" are both grammatical relationships that can be expressed by equative clauses using "be" in English: "The apple is red," and "The cracker is square." Because of the noncorrespondence on this level with the problem that is faced by children learning English, and because of the fact that children learning English have a much wider range of types of utterances available as a base for developing linguistic-conceptual relationships, it was felt in some quarters that it might not be necessary to get independent evidence that the child needs control over "two-term" relationships before we begin to teach. While it was not directly expressed, it was felt by at least some of the participants that requiring the logical structure of two-term relationships to be present before a training program begins might actually place too many constraints on the educator. Rather, single-term relationships such as those presented in the Miller-Yoder paper (this volume) might appear to be a more fruitful place to begin.

It is interesting to note that none of the conference participants raised any of the questions raised by Brown in his recent book (Brown, 1973). Perhaps the major question that Brown asked is whether or not the Premacks' chimps have actually been learning a language. That is, although replacement of certain "sentence" elements does occur when the chimps use the Premacks' system, this replacement is quite restricted, and it is of a scale that in no way approaches the productivity of natural languages. Brown raised the possibility that the responses made by the Premacks' chimps are of the same order as the responses made by pigeons who have been taught to "play" ping-pong through conditioning techniques. Just as the pigeons are not productive, *e.g.,* they do not keep score, the Premacks' chimps do not produce novel "sentences." This in turn raises questions about the relevence of the system in applied situations. Brown's counter-example is Washoe, the chimp that was taught to communicate through use of ASL by the Gardners

(Gardner and Gardner, 1969). Again, unlike Washoe, Sarah never initiated communication, a fact which makes the use of the plastic system in the Premacks' lab distinctly unhuman. Of course, the entire question, at this point, becomes one of the "correct" definition of "language," an assignment too large to undertake here.

Another important question, for the purposes of this volume, is what relevance does the Premacks' work have to the problem of teaching language-handicapped children? This question can be approached by asking if his ideas have had any impact on the teaching of children. Carrier (1973) reported having tried to use an instructional system based on some of the Premacks' ideas and having had some success with it. His most notable failures have been in those cases in which attentional or motivational problems have prevented him from making an input to the child. The fact that he has had some success in a research setting, however, opens up a whole new avenue for investigation that has not previously been available, and it should be pursued vigorously. Most interesting, in Carrier's work, is the fact that he has relied largely on a logical analysis of language rather than a set of developmental sequences as many workers do at present. It should be pointed out, however, that Carrier uses his plastic forms in the context of English grammar, and this fact may eventually turn out to be quite important.

The greatest importance of the Premacks' work, from my point of view, is to be found in the fact that he has concentrated on a functional analysis of the concept of "language." That is, his work points up sharply the fact that a language is basically a tool for expressing cognitive knowledge. In this we see a restatement of an idea that was set forth by the structural grammarians some time ago (*e.g.,* Sapir, 1921, Francis, 1958): that any language is a vehicle for the transmission of information. Perhaps the circle is beginning to close. Many workers who deal directly with children who have language problems are now beginning to find that this conception of language, as opposed to the often expressed notion that language is the whole of cognitive activity, is a much more useful one to have when attempting to make a difference in the functioning of handicapped children. At the least, it makes the task specifiable, and what can be specified can be taught.

The second line of discussion dealt with Moores' paper. In his opening statement, Moores demonstrated some of the variety of manual systems available including fingerspelling, Native Sign, Amerslan, and Signed English. In addition, he mentioned, as possibilities for use with retarded children, other systems such as cued speech, which manually represents features such as point of articulation of speech sounds. Moores stated that his present research involved following the development of deaf children who are growing up using several varieties of Sign Language. He is finding that these children all seem to be developing their language in much the same manner as normal children. This not only includes "manual babbling," but also the development of rules that generate child-specific constructions that are different from the adult language, but which progress toward whatever form the adult language takes. He also stated that his group is finding that Native Sign is capable of expressing grammatical functions like the progressive, but in a way that is much different from English.

One questioner wanted to know if it was possible that exclusive use of Sign, because of the transparent relationship between many signs and the things they signify, might place limitations on the intellectual development of children who grow up using it because of such things as a lack of metaphor. In response, Moores demonstrated some ways in which humor and metaphor are used in Sign, but it was pointed out that these examples were all translations of English. Speaking in terms of Native Sign, it was asked whether or not the expression of such a thing as metaphor is possible. The answer to such a question is not presently available but is likely to come out of work such as that being done by Bellugi and Klima (1972). At least some participants felt that because Sign is a language like any other language, metaphor and other forms normally found in spoken languages will probably be found in Sign.

Interestingly enough, the question of whether deaf children should or should not be allowed to use a manual language never arose, apparently because most participants felt that they should. This is not a feeling limited to the conference participants. In a statement made elsewhere, for example, Hollis and Carrier (1973) have said that nonspeech language systems should be considered as being prosthetic devices for the lack of a spoken language, just as an artificial leg is a prosthetic device for the lack of a real leg. Indeed, the feeling was quite strong among some of the participants that it was imperative to make available alternate language systems to children who might profit from their use. One participant presented three reasons for doing this: 1) that some children find oral language incredibly difficult; 2) that manual systems can be used as oral facilitators (a statement backed up by both clinical and classroom experience); and 3) that in spite of the current sophistication in audiometric testing, there are still children whose eventual skill in using the oral language cannot be predicted and dual systems must be developed for these children so that they will not fall any farther behind their peers than is absolutely necessary.

Some of the participants found Moores' paper valuable because they did not realize that there is a controversy over whether or not a child with a hearing problem should be allowed to use a manual system. Others at the conference were aware of the controversy, and probably the majority, if they were forced to take sides, would find the "manualist" position most comfortable. For these persons, the data being developed by Moores appears to provide some support for this position. Probably the major value of Moores' paper, however, lies in the fact that it is an expression of the very recent movement to get the oral-manual controversy out of the realm of prejudice and guesswork and into the light of hard data. For too long this controversy has raged back and forth supported largely by hot air.

Moores provided an objective report of the relevent research on the use of manual communication with the hearing-impaired, but Lloyd cautioned against overgeneralization from the limited data. For example, it is imperative to note that the "Studies of Deaf Children of Deaf Parents Receiving Early Manual Communication" may also be interpreted as studies of parent reactions to hearing impairment and the resultant emotional problems and related communication difficulties. In other words, the difference in the performance of the deaf children of deaf parents and of hearing parents may be largely related to some systematic difference between the two groups other than the use or lack of use of a manual system. Likewise, when Moores spoke of the richer environment of children of hearing parents, "richer" means more of what? Money, toys, communication, doubt, concerns, frustration, etc. Another concern is that the controversy has been primarily related to oral *vs.* manual and little if any attention has been paid to aural-oral *vs.* manual. The aural aspect may be a critical distinction (see Horton, this volume; Hanners, 1973). In Moores' statement "it may be argued that the history of failure of education of the deaf is a history of failure of the completely oral method" the significant word may be "completely." Moores noted: "As early as 1938 the Russians had decided that the Pure Oral Method was a dismal failure." If any amplification was used prior to 1938 its quality may be seriously questioned. The lack of emphasis on auditory input by most oral programs has been discussed elsewhere by Lloyd (unpublished manuscript). These points are not intended to detract from the significance of nonspeech communication systems but to underscore the need for more hard data and caution in the interpretation of the limited data at this point in time.

Another major issue raised by Lloyd is the practical application of the theory of "Total Communication." While Moores correctly stated that "no present day educator of the deaf advocates a 'pure' or 'rigid' manual position," it seems that many present day educators pay more attention to manual signing and/or spelling than to aural or oral input. It has been previously noted that frequently the so-called total communication approaches have included

> . . . an overemphasis on the manual with a corresponding de-emphasis of the oral-aural aspects. In some cases, total communication has really been a euphemism for the manual method. Those using the manual method usually say they are using the simultaneous method. Unfortunately, the signs and fingerspelling many times communicate a different message than does the oral presentation, if any spoken words are presented. In other words, simultaneous and total communication are often misnomers. Many hearing impaired individuals can overcome such confusions in language input, but when dealing with the retarded (with their adaptive deficiencies) one should not complicate the task by confusing the language input (Lloyd, 1973, p. 61).

There is a need for more research on the combination of manual systems with consistent, high quality auditory input. There may be major problems in the rate and synchronization of these two modes of language input. These problems may be critical to the extent suprasegmental features are critical to language learning. We also need to define what other features of speech and language may be modified by the person who has learned a nonspeech communication system as a second language and then attempts to combine that system with his natural system. Although nonspeech systems have already been found useful with many, questions such as these must be answered if such systems are to realize their full pedagogical potential.

A number of educators and clinicians have found Sign or some other system of nonspeech communication to be extremely important among populations other than the normally intelligent deaf who have not developed their language. Berger (1971, 1972), Hoffmeister and Farmer (1972), and Hall and Talkington (1970), for example, have found Sign to be quite useful among deaf retardates. Hall and Talkington's (1970) data indicated that deaf institutionalized retardates, as a group, learn Sign faster than hearing institutionalized retardates learn spoken words. Possibly this is because the label of "retarded" is often applied to a deaf child who could have been a much higher functioning child if it were not for the communication problem. Berger (1971, 1972) has also found that not only does the learning of signs facilitate communication and even the development of spoken language among institutionalized deaf retardates, it also seems to help decrease the number of behavioral problems in this group. Hoffmeister and Farmer (1972) found that social functioning of institutionalized retardates increased after learning a sign language. The administration in the institution was sufficiently impressed by the results of their study that they placed all the deaf retardates in that institution in signing programs. Other institutions have discovered this as well. At least one has published a manual of signs that is being followed campus-wide (Owens and Harper, 1970).

Many children who are not deaf have language development problems. Bricker's (1972) study of the use of signs to trigger vocalizations in hearing retardates opened up the possibility of the use of signs with this population. The language development of some hearing children may be facilitated by using a manual system. Investigations of this possibility should continue. Others have tried informally to use Sign as the medium of communication among nonvocal hearing children. Reports of success suggest this as yet another possibility for facilitation of language development among some children. This, too, should be followed up.

Cerebral palsied children are often of normal or near-normal intelligence, yet their motoric problems can be of such a magnitude that they appear to be intellectually low-functioning. Seligman (1972), at the Ontario Crippled Children's Centre, reported a great deal of success with the use of Bliss Symbols. These are abstract symbols arranged on a board in a semicircle. The board goes wherever the child goes, and the child can communicate by pointing to a symbol or a combination of symbols on his board. For example, the symbol for "feel" or "feeling" is a heart, and the symbol for "up" is an arrow pointing upward. The combination for "happy" would be to point to the heart and then to point to the vertical arrow, expressing an upward feeling. By extension, the combination for "sad" would be the "heart" and the downward-pointing arrow. Thus, with a small number of symbols a large number of things can be communicated. There are two boards in use: one has 100 symbols, and the other has 340 symbols. Many of the children in the Ontario Centre have been able to progress to the larger set of symbols, which they use to communicate with the staff, their families, and one another. There is no reason to believe that such a system might not be found useful among other children who have difficulty learning to speak a language. One possibility for extending this idea, for example, might be to take symbols from the Rebus program, published by American Guidance Service (Woodcock, 1969), and use them in the same manner.

This was a very difficult discussion for me to put together. Initially I saw the discussion as taking two distinctly different tacks, one dealing with each paper. This comes from the fact that the two papers, like the papers from the conference as a whole, represented two distinctly different research genres. In contrast to the other sessions, however, both genres were present in the same session here, and the result was that it was difficult to integrate the session. Premack is representative of the psycholinguists at the conference. Psycholinguists, like all experimental psychologists whatever their basic data orientation, are primarily interested in the development of theory that will allow them to explain the world. Although their theories do get applied, application of the theory is usually seen as being secondary to the development of the theory itself. Moores, on the other hand, represented the applied linguists at the conference. An applied linguist is primarily interested in the pedagogy of a language or of languages. He will attend to the theories developed by psycholinguists because he may find them useful in his teaching task, and he may even develop some theories himself from time to time. However, theory development, for the applied linguist (if it occurs at all) usually comes about as a result of his attempt to teach and is secondary to his instructional work.

The differences between psycholinguistics and applied linguistics have not received much attention, but the distinction has interesting ramifications that were brought to a head by this session. Not the least of these is that when a mixed group of language researchers get together, if they do not make a conscious attempt to integrate the two orientations, all discussions will include a large number of "either/or" issues. This source of probable noncommunication in conferences such as this, and indeed in the world of language research in general, must be acknowledged and met in any attempt to facilitate interaction and communication between the two groups.

It may be true that a specific theory may have no immediate practical payoff, and it may be just as true that some bit of practical intervention may have no immediate theoretical impact. However, this did not prevent the interchange that can only result both in recognition of commonalities and in mutual assistance for the common good. This is in contrast to the past in which the only interchange between psycholinguists and applied linguists was built around mutual recriminations, and only ill will resulted from the nasty put-down interchanges that we have all seen. Finally, in this conference, we saw something quite different happening. At times communication was difficult, and at times the inevitable misunderstandings arose. But walls built over the years do not come down easily, and this was to be expected. The important thing was the fact that the attempt at communication was made, and this can bring nothing but good. If it continues, and I certainly think it will simply because it must, the gap between the two groups will indeed be narrowed to the mutual benefit of both groups of researchers and the children who need the help that we can give them. It may take a little time to accomplish this, but I have no doubt that it has indeed begun.

REFERENCES

Bellgui, U. and Klima, E. The roots of language in the sign talk of the deaf. *Psychol. Today,* 1972, *6,* 60–64.

Berger, S. L. Systematic development of communication modes: Establishment of a multiple-response repertoire for non-communicating deaf children. In *Proceedings of the Forty-Fifth Meeting of the Convention of American Instructors of the Deaf,* Little Rock, Ark., 1971.

Berger, S. L. A clinical program for developing multimodel responses with atypical deaf children. In J. E. McLean, D. E. Yoder, and R. L. Schiefelbusch (Eds.), *Language Intervention with the Retarded: Developing Strategies.* Baltimore: University Park Press, 1972.

Bricker, D. D. Imitative sign training as a facilitator of word-object association with low-functioning children. *Amer. J. Ment. Defic.,* 1972, *76,* 509–516.

Brown, R. *A First Language: The Early Stages.* Cambridge: Harvard University Press, 1973.

Carrier, J. K. *Application of Functional Analysis and a Non-speech Response Mode to Teaching Language.* Parsons: Kansas Center for Research in Mental Retardation and Human Development, Report 7, February, 1973.

Francis, W. N. *The Structure of American English.* New York: Ronald Press, 1958.

Gardner, R. A. and Gardner, B. T. Teaching sign language to a chimpanzee. *Science,* 1969, *165,* 664–672.

Hall, S. M. and Talkington, L. W. Evaluation of a manual approach to programming for deaf retarded. *Amer. J. Ment. Defic.,* 1970, *75,* 376–378.

Hanners, B. A. The role of audiologic management in the development of language by severely hearing impaired children. Paper presented at the Academy of Rehabilitation Audiology annual meeting, Detroit, Michigan, October 12, 1973.

Hoffmeister, R. J. and Farmer, A. The development of manual sign in mentally retarded deaf individuals. *J. Rehab. Deaf,* 1972, *6,* 19—26.

Hollis, J. H. and Carrier, J. K. Prosthesis of communication deficiencies: Implications for training the retarded and the deaf. Kansas Center for Research in Mental Retardation and Human Development, Parsons, Working Paper 298, July, 1973.

Lloyd, L. L. Mental retardation and hearing impairment. In *Deafness Annual,* Vol. 3. Silver Spring, Md.: Professional Rehabilitation Workers with the Adult Deaf, 1973, pp. 45—67.

Lloyd, L. L. Perspectives on oral education of the hearing impaired. Unpublished manuscript.

Owens, M. and Harper, B. *Sign Language: A Teaching Manual for Cottage Parents of Non-verbal Retardates.* Pineville, La.: Pinecrest State School, 1970.

Sapir, E. *Language.* New York: Harcourt, Brace and World, 1921.

Seligman, J. A new approach to communication for the severely physically handicapped child. Paper presented at the ASHA National Convention, 1972.

Woodcock, R. *Rebus.* Circle Pines, Minn.: American Guidance Service, 1969.

VI EARLY LANGUAGE INTERVENTION

CHAPTER SEVENTEEN

AN EARLY LANGUAGE TRAINING STRATEGY

William A. Bricker and Diane D. Bricker

John F. Kennedy Center for Research on Education and Human
Development, and Infant, Toddler and Preschool Research and
Intervention Project, George Peabody College, Nashville, Tennessee
37203

Within the context of current psycholinguistic conceptions of language development, a discussion of intervention approaches to the language learning of young children is not greatly different from arguing for birth control and abortion in a convent. This analogy has not been hastily drawn in order to stimulate an introductory chuckle. The basis of this remark stems from several years of work during which we have attempted to integrate operant, linguistic, cognitive, and psycholinguistic approaches to language acquisition and language training for children whose language is moderately to severely developmentally delayed. This chapter is another attempt to integrate further these apparently divergent approaches. A quick review of references indicates the extent to which this integration has been tried. Unfortunately, space does not permit a presentation of all of the available references. For example, Menyuk (1971) has written a book about language acquisition and language training and referenced an impressive 235 items. The list quickly establishes Menyuk's position as a psycholinguist and is notable for the almost total exclusion of both operant and cognitive material. In the interest of equal time, an examination of the reference list for Risley, Hart, and Doke's (1972) chapter on language from an operant position lists 25 items of which none refers to linguistic, psycholinguistic, or cognitive material. These examples are not unusual. A similar situation has been noted in the field of experimental psychology by Krantz (1971). From our perspective in the middle, there is a ringing discord where the more "nativistic" theorists refer to the behaviorists as "mindless mechanics." The reference in the opposite direction is "muddle-headed mentalists." This seems to be simply a manifestation of what we have to call "The Language Game."

The Language Game is a yearly sequence of events notable for the lack of well defined leagues, established rules, a regular season, or a method for determining a winner. If we examine the research and theoretical writing of the linguists, psycholinguists, speech clinicians, cognitive psychologists, and behaviorists, analogies between the Language Game and any professional sport could be drawn endlessly. For example, the distinction between language as either a learned form of behavior or an acquired process dependent upon innate structures is not different from deciding on a game that has a time span of some duration with a pattern of actions leading to a final score or a game that is over before it starts. The development of such analogies could be fun except that the Language Game has an immediate and serious purpose which should take precedence over the sporting and competitive nature of any game. Effective language, like good health, should be a human right and not treated as a research toy. Thousands of people are difficult to understand, others have noticeable hesitancies in their speech pattern, many have no effective language, and each suffers because language is the focus for an unruled game. This becomes an interesting contradiction since language is often viewed as the primary example of a rule-based system. For the present writers, the problem is not so much how the game is played as one of determining the reasons for playing the game in the first place. We believe effective language intervention provides a reasonable purpose for it all.

There are several approaches to early language intervention. One of the simplest can be taken from a quote by Chomsky and Miller (1963). They stated:

> A description of this (language learning) device would represent a hypothesis about the innate intellectual equipment that a child brings to bear in acquiring language. Of course, other input data may play an essential role in language learning. For example, corrections by the speech community are probably important. A correction is an indication that a certain linguistic expression is not a sentence. This device may have a set of nonsentences, as well as a set of sentences, as an input, Furthermore, there may be indications that one item is to be considered a repetition of another, and perhaps other hints and helps. What other inputs are necessary is, of course, an important question for empirical investigation (p. 276).

From this viewpoint, a language intervention approach would involve a systematic method for analyzing the production of a child and for determining the types of inputs that might facilitate the acquisition of more complex language. As indicated by Lynch and Bricker (1972), the experimental analysis of behavior (Skinner, 1957; 1966; 1969) may provide the most appropriate method for determining what interventions might be maximally useful in stimulating language development. Exceptions might be taken to this statement by linguists and psycholinguists, but a defense of the position here is premature. The problem with the Chomsky and Miller position is that it ignores the possibility of "other inputs" that might stimulate the development of *prerequisite* processes that form the basis for productive language. The infant and prelinguistic child are not simply sitting around listening to well formed sentences. They are exploring their environment and synthesizing a sensorimotor account of it all (Bruner, 1964; Piaget, 1967; Piaget and Inhelder, 1969; White, 1969). Consequently, an early intervention program in language should begin during early infancy rather than in the middle of the 2nd year of life. In addition, methods for language training should be understandable to most parents and infant caretakers if the training routine is to have broad acceptance and use.

An early language intervention program is interesting from another perspective. The application of the program can serve more frequently in a preventative rather than a corrective capacity. If parents are sensitive to the requirements of important facets of infant stimulation, then the parents will also be sensitive to failures in the system and will be able to take corrective action before important error patterns or deficiencies in comprehension or production become problems requiring professional help. In addition, the program must be structured as a system of graded intervention techniques which involve informal application of stimulation approaches if the child is developing normally. However, if error patterns or delays in acquisition become apparent, then provisions should be available for increasingly more formal and more precise techniques culminating with professional intervention if the error pattern or the delay becomes sufficiently severe. How this can be done is reserved for the final section of this chapter after the bases for an intervention program have been developed.

PSEUDO ISSUES FOR A LANGUAGE INTERVENTION PROGRAM

There are several issues frequently used in the Language Game as a means for differentiating the various leagues in which the game is played. Some issues are critical and must be considered if an effective language intervention program is to be developed. Others are complex but they can be shown to be pseudo issues in the processes of language development and language intervention. Among the latter issues are the role of innate processes in language acquisition, the adequacy of a behavioristic approach to language, the necessity of reinforcement in language learning, and the function of imitation in language training. Since these issues generate tremendous friction among the participants in the Language Game, the writers have attempted to explore the parameters of each of these issues. We have also attempted to indicate reasons they can be put aside temporarily in order to facilitate the development of effective language intervention procedures. We have done this with the greatest reluctance. We know that we are inviting important criticisms of our proposals from practically all the leagues currently involved in the Language Game. However, we feel that prior discussion of these matters is the only basis for an ultimate synthesis among the various approaches to language in service to those children who have major language problems.

Language Acquisition as an Innate Process

This issue has been discussed increasingly since Chomsky (1959) reintroduced psychology to mentalism as an explanation of complex human behavior. The defense of this mentalistic view has been explicitly made by several writers since that time (Chomsky, 1966; Fodor, 1966; Katz, 1964; Lenneberg, 1967; McNeill, 1970). However, one of the most forceful statements in support of innate knowledge has just appeared (Weimer, 1973). Basing his scholarly discussion on two of Plato's paradoxes as represented in the *Meno,* Weimer believes that knowledge of abstract entities and the ability for "productive" or "creative" behavior must be innate. In reference to abstract entities, Weimer indicated the impossibility of recognizing a member of a concept class unless one has prior knowledge of the concept itself. As he stated:

> Factual relativity guarantees that one cannot simply go out into the world and neutrally collect facts. Without a prior conceptual framework, that is, a point of view from which to impose order upon reality, there is only the changing phenomenal flux of experience, the 'blooming, buzzing confusion' of William James. The data of sensation do not come with little tags attached proclaiming their factual status. Observation is not merely focusing one's attention on the data, but rather assimilation of data into the conceptual scheme of the observer (p. 20).

This leads to a restatement of Plato's paradox, namely: "We cannot learn (come to know) anything unless we already know (have learned) it." Weimer then turned to linguistic theory to supply the basis for the second paradox, which involves creative production. In Chomsky's linguistic position, a theory of language must provide a suitable explanation of the novel but appropriate use of language. This involves " ... the speaker's ability to produce new sentences, sentences that are immediately understood by other speakers although they bear no physical resemblance to sentences which are 'familiar' (Chomsky, 1966, p. 11)." The second paradox derives from this point and asks the question: ". . . how can one exhibit knowledge for which one's prior learning history has given no preparation (Weimer, 1973, p. 25)?"

Weimer presented several attempted solutions to these paradoxes, including Aristotle's doctrines of nominalism and associationism. Weimer (1973) described these as follows:

> Abstract entities play no essential role in our knowledge, for all learning is the learning of particulars and their recombination, and abstract concept formation is a derivative result of this process of recombination. . . . The problem of productivity likewise vanishes: it is an illusion resulting from overlooking the recombination of old particulars. Productive thinking is nothing but the association of new combinations of elements (p. 18).

For Weimer, this has been the dominant view in psychology and he noted the fact that not one learning theory has "failed to base its account on associative principles." Weimer then developed several lines of evidence contradictory to the associationistic position leading him to the conclusion that: ". . . associationism marries only universals. Yet, if the doctrine must presuppose universals in order to explain them, then its claim to explain universals in terms of particulars is false (1973, p. 24)." Having apparently destroyed associationism, Weimer went on to state:

This article has argued that his [Plato's] insight was better than that of his successors, from Aristotle down to the neobehaviorists. In 20-odd centuries we have managed to learn nothing at all 'new' about the nature of knowledge and learning. And that does not augur well for the future of psychology (p. 32).

One final point pertaining to Weimer's position is interesting in relation to language acquisition, and that is his view about the "carrier" of the innate entities. Plato used the concept of a reincarnated soul as the seat of universal knowledge which was passed from one generation to the next. Weimer discounted this construction of the transmittal mechanism and substituted a Lamarkian doctrine of inheritance as the basis for linguistic and other abstract universals. He recognized his vulnerability on this point by stating:

Lamarckian biology is indeed in disrepute: there is no evidence for the inheritance of acquired physical characteristics. But the inheritance of behavioral characteristics is well documented, as the discipline of behavior genetics discloses. And the inheritance of capacity to respond, that is, competence as a structural concept underlying the functional notion of disposition to respond, is all the contemporary Platonist needs to maintain his thesis (1973, p. 28).

Thus, Weimer informed the psychologists that their next move should be a 2,500-year return in scientific history to the basics of Plato's thinking and this time proceed from that point with clear recognition of innate abstract entities. It is of interest that Weimer's article was in the *American Psychologist* without editorial comment.

A simple form of defense is to ignore the argument. A more difficult task is to attempt to question it through appropriate evidence. If this position is allowed to stand or to gain support (through increased bandwagon riders), then programs of language training especially for children who do not give evidence of suitable innate structures could be logically phased out as futile gestures. Schlesinger described another outcome by stating:

It has even been argued that all universals of language are innate. . . . Explaining human behavior by invoking instincts has long ago become disreputable in psychology, because it does not constitute an explanation at all. But it seems that we are again faced by an invasion of noun-phrase instincts, verb-phrase instincts, and many others. Such is the outcome of a wholesale renunciation of empiricism (1971, p. 100).

In the same book (Slobin, 1971) one finds a different paradox in McNeill's description of Staats' theory as follows:

Staats offers us what appears to be a contradiction: a finite-state grammar that copes with embedded sentences. However, there is an explanation, and it is that Staats is a nativist! In fact, he is the outstanding nativist here represented (McNeill, 1971, pp. 36–37).

Here we can see the Language Game at its most impressive level of activity in which radical behaviorists are described as extreme nativists and terms such as "association" and "generalization" are said to involve "mentalistic" approaches to language. In our view, innate structures, rather than being ignored, must be seriously considered in order to prevent this interesting position from slowing progress in the development of effective intervention programs.

One way out of this apparent dilemma is to define the innate endowments of an infant more precisely. The key to doing this adequately is to consider the concept of "interaction" in some detail. As indicated recently by Dobzhansky (1972), the full range of biological and behavioral structures and their functions are determined by an inevitable and unceasing interaction between genetic determiners and the full range of environments encountered by the organism. In concluding his discussion of this matter, Dobzhansky stated:

> In flies, as well as in men, the genetic endowment determines the entire range or reactions, realized and unrealized, of the developing organism in all possible environments. A much less happy formulation, often met with in the literature, is that the genotype determines the limits, the upper and the lower extremes, which a character, say a geotactic response, or stature, or IQ, can reach. This would make sense only if we were able to test the reactions of a genotype in all possible environments. Environments are infinitely variable, however, and new ones are constantly invented and added. . . . It would require not a scientific but something like a divine knowledge to predict how much the stature, or IQ, or mathematical ability of any individual or population could be raised by environmental or educational modifications or improvements (1972, p. 530).

When this statement is compared to a recent statement by Piaget (1970), the comparison leads to an interesting basis for questioning Weimer's thesis as well as those of other advocates of a purely nativistic position. Piaget said:

> The establishment of cognitive or, more generally, epistemological relations, which consist neither of a simple copy of external objects nor of a mere unfolding of structures performed inside the subject, but rather involve a set of structures progressively constructed by continuous interaction between the subject and the external world (p. 703).

Piaget went on to state: "We begin [a discussion of his theory] with the last point [quoted above], on which our theory is furthest removed both from the ideas of the majority of psychologists and from 'common sense'." This seems to be confirmed in that no reference is made to Piaget in Weimer's paper, and he is mentioned only indirectly through a reference to Sinclair-de-Zwart by McNeill in the entirety of the Slobin book (1971). It is also true that references to Piaget in the behavioristic literature are extremely rare. Perhaps his position represents the synthesis that investigators and theorists at either extreme might find suitable. If so, this would not be an accident since Piaget, as described by Furth (1970):

... chartered his course like a skillful navigator avoiding the Scylla of nativistic apriorism on the one side and Charybdis of positivistic empiricism on the other side. From his biological perspective he was in a favorable position to avoid both of these extremes and produce a higher synthesis of previously antagonistic views (p. 241).

Discussion of his theory is presented later as the major vantage point for teaching prelinguistic forms of behavior that are the critical prerequisites to language learning in our view. However, Piaget's view on the role of interaction in the development of knowledge about the world appears to meet the objections of Weimer and those of many behaviorists. From this position, the belief in innate abstract entities as explanations can be clearly seen as a pseudo issue in language acquisition and language intervention.

Language as a Learned Behavior

This too is a pseudo issue in that the major criticisms about behavioristic approaches to language refer to learning theory and not to the methods of behavior analysis as represented in the experimental analysis of behavior (Baer, Wolf, and Risley, 1968; Skinner, 1966, 1969). In one sense, the so called "Skinnerian" model is not a learning theory. The model does not deal with learning at all. Learning involves an inference made from observing changes in the behavior of an organism across time. In an experimental analysis of behavior such inferences add little to the observations that generate them. The experimental analysis of behavior is a method for seeking and documenting functional relationships between and among antecedent events, behavioral movements, and subsequent events. Consequently, the experimental analysis focuses on how the environment impinges on the organism and how the behavior of the organism in turn acts on the environment in a stream of interaction that frequently results in progressively more sophisticated adaptions to progressively more complex environments (not totally unlike Piaget's view of behavior development). The experimental analysis of behavior is an open system for collecting facts about the environment-organism interaction and not a semiclosed theory which is structured to generate predictions such as the one formulated by Hull (1951). MacCorquodale (1969) has indicated that the criticisms Chomsky and other linguists make of behaviorism are related more to the hypothetico-deductive systems of Hull (and perhaps even Staats, 1971) than to the experimental analysis of behavior. MacCorquodale described the nature of Skinner's position on language by stating:

... *Verbal Behavior* is best conceived as a hypothesis that speech is within the domain of behaviors which can be accounted for by existing functional laws, based upon the assumption that it is orderly, lawful, and determined, and that it has no unique emergent properties that require either a separate causal system, an augmented general system, or recourse to mental way-stations (1969, p. 832).

The problem is probably not with the system as such but with the terms used within the system to describe both the independent and the dependent variables. Objections are raised against the use of such terms as stimulus, response, reinforcement, discrimination, stimulus control, generalization, and others. The system does not *require* such terms, but they are used as convenient references to operations that are defined by their effects. They are probability statements about observed and carefully indexed relationships between defined independent and dependent variables occurring in the on-going stream of interaction between the organism and its environments. They refer to publicly available relationships that can be systematically replicated. For this reason, these terms are convenient even though they are not necessary for a science of behavior. Lindsley (1964) has indicated that the description of antecedent events, movements, and subsequent events can be made in an objective way and that terms such as stimulus, response, reinforcement, and other forms of technical jargon become applicable only as the appropriate (predefined) effects obtain. Thus, the experimental analysis of behavior is a method for looking at behavior and not, necessarily, a basis for explaining it (at least not at this point in history). This can be seen in the following discussion of another pseudo issue, the role of reinforcement in language learning and language training.

Language as a Reinforced Behavior

In operational terms, a reinforcement is in the class of subsequent events that are associated with an increase in the rate or probability of the behavioral events. In addition, such subsequent events are necessary for the continuation of existing rates or probabilities of the behavioral events that they follow. For example, one of the first applications of this relationship to a human problem was provided by Fuller (1949), who used a sugar solution as a subsequent event and the arm movements of a "vegetative" adolescent as the behavioral event. At first, the sugar solution was given to the boy following the least movement of the arm and was then withheld until he produced greater and greater movements of the arm. The outcome was a high probability of a 90-degree movement of the arm from horizontal to vertical position which was definitely controlled by the presence and delivery of the sugar solution. This relationship fulfilled the operational definition of the sugar solution as a "reinforcer." Another early study investigated social deprivation and social consequences and demonstrated the defined effects that allow the consequences to be called (because of the social nature of the consequences) social reinforcers (Gewirtz and Baer, 1958). Other studies of this type have investigated hierarchies of reinforcement for young children (Bijou and Sturges, 1959) and token systems with autistic-like children (Ferster and De Myer, 1965). In one of the earlier examples of complex behavior modification (Wolf, Risley, and Mees, 1964), a young boy was deprived of food for periods of time so that meals could be used to shape several forms of behavior including wearing a medically required pair of glasses. Edibles, tangibles, and "conditioned" subsequent events have been used to accelerate particular forms of language by a number of investigators (Baer and Sherman, 1964; W. Bricker, 1967; W. Bricker and D. Bricker, 1970b; Guess, 1969; Guess, Sailor, Rutherford, and Baer, 1968; Lovaas, 1968; MacAulay, 1968; Risley and Wolf, 1968; Stremel, 1972). In each of these investigations, the operational definition of reinforcement has been met. However, this does not relieve the principle from some important criticisms.

One form of criticism has come from the psycholinguistic literature. A clear example of this is reported by Brown and Hanlon (1970) in which they used data provided by Sarah, Adam, and Eve that questioned the efficacy of reinforcement in language acquisition. They indicated that social approval or disapproval relating to the morphological and syntactic productions of the children was extremely rare and did not seem to be distributed according to the correct or incorrect grammatical performances of the children. Brown and Hanlon stated that the approval or disapproval of the parents was related more directly to the "truth value" of the children's productions. However, if reinforcement is operationally defined, then the Brown and Hanlon data would not constitute an adequate refutation since they did not establish the reinforcement or punishment value of approval or disapproval, respectively, in relation to any behavior. In the behavior modification literature, such examples of subsequent events that were labeled approval or disapproval would have to be defined as neutral stimuli. In fact, if reinforcement is defined operationally rather than *a priori*, its use or function in language acquisition becomes almost impossible to reject. However, the use of edible or tangible subsequent events has been criticized from within the operant system on a more important basis.

Ferster (1972), who is noted for his scientific contributions to the experimental analysis of behavior, has criticized the use of tangible reinforcement when working with children and has proposed greater use of natural reinforcers. As he stated:

> The distinction between arbitrary and natural reinforcement suggests that the term "control of behavior" can be profitably disentangled from the pejorative sense of coercive control. A full description of the complex natural environment requires that we understand the functional relation between conduct and the way it acts on the social and physical environment. Good or bad, this functional relation is best described as control. The full complexity, humanism, or freedom of behavior need not suffer from recognition of the environment that generated it (p. 109).

Examples of natural reinforcement given by Ferster range from the simple turning of a doorknob in order to move from one environment to another to a complex interaction of using the schoolroom as a place to plan, order materials, and measure materials for the construction of a small cabin that the children were building behind the school. The construction provided the reinforcement for the academic activities occurring in the classroom but in a natural rather than artificial way. The effects of measurements and other preparations were available in the resulting development of the cabin. Planned education that is provided in a way that maximizes natural reinforcement is not new to education, as seen in the writing of John Dewey and others. What is new is that the planning can be done in a system that provides explicit reference to the events that control or influence behavioral development. In addition, the system can be shifted to one based on arbitrary subsequent events in order to shape response forms that are not in a child's repertoire but which are required in a natural interaction with the environment. For example, Ferster indicated that speaking that is reinforced by food consequences (as in many of the studies cited above) will cease once it no longer produces food. This statement by Ferster generated an Editor's Note as follows:

> This is a key point. Behavior therapists may properly use arbitrary reinforcers as part of a therapeutic strategy, but the strategy is doomed unless there is a viable plan for natural reinforcers to take over and maintain the new response patterns (Ferster, 1972, p. 106).

This point is sometimes not fully considered in behavioral approaches to language training. Nor is the *possibility* of such shifts in reinforcement support for behavior development recognized by the psycholinguists.

Another approach to reinforcement has been proposed recently by Estes (1972), who suggested that in human learning reinforcement appears to operate as information which is used by the learner to determine subsequent responses rather than as a mechanical event that strengthens the stimulus-response association. The informational properties of reinforcement have been demonstrated empirically not only by Estes but also in the area of child behavior by Spradlin, Girardeau, and Hom (1966). The construct of contingency awareness proposed by Watson (1966) in reference to early learning in infants seems to be a case where reinforcement contingencies are response-environment interaction systems that have to be taught, a consideration that is implied in Estes' proposal.

Our view is that natural forms of environmental control, especially appropriate social responses to the child's language, are desirable types of reinforcement to be used in a language intervention program. However, our experience during the past several years indicates that some forms of behavior that are necessary for productive language, such as verbal imitation and symbolic match-to-sample performances, cannot be easily generated through natural consequences. When natural consequences fail to maintain behavior, tangible consequences such as ice cream, cokes, cheese, raisins, and sugared cereals are used to "pay" the child to work in a difficult area. Tangible reinforcement is used with the belief (and supporting data) that repertoire development in an area such as verbal behavior will make the child intelligible in the natural environment and will make verbal production a socially effective behavior that does not require sustained extrinsic or arbitrary reinforcement. Since there is nothing in this system which states that reinforcement causes learning or is even a necessary condition for learning (learning being an unnecessary inference in the first place) and since operations that define the concept of reinforcement as it is used in behavior modification technology have been shown to accelerate the rate of development in verbal behavior by children, the rejection of the concept on the basis of theoretical opposition alone or on the basis of inadequate data seems unjustified. Thus, debate about the role of reinforcement in language acquisition seems to be a distracting pseudo issue in a search for means to ameliorate language delays and language deficiencies.

Imitation in Language Acquisition

Another apparent pseudo issue is the role of imitation in language acquisition. For the behaviorally oriented language trainer, imitation has been used frequently as the basis for speech sound and word production training (W. Bricker and D. Bricker, 1972b; MacAulay, 1968; Raymore and McLean, 1972; Stremel, 1972) and is considered a powerful language training tool. McNeill (1970), Menyuk (1963), and other psycholinguists have argued that imitation does not seem to be involved in the language acquisition of normal children since many of the utterances produced by young children do not have counterparts in adult spoken language. If agreement can be reached that verbal imitation is a potentially useful tool for language intervention and that it may *not be* a necessary condition in normal language acquisition, then this too becomes a pseudo issue for a language intervention program.

RELEVANT BASES FOR A LANGUAGE INTERVENTION PROGRAM

To some extent, the issues discussed above constitute a detour from the primary topic in this chapter. However, often these issues are not discussed at length since the alternative positions represented are either accepted or flatly rejected, depending on the approach to language taken by a given investigator. If our proposed resolutions are acceptable to the reader, then early language intervention may be viewed as a useful topic to discuss. We may implement language intervention with a wide range of children who are language-deficient as a consequence of brain damage, behavior disorders, developmental retardation, or poor learning environments. The proposed system of intervention is structured developmentally and is deliberately imbedded in a discussion of normal infant and toddler progress in language and aspects of behavior directly related to language. The time span covered by this discussion is birth to 3 years, although some data are described that were gathered from developmentally retarded children whose chronological age exceeded 3 but whose language comprehension or production was within the specified range.

We would like to be able to say that the system of intervention described in this chapter is an extension of the system proposed earlier (W. Bricker,

1972; W. Bricker and D. Bricker, 1970a). This is not entirely the case. The system generated earlier was based on 8 years of research with institutionalized moderately and severely retarded children who were between 6 and 15 years of age. In addition, the systematic approach represented in the earlier program was supported by the existing data on language processes of retarded children and language intervention procedures generated by other investigators (*cf.* McLean, Yoder, and Schiefelbusch, 1972; Schiefelbusch, 1972). An analysis of this research indicates that most of our cumulative knowledge about the language of developmentally retarded people has been drawn from populations older than 6 years who reside in large institutions. This is understandable from two perspectives. First, formal educational processes for many decades were based on a maturational model of readiness for learning that was defined in terms of the mental age of the child. Consequently, most moderately and severely retarded children were viewed as not being "ready" for formal education or language therapy until they reached the age of 6 years chronologically. J. McV. Hunt's book, *Intelligence and Experience* (1961), was one of the first major attempts to repudiate the maturational model. While data gathered during the past 10 years clearly support earlier education, especially for those who are developmentally delayed, the age of school enrollment and the delivery of professional therapeutic services such as speech therapy are being changed very slowly.

The second reason for our inadequate understanding of retarded language development is that research in this area has been done with convenient and suitable populations typically found only in larger institutions. As Ellis (1971) pointed out:

> In the main, the contents of these volumes [the five *International Review of Research in Mental Retardation* volumes] indicate that most research still focuses on institutionalized retardates who fall into the 'educable' range. An inordinately small amount of research is conducted on the retardate living at home and attending special classes in public schools. Perhaps, they are much less available as subjects for research. At the same time the behavior of the profoundly and severely retarded receives little attention (p. xi).

These factors as well as our own interaction with institutional environments over a period of 8 years led us to establish an alternative structure in which language and related processes of development could be observed and stimulated with both normal and delayed young children. This program was started in September 1970 and is now known as the Infant, Toddler, and Preschool Research and Intervention Project (D. Bricker and W. Bricker, 1971, 1972, 1973).

The program is structured to provide educational and counseling services to approximately 70 children and their families. These children range in age from 6 months to 6 years. Approximately 40 of the children are moderately to severely retarded, *e.g.*, Down's syndrome, while the remaining 30 children are nonretarded. These children each receive 4 half-days of classroom instruction each week in one of five classroom divisions: a crib unit, two toddler units, and two preschool units. The nondelayed children are included in order to provide models for the retarded children and data on the normal acquisition of cognitive and language processes. A parent-training component provides parent counseling and instruction in self-help skills, toileting procedures, language training, motor development, principles of child development, and methods for eliminating undesirable behavior. The parent-training system allows for maximal coordination of the classroom program with the programs of instruction and care provided in the home.

The nature of the program is ideal for the investigation of language processes in young developmentally retarded children for the following reasons: 1) The program covers the developmental spectrum during which most of the important events in language acquisition and language learning occur. The program focuses on the major areas of development including motor and cognitive processes, social development, and language, so that interrelationships among these processes can be studied. 2) The program can take the developmental model seriously since each form of behavior in infancy or early childhood can be related to subsequent events and improvements within the longitudinal structure of the project. Many children who enter during infancy may be with the program for as many as 5 years. 3) The classroom program, the parent-training program, and the research program are coordinated by Diane Bricker, thereby insuring access to the children for research programs as well as providing a coordinated structure to interrelate the research and service components. The contributions of various disciplines included within the program such as special education, physical education, speech pathology, physical therapy, social work, and psychology can be synthesized in a systematic manner for the benefit of the children. 4)The program integrates moderately and severely retarded children with an equal number of nondelayed children of approximately the same developmental level. This integration establishes the basis for the peer-modeling effects which have been observed in so many different situations during childhood. The nondelayed peers also make the teachers and researchers sensitive to the similarities between delayed and nondelayed children and provide specific indications of the ways in which differences between the two groups could be reduced. To date, children as old as 5 years have been effectively taught in the integrated environment of the program. These four points lead to the conclusion that the structure of the project and number of children in the project allow investigations of language to occur at the appropriate time in the child's developmental history and to provide an exciting contrast to the existing literature which forms the source of much of our knowledge about language, language learning, and language training of mentally retarded children.

At the time of this writing, our experiences with the children and a more extensive review of the recent literature over the past 2½ years indicate the importance of the prelinguistic forms of behavior for subsequent language acquisition. Indeed, the possibility exists that these processes, which are not linguistic in a formal sense, and certainly not verbal, constitute the necessary basis for the development of functional language. Several writers have stated this possibility (Bowerman, in press; Schlesinger, 1971) although Piaget established prior claim to this relationship some years earlier (1962). If this general position can be empirically validated, then entirely new modes of instructional activities can be started during the infancy of children who have high probabilities of being moderately or severely retarded. The remainder of this chapter is devoted to an exploration of what these instructional activities might be and how they would be used to stimulate forms of behavior of which language is a logical outcome.

AN EARLY LANGUAGE INTERVENTION SYSTEM

An early language intervention program starts at birth. It starts when the first pediatric examination of the infant determines the health status of the infant (Apgar, 1953) and detects problems that stem from prenatal disease, drug effects, and atypical growth or physical development. The examination also indicates abnormalities resulting from the birth process including possible brain damage, anoxia, or prematurity. Finally, there are the genetically determined problems such as Down's syndrome, phenylketonuria, and Hurler's syndrome. Each problem which is potentially detectable at birth suggests that some special effort might be necessary to provide adequate environmental stimulation of developmental processes. These are special babies, and they and their parents will need special help from the beginning. Given a firm diagnosis of a problem that has a high probability of a resulting developmental delay, the parents must be fully informed and directed to someone who understands the condition, the prospects for future development, and methods the parents can use for special stimulation and careful evaluation. If the parents appear unable to provide stimulation and evaluation of their child's development, then someone (probably a community health nurse or child development consultant) with professional training should be included to help the family.

Other children needing special help are those who are medically unremarkable at birth but who evidence developmental delays by the 6th month. This includes autistic-like children (Rimland, 1964) and other children who are delayed for unknown reasons. These infants are also in need of special support services and should be referred to a professional who is sensitive to development of young children as well as to the various techniques of developmental stimulation. Hopefully, this would not be a person who would assume that the baby might "grow out of the problem" and therefore be willing to wait until the child is 3 or older before doing something special. Too often, when the child does not "grow out of it," the "something special" involves labeling the child mentally retarded. The child may then be considered for institutional placement. The alternative approach is to determine precisely the child's developmental status in certain important areas of development and then, through careful analysis of the infant or toddler's behavior during assessment, construct a program of instruction that would stimulate developmental progression. This is not a fixed mechanical process. It is adapted to the constantly changing moods and "intentions" of the young child. This process can be described most easily in terms of its application in the Infant, Toddler, and Preschool Research and Intervention Project.

The system is based on the sensorimotor lattice structure which indicates the primary sequential forms of behavior and the prerequisite behavior for each. The lattice covers development from the point of certain reflexive responses of infants to intentional and preoperational behavior. A screening instrument has been developed to locate the child within this developmental structure in the various areas that appear most related to important cognitive and prelinguistic structures. This instrument was constructed from several available scales including the Uzgiris-Hunt Provisional Instrument (Uzgiris and Hunt, 1966), and Albert Einstein Scales (Escalona and Corman, undated), and Bayley Scales (Bayley, 1969), the Gesell Developmental Schedule (Gesell and Amatruda, 1949), and other items which are based on Piaget's description of the sensorimotor period. For example, in the area of visual tracking and visual search for objects, there are 12 steps moving from visual fixation on objects to active dropping of the object by the child as he observes the trajectory. There are 8 steps in prehension and visually directed reaching, the importance of which has been described by White (1969) and by Bruner (1969, 1973). There are 5 major steps in the object permanence area, starting with searching for a partially hidden object to searching for an object in a systematic way when the placement of the object was not viewed by the child. Other areas covered include means-ends relationships, objective causality, imitation, functional classification of objects, functional object grouping, and seriation. The screening instrument is not given in one sitting but generally requires many sessions with the child. The purpose of the screening is not to establish a formal score or age placement for the child, but rather to locate the child in developmental space and to prepare for the test-teach system which is the basis of our curriculum. Both the screening and the test-teach system are applicable to normally developing children up to about the age of 4 years and retarded children who could be as old as 15 years but still behaving within the defined developmental space (W. Bricker and D. Bricker, 1972a, Chapt. 8).

The screening instrument has been administered a number of times in the project by Cordelia Robinson and her colleagues (Chatelanat, Spritzer, and Robertson). A group of 29 moderately and severely retarded young children ranging in age from 8 months to about 6 years have provided some exciting results which are currently being formally analyzed. In addition, 13 nondelayed children ranging in age from 10 to 27 months have been tested. The average length of the measurement process was 1½ hr distributed over three or more sessions. The responses of the children were recorded by the tester and by an observer. Interrater reliability for the 31 items in the screening instrument ranged from 0.89 to 1.00 across six observer pairs. While test-retest reliabilities have not yet been established, an odd-even reliability estimate yielded a correlation value of 0.94. While we are optimistic about the probable utility of this screening instrument, we are sufficiently fore-warned about the difficulties surrounding the measurement of infant and young children's behavior to move cautiously.

The test-teach system begins with materials and events that are immedi-ately relevant to the development of the child provisionally indexed by the screening instrument. For example, the object permanence domain specifies a sequence of progressive developments from the point where the child ignores any object that is not physically present to the point where he indicates that he wants an object that is not present and proceeds to initiate a search for the object. This specific sequence has been latticed by Robinson (1972). Coexist-ing with the lattice is a description of the range of situations and materials that can be used to change the developmental status of the child within the object permanence hierarchy. Specific situations and specific materials are used only as examples of the range of events possible with this system. These may be varied from child to child simply because each one brings a previous history that has individualized his repertoire in terms of specific manipula-tions. The objects which are to be sought by the child must fulfill the operational requirements of a positive reinforcer, and this can be indexed by observing that the child will engage in some form of behavior to get and to manipulate particular objects. These objects are then hidden in a relatively systematic way in order to answer the following questions: 1) If the object is only partially hidden from the child, will he work to uncover it? How much of the object must be visible before the child will attempt to get it? 2) If the child readily obtains objects that are only partially hidden, will he attempt to find objects that are completely hidden? Does the child do this only when he sees the object being hidden or will he also search for the object if it is hidden when the child's back is turned to the object? 3) Does the child look where the object was last found or does he look where it was last seen? 4) If the child does not see the object being hidden, and there are several different locations in which the object might be placed, does the child search in a sequential and nonredundant manner? The detailed answers to such questions across repeated testings involving the systematic variation of the materials being hidden and the places where they are hidden provide reasonable data for determining plausible instructional arrangements. Robinson (1972) pre-sented some data reflecting the application of this procedure.

While our data on means-ends repertoire and the objectification of physi-cal causality remain tentative but promising at the present time, we have reasonably well defined routines in motor and verbal imitation, functional classification of objects, and the functional interrelationships that young children use with various objects. The last two, resting on the developments in the first, provide an interesting basis for language. A part of the relevance can be seen in a recently completed study (Chatelanat, Henderson, Robinson, and W. Bricker, 1971) which dealt with objects in relation to a child's set of schemes.

Ten delayed children (8 of whom had Down's syndrome and all of whom were between 2 and 3 years of age) were individually presented 15 objects in a varied order. When the object was presented, the child was verbally encouraged to take it and to play with it. The other objects were out of reach but within view so that the child could indicate some degree of alternative preferences or evidence of wanting to use one toy in relation to another. The child was allowed to manipulate the toy for as long as he wanted. What the child did with the object was recorded by two observers. The task was then repeated with each of 10 nondelayed children of approximately the same ages who were also enrolled in the project. There were 18 forms of behavior that the children typically emitted in relation to the objects. These are listed in Table 1 along with the number of children in each group who evidenced three

Table 1. Number of Delayed and Nondelayed Children Who Exhibited Three or More Instances of Each Object-independent Scheme

Scheme	Occurrences for nondelayed ($N = 10$)	Occurrences for delayed ($N = 10$)
1. Holds object more than 30 sec	3	7
2. Brings object to mouth	2	4
3. Holds object while looking at it more than 30 sec	1	2
4. Hits object with hand	0	0
5. Hits object on table top	0	5
6. Shakes or waves object	3	5
7. Hits two objects together	0	0
8. Gently pats object	1	0
9. Turns object for visual and tactual examination	4	1
10. Slides object on table top	0	1
11. Stretches object	0	0
12. Tears object	0	1
13. Drops object systematically	1	0
14. Throws object	4	9
15. Puts one object into another	1	0
16. Shows object to another person	6	0
17. Points to another object in association with first object	9	1
18. Names the object	2	1

or more instances of each object-independent scheme. In a general sense, the delayed children tended to use more actions independent of the objects (*i.e.,* equally applicable to each object such as throwing or mouthing). All but 1 of the nondelayed children tended to use the object functionally in relation with another object in a manner that could be called representational play. While the evidence here is not overwhelming for either group of children, several children in each group indicated motoric recognition of the objects, and little difference was noted in the behavior of the children even though the delayed toddlers did not have receptive vocabularies relating to these objects (D. Bricker, Vincent-Smith, and W. Bricker, 1973).

This investigation was repeated with a new group of objects which were more homogeneous in terms of the phonetic properties of the object names and more likely to be a part of a young child's repertoire. The children in both groups were tested for functional classification, receptive vocabulary, and expressive naming of the objects. The data from this second investigation are presented in Table 2. These data indicate that the children in the nondelayed group had repertoires in all three areas while the delayed groups demonstrated some degree of sophistication in only the functional classification task. While tentative, the data indicate the possibility of motoric classification of the environment prior to either demonstrated receptive or expressive language in relation to these objects.

Many of the observations made indicated that the children not only performed the responses that were relevant to the functional uses of the object, but also did so in terms of one object in relation to another. For example, a child may not only crumple a paper towel and then use it to wipe his mouth, he may also put it beside his head and pretend to sleep and then place it under a doll's head as he would a pillow. These are the symbolic functional relations among actions and objects to which Sinclair-de-Zwart (1969) seemed to be referring as the basis for sequenced verbal behavior of the children. At least, the children do perform these tasks before we can find

Table 2. The Mean Number of Correct Responses Made on Functional, Receptive, and Expressive Tasks by Developmentally Nondelayed and Delayed Toddlers

Groups	Number of correct responses*		
	Functional	Receptive	Expressive
Nondelayed (*N* = 9) mean	18.5	18.5	19.3
Delayed (*N* = 9) mean	12.3	2.5	5.0

*Possible of 21 correct.

any evidence for either receptive or expressive vocabulary. However, such analyses do provide an important basis for determining the types of words that might fit the child's functional classification of objects as well as the actor-action-object sequences that he employs in his play. These processes must be considered to be potentially important prerequisites of the language acquisition sequence. Even more important, these actor, object, and action schemes can be seen as a phase of a developmental hierarchy on which the behavior of even the lowest functioning child in our project can be located. Each behavioral level is related to a set of stimulation activities that can be used "naturally" to shape the next step in the sequence.

FORMAL LANGUAGE TRAINING PROCEDURES

Once the child is able to classify functionally at least some of his environment, we are able to begin using some of the training procedures that we found useful with the older institutionalized children (W. Bricker, 1972; W. Bricker and D. Bricker, 1970a). These training areas are contained in the language lattice in Figure 1 and are auditory assessment, receptive vocabulary, verbal imitation of sounds and words, object and event naming, and, finally, syntactic comprehension and production.

A screening procedure is used in each area of assessment to determine if the child has a minimal repertoire of the type required in the area and knows "how to play the game" before he is given the full assessment procedure in an area. In most of the areas, the assessment procedure provides the pre- and posttest data that typically serve as the target dependent measure. In addition, each assessment procedure is linked directly into the training strategy so that a discussion of the assessment procedures can lead directly into the implications for training and establish the rationale for the procedures being used.

Receptive Processes

One of the first assessments made is in the area of audiometry. This establishes the hearing level of each child. Interventions in receptive or expressive language should be predicated upon the sensory abilities of the children. This presents no problem with older normal children and adults because simple standardized assessments of vision and hearing are readily available. However, sensory assessment of very young children or moderately and severely retarded persons is neither simple nor standardized. Many researchers in the field have commented on the difficulty of producing accurate audiometric assessment with low-functioning children (D. Bricker and W. Bricker, 1969; Fulton, 1972; Fulton and Lloyd, 1969; Lloyd, Spradlin, and Reid, 1968). However, these investigations have produced a set of procedures that can be used with even very severely retarded children. We have been extending these

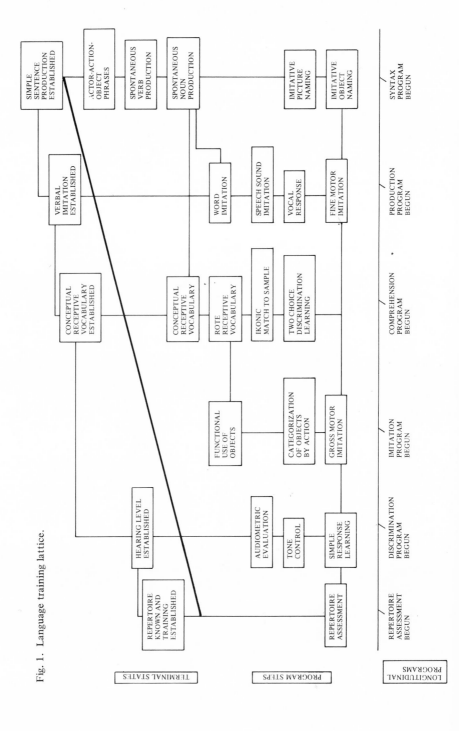

Fig. 1. Language training lattice.

procedures to very young children. Several problems were encountered in this extension (D. Bricker and Vincent-Smith, 1972). First a younger child living in his own home is rarely deprived of food, social attention, toys, or other potentially reinforcing stimuli so that effective consequences are difficult to find. Second, the one-button procedure employed necessitated intervals between successive presentations of the tone during which the child should not respond. This was aversive to many of the children. These problems have been partially solved by moving to a two-button situation that allowed for continual responding by the child and a reinforcement system that involved a bank of colored lights which the child could turn on under some conditions of responding and which turned off when a preferred edible was delivered.

The next major area in the language program is conceptual receptive vocabulary. While the comprehension of language is considered to be prerequisite to expressive language, there has been surprisingly little work in the area. Friedlander (1970) indicated that research on receptive language with normal infants and toddlers has been virtually ignored. One of the reasons for this disregard may be attributed to the difficulties involved in assessing receptive processes. We have recently described some of the problems involved in assessing receptive vocabulary (D. Bricker, Vincent-Smith, and W. Bricker, 1973), and Bellugi (1972) has described similar problems in assessing comprehension of grammatical structures. As she stated:

> To test adequately for comprehension of some grammatical rule, we need to eliminate all other cues. We set up a situation in which the child may perform correctly only by understanding the difference between two pairs of sentences which differ in some minimal grammatical aspect only. It is important to eliminate situational and contextual cues so that the child must rely on his knowledge of syntax (p. 36).

Consequently, problems of assessment in the area of receptive language precede evaluation of training strategies in this area.

D. Bricker (1967) had delineated the utility of employing a two-choice discrimination paradigm to assess receptive processes and to investigate receptive language acquisition. The two-choice situation allows the use of the binomial expansion as a method for determining the probability of chance responding on the part of the child and the point in testing and training where performance is reliably above chance. The paradigm also allows analysis of errors in terms of the other facets of the situation that might control the child's behavior. As indicated by D. Bricker, Vincent-Smith, and W. Bricker (1973), the selection strategies of the child could include position preference, position avoidance, object preference or avoidance, or position patterning, each of which can be manipulated in a two-choice situation first to detect inappropriate strategies and then to eliminate these strategies by bringing the behavior under the control of the relevant dimension. In receptive vocabulary, the relevant stimulus dimension is the word that names one of the two objects which are presented to the child as choices. This process of assessment can be further differentiated in terms of a distinction between rote and conceptual receptive vocabulary.

Studies in the area of rote receptive vocabulary training have employed specific sets of objects with only one exemplar per form class. For example, a "car" choice-item of a specific color, shape, size, and weight was always presented in the presence of the verbal label "take car." The response reinforced in this case is either pointing to or picking the object named by the experimenter from among various stimuli. This specific exemplar of a class of objects called "car" has certain attributes which are relevant for class inclusion and other attributes such as color which are irrelevant. Both the relevant and irrelevant dimensions of the single exemplar could possibly operate to control discrimination learning in the rote receptive vocabulary task.

In a study by W. Bricker and D. Bricker (1970b), which followed the discrimination learning framework presented earlier, a learning across pretest phenomena was observed. One-half of the subjects showed a significant increase in number of correct responses from the first to the second half of the pretest. For these "learners" the standard two-choice training procedures served to maintain but not increase their performance. For those subjects who were "nonlearners" on pretest (showed no significant increase in the number of correct responses from first to second half of pretest), continued two-choice training did not facilitate the acquisition of word-object associations. These subjects remained at chance performance (50% correct) from pretest to posttest.

On the basis of these results, we posited that the use of a distinctive motor movement with each object name might serve as a mediator and thus facilitate the performance of the nonlearners. Support for the training paradigm comes indirectly from two-choice discrimination literature. While pretraining using verbal labeling of objects has been found to facilitate the acquisition of a two-choice discrimination with normal school-aged children and mentally retarded adults (Ellis and Porter, 1966; Girardeau and Spradlin, 1963), pretraining involving a gestural cue or motor mediator has generally been found to be more effective in facilitating the performance of preschool and young retarded children (Jeffrey, 1958; Smith and Means, 1961). The young retarded child may be unable to use verbal labels, which are symbolic cues, as an initial means of determining his choice in a two-choice situation, but may be able to use effectively a motor cue or act, which according to Bruner (1966) and Piaget and Inhelder (1969) is a lower level or less complex behavior. Thus in a training paradigm, the teaching of distinctive motor cues or movements to each object might be used as a bridge to the verbal labels for the objects. The distinctive motor movement involved in functional classification could be used as the stimulus dimension upon which the child is taught a verbal label for an object.

D. Bricker (1972) explored the possibility of using a motor mediator to facilitate rote receptive vocabulary performance with 22 severely retarded children (chronological age range 9–15 years). Subjects were matched on the basis of pretest scores and assigned to one of two groups, experimental (training) or control. For each of the 30 objects on which experimental subjects were to be trained, the child was first taught a distinctive motor movement (imitative sign). Then the word was introduced and the child was taught to make the motor movement to the word (sign-word). Finally the object was introduced in conjunction with the word and the child was taught to make the movement to the object (sign-object). The results indicated that the imitative sign training facilitated the learning of word-object associations in these subjects. Analysis of the pretest and posttest data indicated that the experimental subjects showed significantly greater gains than the control subjects.

Support for the use of motor acts or mediators which involve the actual objects being trained comes from the theoretical writings of Bruner (1966) and Piaget and Inhelder (1969). As indicated earlier, for the young child, an object is what it does or what he can do with it. The child's development from inactive knowledge to symbolic knowledge about his world emerges from his direct interaction and action on his environment. Both Bruner (1966) and Piaget and Inhelder (1969) posited that before a child can manipulate symbols, language being one form of symbols, he must be able to manipulate the objects these symbols represent. For Piaget, as the child moves from simply waving or banging objects indiscriminately to using the same objects in discriminative, functional ways, he is learning the action-relevant nature of his world. From the viewpoint of discrimination learning the child who uses all objects in the same way (*e.g.*, banging) is not attending to the relevant attributes of each object. The attributes which make objects different can be made discriminative if he is reinforced for making differential choices. However, training a child to manipulate different objects in different ways may be seen as a possible training step preceding training in rote receptive vocabulary. Furthermore, training rote receptive vocabulary *via* a functional mediator or motor movement may facilitate the acquisition of conceptual receptive vocabulary.

Imitative Processes

For the behaviorist, imitation has been used as the basis of speech sound and word production training (W. Bricker and D. Bricker, 1972b; MacAulay, 1968; Raymore and McLean, 1972). Imitation is one of the more powerful language training tools, and the parameters need to be studied if this process is to be used efficiently in training.

One method for studying imitation has been to examine the speech sound production of children. For example, W. Bricker (1967) employed an imitation procedure in which 22 consonant-vowel syllables were presented four times each. Analysis of error frequencies indicated a statistically reliable decrease in number of errors produced between 3- and 4-year-olds and

5-year-olds. The sounds were ranked from least to most errors and correlated with the frequency data provided by Irwin (Irwin, 1947a, 1947b, 1948; Irwin and Chen, 1946) and with the frequencies in adult usage taken from Voelker as reported by Miller (1951). The multiple correlation indicated that 80% of the variance in the speech sound errors of the preschool children could be accounted for by the combination of the infant data and the adult frequencies. In addition, the error patterns of the 3-year-old children were much more variable than those of the 5-year-old children, indicating that particular errors become more consistent and persistent with age. This leads to the conclusion that the earlier speech sound training is begun the easier it will be to eliminate the errors. Finally, an analysis of the component features of the errors indicated that the children in all three age groups tended to preserve some of the components of the modeled sound. For example, voiced stimuli were imitated with voiced responses. The most frequent form of error involved a change in the place of articulation. These findings would support the use of motor imitation training as a prerequisite to speech sound training since place of articulation often involves visible changes in the placement of the articulators.

Imitation as a testing device for determining the speech production errors of young children has been employed by several other investigators. Scott and Milisen (1954) found that children produced fewer errors when isolated sounds and nonsense syllables were used as stimuli in comparison with word stimuli. Smith and Ainsworth (1967) using three conditions of assessment— pictures, word imitations, and a combination of pictures and imitations— found smaller error frequencies with the combined stimulus presentation and greatest number of errors produced with picture stimuli. However, Templin (1947) found no differences in error frequencies when she compared imitation procedures with spontaneous production and thus concluded that method of testing did not greatly alter the error pattern. From an operant standpoint, pictures as stimuli for word emission may confound the speech production abilities of the young child since a child might correctly articulate a sound for one word but miss it in another context, indicating that the sound does not have a status that is independent of context (Winitz, 1969). Such independence is critical in speech if the child is to learn to say other words containing that sound. This is similar to the situation in reading where a child may have a reasonable sight vocabulary but lack grapheme-phoneme relationships and, therefore, cannot generalize his repertoire.

A survey by Telford and Sawrey (1967) indicated that 5% of the school-aged children they studied had some form of deviant language and that of this group 81% had articulation errors. As indicated by Yoder and Miller (1972), between 70 and 90% of all moderately and severely retarded children have articulation defects, many of which are omission errors. An investigation by W. Bricker and D. Bricker (1972b) with institutionalized severely retarded children who ranged in age from 6 to 15 years was conducted using the procedure employed with normal preschool children by W. Bricker (1967). The frequency of errors for the mentally retarded children was almost twice that of the 3-year-old normal group of children. However, ranking the error frequencies indicated that the types of errors produced and the stimulus sounds with which they were associated were almost identical between the two groups. Thus, the retarded children made more errors, but these errors were similar to the errors produced by the normal children and reproduced the hierarchy of sound difficulty established by the normal group. The conclusion reached by the investigators was that speech sound production and articulation training are extremely important areas for amelioration with moderately and severely retarded children. In addition, the methods used with normal children for assessing speech sound production and determining types of errors are also applicable to severely retarded young children.

While some speech production programs start with verbal imitation (Raymore and McLean, 1972), a number have been started in the area of motor imitation (Baer, Peterson, and Sherman, 1967; W. Bricker and D. Bricker, 1970a; Kent, Klein, Falk, and Guenther, 1972). Based on these research findings, motor imitation appears to be an important prerequisite for speech imitation when the children are severely retarded because any form of imitation including the imitation of gross motor acts may be absent from the children's repertoire. W. Bricker and D. Bricker (1970a) have pointed out that motor imitation provides a convenient starting point since the child's body parts can be physically guided through the required movements and he can be reinforced for any voluntary motor imitation. Teaching the child the general gross motor imitation "game" is easier than attempting to manipulate the child's lips or tongue. The gross motor imitation training can be shifted to finer movements until, in the last stage, motor imitation of articulator placement is the goal.

In various studies reported in the literature, specific responses were shaped through successive approximations until they resembled the modeled response. As new forms were shaped into the repertoire, the acquisition process became increasingly more rapid until the child imitated a new sound without additional training. This terminal state basically defines generalized verbal imitation or echoic behavior (Skinner, 1957). However, several procedural alternatives are available for training this class of behavior, depending on the view of imitation held by the investigator-trainer. For example, Baer, Peterson, and Sherman (1967) originally maintained that the similarity between the modeled and imitated responses became discriminative for reinforcement to the subject. In this light, the order in which responses were trained or the structure of the responses used in training did not matter. Responses that taught the discrimination of similarity were adequate. Another view presented by Gewirtz and Stingle (1968) assumed that imitation involved a class of responses under the control of intermittent extrinsic reinforcement. Here again, the order or content of training did not influence either the attainment of the defined terminal state or the efficiency of training. However, a third approach to imitation based on a linguistic account of speech sound development does effect order and content of training. This approach is seen in the distinctive feature model of phonology initially presented by Jakobson, Fant, and Halle (1963) and elaborated more recently by Chomsky and Halle (1968). The assumption of this position is that speech sounds are compounds or bundles of component features. When a child learns one of these compounds, he is learning to emit features. If he learns a small number of compounds which contain all relevant features, he will be able to generalize to all novel responses constructed from those features, thus acquiring a generalized repertoire. There are some descriptive data available to support this approach, including the work of Miller and Nicely (1955) and McReynolds and Huston (1971). While there may be no differences among the three approaches in terms of how a single stimulus-response form of behavior is trained, variations in the sequence and structure of content to be taught do exist. These variations may relate to the validity and efficiency of training.

Syntactic Processes

The syntax of a language can be referred to as the set of rules which allow for the production or generation of grammatically correct sentences and the differentiation of these from ungrammatical strings of words. A syntax identifies the relationship of the various parts of a sentence such as the subject of the verb or the object of the verb. Through relationships among words, determined by the syntax of the language, the speaker can convey to the listener, at least in part, his meaning or intentions. The initial phase of syntactic behavior begins when a child puts two words together that have an underlying relationship. As the child acquires new response units, he learns the grammatical rules for using and understanding how these units may or may not be correctly sequenced. For years, knowledge of language development and language behavior of young children was based primarily on descriptive cross sectional investigations (see McCarthy, 1954) and a few longitudinal studies (Bayley, 1933; Braine, 1963; Brown and Bellugi, 1964; Bullowa, Jones, and Bever, 1964; Lenneberg, 1964; Menyuk, 1964; Miller and Ervin, 1964; Shirley, 1933). More recently, data on grammatical development have been appearing in the literature (Bloom, 1970; Cazden, 1968; Chomsky, 1969; McNeill, 1970). Interpretation of the available data on grammatical development remains tentative, and mapping the developmental progression of syntactic behavior is still one of the foremost problems facing the linguist.

While information on the development of syntax with normal children is limited, information on the syntactic behavior of young language-delayed children is almost nonexistent. The research literature is confined almost exclusively to older institutionalized populations (Buddenhagen, 1971; J. Graham and L. Graham, 1971; Guess, 1969; Guess, Sailor, Rutherford, and Baer, 1968; Mein, 1961; Newfield and Schlanger, 1968; Schumaker and Sherman, 1970; Semmel and Dolley, 1971; Stremel, 1972; Talkington and Hall, 1970; Wheeler and Sulzer, 1970). These studies have focused on the description of existing syntactic repertoires and the remediation of deficient repertoires.

The most recent literature has approached the analysis of the syntactic development of mentally retarded children from a theoretical transformational grammar position. Semmel and Dolley (1971) studied comprehension and imitation of sentences in 40 Down's syndrome children from 6 to 14 years of age, with a mean IQ of 34.3. The sentence types employed were kernel, negative, passive, and negative-passive. Comprehension of passive and negative-passive sentences as measured in a two-choice test situation was at chance level, while the comprehension of kernel sentences was significantly above chance, and the comprehension of sentences containing the negative transformation was significantly below chance. In the imitation task, the passive and negative-passive sentences were truncated to roughly equate all sentence types in length. The kernel sentences were correctly imitated significantly more than transformed sentences, as would be predicted by transformational theory.

J. Graham and L. Graham (1971) made a transformational analysis of the speech samples of nine institutionalized males ranging in chronological age (CA) from 10 through 18 and in mental age from 3½ through 10 years. All sentences in the language sample of each subject were rewritten as a kernel construction. A set of transformational rules are then derived to recover the surface structure. A deletion error rate was computed for required lexical items omitted in each subject's speech sample. Spearman *rho* correlations were found as follows: a) 0.90 between mental age (MA) and percentage of sentences with no transformations; b) 0.95 between MA and percentage of sentences with three transformations or more; c) 0.87 between MA and number of generalized transformational rules used; and d) 0.85 between MA and percentage of correct constructions.

Newfield and Schlanger (1968) compared the acquisition of morphological rules by institutionalized educable retarded children and a group of normal children randomly selected from kindergarten and 1st and 2nd grades. Subsequent Peabody Picture Vocabulary Tests (PPVT) indicated a mean MA of 5–10 for the retarded group and 7–9 for the normal group. All children were given the Berko test of nonsense words and a parallel test of lexicon (real word) stimuli, designed to test for plurals, third person singular inflection of verbs, progressive and past tense, the two possessive forms, and comparative and superlative inflections of adjectives. A significant difference in performance favored the normal children on all measures of morphology in both tests. However, the order of acquisition of morphological rules in the retarded children paralleled that of the normal children. The retarded children had greater difficulty in generalization from correct inflections of familiar words to use of the same rules with unfamiliar words. Mental age was significantly related to a majority of the nonsense word measures for normal children and to the lexicon measures for retarded children.

The introduction of transformational analysis has led to an interesting debate concerning the innate learning of language. This debate is responsible for a series of investigations demonstrating the development of specific generative rules in mentally retarded children as a function of environmental manipulations. Three of these studies were concerned with the acquisition of morphological rules. Guess, Sailor, Rutherford, and Baer (1968) used an experimental behavior analysis design in teaching discriminative use of the plural morpheme to a 10-year-old institutionalized retarded girl. She was trained to emit singular responses to the presentation of a single object and to add the phoneme [s] or [z] upon presentation of a pair of like objects. This behavior generalized to the labeling of three like objects using a plural inflection. The subject also applied the generalized rule to words requiring irregular plurals. A second study by Guess (1969) used a similar design in training two institutionalized Down's syndrome boys in a receptive and an expressive task employing plural morphemes. Receptive comprehension was found to function independently of expressive labeling. When reinforcement contingencies were reversed for the receptive task, but not for the expressive, the discriminative behavior of the two boys reversed for the receptive task and not for the expressive one. Schumaker and Sherman (1970) reported a similar investigation in which three retarded adolescents were trained to use past and present progressive verb tense forms appropriately. The experimental procedure employed imitation and differential reinforcement. Each of the subjects was trained using specific verbs, but each was tested with a series of novel or untrained verbs. The data indicated that the subjects learned to apply appropriate generative inflectional rules to untrained verbs as well as to trained verbs. The results of these three investigations support the position that at least limited generative grammatical rules can be acquired by retarded subjects through the manipulation of environmental contingencies.

Although structured within the operant framework, Stremel (1972) developed a more molar language training program than those reported by Guess et al. (1968), Guess (1969), and Schumaker and Sherman (1970). Three moderately to severely retarded children were trained sequentially on verb production, subject-verb production, and finally subject-verb-object production. According to Stremel, the posttest evaluation of the three subjects indicated an increase in the number of subject-verb-object responses to pictures over their pretest performance.

Although these studies are not the only ones involving moderately to severely retarded children, their results are representative of the information currently available on training procedures and descriptions of grammatical behavior of moderately to severely retarded children. The major conclusions to be drawn from this literature are: 1) the retarded person is clearly deficient in the comprehension and production of appropriate morphological and syntactic constructions; and 2) programmed training procedures have produced encouraging results. However, as pointed out earlier, all of these studies have employed older institutionalized retarded children, and the efficacy of extending their conclusions to younger noninstitutionalized delayed children has not been demonstrated.

While a few investigators have examined the syntactic behavior of young noninstitutionalized delayed children (Gray and Fygetakis, 1968a, 1968b; Lee, 1966; Menyuk, 1964), the delay for these children was linguistic rather than intellectual. On standardized intelligence tests they performed within the normal range, while on language assessments they tested at least 1 year behind. Both Menyuk (1964) and Lee (1966) found that the language-delayed children they studied not only were developing normal grammatical structures at a slower rate, but also were missing certain structures. Menyuk pointed out that the language-delayed child, like the normal child, was forming hypotheses about grammatical production, but these hypotheses were incorrect. However, any conclusions drawn from this research must remain tentative because of the limited sample sizes employed and the lack of longitudinal data on individual children. In addition, the Lee and Menyuk studies attempted no amelioration and so can offer no clues as to appropriate training procedures.

Although many instruments have been developed to assess the various aspects of syntactic responses of young children (Berry, 1969; Carrow, 1969), most have problems which make them relatively nonfunctional for research purposes with a population of young (15–50 months) developmentally delayed children. Many of these assessment instruments do not employ repeated measures. Consequently, how much of the child's performance can be accounted for by guessing alone (the chance factor) cannot be determined. In the Northwestern Syntax Screening Test (Lee, 1969) a child can be correct one-fourth of the time by chance while in the Auditory Test of Language Comprehension (Carrow, 1969) a child could be correct one-third of the time by chance. Other tests employ inappropriate stimuli for young children, such as the Preschool Language Scale (Zimmerman, Steiner, and Evatt, 1969) which uses pictures which are too small and numerous. Finally, none of these tests is tied directly to a relevant training program. At best a percentile ranking or age placement is possible which provides the teacher or parent with little assistance of remediating deficits.

We have piloted various syntactic measurement procedures in order to develop an instrument that overcomes some of the problems noted above. The procedure currently being used is based on the Fraser, Bellugi, and Brown (1963) model which examined the imitation, comprehension, and production skills of children in relation to a set of syntactic rules. Fraser *et al.* (1963) tested 12 children between the ages of 37 and 43 months and found that imitation preceded comprehension, which in turn preceded production. Interpretation of these findings must remain tenuous because of the limited number of subjects and the restricted age range used in this investigation. Fernald (1972) has presented further evidence that the findings reported by Fraser *et al.* (1963) of comprehension preceding production should be evaluated carefully in that the results could be an artifact of the manner in which the responses were scored.

The initial evaluation conducted in our laboratory followed the Fraser model in that imitation, comprehension, and production of sets of two- and three-word utterances were tested. Since the population was younger and delayed, simple grammatical rules of actor-action, action-object, and actor-action-object sequences were examined. A two-choice paradigm was employed for picture stimuli presentation. A repeated measure evaluated the chance factor. Approximately 15 delayed and 18 nondelayed children have been tested with this pilot instrument with encouraging results.

However, the instrument needs to be expanded in several ways. First, more delayed and nondelayed children need to be included in the sample. Second, the construct validity of the test needs to be checked by taking samples of the verbal behavior of the tested children in other settings. Third, the effect of using objects rather than pictures as test stimuli needs to be examined. Fourth, the content of the test needs to be expanded in terms of assessing both more simple structures (*i.e.*, more examples of action-object and actor-object sequences) and more complex structures such as negation, pluralization, and tense.

Coinciding with the development of an adequate assessment instrument, research must be done on the variables which influence natural language production. The reference (context) and structure that produces the strings of words generated by young delayed and nondelayed children must be examined. Many linguists are currently concerned with the environmental context in which an utterance was produced to determine the intention of the utterance before deciding what syntactic structure a child was employing (Bloom, 1970; Bowerman, in press; Schlesinger, 1971). The linguist realizes that when the child says, "baby car," he may mean either baby wants to go riding in the car, the car is his, or even give me the car. The only way to determine the child's intent is to examine the context in which the sentence is uttered. To date little experimental effort has been expended in this area.

A second variable in language production which needs to be examined along with context is structure. Structure refers to the content and sequence of content. Several years ago a child's initial two-word utterances would have been described in terms of a pivot-open grammar (Braine, 1963; Brown and Bellugi, 1964; McNeill, 1970). Explanations of two-word utterances based on a pivot-open grammar are now being questioned. As Bloom (1970) has pointed out, pivot-open grammar cannot adequately differentiate certain syntactic structures. The current structure on which several training programs are built is the actor-action-object sequence (Miller and Yoder, 1972; Stremel, 1972). Although this training sequence has been found to be effective, little data exist that would enable one to determine if the actor-action-object sequence is one of the initial structures employed by a child.

CONCLUSIONS

For some children, language acquisition is a slow and difficult process requiring hours of careful training and systematic reinforcement in order to motivate the child. We do not yet know whether such efforts will achieve any major "breakthroughs" in ameliorating the language deficiencies exhibited by many children. If, as Dobzhansky indicated, environments are infinitely variable, we may stumble on intervention strategies that work. At the brink of a cliché, we must recognize that the sin is not to try and fail but not to try at all. However, attempts at amelioration should represent the culmination of a synthesis of all available styles of play in the Language Game and not the Game itself. We do not object to the Game because in the diversity and the competition of its manifestation we discover alternative leads, new conceptions of the nature of language, and new procedures that have been shown to be effective with young children. We need the Game (i.e., the science of language) more than ever. We need the dedicated, time-consuming, and mind-consuming activities of the scientists and the theoreticians if we are to evolve a truly effective language intervention. In this way, we may be able to provide special help for those children who suffer most from our inadequate understanding of language.

ACKNOWLEDGMENTS

The authors wish to express their gratitude to the staff and children of the Infant, Toddler, and Preschool Research and Intervention Project for their assistance, without which this chapter would never have been conceived or completed.

The research reported herein was supported in part by the Joseph P. Kennedy, Jr. Foundation, the Center Grant (NICHHD Grant HD-04510), the Institute on Mental Retardation and Intellectual Development (NICHHD Grant HD-00973), the Mental Retardation Research Training Program (NICHHD Grant HD-00043), and the Parental Teaching Style Assessment Program (NICHHD Grant HD-07073).

REFERENCES

Apgar, V. A proposal for a new method of evaluation of the newborn infant. *Curr. Res. Anesth. Analg.*, 1953, *32*, 260.
Baer, D. M., Peterson, R. F., and Sherman, J. A. The development of

imitation by reinforcing behavioral similarity to a model. *J. Exp. Anal. Behav.*, 1967, *10*, 405–416.

Baer, D. M. and Sherman, J. A. Reinforcement control of generalized imitation in young children. *J. Exp. Child Psychol.*, 1964, *1*, 37–49.

Baer, D. M., Wolf, M. M., and Risley, T. R. Some current dimensions of applied behavior analysis. *J. Appl. Behav. Anal.*, 1968, *1*, 91–97.

Bayley, N. Mental growth in the first three years. *Genet. Psychol. Monogr.*, 1933, *14*, No. 1, 1–92.

Bayley, N. *Bayley Scales of Infant Development*. New York: Psychological Corporation, 1969.

Bellugi, U. Development of language in the normal child. In J. E. McLean, D. E. Yoder, and R. L. Schiefelbusch (Eds.), *Language Intervention with the Retarded*. Baltimore: University Park Press, 1972.

Berry, M. F. *Language Disorders of Children*. New York: Appleton-Century-Crofts, 1969.

Bijou, S. W. and Sturges, P. T. Positive reinforcers for experimental studies with children-consumables and manipulatables. *Child Develop.*, 1959, *30*, 151–170.

Bloom, L. *Language Development: Form and Function in Emerging Grammars*. Cambridge, Mass.: M.I.T. Press, 1970.

Bowerman, M. F. Cross-linguistic similarities at two stages of syntactic development. In E. Lenneberg and E. Lenneberg (Eds.), *Foundations of Language Development: A Multidisciplinary Approach*, in press.

Braine, M. D. The ontogeny of English phrase structure: The first phrase. *Language*, 1963, *39*, 1–13.

Bricker, D. D. (Ed.) *Cumberland House Studies in Behavior Modification*. Interim reports on the Re-Education of emotionally disturbed children, The Department of Mental Health, The State of Tennessee, Nashville, 1967.

Bricker, D. D. Imitative sign training as a facilitator of word-object association with low-functioning children. *Amer. J. Ment. Defic.*, 1972, *76*, 509–516.

Bricker, D. D. and Bricker, W. A. A programmed approach to operant audiometry for low-functioning children. *J. Speech Hear. Disord.*, 1969, *34*, 312–320.

Bricker, D. D. and Bricker, W. A. *Toddler Research and Intervention Project Report: Year I*. IMRID Behavioral Science Monograph No. 20, Institute on Mental Retardation and Intellectual Development, George Peabody College, Nashville, 1971.

Bricker, D. D. and Bricker, W. A. *Toddler Research and Intervention Project Report: Year II*. IMRID Behavioral Science Monograph No. 21, Institute on Mental Retardation and Intellectual Development, George Peabody College, Nashville, 1972.

Bricker, D. D. and Bricker, W. A. *Infant, Toddler, and Preschool Research and Intervention Project Report: Year III*. IMRID Behavioral Science Monograph No. 23, Institute on Mental Retardation and Intellectual Development, George Peabody College, Nashville, 1973.

Bricker, D. and Vincent-Smith, L. Operant audiometry. In D. D. Bricker and W. A. Bricker (Eds.), *Toddler Research and Intervention Project Report: Year II*. IMRID Behavioral Science Monograph No. 21, George Peabody College, Nashville, 1972.

Bricker, D. D., Vincent-Smith, L., and Bricker, W. A. Receptive vocabulary: Performances and selection strategies of delayed and nondelayed toddlers. *Amer. J. Ment. Defic.*, 1973, *77*, 579–584.

Bricker, W. A. Errors in the echoic behavior of preschool children. *J. Speech Hear. Res.*, 1967, *10*, 67–76.

Bricker, W. A. A systematic approach to language training. In R. L. Schiefelbusch (Ed.), *Language of the Mentally Retarded*. Baltimore: University Park Press, 1972.

Bricker, W. A. and Bricker, D. D. A program of language training for the severely language handicapped child. *Except. Child.*, 1970a, *37*, 101–111.

Bricker, W. A. and Bricker, D. D. Development of receptive vocabulary in severely retarded children. *Amer. J. Ment. Defic.*, 1970b, *74*, 599–607.

Bricker, W. A. and Bricker, D. D. The use of programmed language training as a means for differential diagnosis and educational remediation among severely retarded children. Final Report, George Peabody College, Contract OEG2-7-070218-1629, U. S. Office of Education, September, 1972a.

Bricker, W. A. and Bricker, D. D. Assessment and modification of verbal imitation with low-functioning children. *J. Speech Hear. Res.*, 1972b, *15*, 690–698.

Brown, R. and Bellugi, U. Three processes in the child's acquisition of syntax. *Harvard Educ. Rev.*, 1964, *34*, 133–151.

Brown, R. and Hanlon, C. Derivational complexity and order of acquisition in child speech. In J. R. Hayes (Ed.), *Cognition and the Development of Language*. New York: Wiley, 1970.

Bruner, J. S. The course of cognitive growth. *Amer. Psychol.*, 1964, 19, 1–15.

Bruner, J. S. *Toward a Theory of Instruction*. New York: Norton, 1966.

Bruner, J. S. Eye, hand, and mind. In D. Elkind and J. Flavell (Eds.), *Studies in Cognitive Development*. New York: Oxford University Press, 1969.

Bruner, J. S. Organization of early skilled action. *Child Develop.*, 1973, *44*, 1–11.

Buddenhagen, R. G. *Establishing Vocal Verbalizations in Mute Mongoloid Children*. Champaign, Ill.: Research Press Company, 1971.

Bullowa, M., Jones L. G., and Bever, T. G. The development from vocal to verbal behavior in children. *Monogr. Soc. Res. Child Develop.*, 1964, *29* (1, Whole No. 92), 9–34.

Carrow, E. *Auditory Test for Language Comprehension*. Austin: Southwest Educational Development Corporation, 1969.

Cazden, C. B. Some implications of research on language development for pre-school education. In R. D. Hess and R. M. Bear (Eds.), *Early Education: Current Theory, Research and Action*. Chicago: Aldine, 1968.

Chatelanat, G., Henderson, C., Robinson, C., and Bricker, W. Early classification skills of developmentally delayed toddlers. In D. Bricker and W. Bricker (Eds.), *Toddler Research and Intervention Project Report: Year I*. IMRID Behavioral Science Monograph No. 20, Institute on Mental Retardation and Intellectual Development, George Peabody College, Nashville, 1971.

Chomsky, C. *The Acquisition of Syntax in Children from 5 to 10*. Cambridge, Mass.: M.I.T. Press, 1969.

Chomsky, N. Review of Skinner's *Verbal Behavior*. *Language*, 1959, *35*, 26–58.

Chomsky, N. *Cartesian Linguistics*. New York: Harper & Row, 1966.

Chomsky, N. and Halle, M. *The Sound Pattern of English*. New York: Harper & Row, 1968.

Chomsky, N. and Miller, G. A. Introduction to the formal analysis of natural languages. In R. D. Luce, R. R. Bush, and E. Galanter (Eds.), *Handbook of Mathematical Psychology*, Vol. II. New York: Wiley, 1963.

Dobzhansky, T. Genetics and the diversity of behavior. *Amer. Psychol.*, 1972, *27*, 523–530.

Ellis, N. R. *International Review of Research in Mental Retardation*, Vol. 5. New York: Academic Press, 1971.

Ellis, N. and Porter, W. The function of stimulus meaning and ability level in discrimination learning. *Psychonom. Sci.*, 1966, *6*, 463–464.

Escalona, S. K. and Corman, H. H. *Albert Einstein Scales of Sensorimotor Development.* Mimeographed, Albert Einstein College of Medicine, no date.

Estes, W. K. Reinforcement in human behavior. *Amer. Sci.*, 1972, *60*, 723–729.

Fernald, C. D. Control of grammar in imitation, comprehension, and production: Problems of replication. *J. Verb. Learning Verb. Behav.*, 1972, *11*, 606–613.

Ferster, C. B. Clinical reinforcement. *Seminars in Psychiat.*, 1972, *4*, 101–111.

Ferster, C. B. and De Myer, M. K. A method for the experimental analysis of autistic children. In L. P. Ullmann and L. Krasner (Eds.), *Case Studies in Behavior Modification.* New York: Holt, Rinehart & Winston, 1965.

Fodor, J. A. How to learn to talk: Some simple ways. In F. Smith and G. A. Miller (Eds.), *The Genesis of Language.* Cambridge, Mass.: M.I.T. Press, 1966.

Fraser, C., Bellugi, U., and Brown, R. Control of grammar in imitation, comprehension, and production. *J. Verb. Learning Verb. Behav.*, 1963, *2*, 121–135.

Friedlander, B. Z. Receptive language development in infancy: Issues and problems. *Merrill-Palmer Quart. Behav. Develop.*, 1970, *16*, 7–51.

Fuller, J. Operant conditioning of a vegetative human organism. *Amer. J. Psychol.*, 1949, *62*, 587–590.

Fulton, R. T. A program of developmental research in audiologic procedures. In R. L. Schiefelbusch (Ed.), *Language of the Mentally Retarded.* Baltimore: University Park Press, 1972.

Fulton, R. T. and Lloyd, L. L. *Audiometry for the Retarded: With Implications for the Difficult-to-Test.* Baltimore: Williams & Wilkins, 1969.

Furth, H. G. On language and knowing in Piaget's developmental theory. *Hum. Develop.*, 1970, *13*, 241–257.

Gesell, A. and Amatruda, C. S. *Gesell Developmental Schedules.* New York: Psychological Corporation, 1949.

Gewirtz, J. L. and Baer, D. M. The effect of brief social deprivation on behaviors for a social reinforcer. *J. Abnorm. Soc. Psychol.*, 1958, *56*, 49–56.

Gewirtz, J. L. and Stingle, K. G. Learning of generalized imitation as the basis for identification. *Psychol. Rev.*, 1968, *75*, 374–397.

Girardeau, F. L. and Spradlin, J. E. Gestural cues in discrimination learning by retarded children. *Amer. J. Ment. Defic.*, 1963, *67*, 584–588.

Graham, J. T. and Graham, L. W. Language behavior of the mentally retarded: Syntactic characteristics. *Amer. J. Ment. Defic.*, 1971, *75*, 623–629.

Gray, B. B. and Fygetakis, L. Mediated language acquisition for dysphasic children. *Behav. Res. Ther.*, 1968a, *6*, 263–280.

Gray, B. B. and Fygetakis, L. The development of language as a function of programmed conditioning. *Behav. Res. Ther.*, 1968b, *6*, 455–460.

Guess, D. A functional analysis of receptive language and productive speech: Acquisition of the plural morpheme. *J. Appl. Behav. Anal.*, 1969, *2*, 55–64.

Guess, D., Sailor, W., Rutherford, G. and Baer, D. M. An experimental analysis of linguistic development: The productive use of the plural morpheme. *J. Appl. Behav. Anal.*, 1968, *1*, 297–306.

Hull, C. L. *Essentials of Behavior.* New Haven: Yale University Press, 1951.

Hunt, J. McV. *Intelligence and Experience.* New York: Ronald Press, 1961.

Irwin, O. C. Infant speech: Consonantal sounds according to place of articulation. *J. Speech Disord.*, 1947a, 12, 397–401.

Irwin, O. C. Infant speech: Consonant sounds according to manner of articulation. *J. Speech Disord.*, 1947b, 12, 402–404.

Irwin, O. C. Infant speech: Development of vowel sounds. *J. Speech Hear. Disord.*, 1948, *13*, 31–34.

Irwin, O. C. and Chen, H. P. Infant speech: Vowel and consonant frequency. *J. Speech Disord.*, 1946, *11*, 123–125.

Jakobson, R., Fant, C. G., and Halle, M. *Preliminaries to Speech Analysis: The Distinctive Features and Their Correlates,* Ed. 2. Cambridge, Mass.: M.I.T. Press, 1963.

Jeffrey, W. Variables in early discrimination learnings. I. Motor responses in the training of a left-right discrimination. *Child Develop.,* 1958, *19,* 269–275.

Katz, J. J. Mentalism in linguistics. *Language,* 1964, *40,* 124–137.

Kent, L. R., Klein, D., Falk, A., and Guenther, H. A language acquisition program for the retarded. In J. E. McLean, D. E. Yoder, and R. L. Schiefelbusch (Eds.), *Language Intervention with the Retarded.* Baltimore: University Park Press, 1972.

Krantz, D. L. The separate worlds of operant and non-operant psychology. *J. Appl. Behav. Anal.,* 1971, *4,* 61–70.

Lee, L. L. Developmental sentence types: A method for comparing normal and deviant syntactic development. *J. Speech Hear. Disord.,* 1966, *31,* 311–330.

Lee, L. L. *Northwestern Syntax Screening Test.* Mimeographed, Northwestern University, 1969.

Lenneberg, E. H. Speech as a motor skill with reference to non-aphasic disorders. *Monogr. Soc. Res. Child Develop.,* 1964, *29* (1, Whole No. 92), 115–127.

Lenneberg, E. H. *Biological Foundations of Language.* New York: Wiley, 1967.

Lindsley, O. R. Direct measurement and prosthesis of retarded behavior. *J. Educ.,* 1964, *147,* 62–81.

Lloyd, L. L., Spradlin, J. E., and Reid, M. J. An operant audiometric procedure for difficult-to-test patients. *J. Speech Hear. Disord.,* 1968, *33,* 236–245.

Lovaas, O. I. A program for the establishment of speech in psychotic children. In H. Sloane and B. MacAulay (Eds.), *Operant Procedures in Remedial Speech and Language Training.* Boston: Houghton Mifflin, 1968.

Lynch, J. and Bricker, W. A. Linguistic theory and operant procedures: Toward an integrated approach to language training for the mentally retarded. *Ment. Retard.,* 1972, *10,* 12–17.

MacAulay, B. D. A program for teaching speech and beginning reading to nonverbal retardates. In H. N. Sloane and B. D. MacAulay (Eds.), *Operant Procedures in Remedial Speech and Language Training.* Boston: Houghton Mifflin, 1968.

MacCorquodale, K. B. F. Skinner's Verbal Behavior: A retrospective appreciation. *J. Exp. Anal. Behav.,* 1969, *12,* 831–841.

McCarthy, D. Language development in children. In L. Carmichael (Ed.), *Manual of Child Psychology*, Ed. 2. New York: Wiley, 1954.

McLean, J. E., Yoder, D. E., and Schiefelbusch, R. L. (Eds.), *Language Intervention with the Retarded*. Baltimore: University Park Press, 1972.

McNeill, D. The development of language. In P. H. Mussen (Ed.), *Carmichael's Manual of Child Psychology*, Vol. 1, Ed. 3. New York: Wiley, 1970.

McNeill, D. The capacity for the ontogenesis of grammar. In D. I. Slobin (Ed.), *The Ontogenesis of Grammar*. New York: Academic Press, 1971.

McReynolds, L. V. and Huston, K. A distinctive feature analysis of children's misarticulations. *J. Speech Hear. Disord.*, 1971, *36*, 155–166.

Mein, R. A study of the oral vocabularies of severely subnormal patients. II. Grammatical analysis of speech samples. *J. Ment. Defic. Res.*, 1961, *5*, 52–59.

Menyuk, P. A preliminary evaluation of grammatical capacity in children. *J. Verb. Learning Verb. Behav.*, 1963, *2*, 429–439.

Menyuk, P. Comparison of grammar of children with functionally deviant and normal speech. *J. Speech Hear. Res.*, 1964, *7*, 109–121.

Menyuk, P. *The Acquisition and Development of Language*. Englewood Cliffs, N. J.: Prentice-Hall, 1971.

Miller, G. A. *Language and Communication*. New York: McGraw-Hill, 1951.

Miller, W. and Ervin, S. The development of grammar in child language. *Monogr. Soc. Res. Child Develop.*, 1964, *29* (1, Whole No. 92), 9–34.

Miller, G. A. and Nicely, P. A. An analysis of perceptual confusions among some English consonants. *J. Acoust. Soc. Amer.*, 1955, *27*, 338–352.

Miller, J. F. and Yoder, D. E. A syntax teaching program. In J. E. McLean, D. E. Yoder, and R. L. Schiefelbusch (Eds.), *Language Intervention with the Retarded*. Baltimore: University Park Press, 1972.

Newfield, M. U. and Schlanger, B. B. The acquisition of English morphology by normal and educable mentally retarded children. *J. Speech Hear. Res.*, 1968, *11*, 693–706.

Piaget, J. *The Language and Thought of the Child*. New York: World Publishing, 1962.

Piaget, J. *Six Psychological Studies*. New York: Random House, 1967.

Piaget, J. Piaget's theory. In P. H. Mussen (Ed.), *Carmichael's Manual of Child Psychology*, Vol. 1, Ed. 3. New York: Wiley, 1970.

Piaget, J. and Inhelder, B. *The Psychology of the Child*. New York: Basic Books, 1969.

Raymore, S. and McLean, J. E. A clinical program for carry-over of articulation therapy with retarded children. In J. E. McLean, D. E. Yoder, and R. L. Schiefelbusch (Eds.), *Language Intervention with the Retarded*. Baltimore: University Park Press, 1972.

Rimland, B. *Infantile Autism*. New York: Appleton-Century-Crofts, 1964.

Risley, T. R., Hart, B. M., and Doke, L. Operant language development: The outline of a therapeutic technology. In R. L. Schiefelbusch (Ed.), *Language of the Mentally Retarded*. Baltimore: University Park Press, 1972.

Risley, T. and Wolf, M. Establishing functional speech in echolalic children. In H. Sloane and B. MacAulay (Eds.), *Operant Procedures in Remedial Speech and Language Training*. Boston: Houghton Mifflin, 1968.

Robinson, C. C. Analysis of stage four and five object permanence concept as a discriminated operant. Unpublished doctoral dissertation, George Peabody College, Nashville, 1972.

Schiefelbusch, R. L. (Ed.) *Language of the Mentally Retarded*. Baltimore: University Park Press, 1972.

Schlesinger, I. M. Production of utterances and language acquisition. In D. I. Slobin (Ed.), *The Ontogenesis of Grammar.* New York: Academic Press, 1971.

Schumaker, J. and Sherman, J. A. Training generative verb usage by imitation and reinforcement procedures. *J. Appl. Behav. Anal.,* 1970, *3,* 273–287.

Scott, D. A. and Milisen, R. The effectiveness of combined visual-auditory stimulation in improving articulation. *J. Speech Hear. Disord.,* 1954, No. 4, 51–56.

Semmel, M. I. and Dolley, D. G. Comprehension and imitation of sentences by Down's syndrome children as a function of transformational complexity. *Amer. J. Ment. Defic.,* 1971, *75,* 739–745.

Shirley, M. M. *The First Two Years: A Study of Twenty-five Babies,* Vol. II. *Intellectual Development.* Institute of Child Welfare Monograph Series No. 7. Minneapolis: University of Minnesota Press, 1933.

Sinclair-de-Zwart, H. Developmental psycholinguistics. In D. Elkind and J. H. Flavell (Eds.), *Studies in Cognitive Development: Essays in Honor of Jean Piaget.* New York: Oxford University Press, 1969.

Skinner, B. F. *Verbal Behavior.* New York: Appleton-Century-Crofts, 1957.

Skinner, B. F. Operant behavior. In W. K. Honig (Ed.), *Operant Behavior: Areas of Research and Application.* New York: Appleton-Century-Crofts, 1966.

Skinner, B. F. *Contingencies of Reinforcement: A Theoretical Analysis.* New York: Appleton-Century-Crofts, 1969.

Slobin, D. I. (Ed.) *The Ontogenesis of Grammar.* New York: Academic Press, 1971.

Smith, M. W. and Ainsworth, S. The effects of three types of stimulation on articulatory testing results. *J. Speech Hear. Disord.,* 1967, *10,* 348–353.

Smith, M. and Means, J. Effects of type of stimulus pretraining on discrimination learning in mentally retarded. *Amer. J. Ment. Defic.,* 1961, *66,* 259–265.

Spradlin, J. E., Girardeau, F. L., and Hom, G. L. Stimulus properties of reinforcement during extinction of a free operant response. *J. Exp. Child Psychol.,* 1966, *4,* 369–379.

Staats, A. W. Linguistic-mentalistic theory versus an explanatory S-R learning theory of language development. In D. I. Slobin (Ed.), *The Ontogenesis of Grammar.* New York: Academic Press, 1971.

Stremel, K. Language training: A program for retarded children. *Ment. Retard.,* 1972, *10,* No. 2, 47–49.

Talkington, L. W. and Hall, S. M. Matrix language program with mongoloids. *Amer. J. Ment. Defic.,* 1970, *75,* 88–91.

Telford, C. W. and Sawrey, J. M. *The Exceptional Individual: Psychological and Educational Aspects.* Englewood Cliffs, N. J.: Prentice-Hall, 1967.

Templin, M. C. Spontaneous versus imitated verbalization in testing articulation in preschool children. *J. Speech Hear. Disord.,* 1947, *12,* 293–300.

Uzgiris, I. C. and Hunt, J. McV. An instrument for assessing infant psychological development. Unpublished manuscript, University of Illinois, Chicago, 1966.

Watson, J. S. The development and generalization of "contingency awareness" in early infancy: Some hypotheses. *Merrill-Palmer Quart. Behav. Develop.,* 1966, *12,* 123–135.

Weimer, W. B. Psycholinguistics and Plato's paradoxes of the *Meno. Amer. Psychol.,* 1973, *28,* 15–33.

Wheeler, A. J. and Sulzer, B. Operant training and generalization of a verbal response form in a speech deficient child. *J. Appl. Behav. Anal.*, 1970, *3*, 139–147.

White, B. L. The initial coordination of sensorimotor schemas in human infants—Piaget's ideas and the role of experience. In D. Elkind and J. H. Flavell (Eds.), *Studies in Cognitive Development.* New York: Oxford University Press, 1969.

Winitz, H. *Articulation Acquisition and Behavior.* New York: Appleton-Century-Crofts, 1969.

Wolf, M. M., Risley, T. R., and Mees, H. I. Application of operant conditioning procedures to the behavior problems of an autistic child. *Behav. Res. Ther.*, 1964, *1*, 305–312.

Yoder, D. E. and Miller, J. F. What we may know and what we can do: Input toward a system. In J. E. McLean, D. E. Yoder, and R. L. Schiefelbusch (Eds.), *Language Intervention with the Retarded.* Baltimore: University Park Press, 1972.

Zimmerman, I. L., Steiner, V. G., and Evatt, R. L., *Preschool Language Manual.* Columbus, Ohio: Charles E. Merrill, 1969.

CHAPTER EIGHTEEN

INFANT INTERVENTION AND LANGUAGE LEARNING[1]

Kathryn Barth Horton

Bill Wilkerson Hearing and Speech Center and Vanderbilt University, Nashville, Tennessee 37212

The ever-present concern regarding language insufficiency of retarded children is self-evident and does not require elaborate reiteration. It suffices to say that a significant differentiating characteristic between intellectually normal and retarded children is language efficiency or deficiency. Inadequate speech is only one related manifestation. Work directed toward narrowing the gap between the linguistic proficiency of normal and retarded children has been extensive. Testimony to this fact is the number of research reports concerned with language and retardation, yet a review of these works does not lead to the conclusion that all of the questions have been answered, or even that all the questions have been asked.

The pace at which research efforts resolve the questions of language learning or map the unplotted territories of general learning for retarded children has not been an urgent concern until recently. Now, however, concern for the deficient and dependent members of our society is assuming serious proportions. The vastly increasing complexity of our society, with its phenomenal expansion of technology, makes difficult the assimilation or acceptance of persons without marketable skills. In other words, what is the future of the retarded in the 21st century? Consideration of this question is an essential prerequisite to serious deliberations regarding habilitation of the retarded.

Efforts to study and ultimately facilitate language development in retarded children are made difficult by an inadequate base of information about the early stages of language development in its normal course. The field lacks a natural history of language acquisition derived in natural milieus from a large number of children of different backgrounds. The absence of normal perspectives of language acquisition impedes efforts to study and develop intervention programs for children whose language acquisition is deficient and deviant.

[1] The preparation of this paper was partially supported by United States Office of Education Grant 0-70-4709-(618) and National Institute of Mental Health Grant MH 20638-01.

It is particularly appropriate that this effort include sections concerned with the earliest stages of postnatal development. The infant years 0–2 may represent a new and a last frontier opportunity to explore in trying to achieve the objective of habilitating each retarded child.

My approach in this exploration is that of a clinician first and of a researcher second. What I have to say and to suggest interweaves "hard" facts substantiated by research documentation and "soft" facts gained from 20 years of clinical experience with language-impaired infants, children, and adults.

THE POTENTIAL OF INFANCY

Animal research and experimental manipulation have illustrated that events in early life may effect major changes of a permanent nature. This general principle has been extended to man. It suggests significant and practical implications for shaping infant and preschool years to maximize the developmental potential of the human. But just as the plasticity of the human organism allows for shaping to maximize potential, so too can the early experiences of an infant limit development.

Mason (1970) summarized the effects of deprivation in early experience from animal research. Early sensory deprivation in apparently critical developmental periods leads to demonstrable physiological effects, such as the disintegration of established biological systems—vision and audition—as well as to significant and chronic deficiencies in behavioral adjustments. There is strong evidence that many basic sensorimotor skills are dependent upon environmental inputs and on the opportunity to utilize, integrate, and perfect these skills. Early deprivation has also been related to less obvious, yet nonetheless neurologically based, effects on behavior such as excessive arousal, when the organism is faced with novel or increased levels of stimulation. These characteristics persist even after prolonged periods of interaction with a nondeprived environment. Isolation rearing of birds, monkeys, and chimps has resulted in enduring patterns of behavior which deviate significantly from species norms, but which are not directly interpretable in terms of neurological or biological impairment. These chronic behavior patterns include deviant sexual behavior, development of different song patterns, hyperaggressiveness, and a complete absence of maternal behavior.

Since man must be viewed primarily as a biological organism, it is logical to apply principles growing out of animal research. The experiences and stimulation, or lack of it, during the early (and apparently critical) periods of development can result in profound and enduring effects upon the neurological, physiological, and behavioral capabilities of the human.

If deprivation is severe enough, it can lead to radical and permanent impairment of information-processing systems. Although even these extreme forms of deprivation continue to be a problem to man, they are less common, more easily remedied, and certainly less difficult to appraise, than those more subtle forms of deprivation that for all practical purposes leave the organism functionally intact, but unprepared to move on to the higher order achievements of which it is potentially capable (Mason, 1970, p. 47).

Our ultimate concern must center on how to structure the early years of life to facilitate development of language in individuals whose competencies in language are universally at risk. The achievement of this goal is dependent upon the application of knowledge in two basic areas: 1) the dimensions specified in qualitative and quantitative terms of language competence; and 2) the interrelationships between early experience and the development of language competence.

RECEPTIVE LANGUAGE DEVELOPMENT

Practically any treatise on language development voices the generalization that understanding precedes expression or, stated another way, that comprehension paces production. These statements are clichés. Review of research in language development or remediation reveals that comprehension as a forerunner of language production is largely ignored by both theoreticians and practitioners. The major stress is on production. Most psycholinguistic data are limited to those stages of language acquisition following production of utterances classifiable as "first words."

Examinations of psycholinguistic models and theory also reveal the consistent distinction made between prelinguistic and linguistic stages of development. As is the case with receptive language, prelinguistic development has had limited exploration in terms of both theory and behavioral observation. First considerations center predominantly on production of language.

Friedlander (1968, 1969, 1970), one of the few investigators who has concentrated heavily on the study of receptive language, made the following statement:

> Judging by the theoretical and speculative literature as it stands today, receptive language development in infancy is a minor topic of marginal significance. Issues related to infant listening and receptive processes are virtually ignored in the new wave of language studies that assumed torrential proportions in the early 1960's (Friedlander, 1970, p. 7).

It is clear that there has been limited research on how infants learn to recognize the semantic, lexical, syntactic, phonological, and prosodic aspects of language. This may be at least partially explained by the complexities involved in measuring comprehension. For the person interested in the habilitation of language-delayed and deviant persons, including mentally retarded children, these areas of investigation represent a problem group of major significance. For those concerned with infant intervention, these questions represent the priority area of investigation and application. However, our knowledge of the processes involved is so scant that stringent limitations are placed even in categorically organizing the topic.

Carroll (1964) suggested three interrelated developmental sequences necessary in language learning. First, cognitive structures which allow the child to recognize, discriminate, to some degree classify and manipulate the features and processes of his world undergird all language development. Second, the child must develop the capacity to discriminate and comprehend the patterns of speech to which he is exposed in his environment. And third, the child must develop the ability to produce the sounds of speech which conform to adult speech. The third is dependent on the second, and both are dependent upon the first. The child's ability to produce volitionally the sounds of speech is dependent on his ability to recognize and discriminate them. His ability to recognize and discriminate the patterns of language he hears is dependent on the development of undergirding cognitive structures which allow him to establish semantic referents.

The availability of substantive information on these three aspects of language learning is inversely related to the importance of each of these aspects in terms of the total process of language development.

Cognitive Basis of Language

"Language is useless without thought and thought without language is nebulous." In this statement Saussuere (1959) summarized the case for considering the cognitive basis of language. The study of language development in the retarded child requires examination of its cognitive prerequisites.

Macnamara (1972) and Bloom (1970, 1971) spoke to the nonlinguistic cognitive principles of language acquisition.

> ... infants learn their language by first determining, independent of language, the meaning which a speaker intends to convey to them and by then working out the relationship between the meaning and language. . . . The infant uses meaning as a clue to language, rather than language as a clue to meaning. . . . Meaning and the linguistic code are best treated as though they were elements of a compound much in the way that oxygen and hydrogen are the separate elements which combine to form molecules of water. That is the two are not usually experienced separately though they are distinguishable (MacNamara, 1972, pp. 1 and 3).

This position suggests that (in the early periods of development) thought is developed to a greater degree than is the linguistic capability to translate thought. Implicit is the notion that without such cognitive development, language cannot and will not develop.

Research on the cognitive structures prerequisite for the emergence of language is limited. However, we may isolate these cognitive principles by identifying the specifics of children's emerging language and then working backward. Macnamara (1972) suggested that the lexicon of the child emerges in the following order: names for entities, names for their variable states and actions, and then names for their permanent attributes. Bloom (1971) described the sequence of emergence in a similar way. Early syntactic utterances relate to the existence, nonexistence, and action on a referent. Children attend first to agents, actions, and objects before they attend to the attributes of objects. Bloom (1970) and McNeill (1970) suggested that these early single words are used by the child to express a variety of semantic structures. In considering the child's strategies for learning the syntax of his language, Macnamara (1972) suggested that the child must discriminate the structures of syntax and then relate them to semantic structures.

> . . . how does the infant use meaning as a clue to certain syntactic devices. The most likely avenue to explore here is the prior learning of vocabulary, principally nouns, verbs, and adjectives. . . . Children initially take the main lexical items in the sentences they hear, determine referents for these ideas, and then use their knowledge of the referents to decide what the semantic structures intended by the speaker must be (p. 7).

Efforts directed at stimulating language development of normal infants, including those from environments classifiable as "deprived," operate on the assumption that the cognitive undergirdings necessary for language learning are established or establishable. We cannot make these same assumptions when conceptualizing programs for retarded infants. We must first establish the presence or absence of requisite cognitive structures which have as yet to be completely defined.

The Relationship of Early Vocalization and Speech Development

There is a sizable body of descriptive data available on early vocal behavior (Ramey and Hieger, 1971–72). However, the relationship of early vocal experience on speech development has not been studied extensively. What is known concerning the linkage between kinesthesis and audition in feedback functions suggests the importance of early vocal experience as it undergirds fluent and articulate speech development. Neonatal vocalization is thought of as being reflexive in that it represents a set of unconditioned responses to some stimulus or stimuli, either internal or external. As development proceeds, however, the purposive aspects of infant vocalization become more apparent. Infants move into a stage of vocal behavior typically referred to as babbling which apparently is produced and maintained by the kinesthetic feedback associated with the vocal production. The developmental process in vocal behavior (and its feedback systems) may be represented as a layering process in which additional feedback systems come into play and assume priority for a period of time in influencing vocal productivity. At 5-6 months of age the auditory feedback system appears to assume a primary role in serving as a stimulator of vocal play. It is at this point that the vocal productivity of hearing-impaired babies starts to decrease in quantity as a consequence of their reduced auditory sensitivity. Thus their early vocal experiences, in quantity and quality, start to deviate substantially from those of normal-hearing children. A result is that hearing-impaired children do not have the same experiential base from which the highly developed vocal-kinesthetic feedback and monitoring systems of fluent and articulate speech emerge.

The same statement is applicable to babies who are ultimately found to be intellectually retarded. Analysis of case history information of retarded children reveals frequent reports by parents that these babies were quiet and vocalized minimally during the early months. For these children also, we must assume that their experiential bases on which the regulating feedback systems of articulate speech are built are limited and probably inadequate.

Vocalizing behavior of infants can be controlled quantitatively by contingent reinforcement, including both social and nonsocial reinforcers (Weisberg, 1963; Todd and Palmer, 1968; Rheingold, Gewirtz, and Ross, 1959). Seigel (1969) provided a comprehensive review of pertinent research in this area and pointed out the need for basic descriptive studies of infant vocal behavior. Routh (1969) presented evidence that vocalizations can be selectively controlled by differential reinforcement in infants between 2 and 7 months of age. Thus the combination of these efforts demonstrates that not only the quantity and rate of vocal production can be controlled using contingent reinforcement methods but also the type of specific utterances can be controlled.

If one accepts the premise that early vocal experience does influence speech development in the dimensions of articulatory competence and fluency, then it is reasonable to conclude that the vocal behavior of babies known to be at risk in intellectual and/or sensory function should be experimentally controlled so as to maximize the quantity and variety of prelingual utterances. In other words, contingent reinforcement principles should be applied as suggested by the studies cited earlier. The maintenance of a maximal quantity and variety of vocal play during the early months of life is an important first step in optimizing capacity for speech development.

Auditory Organization and Early Language Learning

Evidence attesting to the auditory discriminative capacities and the importance of listening for infants during the first 2 years of life is being accumulated by a number of investigators. Butterfield (1972), Eimas (1971, this volume, in press), and Morse (1972, this volume) have demonstrated that infants make discriminative responses between consonant-vowel combinations with Eimas and Morse suggesting that infant speech perception is linguistically relevant. Friedlander, directing his work at babies in the 8- to 15-month range, has shown them to make discriminations and exhibit preferences for vocal factors of familiarity, intonation, rhythm, and loudness and for message factors of length, redundancy, and amount of information. His work suggests the presence of an experiential continuum on which some of these variables may be placed.

Eisenberg's (1970) extensive review of the literature regarding developmental auditory behavior, its relation to adaptive and to hearing processes, and its relevance to infrahuman and adult hearing behavior supports and elaborates Friedlander's findings. Eisenberg suggested a biologically based conceptual model to which hypotheses of developmental audition can be related and against which they may be tested.

Whereas the concerns of developmental linguistics and psycholinguistics have been with the active process engaged in by the child in language learning, the efforts of Eisenberg (1964a and b, 1965, 1966, 1967, 1969, 1970) and of Friedlander (1968, 1969, 1970) have been directed at filling the void of available information concerning the nature of the passive side of auditory and language learning—the input functions. Eisenberg's work has been directed at delineating and defining the hierarchy of auditory specializations that undergird man's use of verbal codes. Friedlander has studied infant hearing as a sensitivity measurement function and infant listening as a psycholinguistic function. Disciplines concerned with language development generally accept the principle that output or expression of language is dependent upon and follows input or reception of language. Translation and extension of this principle imply that the organization of effective listening is indispensable for the development of speech and language competence.

Thus the knowledge of the parameters of organization of the developing auditory system must be applied in designing a learning environment for the retarded infant.

Ruder (1972) reiterated the importance of increasing our knowledge of the prelinguistic stages of development. In the model of psycholinguistic acquisition which he suggested, he referred to the entirety of the complex of prelinguistic and receptive competencies as "knows gross speech patterns." Some of the more precise dimensions of this broad complex of competencies have been documented. Eisenberg's (1964a and b, 1965, 1970) extensive studies on neonatal auditory behavior have demonstrated the perceptual discriminative capacity of the infant. She reported that signals below 4000 HZ tend to evoke responses two or three times more frequently than signals in the higher frequency ranges. Acoustic signals which fall into the speech-hearing frequency range are particularly effective in evoking responses (Eisenberg, 1965). Both Eisenberg (1970) and Hutt, Hutt, Lenard, Bernuth, and Muntjewerff (1968) have demonstrated the greater stimulus value of patterned signals over nonpatterned signals. The work of Eisenberg (1970), Butterfield (1968), Moffett (1971), McCaffrey (1970) and Morse and Eimas (this volume) substantiate the capacity of infants to make fine discriminations between acoustically similar consonant sounds. All these studies combine to highlight the level of perceptual-cognitive sophistication in auditory function that is partially present at the neonatal stage and continues to be refined rapidly within the first 15 months of life.

The most important dimension in auditory perception lies in the temporal qualities of acoustic experience. Specialists in psychoacoustics inform us that the human auditory system is especially attuned to sounds of different duration. For instance, vowels presented in sequences can be discriminated almost entirely by their duration. Another variable in the temporal dimension affecting auditory perception is the ability to distinguish sequences of sound events. Normally a time separation of more than 1 msec is required to perceive two acoustic events as separate (Hirsh, 1966). We must ask this question: if the temporal variable involved in perceiving speech were altered, would mentally retarded children with language deviancies perform better in speech perception and comprehension? Do their central nervous systems require a slower rate of input? Woodcock and Clark (1968) found that children with lower IQ's performed better at listening rates which were slower than the rates found to be most efficient for higher IQ subjects. Woodcock's (1969) work in the application of rate-controlled recordings has relevance to the linguistic management of language-retarded children. He found the combination of auditory and visual stimuli to be more efficient and effective as a medium for learning for retention of verbal material than listening alone, and he found listening to be superior to reading. His subjects achieved the highest scores in retention when they listened at expanded rates of 75–100 words per minute. In analyzing the relationship of performance on these tasks to intelligence, he found mental age to be a highly significant variable. If one attempts to apply Woodcock's findings in developing methodology for mentally retarded children, the logical next step would seem to be the use of controlled presentation for linguistic stimuli at rates substantially lower than the normal speaking rate of 150–175 words per minute.

Relationship between Auditory Organization and Vocalization

The interrelationship and interdependence of sensory and motor functions suggests that vocal production and auditory perception cannot be separated as language and speech development is studied. The role of audition as a basic sensory channel through which speech is learned cannot be denied. The findings of Chase et al. (1969) support the contention that disruptions in auditory feedback in the infant significantly affect prelingual vocal production and consequently later speech behavior. Research in auditory perception has demonstrated that audition and kinesthesis are importantly linked in the perception of speech (Liberman, 1957; Twaddell, 1952). Cherry (1957) and MacNeilage (1963) suggested that if there is an order in the auditory and kinesthetic events associated with sound perception then we perceive sound sequences only after the neuromuscular patterns of articulation have been mediated (kinesthetic feedback). Eisenberg's (1970) review of the research on developmental audition noted the evidence of intrinsic audiovocal neural relays, of acoustic preferences as they are developmentally influenced, and of plasticity in the mechanisms of auditory feedback. The importance of considering vocal, verbal, and auditory functions as intricately meshed and interdependent systems is obvious and underscores the necessity of maximizing the quality and quantity of the vocal and verbal behavior of the very young child.

PARENTAL INFLUENCE ON DEVELOPMENT

The notion that "parenting" is important is not new. Education for parents dates back to the early 1800's in the United States. We have developed several theories on the parent's role in shaping children's development, but we have done little to put our theories into practice. Too many programs serving children have given only lip service to parents' and families' emotional stability, their economic circumstances, their attitudes, their expectations. These factors all exert critical influences in their children's patterns of development.

For the past several decades systematic observational and research efforts have been on the increase, as have efforts to educate and involve parents in the developmental and educational process. The focus of the 1960's on the "disadvantaged child" gave further impetus to the investigation of the influence of the mother on cognitive and language development. Despite the acceleration of interest on this topic, much remains to be done. Viewing mothering as a greatly underrated occupation, Bruner (1970) summed up the current situation in the following statement.

> . . . there is an enormous influence exerted by the caretaker, be it mother, teacher, or whoever the person who is usually there. Is it the role of an accessible model, or as John Bowlby (1969) has recently proposed, is it that the caretaker provides a basis for reciprocal relationship that allows the infant to develop rules for getting on generally? While the importance of reciprocity is universally granted, most contemporary theories of intellectual or cognitive development leave the mother out of account. I include my own theories in this condemnation! (p. 113).

Bruner's opinion as to the importance of the caretaker is shared and documented by numerous investigators including Bayley (1955), Schaefer, (1968), Wachs, Uzgiris, and Hunt (1971), White (1971a,b), Bayley and Schaefer (1964), Levenstein (1970, 1971), Gordon (1969), Klaus and Gray (1968), and Weikart and Lambie (1968, 1969).

Studies specifying maternal or parental characteristics that seem to be significantly positive in influencing development include those of White (1971a,b), Wachs, Uzgiris, and Hunt (1971), Bayley and Schaefer (1964), Hess, Shipman, Brophy, and Bear (1969). Those factors which have consistently emerged as influential include parental affection, permissiveness, methods of control, teaching style, and language style.

Parental Language

The style of maternal language input to and interaction with the child is a significant variable in both cognitive and linguistic development. Rarely will one encounter a reading on language acquisition that does not describe it as a by-product of the socialization process, especially between mother and child. Language may be learned at or on mother's knee; however, the parameters of this learning have evoked only recently the interest of developmental psychologists and psycholinguists. They are now just beginning to attract attention in the ranks of audiology and speech pathology.

Olim (1970) suggested that maternal language style is one of the major variables in the creation and maintenance of poverty. His contention is that the deprivation is based in the communication process between mother and child, specifically in the characteristics of lack of cognitive meaning and cognitive and linguistic elaboration. This same contention has both direct and indirect relevance to the condition of mental retardation.

Olim (1970) investigated the styles of language interaction of 163 black mothers from three socioeconomic levels and their relationships with the cognitive development of their 4-year-old children. He found statistically significant differences in language style between the three socioeconomic levels. The mother's language proved to be a better predictor of the child's cognitive performance than the IQ of either the mother or the child.

General and verbal IQ's of three groups of preschoolers were compared by Levenstein (1970) before and after the exposure of the experimental group to 7 months of sessions carried out in homes designed to stimulate verbal interaction in mother-child dyads. The experimental group demonstrated significant gains in comparison to the two contrast groups.

Bernstein (1961) has described what he refers to as the "restricted" and "elaborated" linguistic codes and their application to the study of maternal-child interaction. He has related 10 characteristics to the restricted code and 8 to the elaborated. These concepts have potential for application to very young children. The use of the concept of linguistic code, as applied by Bernstein, concerns those principles, derived culturally, which operate to regulate the selection and organization of speech events. The restricted and elaborated codes are defined in terms of the relative ease or difficulty of predicting the range and flexibility of syntactic alternatives a speaker may adopt to organize or convey meaning. Bernstein's description of the restricted and elaborated codes includes such characteristics as degree of articulatory cues, speed, fluency, continuity of meaning, condensation levels of syntactic and vocabulary selection, degree of reliance on implicit or explicit meaning, levels of causality, explication and specification of meaning, person or group orientation, and degree of reliance on the verbal or extraverbal channels. The work of Deutsch (1964) suggests that characteristics which mark impoverished conditions for language learning include a lack of feedback from an adult. Deutsch's suggestions for optimizing the language learning environment between adult and child are similar to those of Kupriyanova and Fedoseyeva (1965). Words should be used within meaningful contexts; the speaker should feedback and expand the child's productions; objects should be given verbal labels; and objects and events or experiences should be verbally related.

Wachs, Uzgiris, and Hunt (1971) investigated variables related to levels of cognitive development. Assessing mental representation of objects, understanding means-ends relationships, the variety of ways and frequency of using objects, vocalizations, ability to anticipate consequences of actions, exploratory and social behaviors, and fear reactions, they found variables directly mediated by the parents especially important at 15 months of age. Such strategies as vocalizing and talking to the child, naming objects, and playing games were positively correlated with infant vocal behavior, developmental schemas, means-ends relationships, and foresight skills.

Talking to children has been both theorized and demonstrated as important in shaping development. Perhaps the clearest examples of application of this assumption are evidenced in the management of hearing-impaired children. Teachers in training are taught and parents are advised to "talk, talk, talk." Implicit is the notion that quantity of talking is the key. Children during the first several years of life are presented with tremendous variety of utterances, not sequenced in any known way, ordered along any defined continium of complexity, or even reinforced on a systematic schedule. Yet they learn. However, language that is addressed to young children has been shown to be significantly different from the mainstream of language they incidentally experience in their environment. Broen (1972) has addressed her research specifically to this topic. Broen focused on a number of dimensions of language style of "successful" mothers and compared the differences when language was directed to younger and older children and to adults. In talking to younger children, mothers relied heavily on single words as complete remarks. Sentences produced tended to be complete in the sense of intonational contour and expression of a complete thought but grammatically incomplete. When talking to older children and to adults, there were fewer instances of single word usage, more pauses, more broken sentences and extraneous conjunctions and a greater incidence of dysfluency. The commonality of sentence pattern usage and speech style among the mothers in talking to their younger children was notable.

Brown and Bellugi's (1965) observations also revealed the use of short, grammatically simple, and correct sentences by mothers with their young children. The mother's sentences were interpreted to be repetitious of the child's utterances coupled with expansion through the addition of words and intonation. The use of these expansions occurred about 30% of the time.

In contrast, speech observed among adults is rapid. Adult speech ranges from 120 to 180 words per minute and is characterized by frequent incomplete and broken sentences, dysfluencies, and pauses unrelated to grammatical structure.

Interesting questions are suggested by these contrasting findings. In the first place, in large groups of mothers how much variation in language style exists? Secondly, how do differences of maternal input effect the speech, language, and cognitive development of the children? Thirdly, we must ask: Do parents of children known (or later determined) to be retarded talk differently to these children than to their normal children? How does knowledge of retardation in their child affect the vocal and verbal behavior of the parents to the child?

Siegel (1967), in his review of studies of interpersonal research with retarded children, summarized the general findings that the vocal and verbal behavior of normal adults in relating with retarded children is influenced by the vocal or verbal level of the child and specifically that there is a direct relationship between the child's verbal level and adult's type-token ratio. Siegel (1967) and Spradlin and Rosenberg (1964) stated the need to differentiate adult verbal behavior in interactions with retarded children beyond broad generalizations regarding "simplicity" of language. The need exists to extend similar investigations to the verbal interaction patterns of parents with their retarded infants and toddlers.

The next logical question to entertain is: How amenable to alteration is the language style of parents or caretakers? Horton (1971) is investigating the alteration of maternal language style along the dimensions of the mother's use of reinforcement, redundancy, corrective feedback, expansion, and relevancy. Single concept video-tape training programs are being developed and researched for their effectiveness in changing the behavior of mothers interacting with their 4- and 5-year olds along the parameters of language input and interaction cited above.

INFANT INTERVENTION PROGRAMS

Infant education efforts have been on the increase over the last 2 decades, having been given special impetus by our attempts to abolish poverty and its deleterious effects on children's development. There have not been, however, emphases on or priorities afforded to early intervention across the various types of handicapping conditions. Review of the recent writing on mental retardation (Dunn, 1973; Lillywhite and Bradley, 1969; McLean, Yoder, and Schiefelbusch, 1972, Schiefelbusch, Copeland and Smith, 1967; Schiefelbusch, 1972a and b) reveals that no major consideration is given intervention in the 0- to 2- or 3-year period.

The Handicapped Children's Early Education Program of the Bureau of the Education of the Handicapped has stimulated early programming for developmentally delayed infants. However, of the more than 100 presently funded projects, apparently only 8 are directing their efforts exclusively at retarded children.

An extensive research and development effort is currently ongoing at Peabody College. The Toddler Research and Intervention Project developed by Diane and William Bricker (1971; 1972; this volume) includes developmentally delayed and nondelayed children between 1 and 4 years of age. The project, discussed in detail in the preceding chapter, is viewed as an operational demonstration of the operant approach to learning and cognitive and linguistic theory in action. It contains the distinctive features of integrating developmentally delayed and nondelayed children and parents into the program.

A project focused on preventing mental retardation through infant intervention has been in operation for about 8 years in Milwaukee. Heber's (1972) effort involves babies who were considered to be at risk intellectually by virtue of the fact that their mothers demonstrated IQ's under 75. This researched effort has the advantage over many of having substantial longitudinal data now available which makes possible an in-depth analysis of its long range effectiveness.

Heber's program seeks to determine whether it is possible to mitigate or prevent intellectual deficits in high risk, cultural-familial retardates through a combination of family intervention and direct child intervention. Infant intervention was initiated at 3 months and terminated at 6 years. His results thus far are reported to demonstrate a continued differential development in IQ and language development in favor of the experimental group. Heber's experimental subjects from chronological age points of 36 months to 66 months have maintained 12 months or more in mental age advantage over the control subjects. Language performance of the children was assessed in the areas of imitation, comprehension, and production. From 18 to 35 months, the experimental children exhibited statistically significant differences in the use of a greater number of lexical items in more utterances as compared to the controls.

From 36 to 56 months, free speech measures failed to discriminate. However, performance on all three standardized language assessment tools revealed differences between the experimental and control groups of 12–18 months.

Infant detection and treatment for the hearing-impaired child has a well established tradition in the field of deaf education as being essential to optimizing language and speech development and ultimate educational achievement. Recognition of the importance of infancy has in turn created a focus on the course of action which should be followed with the family of a deaf infant. The goal is not only to detect hearing impairment early and measure it but also to capture the auditory residual and maximize its contribution to early language acquisition. Those interested in aural and oral language development in the deaf child recognize the critical nature of the first 2 years of life in establishing the prerequisites for speech and inter-sensory patterning.

During the 1960's, a number of programs directed at early intervention through parents were initiated. One of these, The John Tracy Clinic in Los Angeles, was a forerunner in introducing a new format for early intervention through parent training. Rather than using the classroom or clinic as the locus in which to teach parents what to do at home to facilitate the development of their hearing-impaired children, the parents were taught in a simulated home, and the everyday activities of the household became the vehicles for teaching. A number of other centers soon followed this model including Central Institute for the Deaf in St. Louis, the University of Kansas Medical Center, and The Bill Wilkerson Hearing and Speech Center in Nashville.

The Home Teaching Program for Parents of Very Young Deaf Children (Horton, 1968, 1973; McConnell and Horton, 1970; Horton and McConnell, 1970; Horton and Sitton, 1970; McConnell, 1970) researched the effective-ness of this early intervention approach over a 3-year period during which 94 deaf children and their families participated. The measure of success of the project was demonstrated in the assessment of language growth and auditory development in children. Over a 28-month period, the children showed an increase in language quotient of 21 points as compared to the expected linear growth in performance quotients. Their levels of awareness for speech using amplification improved more than 10 dB (statistically significant at the 0.001 level) over the period of training.

Eighteen of the early participants in this project, now at school age, have been able to enter regular 1st and 2nd grades and perform successfully—a truly significant accomplishment for any deaf child. Several studies (Rushing, 1973; Liff, 1973) have recently been completed or are in progress, directed at analyzing the language performance of these children as compared to normals and other deaf children who were not identified before 2 years of age. Significant differences exist among the three groups using Lee's Develop-mental Sentence Scoring (Lee and Canter, 1971) in the direction of the children with whom intervention was early, showing language approximating that of normals.

In this project the key to successful early intervention lay in using parents as agents of change. The premises of the program and others similar to it in goals are very early detection, preferably within the 1st year of life, and early intervention involving, first, maximizing the child's opportunity to develop functionally his auditory residual through binaural hearing aid use and, second, upgrading his auditory and linguistic environment through intensive parent training. For the last 3 years, the program has been extended to include, in addition to hearing-impaired infants, language-delayed infants including those with general developmental delay.

Program objectives fall into five general categories: 1) to teach parents to optimize the auditory environment for their child; 2) to teach parents how to talk to their child; 3) to familiarize parents with the principles, stages, and sequence of normal language development and how to apply this frame of reference in stimulating their child; 4) to teach parents strategies of behavior management; and 5) to supply affective support to aid the family in coping with their feelings about their child and the stresses that a handicapped child places on the integrity of the family.

Auditory training is given emphases for both the hearing-impaired and normal-hearing children. In order to teach the parents how to orient their child to sound, they are provided specific instruction on 1) how to select environmental sounds to which to call their child's attention; 2) how to respond visibly and appropriately to the occurrence of sound, thereby stimulating the child's response; 3) how to associate consistently all sounds and their sources; and 4) how to reinforce positively the child's responses to sound. For the hearing-impaired children, the families are given specific assistance by both the audiologists and the teaching staff in helping their children to adjust to full time binaural hearing aid use.

The focus of the program objectives is on developing receptive language and establishing and/or strengthening the undergirding vocal functions for expressive language. Parents are taught to optimize their linguistic input to their child. The specifics of this teaching are housed in our Rules of Talking (Lillie, 1972). These 27 rules are presented in sequenced clusters and reflect the following parameters: 1) nonverbal and 2) verbal *reinforcement* of the child's vocal and/or verbal behaviors, 3) *relevancy* to the immediate situation, interest, and experiential background of the child; 4) *redundancy* in lexical, syntactic, and semantic input; 5) *feedback,* lexical, syntactic, and semantic; 6) *expansion,* lexical, syntactic, and semantic; and 7) appropriate use of *intonation* and *stress.*

After a perspective of almost 8 years, we have seen a "new breed" of deaf child emerge from these efforts—a child whose linguistic characteristics are more like his normal-hearing peers than his deaf peers without early detection and intervention. Similarly exciting results have been witnessed by a number of other programs engaging in similar efforts. Early identification, early amplification, and early parent training for many of these children has meant the difference between special education and education in the mainstream.

NEEDS

The unanswered and yet-to-be-asked questions involved with infant intervention with the retarded are vast in number. They bear on the most basic aspects of development—cognitive, affective, and linguistic. It is impossible to parcel out one aspect of behavior in the infant, such as language, and examine it in isolation from the totality of early development. Thus we are required in any serious intervention effort to look at the infant from all perspectives, regardless of our competencies as defined by our professional training, experience, and interest.

Schaefer (1970) suggested the need for the development of UR-education, a new discipline which focuses on the earliest and thus most basic education of the child as a means of developing more effective early childhood education approaches beginning at birth. He envisions this discipline as comprising not only the more academic education disciplines but also the behavioral and growth sciences and also as giving high priority to the study of parent-child relationships. Certainly this concept has import for all endeavors directed at habilitating handicapped children, including the retarded.

Early Identification

Early intervention requires early identification. Currently, in almost all communities, developmental screening of the juvenile population on a consistent or pervasive basis does not occur until the entry of this population into the public educational system at 5 or 6 years. Detection of retardation or any other impairment during the infant and preschool years occurs on an individual and serendipitous basis. Parents who observe delayed development in their child may seek professional help on their own, but usually such help-seeking behavior does not occur until the 3rd or 4th year of life, and in cases of mild or moderate retardation may not occur at all. Systems to detect retardation reliably in the infant and preschool years have not been implemented on any significant scale. As a result, optimal utilization of intervention strategies cannot be achieved. This problem is, in part, the result of the failure of communities to establish systems for health care and educational management which transcend the divisions between public and private health services and between boundaries separating professional "territorial rights." Before effective intervention will be achieved, unified cooperative service delivery systems must be established to detect retardation very early in life.

The Language of the Retarded

Delayed or arrested language development is evidenced as one of the most universal characteristics of mental retardation. Review of the literature on language and retardation confirms that there seems to be a general acceptance that the retarded represent a homogeneous group with reference to their linguistic characteristics. At best the differences are depicted as falling on a continuum representing the degree of language deficiency. But are the retarded homogeneous with reference to their language or any other behavior? In my experience, the answer to this question is, "No." Evaluation of the linguistic characteristics associated with the various conditions resulting in retardation must include primarily an analysis of the information processing, storage, and retrieval characteristics of the individuals involved. It cannot stop with ascribing some "language age" equivalent measure, or analyzing the misarticulations, or possibly assessing the physiological capabilities of the oral mechanism and the imitative abilities of the person. We must have not only an understanding of the commonalities of language problems in a retarded population but also an appreciation of the specific differences that exist within that population.

Weiner (1971) has found language-disordered children with nonverbal IQ's within the normal range to be significantly different in their information-processing abilities at both the perceptual and conceptual levels in the auditory sphere. Clinical experience verifies that language disorders are, in the main, auditory disorders. How consistent is this characteristic within a large group of retarded individuals? If it represents a consistent component of the problem, what are the clinical and educational implications?

Berry (1969) and Wyatt (1969) both reported significant perceptual-motor disturbances in language-disordered children, retarded and normal. What are the implications of this finding regarding early development? Freedman (1971) noted the significance of reduced or absent early handling of the infant by the mother and its contribution to the failure to develop awareness of body parts. Animal research verifies the importance of early movement on both affective and cognitive aspects of development. What are the experiences of retarded or at risk babies in this realm? How do they relate to the development of kinesthetic feedback systems that undergird the production of oral language?

What is the role of reinforcement in learning language? Siegel (1972) suggested that the reinforcement parameters involved in language and speech learning are highly complex and go far beyond a consideration of amount. Stark (1973) raised a similar question regarding reinforcement. What is its role beyond establishing the conditions under which language learning can occur? Enthusiasts for the application of operant models to language learning have sometimes represented that approach as a panacea. What they overlook is that we must consider not only the how of learning but also the relevance of what is being learned. Lynch and Bricker (1972) and Bricker and Bricker (this volume) suggested the alliance of often diametrically opposed approaches to the language learning process.

What is needed is a comparison of different approaches to language disorders along with a study of their longitudinal effects. This kind of research will shed light on the question of whether normal language acquisition processes and sequences should provide the basis for designing treatment methods.

Parental Roles

What are the parameters of parent-child interaction and how do they affect the language learning of the child? What are the optimal behaviors of the parent at what times in development to facilitate language development? Can parental language style be altered?

Normal Language and Cognitive Development: Their Relationship

The existence of generally divergent and often diametrically opposed approaches to the maximization of language development in the mentally retarded child can be considered the result of premature experimentation in this area. Stated simply, we have engaged in direct, applied research on language and cognitive development in the mentally retarded child without having a clear, empirically based understanding of language and cognitive development in the normal child. LaCrosse, Lee, Letman, Ogilvie, Stodolsky, and White (1970), in their report on research and educational practices during the first 6 years of life, discussed in depth the deficits in our understanding of language and cognitive development in normal, preschool age children. While the findings of LaCrosse *et al.* are too lengthy to be discussed here in depth, a number of interesting points were made. First, in terms of both cognitive and language development, there is little research in the 1–3 age range. Second, there is a serious lack of basic research into the development of language and cognition. Most of the research being done is of an applied, interventionist nature. Third, longitudinal studies on either cognitive or language development in normal children are seldom carried out, with the result that little is known about either, although a general increase in longitudinal cognitive studies has been noted. And fourth, few studies have attempted to deal with the interrelationship between cognitive development and language development.

If a firm, empirically based understanding of the developmental processes in normal children of preschool age has not yet emerged, how can we hope to understand (and develop approaches which will compensate for) those children whose language and cognitive development has been retarded? What is desperately needed for the growth of successful intervention projects in the area of language development in mentally retarded children is basic research on cognitive and language development in normal children. It is only with a firm understanding of how these processes normally develop that meaningful intervention strategies can be formulated and tested.

REFERENCES

Bayley, N. On the growth of intelligence. *Amer. Psychol.,* 1955, *10,* 805–818.

Bayley, N. and Schaefer, E. S. Correlations of maternal and child behaviors with the development of mental abilities: Data from the Berkeley Growth Study. *Monogr. Soc. Res. Child Development.,* 1964 *29,* 6.

Bernstein, B. Social structure, language and learning. *Educ. Res.,* 1961, *3,* 163–176.

Berry, M. F. *Language Disorders in Children: The Bases and Diagnoses.* New York: Appleton-Century-Crofts, 1969.

Bloom, L. *Language Development: Form and Function in Emerging Grammars.* Boston: M.I.T. Press, 1970.

Bloom, L. Why not pivot grammer? *J. Speech Hear. Disord.,* 1971, *36,* 40−51.

Bowlby, J. *Attachment and Loss,* Vol. 1. New York: Basic Books, 1969.

Bricker, D. and Bricker, W. Toddler research and intervention project report−year I. IMRID Behavioral Science Monograph No. 20. Nashville, 1971.

Bricker, D. and Bricker. W. Toddler research and intervention project report−year II. IMRID Behavioral Science Monograph No. 21. Nashville, 1972.

Broen, P. A. The verbal environment of the language-learning child. ASHA Monograph 17. Washington, D. C.: American Speech and Hearing Association, 1972.

Brown, R. and Bellugi, U. Three processes in the child's acquisition of syntax. *Harvard Educ. Rev.,* 1965, *34,* 133−151.

Bruner, J. S. Discussion: Infant education as viewed by a psychologist. In V. H. Dennenberg (Ed.), *Education of the Infant and Young Child.* New York: Academic Press, 1970.

Butterfield, E. C. An extended version of modification of sucking with auditory feedback. Working paper 43. Bureau of Child Research Laboratory, Children's Rehabilitation Unit, University of Kansas Medical Center, October, 1968.

Butterfield, E. C. and Siperstein, G. N. Influence of contingent auditory stimulation and non-nutritional suckle. In Bosma, J. (Ed.), *Oral Sensation and Perception: The Mouth of the Infant.* Springfield, Ill.: Thomas, 1972.

Carroll, L. B. *Language and Thought.* Englewood Cliffs, N. J.: Prentice-Hall, 1964.

Chase, R. A. Delayed feedback audiometry. Final report, Research Grant RD-1899-S. Washington, D. C.: Division of Research-Demonstration Grants, Social and Rehabilitation Services, Department of Health, Education, and Welfare, 1969.

Cherry, C. *On Human Communication.* Cambridge, Mass.: M.I.T. press, 1957.

Deutsch, M. *The Role of Social Class in Language Development and Cognition.* New York: Institute for Developmental Studies, Department of Psychiatry, New York Medical College, 1964 (mimeographed).

Dunn, L. M. *Exceptional Children in the Schools.* New York: Holt, Rinehart and Winston, 1973.

Eimas, P. D. Speech perception in early infancy. In L. B. Cohen and P. Salapatek (Eds.), *Infant Perception.* New York: Academic Press, in press.

Eimas, P. D., Siquelard, E. R., Tusczyk, P., and Vigorito, J. Speech perception in infants. *Science,* 1971, *171,* 303−306.

Eisenberg, R. B. Examination of auditory behavior. *J. Audit. Res.,* 1965, *5,* 159−177.

Eisenberg, R. B. The development of hearing in man: An assessment of current status. Report submitted to the Subcommittee on Human Communication and Its Disorders, National Advisory Neurological Disease and Blindness Council, 1966.

Eisenberg, R. B. Stimulus significance as a determinant of newborn's responses to sound. Paper presented at SRCD Meeting, New York, 1967.

Eisenberg, R. B. Auditory behavior in the human neonate: Functional properties of sound and their ontogenetic implications. *Int. Audiol.,* 1969, *8,* 34−45.

Eisenberg, R. B. The organization of auditory behavior. *J. Speech Hear. Res.*, 1970, *13*, 453–471.

Eisenberg, R. B., Coursen, D. C., Griffen, E. J., and Hunter, M. A. Auditory behavior in the human neonate: A preliminary report. *J. Speech Hear. Res.*, 1964a, *7*, 245–269.

Eisenberg, R. B., Griffen, E. J., Coursen, D. B., and Hunter, M. A. Auditory behavior in the human neonate: A preliminary report. *J. Speech Hear. Res.*, 1964b, *7*, 159–177.

Freedman, D. A. Cogential and peri-natal sensory deprivation: Some studies in early development. *Amer. J. Psychiat.*, 1971, *127*, 115–121.

Friedlander, B. Z. The effect of speaker identity, voice inflection, vocabulary, and message redundancy on infants' selections of vocal reinforcement. *J. Exp. Child Psychol.*, 1968, *6*, 443–459.

Friedlander, B. Z. Identifying and investigating major variables of receptive language development. Paper presented at the meeting of the Society for Research in Child Development, Santa Monica, 1969.

Friedlander, B. Z. Receptive language development in infancy: Issues and problems. *Merrill-Palmer Quart.*, 1970, *16*, 7–51.

Gordon, I. Early Child Stimulation through Parent Education. Final Report. University of Florida, Gainesville, 1969.

Heber, R., Garber, H., Harrington, S., and Hoffman, C. Rehabilitation of families at risk for mental retardation: Progress report. Rehabilitation Research and Training Center in Mental Retardation, University of Wisconsin, Madison, Dec. 1972.

Hess, R. D., Shipman, V. C., Brophy, J. E., and Bear, R. M. The cognitive environments of urban pre-school children: Followup phase. Graduate School of Education, University of Chicago, Chicago, 1969.

Hirsch, I. J. Audition in relation to perception in speech. In E. C. Carterette (Ed.), *Brain Function. III. Speech, Language, and Communication.* Berkeley: University of California Press, 1966, p. 103.

Horton, K. B. Early amplification and language learning—or—Sounds should be heard and not seen. *J. Acad. Rehab. Audiol.*, 1973.

Horton, K. B. Home demonstration teaching for parents of very young deaf children. *Volta Rev.*, 1968, *70*, 97–104.

Horton, K. B. Training maternal language style through multimedia. Applied Research Grant ERP-MH 20638-01, National Institute of Mental Health, 1971.

Horton, K. B. and McConnell, F. Early intervention for the young deaf child through parent training. In *Proceedings of the International Congress on Education of the Deaf, Stockholm*, Vol. I. 1970, pp. 291–296.

Horton, K. B. and Sitton, A. G. Early intervention for the young deaf child. *S. Med. Bull.*, 1970, *58*, 50–57.

Hutt, S. J., Hutt, C. Lenard, H. G., Bernuth, H. V., and Muntjewerff, W. J. Auditory responsivity in the human neonate. *Nature*, 1968, *218*, 888–890.

Klaus, R. A. and Gray, S. W. The early training project for disadvantaged children: A report after five years. *Monogr. Soc. Res. Child Develop.*, 1968, *33*, 4.

Kupriyanova, N. B. and Fedoseyeva, T. N. *Plays and Activities with Children up to 3 Years.* Leningrad: Medicina, 1965 (In Russian)

LaCrosse, E. R., Jr., Lee, P. C., Letman, F., Ogilvie, D. M., Stodolsky, S. S., and White, B. L. The first six years of life; A report on current research and educational practice. *Genet. Psychol. Monogr.*, 1970, *82*, 161–266.

Lee, L. L. and Canter, S. M. Developmental sentence scoring: A clinical procedure for estimating syntactic development in children's spontaneous speech. *J. Speech Hear. Disord.*, 1971, *36*, 315–340.

Levenstein, P. Cognitive growth in preschoolers through verbal interaction with mothers. *Amer. J. Orthopsychiat.*, 1970, *40*, 426–432.

Levenstein, P. Learning through (and from) mothers. *Childhood Educ.*, 1971, *48*, 130–134.

Liberman, A. B. Some results of research on speech perception. *J. Acoust. Soc. Amer.*, 1957, *29*, 117–123.

Liff, S. M. The effects of early intervention on the language of hearing impaired children. In *Early Intervention and Language Development in Hearing Impaired Children*. Nashville: Vanderbuilt University, 1973.

Lillie, S. M. Principles of parent teaching for language handicapped children under four. Division for Children with Communication Disorders, Bulletin IX, 1972, 15 –19.

Lillywhite, H. S. and Bradley, D. P. *Communication Problems in Mental Retardation: Diagnosis and Management*. New York: Harper & Row, 1969.

Lynch, T. and Bricker, W. A. Linguistic theory and operant procedures: Toward an integrated approach to language training for the mentally retarded. *Ment. Retard.*, 1972, *10*, 12–17.

Macnamara, J. Cognitive basis of language learning in infants. *Psychol. Rev.*, 1972, *79*, 1–13.

MacNeilage, D. F. Electromyographic and acoustic study of the production of certain final clusters. *J. Acoust. Soc. Amer.*, 1963, *34*, 461–463.

Mason, W. B. Early deprivation in biological perspective. In V. H. Dennenberg (Ed.), *Education of the Infant and Young Child*. New York: Academic Press, 1970.

McCaffrey, S. Speech perception in infancy. Personal communication, 1970.

McConnell, F. A new approach to the management of childhood deafness. *Pediat. Clin. N. Amer.*, 1970, *17*, 347–362.

McConnell, F. and Horton, K. B. A home teaching program for parents of very young deaf children. Final report, Project 6-1127, Grant OEG 32-52-0450-6007, 1970.

McLean, J. E., Yoder, D. E., and Schiefelbusch, R. L. (Eds.). *Language Intervention with the Retarded: Developing Strategies*. Baltimore: University Park Press, 1972.

McNeill, D. *The Acquisition of Language: The Study of Developmental Psycholinguistics*. New York: Harper & Row, 1970.

Miller, W. and Ervin, S. The developmental of grammar in child language. *Monogr. Soc. Res. Child Develop.*, 1964, *29*, 9–42.

Moffett, A. Consonant cue perception by twenty to twenty-four week old infants. *Child Develop.*, 1971, *42*, 717–731.

Morse, P. A. The discrimination of speech and nonspeech stimuli in early infancy. *J. Exp. Child Psychol.*, 1972, *14*, 477–492.

Olim, E. G. Maternal language styles and cognitive development of children. In F. Williams (Ed.), *Language and Poverty: Perspectives on a Theme*. Chicago: Markham Publishing Co., 1970.

Ramey, C. T. and Hieger, L. The vocal behavior of infants. In *Research Relating to Children*, Bulletin 29, September 1971–February 1972. ERIC Clearinghouse on Early Childhood Education.

Rheingold, H. L., Gerwitz, J. L., and Ross, H. W. Social conditioning of vocalizations in the infant. *J. Comp. Physiol. Psychol.*, 1959, *52*, 68–73.

Routh, D. K. Conditioning of vocal response differentiation in infants. *Develop. Psychol.,* 1969, *1,* 219–226.

Ruder, K. F. A psycholinguistic viewpoint of the language acquisition process. In R. L. Schiefelbusch (Ed.), *Language of the Mentally Retarded.* Baltimore: University Park Press, 1972.

Rushing, K. C. A study of the syntax used by hearing impaired children. Unpublished master's thesis, Vanderbilt University, Nashville, 1973.

Saussure, F. De. *Course in General Linguistics.* New York: McGraw-Hill, 1959.

Schaefer, E. S. Progress report: Intellectual stimulation of culturally deprived infants. Personal communication, July, 1968.

Schaefer, E. S. A home tutoring program. *Children,* 1969, *16,* 59–61.

Schaefer, E. S. Need for early and continuing education. In V. Dennenberg (Ed.), *Education of the Infant and Young Child.* New York: Academic Press, 1970.

Schiefelbusch, R. L. Language disabilities of cognitively involved children. In T. V. Irwin and M. Marge (Eds.), *Principles of Childhood Language Disabilities.* New York: Appleton-Century-Crofts, 1972a.

Schiefelbusch, R. L. (Ed.) *Language of the Mentally Retarded.* Baltimore: University Park Press, 1972b.

Schiefelbusch, R. L., Copeland, R. H., and Smith, J. O. *Language and Mental Retardation: Empirical and Conceptual Considerations.* New York: Holt, Rinehart & Winston, 1967.

Siegel, G. M. Interpersonal approaches to the study of communication disorders. *J. Speech Hear. Disord.,* 1967, *32,* 112–120.

Siegel, G. M. Vocal conditioning in infants. *J. Speech Hear. Disord.,* 1969, *34,* 3–20.

Siegel, G. M. Three approaches to speech retardation. In R. L. Schiefelbusch (Ed.), *Language of the Mentally Retarded.* Baltimore: University Park Press, 1972.

Spradlin, J. E. and Rosenberg, S. Complexity of adult verbal behavior in a dyadic situation with retarded children. *J. Abnorm. Soc. Psychol.,* 1964, *68,* 694–698.

Stark, J., Rosenbaum, R. L., Schwartz, D., and Wisan, A. The non-verbal child: Some clinical guidelines. *J. Speech Hear. Disord.,* 1973, *38,* 59–71.

Todd, G. and Palmer, B. Social reinforcement of infant babbling. *Child Develop.,* 1968, *39,* 591–596.

Twaddell, W. Phonemes and allophones in speech analysis. *J. Acoust. Soc. Amer.,* 1952, *24,* 607–611.

Wachs, T. D., Uzgiris, I. C., and Hunt, J. McV. Cognitive development in infants of different age levels and from different environmental backgrounds: An explanatory investigation. *Merrill-Palmer Quart. Behav. Develop.,* 1971, *17,* 283–317.

Weikart, D. P. and Lambie, D. Z. Preschool intervention through a home tutoring program. In J. Hellmuth (Ed.), *The Disadvantaged Child, Vol. 2.* Seattle: Special Child Publications, 1968.

Weikart, D. P., Lambie, D. Z., *et al.* Ypsilanti-Carnegie infant education project progress report. Department of Research and Development, Ypsilanti Public Schools, Ypsilanti, Mich., 1969.

Weiner, P. S. The cognitive functioning of language deficient children. In J. Hellmuth (Ed.), *Cognitive Studies: Deficits in Cognition.* New York: Brunner/Mazel, Inc., 1971.

Weisberg, P. Social and nonsocial conditioning of infant vocalizations. *Child Develop.*, 1963, *39*, 377–388.

White, B. L. Fundamental early environmental influences on the development of competence. Paper presented at the Third Western Symposium on Learning: Cognitive Learning at Western Washington State College, Bellingham, October 21–22, 1971a.

White, B. L. *Human Infants: Experience and Psychological Development.* Englewood Cliffs, N. J.: Prentice-Hall, 1971b.

Woodcock, R. W. The application of rate-controlled recordings in the classroom. Paper presented at the Second Louisville Conference on Rate and/or Frequency Controlled Speech at the University of Louisville, October 2–3, 1969.

Woodcock, R. W. and Clark, C. R. Comprehension of a narrative passage by elementary school children as a function of listening rate, retention period, and I.Q. *J. Commun.*, 1968, 18(3), 259–271.

Wyatt, G. L. *Language, Learning and Communication Disorders in Children.* New York: The Free Press, 1969.

CHAPTER NINETEEN

DISCUSSION SUMMARY–EARLY LANGUAGE INTERVENTION

Lawrence J. Turton

Institute for the Study of Mental Retardation and Related Disabilities, University of Michigan, Ann Arbor, Michigan 48104

The important implication to be derived from the programs described by Bricker and Bricker and Horton is that language activities for preschool handicapped children are but one facet of a total developmental program. Infant programs should address themselves more to generic developmental behaviors and environmental issues than to specific language structures. The underlying philosophy of the two papers on early intervention can be summarized as follows: Since problems present at birth, or soon thereafter, prevent the child from profiting from normal interactions with the environment, parents and professionals must provide the youngster with appropriate prosthetic equipment and a modified environment. Language systems will be acquired by the youngster when the maximal developmental environment has been attained as a result of the intervention procedures.

DIFFERENCES BETWEEN THE TWO PROGRAMS

The two programs described in this section represent some interesting contrasts in the application of this philosophy. The Horton program is concerned primarily with (apparently) intellectually normal individuals who have a critical sensory deficit, *i.e.,* a severe to profound hearing loss. The Bricker and Bricker project serves youngsters who are severely handicapped cognitively, linguistically, and motorically. While the former program views "mainstreaming" into general education as its ultimate goal, the Brickers' goal is less well defined and measurable, *i.e.,* prevention of institutionalization and maximal developmental progress in whatever areas possible. Regular educational placement for the hearing-impaired child is, of course, predicated upon language and cognitive skills which approximate those found in normal-hearing children.

The clinical and research premises of the two programs represent different approaches to early intervention. The program for hearing-impaired youngsters conducted by Horton and her associates at the Bill Wilkerson Center is concerned with the application of the principles of aural-oral habilitation to infants. Parents are viewed as the primary change agents who have ultimate responsibility for assisting the child in the process of adapting to the natural conditions of the home and modifying the child's environment to maximize language learning. A basic assumption is that parents are most effective when they function as parents and not as quasi-teachers. The program helps the parents modify their communication style in natural parent-child interactions and activities rather than changing the nature of such activities. The child's development is facilitated by the fitting of hearing aids as soon as possible after identification of the hearing loss. The amplification permits the introduction of auditory training procedures which are designed to stimulate the acquisition of the auditory and kinesthetic feedback systems necessary for language. Thus, this program can be viewed as a modification of clinical methodology to a new population, the infants, through the development of new skills by their parents.

In contradistinction to the Horton program, the Bricker and Bricker endeavor can be viewed as an exploration into the effects upon handicapped children of combining the stages of Piagetian theory of development with the technology of behavior modification. The change expected in the handicapped infant is the development of the stages of sensorimotor development, including the prerequisite behaviors for language. In place of prosthetic devices, a prosthetic environment is created which includes the human trainer and the instrumentation necessary to teach the infant new behaviors and to record functional changes.

The research systems superimposed upon the clinical programs are logical extensions of the premises upon which the projects are based. Data on children in the hearing-impaired program are derived from measures administered pre- and posttreatment and/or posttreatment when compared to normal-hearing peers. The model is one frequently used in clinical research wherein the concern is with the cumulative effects of the treatment after all clinical procedures have been implemented.

On the other hand, the Bricker and Bricker research model approximates that of behavioral psychology wherein ongoing changes in the developmental level of the child are of critical interest because 1) they are the criteria for the effectiveness of a treatment procedure at a point in time; and 2) continuation or modification of the procedure is contingent upon the presence of the desired behavior. Thus, intratreatment measures assume greater importance than pre- and posttreatment differences.

There is an apparent contradiction between the use of a developmental model such as Piaget's and a training model such as the functional analysis of behavior. On the one hand, the acceptance of the Piaget model should work from the assumption that there are inherent hierarchies of skills and behaviors which are acquired at certain maturational levels. At the same time, the behavioristic approach assumes that the behaviors can be taught in some sequence independent of the specific age level. Thus the Brickers' program has put itself in the position of accepting a model while challenging that model at the same time.

This apparent contradiction is resolved by the fact that the clinical research program of the Infant, Toddler, and Preschool Research and Intervention Project is designed to ferret out the variables which influence the child's behavior, rather than the specific forms or classes of behaviors *per se*. The intent is to lead the child to the point where he can learn additional skills without subsequent training. The issue is not one merely of challenging a developmental theory with a particular set of training procedures but rather to find behavioral definitions for the patterns and stages described in the Piagetian model.

IDENTIFICATION OF STIMULI RELEVANT TO BEHAVIORAL CHANGES

The incorporation of the Piagetian model in an intervention program requires that behaviors be assessed while in the developmental phase rather than when they have appeared in the repertoire of the child. When superimposing a functional analysis approach on the Piagetian stages, the clinical researcher must isolate the environmental events which stimulate the behavior, those which shape the final behavior, and those which reinforce the child for responding in the appropriate fashion. Essentially, the task is to find those stimuli which are relevant to the infant's behavior in the absence of physical props or imitative processes facilitating the child's functions.

However, this raises the issue of the relevance of the selected stimuli and the generalization process. Since research has not identified a finite set of characteristics which distinguish an object or word from all others in the environment, the intervener must assume that he/she has selected the appropriate behavior for a child and can identify the controlling stimuli.

One solution proposed is to discover the classes which each child has available to him/her and attach a name or label to the classes. This approach intensifies the need to be able to identify the behaviors which the child is in the process of learning so that the class name can be attached to the relevant attributes of the class as quickly as possible.

If one adopts the Piagetian model, however, one must contend with the premise contained therein that children probably do not have definable classes until 6 or 7 years of age. Furthermore, within this model children appear to go through a stage of inappropriately using an object relative to the adult class, then using the object in a fashion accepted by the adults, and then finally using the object in a symbolic but appropriate fashion. The point of concern is whether the criterion for the child having the class is his ability to use it in an appropriate fashion relative to the adult definition or in a symbolic fashion which extends it beyond the adult class. The response to this concern related back to the research philosophy of the Brickers' project, namely, that the task of the professional is to identify those variables which lead to the development of the behavioral repertoire rather than measuring just the repertoire itself. In other words, the criterion should be the identification of the behaviors which lead to the development of the repertoire and which serve as the stimulus control for that particular class of behaviors, not whether adults accept the child's usage of the object.

If the basic premise of the training program is to determine the relevant variables or attributes and the irrelevant ones, the clinical researcher has an obligation to specify how the relevancy was determined. The process employed by Bricker and Bricker is best summarized as one of excluding those variables which apparently do not control the child's behavior when being taught an object or word and which are not overgeneralized by the child.

A problem with the concept of determining relevant attributes is that the relevancy may be restricted to some stage of development because attributes apparently have a high priority on the child's hierarchial order at one point in time and a lower priority at another point in time. The answer to that concern is found in the analysis of the child's errors in that those variables which control his errors are specifically those which must be modified by the trainer so that the appropriate stimulus parameters become relevant to the child. We essentially have a condition where the clinical researcher is the culture for the youngster and defines the relevant set of attributes or stimulus elements which will control his behavior.

THE ROLE OF NORMAL CHILDREN IN EARLY INTERVENTION

One aspect of both projects is the incorporation of nondelayed children with the young handicapped children. Although there is some indication that these children also benefit from the experience as well as contributing to the program for the delayed children, little research evidence is available which would specify the nature of that benefit and the conditions which facilitate it. The presence of the normal children in an early intervention program serves to balance the percepts of the teachers relative to their expectancies for the handicapped children. Behaviors of the nondelayed children also can be used as models for developmental changes in the delayed children. There may also be changes in the attitude of normal children toward handicapped children, but long term research evidence to support this contention is not available.

The ratio of nonhandicapped to handicapped children is apparently a difficult variable to manipulate. Within similar programs, the participants of the conference reported that for some programs a mix of 1 normal to 1 handicapped child appeared to be appropriate but that a 2 or 3 to 1 mix, now being introduced into the Wilkerson program, did not seem to work as well.

The role of the nonhandicapped child appears to be most important in determining the ratio. If they are members of the group receiving the same instructions as the handicapped children, then the ratio is not as critical. If, however, they are used in a tutorial fashion to facilitate the behavior of the handicapped child, that number becomes most important. The integration of handicapped and nonhandicapped children in the hearing-impaired program is important because the ultimate goal of the program is to place the child with hearing problems into a normal classroom. At the present time, the Wilkerson Center program is striving to obtain a mix of 3 handicapped children into a normal classroom with a total class size of approximately 28–30.

THE ROLE OF PARENTS IN EARLY INTERVENTION

The discussion by Horton focused upon the role of parents in the habilitation process of the hearing-handicapped child 0–24 months of age. The program at the Bill Wilkerson Center is, in fact, focused entirely upon parents of the children referred prior to their 3rd birthday. The clinical setting is actually a home which allows the professionals to build a program for the child appropriate to his natural setting and the skills of the parents. Both parents are incorporated into this activity with the assumption that fathers and mothers are of equal value and importance to the development of the child.

The goals of the early intervention program for the parents of the hearing-impaired children are 1) to teach the parents to communicate verbally with their children in a linguistically relevant fashion; and 2) to enhance the role of the parents as reinforcers of the linguistic behavior of the children in terms of stimulating vocal and verbal productivity and shaping those responses. These goals are attained through procedures designed to enhance the functioning of parents as parents and not as substitutes for a clinician.

One task facing the clinician, however, is to define linguistic relevance for the parents. In terms of the hearing-impaired child, the parents must be sensitive to his experiential background as it provides stimuli for language acquisition. They must also be aware of the child's interest in the content of the language and the need for redundancy in their utterances. Furthermore, the vocal and verbal productions of the child must be reinforced by the parents; corrected through feedback; and expanded in terms of lexical, semantic, and syntactic structures. The parents must be cognizant of the child's developmental stage so that they enhance the use of that which has been acquired and shape those language skills which are being acquired. This approach is not unlike that adopted by the Brickers in their attempts to identify object stimuli which are important in controlling the developmental process.

Once parents are entered into the program in a significant fashion, the clinician is faced with the problem of dealing with the affective feelings of guilt and anxiety which are often present immediately after the handicap has been identified. There is an affective domain which must be dealt with in a way to facilitate the parents' role as parent-teachers of more specific behaviors. One approach is to designate a group of professionals, *e.g.*, psychologists and social workers, who are assigned the task of dealing with the affective domain whereas the teachers and clinicians are to deal with the developmental linguistic skills. The experience of the program at the Wilkerson Center, however, was that parents did not recognize this dichotomy between the two groups of professionals. Regardless of the person's programmatic assignment, when the parents were dealing with a professional they would raise issues which were most paramount to them at that point in time. The compromise reached was to hire staff who themselves were parents and to use a parent in staff orientation sessions to make the staff more sensitive to the needs of the parents and to give them ways of handling the problems raised by the parents.

IDENTIFICATION AND ASSESSMENT OF HANDICAPPED INFANTS

The identification of handicaps during infancy is a critical function of any early intervention program. In the area of audiological assessment, technical procedures are now available for evaluating hearing levels of infants and preschoolers. However, a service gap exists between the development of the procedures and the use of such procedures by medical and nonmedical practitioners so that high risk infants can be identified and placed in an appropriate program (AAOO, AAP, and ASHA, 1971; 1974; Downs, 1970; Downs and Hemenway, 1972; Goldstein and Tait, 1971; Meier, 1973). One reason for the service gap is the lack of public and professional information. Another is the concern over the adequacy and reliability of some audiological procedures when used with infants. The discussion on cortical audiometry illustrated this problem. Some clinical facilities report confidence in the degree of hearing loss measured through this procedure with infants, particularly as the results predict eventual hearing level. Others, however, do not share this confidence in cortical audiometry and prefer to utilize behavioral approaches only. (For a current discussion of audiological assessment the reader is referred to books edited by Fulton and Lloyd, 1969; and by Jerger, 1973.)

The important consequence of this disagreement is manifested in the decision to recommend a hearing aid and auditory training procedures. Horton reported successful results with standard pure tone audiometrics when employed over repeated sessions with the children. Thus, the Wilkerson program has adopted a prosthesis/auditory training program based on repeated monitoring of the child and not based on a single measure.

In terms of language assessment, however, we are still faced with the problem of developing reliable and valid language (or prelanguage) measures which can be applied in the infancy years. We must be able to identify those skills which are a necessary part of the total developmental process, including vocal behavior, perceptual skills, and cognitive functions. The clinician must be able to identify also those behaviors which help the infant to go from visual control to physical control to linguistic control over his environment. An infant "language" assessment and training program is thus a developmental process wherein the child's performance level is specified by nonlanguage and prelanguage behaviors and continued development is facilitated by the adults in the environment.

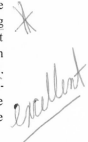

excellent

EVALUATION OF TREATMENT PROGRAMS AND PROCEDURES

In addition to concerns over the appropriateness of assessment procedures, the clinical research must deal with the issue of assessing the effectiveness of the treatment procedures. A second level should concern itself with the evaluation of the terminal behaviors projected by the goals and objectives of the program, *i.e.*, those behaviors and developmental skills identified as being significant by the clinicians. The third level should measure the changes in other behaviors or areas of achievement which are dependent upon the original terminal behaviors, *e.g.*, the degree to which school achievement is influenced by the child's language skills.

Evaluation measures, however, are directly related to the developmental theory and/or learning principles adopted by the clinicians. In the area of language development, the decision-making process involved in selecting the bases for the early intervention generated less than unanimous agreement from the conference participants. Researchers in normal language acquisition have produced a body of data on development and several theories. One can argue that those structures and content first produced by normal children should be employed as the first objectives for the intervention program. However, the explication of a theory does not necessarily mean that it provides a framework for programs for children who have not acquired language through normal processes.

In addition to the content of the program, the learning principles upon which the strategies are based also constitute an area of disagreement. Although the Bricker and Bricker program stresses the operant or instrumental conditioning paradigm, classical conditioning principles are another option available to the clinician. However, a concern was voiced during the discussion that learning theory approaches may result in techniques which are inappropriate to the natural acquisition of language. Normal language development processes may contain procedures and techniques which have not been thoroughly analyzed and made available to the clinician.

When considering a program for the hearing-impaired, the problem of the form of the communication symbol confounds the issue. The Horton program is indicative of an aural-oral approach which places emphasis upon auditory input assisted by hearing aids when necessary and an oral response from the child. An alternative is the "manual" or sign language system which initially emphasizes a gestural mode and later moves the youngster to an oral communication system. One approach to resolving the issue has been to initiate an oral approach but switch to the manual when the child appears to be unsuccessful with the former. However, the alternative could be to initiate communication with either system to get the child interacting with the environment but maintain oral language as the ultimate goal.

Another concept was presented during the discussion, namely, that the content or learning principles are not as significant as the emotional relationship between the youngster and the parents. The professional's role is to guide the parents in their attempts to understand the child's reactions to his problems and how he communicates this reaction to his environment.

The discussion did not culminate in any agreement over these issues. It basically reflected the difficulties which professionals have in adapting the information from one area of study, normal development, and utilizing it in another, early intervention. Some broad conclusions can, however, be derived from the discussion:

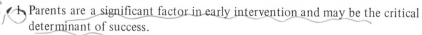

1. Parents are a significant factor in early intervention and may be the critical determinant of success.
2. Continued research is needed to understand the developmental process, particularly those aspects which can be adapted to an early intervention program.
3. The emphasis in early intervention should be on the stimuli and processes which are relevant to the acquisition of skills rather than on the skills themselves.
4. The technology for early identification of communication problems should be utilized in systematic follow-up programs for high risk infants and toddlers. These programs are essential for children who manifest mild to moderate problems which are frequently missed in routine examinations.

REFERENCES

AAOO, AAP, and ASHA, Joint Committee statement on infant hearing screening (November 1970). *ASHA,* 1971, *13,* 79.

AAOO, AAP, and ASHA, Supplementary statement of the Joint Committee on infant hearing screening (July 1972). *ASHA,* 1974, *16,* 160.

Downs, M. P. The identification of congenital deafness. *Trans. Amer. Acad. Ophthalmol. Otolaryngol.,* 1970, *74,* 1208–1214.

Downs, M. P. and Hemenway, W. G. Newborn screening revisited. *Hear. Speech News,* 1972, *40,* No. 4, 4–5, 26, 28–29.

Fulton, R. T. and Lloyd, L. L. (Eds.). *Audiometry for the Retarded: With Implications for the Difficult-to-Test.* Baltimore: Williams and Wilkins, 1969.

Goldstein, R. and Tait, C. Critique of neonatal hearing evaluation. *J. Speech Hear. Disord.*, 1971, *36*, 3–18.

Jerger, J. (Ed.). *Modern Developments in Audiology*, Ed. 2. New York: Academic Press, 1973.

Meier, J. *Screening and Assessment of Young Children at Developmental Risk.* Washington, D.C.: The President's Committee on Mental Retardation, 1973.

VII LANGUAGE INTERVENTION FOR THE MENTALLY RETARDED

CHAPTER TWENTY

AN ONTOGENETIC LANGUAGE TEACHING STRATEGY FOR RETARDED CHILDREN[1]

Jon F. Miller and David E. Yoder

Department of Communicative Disorders, University of Wisconsin, Madison, Wisconsin 53706

To develop communication skills in every mentally retarded child has been a goal [and desire] of parents, educators, and clinicians for many years. The professional literature is replete with descriptions and reports of speech and language teaching programs. These programs have been popular since special education first became recognized in this country and earlier in Europe with the work of Maria Montessori.

With the recent explosion of information related to developmental psychology, cognitive psychology, psycholinguistics, and principles of behavior modification, we are in a much better position to survey the field. We can also make some speculative comments about where we should be going as professionals interested in improving communication behaviors of mentally retarded children.

Within the past 5 years a plethora of programs published under the general rubric of "language development or language teaching for the retarded" have appeared in the professional literature and on the commercial market. What do these so-called language programs really teach? The answer, of course, rests with our individual understanding of language behavior, which undoubtedly also includes some intrinsic or extrinsic criteria for how one goes about teaching language behavior.

In reviewing the literature related to the communication of retarded children, we find a number of studies which demonstrate that retarded children can and do learn linguistic features when the environment is structured to reinforce appropriate and inappropriate behavior differentially.

Most language teaching programs for retarded children are based to some degree on the principles of behavior modification. Some are strictly operant and neo-Skinnerian in character. Others make use of other principles or techniques based on operant theory. Some clinicians employ systematic reinforcement without consistently subscribing to the theoretical framework. They do not base their teaching program on a functional analysis of behavior.

[1] The work reported here was supported in part by Grant MCT-000915-06-0 from the United States Public Health Service and Mental Health Administration.

Most programs using a behavior modification approach can be simplistically summarized in the following way: Where sentence production is the target response, a number of prerequisite behaviors are taught in a sequential order. Receptive vocabulary is taught by reinforcing an act of discrimination based on relevant dimensions and extinguishing the child's responses to the irrelevant components in a two-choice situation. Later in the sequence of behaviors to be taught, motor imitative then vocal imitative behaviors are presented. Then, by combining the previously learned receptive vocabulary with the program on developing imitative behaviors, labeling of objects is taught. Eventually, all past learning culminates in teaching sentence production.

One can be skeptical of the specificity of this approach. No language program can possible teach all the responses a child will need (or could naturally make) simply by a program employing imitation, modeling, and differential use of reinforcement. Such programs only allow the acquisition of echolalic surface structures. Brown and Bellugi-Klima (1971) have commented that, "the processes of imitation and expansion are not sufficient to account for the degree of linguistic competence that children regularly acquire . . ." (pp. 314–315).

One might ask (after reviewing the studies based strictly on operant paradigms) what we have demonstrated other than the fact that retarded children can learn some topographical language responses. Are the behaviors generalizable to a functional communication system which allows a person to solve problems and engage in social interactions?

The previous discussion related to the use of behavior modification in teaching language to retarded children is not meant to depreciate its importance. But we do call into question some of the ways it has been used. The operant or behavioral approach may be more appropriate for some language skills than for others. In many cases, the clinician is confronted by a child with a total absence of language or even vocalizations. It may be necessary to implement a program of shaping behavior to find out whether the individual's vocalizations can in any specifiable sense be brought under operant control. Not restricting a program to production aspects allows the clinician to consider what kind of skills are necessary for the development of communication behavior, to apply a functional assessment to these skills, and to plan an appropriate program to compensate for deficits.

Allowing a child to develop a system to communicate basic needs, wants, and ideas requires more than mere acquisition of linguistic features taught in specified ways and places. Mittler (in press), Morehead (1972), Miller and Yoder (1972a,b), and others have suggested that imaginative and representational play along with appropriate stimulation within living environments forms an important foundation for cognitive and linguistic development. The ability to play or cope in such a way as to make one object or activity stand for another is one precursor of learning that things have names and that language can be used creatively and generatively. To the extent that language development is related to general representation and is dependent upon conceptual development, it may be necessary to assess and attempt to develop certain conceptual functions as an integral part of a communication development program for retarded children.

The importance of planning a language or communication training curriculum in the context of a consistent theoretical and procedural framework is repeatedly stressed in the work of Bricker and Bricker (1970a,b), Lynch and Bricker (1972), and Miller and Yoder (1972a,b). They believe that synthesizing psycholinguistic and behavioral models results in the most effective and efficient communication teaching programs. The psycholinguistic information assists in determining the content of instruction, as well as the processes necessary for acquisition, while behavior management provides the instructional procedures to teach that content most effectively.

As more studies of child language emerge, we change our understanding of what it is that children learn when they learn language. We are now also beginning to understand how the child may be acquiring language, in terms of the processes and strategies employed. As the data on language development are compiled and new analyses are implemented, the theories of acquisition need to be rethought. Such a rethinking process appears to be going on at the present time in child language. A new perspective is emerging regarding the basis for the acquisition process. This is a shift from a syntactic basis to a conceptual-semantic basis.

Theories in child language will continue to change as we strive for a better understanding of the language acquisition process. Therefore, it is important that language teaching programs be constructed to accommodate new data as they emerge. We believe the best way to do this is to develop a set of program criteria and a set of operating principles to implement the program. This results in an approach to programming based on a set of principles with decision rules to be applied to each child. The program will conform to the child's needs and abilities rather than the child conforming to the program. This paper represents the accommodation of new perspectives and data in child language into the general program format set down by Miller and Yoder (1972a).

In our own work with retarded children we have developed the following set of criteria to guide program development. We have found them to be sound reference points from which we can operate to provide a functional communication system for retarded children.

1. A program must be based on a realistic set of communication exit behaviors. Here we base the terminal behavior on linguistic needs which a given child may have, dependent upon the living and educational environment as well as developmental abilities.

2. A program must be based on what is known about normal cognitive and psycholinguistic development.

3. A language program must take into account the kinds of interactions that normally take place between children and persons in their environments.
4. Language programs must help the child become an active participant in linguistic and nonlinguistic experiences which enhance his communication competence.
5. A program must have a systematic approach to teaching the desirable and appropriate language.

Figure 1 is a hierarchical framework within which we believe we can work to effectively bring about our desired communication behavior with the retarded child. The target response as indicated across the top of the diagram is that of communication and all the adjunct subresponses. That behavior is acquired by an individual exposed to a system as indicated under the column "Features" as well as through multiple experiences which would be found under "Situations." We have listed both linguistic and paralinguistic features as important to communication. But we wish to point out that emitted features alone cannot and do not bring about dyadic communication events. Consequently, it is necessary to combine the feature with the situation and then to evaluate the consequence to indicate whether a communicative event has resulted. For example, the child who emits the response "no eat" in the presence of an empty plate is probably indicating that he is finished with the task of eating, whereas the child who emits the same response in the presence of a full plate may be indicating that he does not wish to engage in the act of eating. Not only are we interested in the feature-plus-situation aspect to gain better information about the child's linguistic intentions, but we believe that by using the situation (environments) in which the child spends the majority of his time as experiential and teaching environments we will increase the probability of more closely meeting communication needs of the individual. This procedure will result in teaching him very relevant communication behaviors. We are aware that some very basic prerequisite behaviors may need to be brought under control within structured therapeutic situations before attempting to teach the behaviors in more open and natural situations. A program based on the teaching of such behaviors as auditory skills, discrimination, memory, etc. is not sufficient to develop communication competence in retarded children.

We wish now to direct our discussion to some fundamental ideas which are important in any language and communication teaching program. The ideas which we are developing here are applicable to any child regardless of his level of development. We are limiting our discussion primarily to children at the presyntax stage of development, but the tenets put forth are as applicable to a child at a more advanced level of development.

Fig. 1.

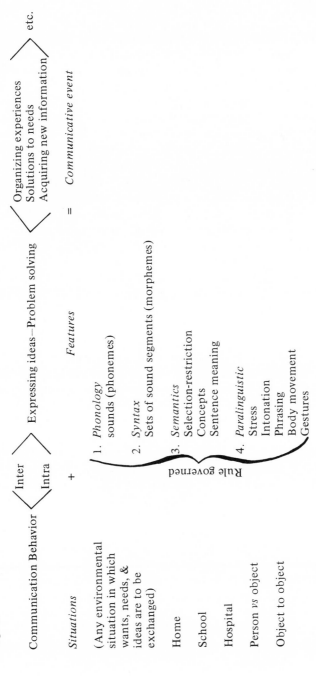

CONTENT

Constructing language training programs involves several component parts. First, it is necessary to have an understanding of what children learn when they are beginning a language. This involves, of course, the knowledge of what language is, its form and functions. With an understanding of what it is that children learn, we will then know what is to be taught (the content). The second component is the order or sequence in which the content should be presented. Content sequence should be based on a rationale which will promote ease of learning. Thirdly, after content and sequence are determined, a teaching technology needs to be selected. The teaching strategy should be implemented according to the content to be taught. The technology employed to teach the content at stage I of language development is likely to differ in the techniques and implementation strategies from those used to teach the content at stage V of language development. Fourthly, the three components of the teaching program are dependent upon the cognitive and linguistic level of the child.

In developing the framework for a language teaching program, the goal will be to develop a set of operating principles which reflect current developmental theory and data. These operating principles will provide the framework for program implementation with individual children and will reflect the flexible and creative nature of language and its basic function—communication.

The language behavior of mentally retarded persons has been studied extensively. However, few studies have been developmental in nature. Most studies have been designed to determine if the language of retarded children is deficient when compared with matched normal children or to report the number of retarded children who have deficiencies. These studies are not very useful to persons who are trying to determine similarities and/or differences in the language acquisition process between retarded and normal children. A review of the literature completed in 1970 (Yoder and Miller, 1972) concluded that retarded children develop the language code in a manner similar to children without intellectual deficits, but at a slower rate. The most recent literature does not alter this general conclusion. However, that conclusion is equivocal in that there are few developmental studies and no longitudinal studies of language development in retarded children at this time. At the present time, then, we will assume that retarded children acquire language in a manner similar to nonretardates except for a rate difference. This assumption provides the basis for the first operating principle dealing with content selection. Since the basic problem is to develop a program to teach language rather than remediate an existing deviant system, the following operating principle is proposed: *I. The content for language training for retarded children should be taken from the data available on language development in normal children* (Miller and Yoder, 1972a,b).

Implicit within this operating principle is the notion that through study of the normal developmental data we will be able to determine what it is that children learn and something about the necessary conditions for language learning. Within the area of normal language development, there have been rapidly changing views (and new insights) regarding the basic elements acquired in initial language learning. These changing views represent a shift from viewing acquisition as based on syntactic units to a recognition that acquisition is probably based on semantic units. This shift was precipitated by Bloom (1970), who studied what children talk about in the early stages of language development rather than studying the form (syntax) of children's utterances alone. Her work produced some different conclusions about what is being learned linguistically. The grammars that resulted from Bloom's study, when semantic intent was taken into account, looked different from previous early grammars, revealing that 1) not all children acquire syntax in exactly the same way, 2) there is a relatively close approximation to adult syntax, and 3) children's utterances are intentional and express semantic functions relative to their experiences.

Subsequent studies of children's early productions (Schlesinger, 1971a; Brown, 1973a,b) paralleled Bloom's findings to the extent that they analyzed utterances in context to determine semantic intent. The Bloom, Schlesinger, and Brown studies differed in the degree to which they relied on syntax as the explanatory basis for characterizing what children know about structural relationships in the early stages of language development. Bloom (1970) and Brown (1973a,b) considered the structural relationships evidenced in child speech to be syntactically based, while Schlesinger (1971a,b) has proposed that the components of the structural relationships expressed by children's utterances are semantic concepts rather than syntactic structures. In Schlesinger's production model, semantic concepts such as agent, action, object, possession, and location are the basic structural components of sentences. These semantic concepts are produced by syntactic devices directly, rather than being derived from basic syntactic information. Children's early utterances, though based on semantic concepts, reflect syntactic knowledge in that the position of concepts in utterances and the grammatical category for each position need to be established for production. The mechanisms Schlesinger proposed to account for position and grammatical category of position are syntactic.

Bowerman (1971), studying two Finnish children and one American child, sought to answer the question, "How can the structural relationships expressed in children's early word combinations best be described?" (p. 1). After evaluating existing proposals, Bowerman concluded that there is little evidence to justify crediting children with knowledge of basic grammatical relations and the constituent structure which they entail. In her view, children initially learn semantic concepts and begin combining words through learning simple order rules. These early word combinations perform functions which are basically semantic, such as "agent," "action," "object acted upon." Only later through experience does the child organize his knowledge according to the more abstract grammatical relationships of his language.

The findings discussed so far have been studies of children's early language production. In order to come to some conclusion as to whether children's early utterances reflect knowledge of basic grammatical relations, subject-verb-object (S-V-O), or reflect ordering strategies based on expression of semantic functions, let us briefly examine studies of children's comprehension behavior. Children must be able to comprehend S-V-O constructions with contrasting word order to be credited knowledge of basic grammatical relations. That is, word order is basically a syntactic phenomenon and if the child has syntactic knowledge he should be able to use word order to determine subject and object in contrasting sentences on a comprehension task. This behavior should be evident during at least the last half of developmental stage I as defined by Brown (MLU—mean length of utterance— 1.0–2.0). The result of one comprehension study with stage I children indicates that word order is not used consistently by these children (deVilliers and deVilliers, 1972 as reported in Brown, 1973). Smith (1972), although not studying word order directly, found that early stage 1 children (MLU 1–1.25) comprehended two-word S-V and V-O constructions at 90% correct, three-word S-V-O constructions and fully grammatical S-V-O constructions at 20% correct; late stage I children (MLU 1.50–2.0) S-V, V-O, and S-V-O and fully grammatical sentences all at 50% correct; while stage II children (MLU 2.0–2.5) comprehended S-V and V-O at 10%, S-V-O at 80%, and fully grammatical sentences at 90% correct. These data indicate a possible shift on the part of the child from a semantically based strategy early to a more general syntactic strategy later in development. All constructions tested were of agent-action-object of action semantic form. Other studies (Owings, 1972; Carrow, 1968) have indicated that children do not master subject-object relations in comprehension until later, ages 5 and 3, respectively. Two other studies in press (Bever, Mehler, and Valian; and deVilliers and deVilliers) which are reported by Brown (1973a,b) provide evidence for use of order at stage I. However, Brown cited two other studies which support knowledge of word order cues at stage I. Subjects were grouped by age rather than developmental stage (Fraser, Bellugi, and Brown, 1963; Lovell and Dixon, 1967). It is unlikely that the subjects in these last two studies were at stage I language development. Wetstone and Friedlander (1973) reported that children in the one- and two-word stages of production development respond as correctly or relevantly to questions and commands with distorted word order as to those with normal word order, responding to both at above chance levels. Finally, a study by Chapman and Miller (1973) investigated the relationship between the child's use of word order as a cue in comprehension and production of subject-verb-object sentences. The three groups of subjects were defined by production stage of development as measured by MLU (group 1, MLU = 1.75; 2, MLU = 2.25; and 3, MLU = 2.75). The pattern of performance for each group was the same. Correct word order for subject and object was observed significantly more often in speaking than as a cue to subject and object in the comprehension task. Chapman and Miller concluded that production precedes comprehension in grammatical acquisition for subject-object structures.

In conclusion, from the available comprehension data, children do not appear to employ syntactic strategies in comprehension when they begin to put words together. Indeed, their use of word order appears to increase as more language is acquired. Comprehension of sentences based on grammatical cues improves only as linguistic knowledge increases and may not be complete until sometime after the child can comprehend and produce sentences of a particular form in context, i.e., appropriate environmental circumstances and experiences.

In reference to the preceding discussion, we draw the following conclusions regarding what a child is learning when he is acquiring his language. Semantic concepts provide the basis for early language acquisition. Through experience with objects and events around him, the child begins to perceive particular objects and relationships conceptually. At the same time he is experiencing the linguistic code of his community spoken around him. Through frequent experiences with particular objects and relations with accompanying linguistic marking of environmental events, the child begins to mark linguistically those objects and relationships he perceives conceptually. When perceived objects and relationships are marked, they become semantic concepts and the child has begun to map aspects of his experience linguistically. Semantic concepts, then, are derived directly from the child's experience, both linguistic and nonlinguistic. After the child attains the concept of object permanency, his expression at the single word level increases in terms of lexicon size, particularly for substantive forms, and also in expressing relationships in new situations (Bloom, 1973). The functions expressed at the single word level then become expressed with two words (see Table 1). Relatively few new functions are expressed as the child moves to two-word forms. This phenomenon would tend to support Bowerman's (1971) notion that early structural relationships are based on simple order strategies that are semantically based and intended to express a specific function. Table 1 shows that children express similar semantic functions all the way through stage I, though the form of their utterances is increasing in length from one to up to seven morphemes (Brown, 1973a,b). Within this framework, syntax can be thought of as a general abstract organizational structure which allows the child to use the numerous semantic concepts acquired in comprehension and production in a manner consistent with his linguistic community.

Table 1. Functions Expressed in Early Production Stage 1*

Relational Functions Single Word Utterance Level		
Recurrence	Request Comment	More
Nonexistence	Existence expected	No
Disappearance	Existence in immediately preceding context	Away A gone
Rejection		No
Cessation	Ongoing event ceased	Stop
Existence	Objects or people pointed out, noticed, or found Events that were sudden or startling	There Uh Oh
Substantive Functions		
Comments Greetings	Attaching a linguistic sign or label to the per- ceived event of:	Mama Dada Mimi Baby
Vocatives	To call for someone (less frequent than comments or greetings)	Mama Dada Mimi
Agent	Agent of an intended or immediate action	Mama Dada Mimi Baby
Object	(Infrequent occurrence) object of an action	Mama Dada Mimi Baby
Action	Marking of action or event states	Tumble Back Catch Turn Tire
Possession	Objects associated with: Objects belonging to:	Daddy Mommy

*Sources: Bloom, 1970, 1973; Brown, 1970, 1973a, b; Schlesinger, 1971a, b.

Functional Relations, Two-Word Utterances

Existence	This (a, the, that, it, there) + substantive word
Recurrence	More (another) + substantive word; used as request or comment
Nonexistence	No (away, all gone) + substantive word; used also to express disappearance
Rejection	No + substantive word
Denial	No + substantive word (late)

Semantic Relations

Agent-action	N + V	Daddy hit, Adam put, Eve read
Action-object	V + N	Hit ball, put book, read book
Agent-object	N + N	Mommy sock, Mommy pigtail, Mommy milk
Possessive	N + N	Daddy chair, Mommy lunch, Adam checker
Locative (two forms)	N + N	Sweater chair, book table, bear raisin
	V + N	Walk street, go store
Attributive	Adj + N	Big train, Red book
Experiencer-state	I (me) + hear, want, love, need.

Datives of indirect objects	Give Mommy
Commitatives	Walk Mommy
Instrumentals	Sweep broom

Second Half of Stage 1 MLU 1.50 (Brown, 1973a, b)

Three-Term Relations

Type I

Agent-action-object

Agent-action-locative

Action-object-locative

Appear to be combinations of semantic relations expressed earlier in Stage 1 with repeating term omitted; *i.e.,* agent-action, (Adam hit) + action-object (hit ball)→ agent-action-object (Adam hit ball) with redundant action (hit) deleted (Brown, 1973)

Type II

Noun phrase expansion within two-term relation

Two-term relations expanded from within always express one of the following: attribution, possession or recurrence; example: action-locative (sit chair)→ (sit Daddy chair) locative expanded as possessive (Brown, 1973)

Four-Term Relations

At the end of Stage 1, four-term relations are of the same two types as described for three-term relations.

The need for syntax arises on the part of the child in order to make his expression of semantic concepts understood by others in his community. That is, a consistent form for utterances is necessary for communication to take place. This form, syntax, allows the expression of semantic concepts in a variety of ways that may be unique but fully comprehensible. It would appear that the development of syntax begins at stage II and continues for quite a few years (Chomsky, 1969; Epstein, 1973).

The things that children talk about in their first utterances are remarkably consistent across languages (Brown, 1973a,b; Bowerman, 1971). The functions that children express in stage I (MLU 1.0–2.0) are listed in Table 1. This consistency across language provides further support for the notion that semantic concepts are the basis for language development. The similarity of functions expressed in early development is the result of perceptual-cognitive development which is universally consistent for all human beings. Although all languages can be described syntactically, children acquire syntax over time as a means of mapping the semantic concepts acquired for communication needs in their linguistic community.

In considering the first component of the three (content, sequence, technology) necessary in constructing a language teaching program, we conclude that the basis of early language development is the semantic concept. Semantic concepts or functions, then, are the basic elements to be taught in the teaching program. With the application of the first operating principle, "The content for language training for retarded children should be taken from the data available on language development in normal children," the semantic functions delineated in Table 1 become the basic content for the teaching program for children working through stage I of development.

SEQUENCE

The second component of the teaching program to consider is the order or sequence in which the content should be presented. The ordering of content can be approached logically in two ways. First, order of content can be according to the frequency of occurrence of semantic functions expressed by normal children. Secondly, content order may be according to the sequence in which semantic functions are acquired by normal children.

First, frequency of occurrence in child language probably reflects two factors. 1) At the beginning of stage I it reflects the frequency with which the child comes in contact with particular objects and events in his environment. Since initially single words are used to comment on the child's own or others' actions within a specific context (Bloom, 1973), the frequency with which semantic functions are expressed is dependent upon the frequency of experience with the objects and events marked by semantic functions. 2) Later, as the child talks about the interaction of objects and events and is able to mark new instances of semantic functions in his experience, frequency of occurrence probably reflects communicative value for the child of particular functions as well as a means of solving certain need situations.

The second approach to ordering content for teaching, *i.e.*, recapitulation of the sequence in which semantic functions are acquired by normal children, may reflect the difficulty level of the functions acquired. Those expressed early are assumed to be easier to learn than those expressed later. Referring back to Table 1, the functions expressed early, with single words, are remarkably similar to those expressed later in stage I. There appear to be few new functions expressed as the child proceeds through stage I. What does change, however, is the specificity with which semantic functions are expressed. This increased specificity reflects a change in utterance form through stage I. The general form of utterances, expressed grammatically, is subject-verb-object with the child beginning to expand the forms used by the end of stage I, negative, interrogative, and imperative (Brown, 1970). This second approach to ordering content does not provide much direction for ordering semantic concepts. It does, however, provide a basis for ordering the forms with which semantic functions are expressed. Although an explicit invariant order of utterance forms acquired does not exist, a general ordering of the forms children acquire can be derived for stages I–V from existing developmental data.

The semantic functions listed in Table 1 are not listed necessarily in the order of acquisition within each utterance length category. This could not be done with any degree of confidence because of the limited number of subjects studied, and the stages (in MLUs) the samples were taken for study. The functions listed are in general those most frequently used by the children studied and account for the majority of their utterances.

There are two component parts of the content, then, to be considered in developing a sequence for a language teaching program: 1) the semantic functions and 2) the form to be specified for the expression of the semantic functions. For specifying a teaching order for these two factors the following operating principle is offered: *II. Semantic concepts should be ordered for teaching on the basis of frequency of occurrence (see Table 1), and selection of the utterance form for expression should be determined by the sequence of forms acquired by normal children.*

In applying the operating principle to the functions first expressed at the beginning of stage I with single words, it becomes apparent that most of these functions occur frequently in child speech. It is necessary, then, to choose which of these functions are to be taught first. On what basis can such a decision be made? The factor most directly related to the process the normal children appear to go through is both linguistic and nonlinguistic experience. Experience with objects and events in the child's environment is the basis for early linguistic marking. An inventory of the nonlinguistic experiences and the environmental situation of the child who is to be programmed will reveal those experiences which occur frequently. This analysis will also help to determine the choice of lexical items to be specified for marking particular semantic functions. This procedure individualizes the content and makes it directly relevant to the child's experiences and environmental situation. Although all children share certain common experiences (eating, toileting, dressing), these experiences for retarded children may not be carried out in the same environmental situation. The retarded child may be living in a residential facility, foster home, or residential school. In these situations the child's experience with adults, in eating, toileting, and dressing activities, is likely to be less consistent, because more adults are involved at different times of the day than with the child living at home. Even for a common set of activities, the retarded child may experience many different adults carrying out these activities with and for him. While there may be similar activities experienced, environmental circumstances may differ, as well as the linguistic experience between adults in the environment. The selection of a lexicon, then, should reflect the child's environmental situation and needs, with variation most evident for substantive functions, *i.e.,* names of people, actions of which the child is capable. Functional relationships can be marked with the same lexicon used by normal children since they are not referent-specific or tied to specific environmental events.

The basis for teaching semantic functions lies in the child's experience with objects and events in his environment. It is essential for the child's own unique experiences to serve as the basis of training, thereby maximizing what the child brings to the learning situation in terms of his potential perceptual-cognitive awareness of objects and events around him. Rather than contriving unique situations and experiences for the child and teaching him to mark them, the child is taught to linguistically mark objects and relations through familiar context which will enable him to express these directly in his environment.

PROGRAM FORMAT

The level of language content this program proposes to teach has been described as stage I in normal children (MLU 1.0–2.0). The basic program content is detailed in Table 1. The goal is to develop a functional communication system in the child, regardless of the level of expression employed. With semantic functions as the basis for teaching, first utterances will be communicative within specific contexts. The acquisition of both relational and substantive functions expressed by single words provides the child with the necessary components to move logically to expressing these functions more explicitly with two words. Later this provides the basis for his acquisition of the grammatical regularities of his language. Because several factors may limit language acquisition in retarded children, we will not be able to teach a fully developed language system to every child. With this program, regardless of the level of language at which the child ceases learning, he will be able to communicate within his environment to some extent.

The children for whom this program is intended need only limited capabilities to begin the program sequence. Minimally, the child may be producing approximations to single words or indicate cognitive awareness of one or more relational or substantive functions through gestural or behavioral responses. If awareness of functions is evident but there is no meaningful production, it is essential to establish that the speech mechanism is intact and capable of producing articulated speech. Minimal requirements for entry, then, are: 1) intact speech mechanism and 2) cognitive awareness of one of more relational or substantive functions or 3) production of approximations of single words, imitative or spontaneous. This program is not intended to move the child from vocal behavior (babbling) to verbal behavior (first word). A separate program with specifically delineated steps needs to be developed to move the child from vocal to verbal behavior.

Entry at any point in the sequence of content in stage I is possible, of course, providing that appropriate measures of baseline language functioning are taken. The measures should include mean length of utterance in words or morphemes (see Slobin, 1967, for analysis procedures); evaluation of the corpus to determine the relational and substantive functions expressed, according to utterance form; observation of the child's environmental situation, to chart frequency of occurrence of specific experiences marking functions expressed by children at stage I; observation of the child's behavior to chart indications (gestural, vocal, or verbal) of cognitive-perceptual awareness of stage I functions; and, finally, an indication of the child's level of cognitive development relative to the sensorimotor period and the functions the child's language expresses in stage I (see Mehrabian and Williams, 1971, for tasks relevant to this purpose). Relationship between the child's level of conceptual development and language will be discussed in more detail in a later section. With this information, the appropriate entry point for the content and sequence can be determined for the child.

The major components of a language teaching program like the normal language acquisition situation are: the child's experience, linguistic and non-linguistic, and the child's cognitive-perceptual development. The interaction of these phenomena results in language being acquired. Since the retarded child has not acquired a language system within his environment through this interactive process, the teaching program must intervene. Since to intervene implies a rearrangement of factors, what factor or factors can be manipulated to facilitate acquisition of communication? Of the two basic components, environment and conceptual behavior, only environment can be manipulated directly. Cognition, *i.e.,* what the child brings to the task, falls within the realm of private events. According to Piagetian theory, however, the child's interaction with objects and events in his environment (experiences) does alter conceptual behavior. It remains to be determined whether the conceptual development of retarded children can be facilitated through structuring experiences. Acquisition will be enhanced by altering experience, from a general nonspecific nature to noting specific functional relations with accompanying linguistic marking. By pairing explicit environmental experiences with their linguistic referent, the child will note these relations and begin to express them.

There are two general factors representing interaction with environmental events which may be manipulated for any language treatment program: 1) experience with objects and events and 2) experience with the language of his community. The goal of treatment programs is to control these factors in systematic ways to facilitate learning. For the most part, treatment programs have been concerned primarily with one or the other of these factors and have only minimally recognized the importance of the interaction between the two for the acquisition of language. For example, behavior modification programs have typically concentrated on organizing the child's experience within the learning situation to control the child's behavior (*i.e.,* attention, motivation), to increase the frequency of occurrence of appropriate responses to specific stimuli. These programs, with their exacting technology, are effective in altering and shaping a multitude of behaviors, including verbal behavior. Where these programs have experienced difficulty is in developing spontaneous, creative language which the child can use in his community. The child's language typically consists of stereotypic verbal productions which are responses to specific verbal or nonverbal stimuli within the learning situation. Generally, without additional specific programming related to the sociolinguistic aspects of his language, the child makes little use of these responses outside the learning situation.

It is our contention that these two problems are the result of several factors within behavioral programs and do not conflict with the general tenets of behavioral management. The first is program content; the second is sequence of content; the third is the pairing of experiences (from the child's environment directly with the appropriate linguistic marking by the child); the fourth is contingencies for reinforcement; and the fifth is definition of success or terminal behaviors. By using different operating principles, definitions, and criteria, the problems of stereotypic verbal productions and limited generalization to the natural language situation can be overcome.

The first two factors—the rationale for the content and the operating principles for determining the sequence of the content for teaching—have been detailed in preceding sections. The third factor, the pairing of linguistic with nonlinguistic experiences in the treatment situation is basically an application factor—application, that is, of the principles laid out in the first two factors. Through pairing explicit environmental experiences with their linguistic referent, the child will note these relations and their markers and begin to express them. The starting point should be with those semantic relations frequently expressed in the child's experience and for which he has demonstrated cognitive-perceptual awareness (see Table 1). We are then ready to evoke operating principle III: *Select a single frequently occurring experience demonstrating a particular semantic function. Pair with the appropriate lexical marker, and after child demonstrates mastery, move to multiple experiences expressing the same function.* The child should be taken through the following steps toward mastery of the lexical marking of the semantic relation with the application of operating principle III: 1) exposure to the paired experience with the lexical marking (no verbal production required from the child); 2) indication of comprehension of the lexical marker in relation to the experience; 3) pairing of experience with lexical marker with imitative response requested from the child; 4) beginning to fade child's imitative responses in favor of spontaneous responses by introducing different, familiar experiences expressing the same semantic function and marking them for the child; and 5) stabilizing the child's spontaneous marking of the function through fading the marking of each function expressed experientially. For example, we have found severely retarded children who have begun to use some referential words to label objects, engaging in what we considered limited communication, if one could even call it communication at all, until relational experiences were comprehended. One subject was taught the semantic concept *recurrence* marked by the relational term "more" by programming activities which had high interest and motivational components built in to them. A programmed activity was continued only when the child requested that it continue by emitting the response "more." Since the child was at a verbal imitation stage, it was not difficult to get the verbal response under control. However, with few trials, it was possible to manipulate the situations so that the child emitted a high rate of "more" marking recurrence, and without prompting or being taught its use in other situations soon began to pair it appropriately with other referents and to expand it to two- and three-word combinations. The same experience was encountered in teaching the semantic functions nonexistence and disappearance. Our limited experience with two subjects would indicate that, once the child acquired semantic function (through the experiences offered), he used the appropriate relational term and then generalized it appropriately to manipulate his environment in different ways. This was evidenced on the ward, in a school situation, and in free play activities.

The procedure outlined is not meant to be unidimensional, working, that is, on only one function at a time. We have found that working on one function leads to faster acquisition for the child than beginning with several different functions. After the first function is mastered in one context, other functions can be introduced without decreasing performance. This then allows for work on several functions at different levels of mastery.

When the child is spontaneously marking a function in a variety of experiential settings, expansion techniques should be employed. Expansion of utterance form can be initiated before the child can express all the functions listed under the single word level in Table 1. Normal children begin to express certain functions with two words while others are expressed with a single word. The levels of semantic functions listed in Table 1 are by no means static.

Which type of single word utterance should be expanded first? For most children studied, utterances expressing relational functions are expanded first, "more" "more milk" (Brown, 1970). In analyzing closely what is being expressed additionally in early expansions, it appears that with relational functions—recurrence, existence, nonexistence, etc.—the expansion marks the referent within a specific context. At the two-word level these are called functional relations by Bloom (1970). The expansion appears to be a rather straightforward operation of designating the specific referent for which the relationship holds in context. For expansions of substantive forms (agent, action, possessive, object), the child moves to expression of relationship between two substantive functions in a particular situational experience (agent-action, action-object, agent-object, and possesses-possessed, etc.). These utterances have been termed semantic relations by Brown (1973a,b) where the relationship is expressed by the two co-occurring substantive forms in context.

According to Brown (1970), functional relations occur in child speech before semantic relations. This may be a result of their being cognitively more obvious than relationships expressed by two co-occurring substantive words. Indeed, with retarded children we have found greater ease of learning trials to appropriate expression for functional relations over semantic relations. After some functional relations are expressed, however, semantic relations are learned more rapidly than before. Therefore, when expansions are indicated after several frequently occurring relational functions and substantive functions have been acquired, first expansions should be of relational functions. This leads to operating principle IV: *First expansions of single word utterances should be of relational functions previously expressed.*

Expansion forms used to mark specific functions at the two-word level can be noted in Table 1. Expansions are generally a matter of introducing new forms to the child to mark functions within the child's repertoire. This procedure reflects half of the operating principle expressed by Slobin (1970) for normal children acquiring language: "New forms first express old functions." The second half of this principle "New functions are first expressed by old forms" (p. 2), provides a basis for determining the lexical markers for new functions to be taught. One need only look at Table 1 to see numerous examples of the last half of Slobin's operating principle, particularly at the single word level. Modeling procedures should be employed as a way of introducing primarily new forms to the child. Occasionally, however, new functions can be introduced through modeling as comments about a particular experiential situation. The uses of imitation, expansion, and modeling in language training were discussed in a previous program. We will not discuss them further as their use has not changed since the advent of that program. For further details, see Miller and Yoder (1972a).

The other point yet to be discussed in relation to factor 3 is the general nature of linguistic input to the child. The linguistic input to the child should be structured to maximize comprehension on the part of the child as well as to explicitly mark the function experienced. Therefore, keeping in mind the preceding discussion of the interaction of form and function, the linguistic input to the child should in general be one step more advanced than the child's stage of language production as measured by MLU, except at the initial stages of single word utterance development. Input to the child would initially be single words only, marking specific functions; later two- and three-word markings through expansions; then short, simple, fully grammatical sentences. Toward the end of stage 1 production development, expansions should reflect the order of development of the 14 functional morphemes described by Brown (1973a,b) for stage II of production development. These expansions should be within a fully grammatical sentence form. Besides providing explicit linguistic marking for the semantic functions to be taught, this type of input facilitates comprehension as long as the child's stage of production development is monitored (Shipley, Smith, and Gleitman, 1969; Smith, 1972).

The fourth factor to be discussed relevant to the decisions made in treatment program development is specification of the contingencies for reinforcement. It is important to remember that a single form may be used to express several functions and several forms can express a single function (see Table 1). This concept is particularly important for determining the category of responses to be reinforced. For example, we have one youngster to whom we have taught the semantic function *action* marked by "eat." The eat response is now used by the child in multiple situations to express multiple functions. He will say eat in the presence of the food to be eaten. "Eat" is used to label the utensils with which he will eat the food. "Eat" is emitted to indicate the act of eating as well as to indicate that he is hungry and wishes to eat. Observing, then, the situations in which the word "eat" is used allows us to know the intent of the response. The child has communicated appropriately within his environment. It is not always possible to determine the exact function the child is expressing, particularly in the early stages of training and because determination of the function rests on a judgment of an observer taking into account the context. Therefore, reinforcement should be administered when an appropriate form is *emitted* in context. It should be noted that this procedure allows for the reinforcement of so-called "extraneous responses" on the part of the child. This is important because extraneous responses reflect the child's acquisition processes at work and these responses are probably more important to reinforce than those specified in the program because they are reflecting what the child brings to the task and are more natural for him. In examining extraneous responses resulting from several programs for retarded children, there is great similarity in their form when compared to the forms produced by normal children in the early stages of language development (Kent, 1970). The reinforcement of the appropriate form emitted in context results in the potential reinforcement of a class of forms all expressing the same function as well as a single form expressing several functions. This procedure also allows for a flexible system which is adaptable to the comprehension and production abilities of the individual child.

The fifth factor to be discussed involves the definition of success or terminal behaviors. The terminal behavior intrinsically specified in this program is a functional creative language system which the child can use for communication in his community. This does not mean that the goal of this program is to teach the fully developed adult system to every child. The implication here is that the child may cease to acquire language at some point on the developmental scale, as judged by a flattening of his learning curve. He should, however, be able to communicate his intentions with the language he has acquired. His language system may never attain grammatical status compared with an adult system. Success, then, is a judgment made by observing the child in the natural language situation rather than the laboratory.

POTENTIAL LIMITING FACTORS ON COMMUNICATION ACQUISITION

Several factors related to either retarded children or the language acquisition process have been identified as potentially restricting to language learning or to the level of linguistic attainment. These factors can be considered extralinguistic behaviors since they are related to behaviors which are not language-specific.

Attending Behaviors

Zeaman and House (1963) reported that moderate to severely retarded individuals evidenced an attentional deficit in discrimination learning, but, once the relevant cues were attended to, appropriate responses proceeded at a rapid rate. More recently, Crosby (1972) distinguished between the ability to maintain attention to relevant stimuli and the ability to inhibit responses to irrelevant stimuli. The latter was defined as distractibility. He found that the retarded were prone to distractible responses but their performance was not more affected by distraction than normals. A wide range of individual differences was noted. Crosby concluded that distractibility should be considered an individual rather than a group characteristic. Management within the treatment program should be determined by the individual child's behavior. The shaping of attending behaviors can best be accomplished within the context of the program, at the first stages of the program sequence. Behavior modification procedures of the form described by (Bricker, 1972) have been most successful in shaping attending behavior.

Motivation

Zigler (1966) reported that two factors—1) motivational variables associated with institutional living and 2) a history of failure experiences—will either together or independently affect cognitive behavior. Both of these factors directly affect language acquisition. Increasing motivation is an inherent component of behavior modification procedures; through implementation of the proposed program, successful learning experiences will supplant any history of failure experiences for the child.

Cognitive Behavior

It has been proposed by many investigators that language is dependent upon conceptual development (Bloom, 1970; 1973; Brown, 1973a,b; Morehead, 1972; Church, 1971; Mehrabian and Williams, 1971; Sinclair, 1970; 1971; Schlesinger, 1971a,b; Bowerman, 1971; Slobin, 1970). The learning of language by retarded children may well be limited by the extent of their cognitive competence. The critical question here is whether or not cognitive abilities can be enhanced by careful organization of the child's experience. Specifically, can the cognitive precursors to early language be developed in children when they do not exist? We believe that the organization of this program provides a clear method to test this hypothesis.

The rationale and organization of this program prompt further research in several areas. It is clear that we need more direct information about the retarded child as a language learner in his community. This information includes prerequisite behaviors, processing strategies, and experimental manipulation of treatment strategies designed to enhance learning. Specifically:

1. Do retarded children produce semantic functions similar to those expressed by normal children in the the early stages of language development in their community?

2. What is the nature of the retarded child's cognitive behavior as it relates to his language behavior during stage I (the sensorimotor period)?

3. What processing strategies do retarded children employ in comprehending sentences at the early stages of production?

4. Does a program based on teaching semantic concepts enhance language development to the extent that a communicative system results regardless of the level at which language learning ceases?

In summary, this program is based on the notion that semantic concepts form the basis of what is learned by children acquiring language. Through evoking the operating principles within the context of a behavior modification paradigm, a functional and creative communication system will result.

Operating Principles

I. The content for language training for retarded children should be taken from the data available on language development in normal children.

II. Semantic concepts should be ordered for teaching on the basis of frequency of occurrence, and the selection of utterance form for expression should be determined by the sequence of forms acquired by normal children.

III. Select a single frequently occurring experience, demonstrating a particular semantic relation; pair with appropriate lexical marker; and after child demonstrates mastery, move to multiple experiences expressing the same function.

IV. First expansions of single word utterances should be of relational functions previously expressed.

This program specifies the relationship between form, function, and experience and provides for the shaping of attending behavior and increasing motivation in retarded children. It also provides a method for testing the relative contribution of programmed experience and linguistic marking in enhancing cognitive-perceptual awareness of objects and events in the child's environment that are the basis of language development.

REFERENCES

Bloom, L. *One Word at a Time.* The Hague: Mouton, 1973.
Bloom, L. M. *Language Development: Form and Function of Emerging Grammars.* Cambridge, Mass.: M.I.T. Press, 1970.
Bowerman, M. Structural relationships in children's utterances: Syntactic or semantic? Paper presented at the Conference on Language Development, University of New York, Buffalo, Aug., 1971.
Bricker, W. A systematic approach to language training. In R. Schiefelbusch (Ed.), *Language of the Mentally Retarded.* Baltimore: University Park Press, 1972.
Bricker, W. and Bricker, D. A program of language training for the severely language handicapped child. *Except. Child.,* 1970a, 101–111.
Bricker, W. and Bricker, D. Development of receptive vocabulary in severely retarded children. *Amer. J. Ment. Defic.,* 1970b, *74,* 599–607.
Brown, R. and Bellugi-Klima, U. Three processes in the child's acquisition of syntax. In A. Bar-Adon and W. Leopold (Eds.), *Child Language; A Book of Readings,* Chap. 49. 1971, pp. 307–318.
Brown, R. The first sentences of child and chimpanzee. In R. Brown (Ed.), *Psycholinguistics.* New York: The Free Press, 1970.
Brown, R. Development of the first language in the human species. *Amer. Psychol.,* 1973a, 97–106.
Brown, R. *A First Language: The Early Stages.* Cambridge: Harvard University Press, 1973b.
Carrow, S. M. A. The development of auditory comprehension of language structures in children. *J. Speech Hear. Disord.,* 1968, *33,* 99–111.

Chapman, R. S. and Miller, J. F. Early two and three word utterances: Does production precede comprehension? Paper presented at the Fifth Annual Child Language Research Forum, Stanford University, Stanford, April, 1973.

Chomsky, C. *The Acquisition of Syntax in Children From 5–10.* Cambridge: M.I.T. Press, 1969.

Church, J. Methods for the study of early cognitive functioning. In R. Huxley and E. Ingram (Eds.), *Language Acquisition: Models and Methods.* Academic Press: New York, 1971.

Crosby, K. Attention and distractibility in mentally retarded and intellectually average children. *Amer. J. Ment. Defic.,* 1972, *77,* 46–53.

Epstein, H. The child's understanding of causal connectives. Paper presented at the Fifth Annual Child Language Research Forum, Stanford University, Stanford, April, 1973.

Fraser, C., Bellugi, U., and Brown, R. Control of grammar in imitation and comprehension and production. *J. Verb. Learning Verb. Behav.,* 1963, *2,* 121–135.

Kent, L. Personal communication, April, 1970.

Lovell, K. and Dixon, E. The growth of the control of grammar in imitation, comprehension and production. *J. Child Psychol. Psychiat.,* 1967, *8,* 31–39.

Lynch, J. and Bricker, W. Linguistic theory and operant procedures: Toward an integrated approach to language training for the mentally retarded. *Ment. Retard.,* 1971, 12–17.

Mehrabian, A. and Williams, M. Piagetian measures of cognitive development for children up to age two. *J. Psycholing. Res.,* 1971, *1,* 113–126.

Miller, J. F. and Yoder, D. E. A syntax teaching program. In J. E. McLean, D. E. Yoder, and R. L. Schiefelbusch (Eds.), *Language Intervention with the Retarded: Developing Strategies.* Baltimore: University Park Press, 1972a.

Miller, J. and Yoder, D. On developing the content for a language teaching program. *Ment. Retard.,* 1972b, 9–11.

Mittler, P. Language and communication. In A. Clarke and A. Clarke (Eds.), *Mental Deficiency: The Changing Outlook,* London: Methuen, In press.

Morehead, D. Early grammatical and semantic relations: Some implications for a general representational deficit in linguistically deviant children. *Lang. Disord. Child.* 1972 (special issue, No. 4).

Owings, N. O. Internal reliability and item analysis of the Miller-Yoder test of grammatical comprehension. Master's thesis, University of Wisconsin, Madison, 1972.

Schlesinger, I. M. Production of utterances and language acquisition. In D. I. Slobin (Ed.), *The Ontogenesis of Grammar.* Academic Press: New York, 1971a.

Schlesinger, I. M. Learning grammar: From pivot to realization rules. In R. Huxley and E. Ingram (Eds.), *Language Acquisition: Models and Methods.* Academic Press: New York, 1971b.

Shipley, E., Smith, C., and Gleitman, L. A study of the acquisition of language: Free response to commands. *Language,* 1969, *45,* 322–342.

Sinclair, H. Transition from sensori-motor behavior to symbolic activity. *Interchange,* 1970, *1,* 119–126.

Sinclair, H. Sensori-motor action patterns as a condition for the acquisition of syntax. In R. Huxley and E. Ingram (Eds.), *Language Acquisition: Models and Methods.* Academic Press: New York, 1971.

Slobin, D. (Ed.) *A Field Manual For Cross-Cultural Study of Communicative Competence.* University of California, Berkeley, 1967.

Slobin, D. I. Suggested Universals in the Ontogenesis of Grammar, Language-Behavior Research Laboratory: Working Paper 32, April, 1970.

Smith, L. L. Comprehension performance of oral deaf and normal hearing children at three stages of language development. Doctoral dissertation, University of Wisconsin, Madison, 1972.

Wetstone, H. and Friedlander, B. The effect of word order on young children's responses to simple questions and commands. Paper Presented at Annual Meeting of the Society For Research in Child Development, Philadelphia, April, 1973.

Yoder, D. E. and Miller, J. F. What we may know and what we can do: Input toward a system. In J. E. McLearn, D. E. Yoder, and R. L. Schiefelbusch (Eds.), *Language Intervention with the Retarded: Developing Strategies.* Baltimore: University Park Press, 1972.

Zeaman, D. and House, B. The role of attention in retardate discrimination learning. In N. R. Ellis (Ed.), *Handbook of Mental Deficiency.* New York: McGraw-Hill, 1963.

Zigler, E. Personality structure in the retardate. In N. R. Ellis (Ed.), *International Review of Research in Mental Retardation,* Vol. 1. New York: Academic Press, 1966.

CHAPTER TWENTY-ONE

TO TEACH LANGUAGE TO RETARDED CHILDREN[1]

Doug Guess, Wayne Sailor, and Donald M. Baer

Research Department, Kansas Neurological Institute, Topeka, Kansas 66604, and Bureau of Child Research and Department of Human Development, University of Kansas, Lawrence, Kansas 66045

The most effective teaching and training programs for the retarded during the past few years have been intensive, consistent, organized, and well maintained efforts requiring much effort, skill, and time. Some persons responsible for such programs assumed that the retarded child needed to be saved from the morass of total institutional dependency. So they taught self-help skills such as washing, dressing, toileting, and eating. They freed the child from self-destructive and aggressive behaviors and helped him acquire techniques for socializing with his fellows. The child may have remained in an institution, but it would be a better institutional environment for him. Other teachers and trainers assumed that their goal was not to make institutional life better but rather to free the retarded child from the institution altogether. Working under that assumption, it was necessary to teach the retardate to speak a reasonable version of the language used in the outside world to which he was to return.

The outside world operates with a heavy reliance on spoken and written words. While it can make some allowances for persons not well skilled in the use of words, it will not make many allowances, or extensive ones. Thus, of all the skills to be taught to an outward-bound retardate, language was given high priority. The results were less than adequate for the goal sought. Retarded children are not flowing in a steady stream from society's institutions and speaking to the outside world well enough to live there. Nevertheless, the logic which makes language a major component of their curriculum is unaltered, as is the determination of some teachers to see if it can be done. Thus, the development of teaching programs meant to produce useful language continues even in children so retarded at the outset as to be without any recognizable language skills. This chapter is meant to provide some review

[1] Preparation of this article and of much of the research it reports were supported in part by Grant 00870 from the National Institute of Child Health and Human Development to the Bureau of Child Research, University of Kansas.

of past and current efforts, some argument about what may be lacking in those efforts, some guesses about where help could be found, and (consequently) a proposal for a different language training program.

REVIEW

This review is separated into two major sections. The first surveys studies which deal primarily with normal speech and language development. This aspect of the review will concentrate on some consistent findings from the field of developmental linguistics. These findings have direct applicability to the construction of a speech training program for deviant children. The second portion of the review pertains to those studies which have used operant procedures, or behavior modification, to teach speech and language skills to children with observable speech and language defects. Emphasis will be on the procedures and techniques for training.

Some Highly Selected Contributions from the Field of Psycholinguistics

Phonological Acquisition. Milisen (1972) has pointed out that of all variables related to speech acquisition, the "ones probably most extensively studied and the ones most highly correlated with speech development are the frequency and variety of production of speech sounds . . ." (p. 662). Certainly, Irwin (1949) has provided a wealth of normative data, even to the point of percentile rankings for the frequency and variability of phoneme types among infants. He and his co-workers have shown that frequency of sounds and variety of phoneme types (Irwin and Chen, 1946) increase to about 30 months of age. Additional comparisons have found that boys tended to be inferior to girls (after the 2nd year) in the variety of sounds produced (Irwin and Chen, 1946) and that mental retardates (Irwin, 1942a,b) and cerebral-palsied children (Irwin, 1952) were delayed in both frequency and variety of sounds produced.

Some investigators (Jakobson, Fant, and Halle, 1963) hypothesized that phonemic development is patterned according to a system of phonemic contrasts. Phonemes which are maximally contrasting (*e.g.,* vowel-consonant) in articulation appear first in the infant. Later development includes those sounds which have smaller contrasts, such as labial and nonlabial consonants, etc. The *distinctive features approach* resulting from these investigations is a combination of the traditional mode and of articulation description plus the more recent knowledge of acoustic phonetics (Chomsky and Halle, 1968). Results of this research have specified that each English distinctive sound is composed of small elements called features, the systematic presence or absence of which determines the shape of an English sound segment. In the simplest terms, the shape of an English sound can be put together by adding certain features and omitting others.

Acquisition of Grammar. It would be difficult to review completely the vast amount of available literature relevant to the acquisition of grammar among normal children. This section will be limited to the studies which are most applicable to the conduct of a language training program for nonverbal children, with a minimum of discussion of theoretical issues surrounding the causative nature of linguistic development.

However, before discussing the contributions of developmental linguistics to this proposal, it might be helpful to summarize briefly the basic methodological approaches used by various investigators to obtain data relevant to the acquisition of language. Obviously, the methods of data collection are important when reviewing the results of these investigations.

The methodological approaches have been divided into four categories, with a sample of studies exemplifying the various approaches. It is realized, of course, that overlap between categories may occur for some investigations, and that a few studies may not fit well in any of the categories.

Inductive Grammar Approach. This approach appears to have evolved from the earlier diary reports of children who were acquiring speech (*cf.* Leopold, 1939) and involves essentially longitudinal observations and verbatim recording of utterances produced by children at various points in time. Typically, these studies include only a small group of children (Braine, 1963; Brown and Fraser, 1964; Miller and Ervin, 1964). Sample observations of the child's spontaneous speech are tape-recorded at weekly or monthly intervals, with notations made of the particular context in which each utterance was produced. From the complete *corpus* of each child's speech, attempts are made to write or "induce" (Brown and Fraser, 1964) a grammar, which is accomplished by performing a distributional analysis of the words comprising the utterances. The analysis is used to reveal words which are used most frequently and the combinations of these words with other words which occur less frequently.

Specific Grammar Approach. This approach again makes longitudinal observations of the child's utterances at various points in time. However, only the absence, presence, or increasing complexity of specific grammatical systems are recorded from the speech *corpus.* A study of Bellugi (1964) exemplifies the specific grammar approach as used to observe the development of negation.

Evoking Stimulus Approach. As pointed out by McNeill (1970), the spontaneous utterances of a child may indicate his level of *performance,* but these utterances may not necessarily reflect his linguistic *competence.* Competence in this case is a theory about what the child actually knows. Therefore, rather than relying on the spontaneous speech of a child, some investigators have used a variety of stimulus materials, objects, and procedures to elicit specific grammatical utterances from children. For example, Berko (1958) used nonsense syllables and unusual drawings to observe the development of morphological inflections at various age levels. Puppets were used by Brown (1968) to study the ability of children to transform sentences. In one part of the study, children were expected to model the sentence pattern of puppets which spoke in either the active or passive voice. Fraser, Bellugi, and Brown (1963) utilized a verbal imitation task and pictures illustrating grammatical contrasts to study the emergence of comprehension among 3-year-old children.

Deviant Group Approach. The deviant group approach may involve any one of the above methodologies. The major point of departure is the subject population. The underlying assumption of this approach is that the study of various deviant groups may provide information and insights relevant to normal speech and language development; *i.e.,* observing malfunctions and irregularities in language development among biologically deviant groups enables one more accurately to describe and clarify variables operating in normal development. Lenneberg, Nichols, and Rosenberger (1964) observed articulation skills, vocabulary expansion, and the understanding of sentence patterns among children with Down's syndrome over a 3-year period. Semmel and Dolley (1971) studied the ability of Down's syndrome children to comprehend and imitate verbally presented sentences of varying complexities. Lovell and Bradbury (1967) used the procedures developed by Berko (1958) to observe morphological inflections among retarded children.

In summary, the majority of studies in early language acquisition have used methodological approaches which observe and record the emergence of various grammatical skills as a function of chronological age, or in some cases, as a function of defective organisms. Experimental manipulations have involved primarily the alteration of stimulus materials or tasks to evoke specific grammatical utterances from children. Conspicuously absent from these studies are attempts to alter directly the speech and language performance of children (while systematically manipulating those variables responsible for the behavioral change) and studies which teach directly new linguistic skills, again manipulating those variables which constitute the training procedures—an important consideration when working with nonverbal children. Nevertheless, the observational studies reported have provided valuable information pertaining to the sequence of linguistic development among children, and they have contributed to the development of numerous procedures and instruments to observe (but not change) a child's linguistic performance. The following section will review some of the more consistent findings which have resulted from these investigations.

Early Developmental Sequences of Language Skills. McNeill (1970) has described and examined three universal stages or points in the early development of grammar, starting with the initial utterances (referred to as the holophrastic period) to the combination of single words (pivotal grammar) and, finally, the emergence of early phrase structure, described as resembling "telegraphic" speech. Each of these periods or stages is sufficiently distinct to warrant separate discussion.

The emergence of single morphemes (or words) usually occurs at about the age of 1 year. In the opinion of many investigators (*cf.* McCarthy, 1954), these single-word utterances may convey a variety of meanings for the child and may be equivalent in meaning to full sentences used by adults. As defined by McNeill (1970) " 'holophrastic speech' refers to the possibility that single-word utterances of young children express complex ideas, that *ball* means not simply a spherical object of appropriate size, but that a child wants such an object, for example, or that he believes he has created such an object, or that someone is expected to look at such an object" (p. 20).

At some point around 18 months, most children begin to use word combinations in their speech. The pattern and structure of these early utterances have been the focus for several investigations (Braine, 1963; Brown and Fraser, 1964; Miller and Ervin, 1964). Each study was based on longitudinal observations of normal children who were acquiring word combinations. Results show that early word combinations consist of two parts. One part includes a small, but frequently occurring number of words which appear in a fixed position in the child's utterances. These words, referred to by Braine (1963) as "pivots," may occur as the initial word in the combination (*e.g., see* doggie, *see* mommy, *see* book, etc.) or as the last word in the combination (*e.g.,* close *it,* hit *it,* find *it,* etc.). All the remaining words in the child's vocabulary are available for combination with the pivot words, and are referred to as the "X-class." Braine maintained that language grows structurally as the child learns the position of new words (pivots), while the child's language grows in vocabulary by adding to the X-class.

Other investigators have used analogous terms to describe pivot and X-class words. Brown and Fraser (1964) used "functors" and "contentives"; Miller and Ervin (1964) have referred to "operators" and "non-operators."

Several investigators have referred to the "telegraphic" nature of utterances produced by young children (Brown and Fraser, 1964; McNeill, 1970; Rebelsky, Starr, and Luria, 1967), referring to the fact that the child's first sentences are abbreviated versions of adult speech. Missing from the child's utterances are words which carry little information, such as articles, auxiliary verbs, copular verbs, and inflections. Slobin (1971) examined data from several studies of child language in many countries and many different languages. He maintained that such "telegraphese" is one of the universals of language learning. Data summarized by McCarthy (1954) show increasing sentence length from early childhood through maturity. At 18 months the child is using one-word sentences and just beginning to combine words. Approximately 1 year later, most utterances average two or three words, and by the age of 3½ years, most children are using complete sentences which average about four words each.

Brown and Fraser (1964) maintained that telegraphic speech is produced by some kind of immediate memory span, which is reflected both in the child's ability to imitate sentences of various lengths and in spontanteous situations where the child is constructing sentences. They related their position to studies which show that the memory span of children increases with age. Brown and Fraser also pointed out, however, that span limitation does not account for the systematic tendency to retain some morphemes, while dropping others. This, of course, is related to studies which have recorded various parts of speech at different age levels. Young (1941) observed 441 children ranging in age from 30 to 48 months. She found pronouns and verbs were most common; nouns occurred next in frequency, followed by adverbs, adjectives, prepositions, infinitives, interjections, and conjunctions, respectively.

In summary, the development of early grammar among normal children progresses from initial one-word utterances to word combinations, and the emergence of simple phrase structure, referred to as telegraphic speech. From there, speech and language acquisition multiplies rapidly in complexity and structure. The sophistication of a child's language corresponds to the development of higher-order grammatical rules, the combination of phrases in utterances, the inclusion of more informative and content words in the sentence structure, etc. At this point, it would indeed be tempting to embark on a more theoretical discussion involving the nature of linguistic development, and certainly the impact of transformational grammar on the field of linguistics (Chomsky, 1965; McNeill, 1970; Bloom, 1970). This progression would inevitably lead to current theoretical disputes concerning the very nature of how a child comes to either *know* (Lenneberg, 1964, 1967) or *learn* (Skinner, 1957) a language, and whether language acquisition is a result of innate biological and maturational factors, or primarily the result of environmental factors. Since the purpose of this chapter is to construct a training program for teaching speech and language skills, it is predictable that emphasis is placed on the conditions under which speech and language behavior can be taught, and variables which may affect acquisition—the topic of discussion in the second section of this literature review.

Operant Analyses of Language Deficiencies

A Chain of Experimental Analyses. Within the past decade, considerable attention has been directed toward the application of learning techniques to the development of language skills among individuals who are deficient or deviant in this important area. Operant techniques in particular have been used to correct inappropriate speech patterns (Risley and Wolf, 1967; Wheeler and Sulzer, 1970), to reinstate speech in currently mute persons who previously spoke (Isaacs, Thomas, and Goldiamond, 1955; Sherman, 1963, 1965), and to develop simple language in children who had never talked (Lovaas, Berberich, Perloff, and Schaeffer, 1966; Sloane, Johnston, and Harris, 1968; Guess, Rutherford, and Twichell, 1969; Bricker and Bricker, 1970; Sailor, 1970; Buddenhagen, 1971). Taken as a class, these studies have shown successful applications with children and adults variously described as mentally retarded, brain-damaged, autistic, and schizophrenic.[2]

Furthermore, a theoretical analysis of language development as a reinforcement-based process has begun to emerge within the same research framework. Skinner (1957) had already affirmed the operant nature of language in 1957; but his analysis was very speculative. However, within 2 years Salzinger (1959) offered a preliminary review of some actual manipulations of language as an operant behavior class subject to experimental programming, and 3 years thereafter co-authored a simple demonstration of children's speech as a reinforceable behavior (Salzinger, Salzinger, Portnoy, Eckman, Bacon, Dentsch, and Zubin, 1962). Meanwhile, Isaacs, Thomas, and Goldiamond (1965) and Sherman (1963, 1965) were presenting their language reinstatement demonstrations, perhaps equally as much testimony to the fundamentally operant nature of language as they were contributions to clinical techniques. Similarly, the Risley and Wolf (1967) demonstrations of how to shape echoic verbalizations into referent-controlled labels were as much a theoretical analysis of the label (as a special case of the discriminated operant) as they were remedial teaching procedures. The language-building programs of Lovaas and his associates (e.g., 1966) played the same dual role, over a steadily widening range of language forms (labels, mands, verbs, pronouns, prepositions, etc.). With time, and with published precedents as stimuli, the language targets of such analyses grew more complex. Thus, grammatical structures which should generalize to untrained instances were studied, first in the simple case of pluralization rules (Guess, Sailor, Rutherford, and Baer, 1968; Guess, 1969; and Sailor, 1971). Schumaker and Sherman (1970) extended this analysis to the generalized use of past and present verb tenses. Baer and Guess (1971) showed similar processes (at the level of receptive speech) in the generalized use of comparative and superlative adjectives, and the productive use of noun suffixes (1973). Sailor and Taman (1972) developed stimulus control procedures to establish the relational skills implicit in the accurate use of prepositions. Following the same general logic, Wheeler and Sulzer (1970) initiated an operant analysis of syntax, by establishing a generalized skill of complete sentence constructions in place of the "telegraphic" speech previously used by a child; Garcia, Guess, and Byrnes (1973) have demonstrated the development of simple syntax through imitations of a "model." Meanwhile, Guess (1969) broached the problem of cross-modality generalization (i.e., transfer of grammatical skills from receptive to productive speech, or vice versa), showing that the grammar

---

[2] These studies are cited as useful and dependable guideposts along a complex route. Many other reports can also be cited in support of the same conclusions, notably, Sherman, 1964; Wolf, Risley, and Mees, 1964; Hewett, 1965; Kerr, Meyerson, and Michael, 1965; Salzinger, Feldman, Cowan, and Salzinger, 1965; Cook and Adams, 1966; Baer, Peterson, and Sherman, 1967; Hartung, 1970; and Sulzbacher and Costello, 1970.

of productive speech need not be affected by receptive training of a relevant rule; whereupon Harrelson (1969) showed that receptive grammar need not be altered by productive rule training. Subsequently, Guess and Baer (1973) replicated both failures of generalization, this time as simultaneous deficits within single subjects, and then developed brief reinforcement procedures to establish both lines of generalization.[3]

Concurrent with this increased complexity and importance of the targets of experimental language analysis, Staats (1968) presented a thorough and detailed revision of its underlying theoretical approach, again displaying its roots in basic learning principles, and also extending it to complex learning processes as well as to those usually segregated (theoretically) as "cognitive."

Consolidation of Some Basic Techniques. Clearly enough, these operant analyses of language had started at extremely rudimentary levels; but, equally clearly, they had moved steadily toward developing more and more complex and comprehensive language skills. At the same time, a certain amount of the total research effort looked not ahead but inward, in an effort to better understand, improve, or perhaps dispense with certain behavioral mechanisms which, so far, seemed basic to the progress made. These studies centered around both imitation (on which every program seemed to rely) and the freeing of speech skills from the mere imitative control under which they had experimentally developed, to make them "expressive."

Vocal Imitations. Two general training techniques were frequently and successfully used in establishing some level of speech proficiency in speech-deficient individuals. In both cases, an initial step was to establish the general behavior of reliably matching a variety of responses demonstrated by the therapist (imitation). The procedure followed in building this complex repertoire included physically helping the patient to imitate responses demonstrated by the model while concurrently reinforcing these "prompted" matching responses. These physical prompts were then slowly removed, step by step, and reinforcers were delivered for closer and closer approximations to the modeled response until only the demonstration was needed to produce the matching response. (These procedures are usually referred to as shaping, fading, and chaining.)

In what seemed to be a logical approach to the training of vocal imitation, some researchers first began with training a number of simple motor imitations. Baer, Peterson, and Sherman (1967) trained over 100 motor imitations (some very complex) before attempting the training of vocal imitations. These experimenters worked with three severely retarded children who showed no speech or imitative behavior prior to training. As subjects learned

---

[3] Guess and Baer (1973), in a recent chapter, have summarized many of these grammar-oriented studies and have argued for the usefulness of such research programs as well as for the theoretical framework of language development and language training implicit in them.

to imitate motor responses, they began to imitate other nontrained motor responses. This suggested that subjects had acquired a general imitative skill ("generalized imitation") which could be used to develop vocal imitation. However, the transition from motor to vocal imitations was not a smooth one, although the chaining of motor and vocal responses together (*e.g.*, raise hand and say "hi") resulted in reliable vocal imitation. Sloane, Johnston, and Harris (1968) also established vocal imitations in six retarded children who were initially nonverbal and nonimitative. These investigators included mouth and tongue imitations among the motor responses. Training again consisted of providing consequences for closer and closer matches to responses demonstrated by a model; motor imitation training preceded vocal imitation training. Vocal training consisted of modeling a combination of the previously learned mouth-tongue movements with vocal sounds. Using these procedures, they were able to establish vocal imitation in all subjects.

Other researchers reporting success in remedial speech training have omitted the motor imitative component. Risley and Wolf (1967) established functional speech in autistic, echolalic children using imitative control procedures. These children did emit vocal and verbal speech sounds, but they did so inappropriately. Consequently, these authors chose to bring vocalizations under imitative control. The method used consisted of the therapist saying a word a fixed number of times each minute and reinforcing the child (with parts of meals, sweets, etc.) for reproducing that word within a few seconds after the therapist. Their results indicated that all children came under the control of the therapist's vocal emission (imitative control). Lovaas (1968) listed four successive steps used to develop imitative speech in autistic children with no mention of motor imitation training. 1) The first step calls for reinforcement of all vocal responses by the child combined with reinforcement of eye contact between therapist and child. 2) The therapist emits a vocal demonstration at 10-sec intervals and reinforces the child for emitting any vocal response within 6 sec after the demonstration. 3) Reinforcement is dispensed only if the child's vocal response is similar to that demonstrated by the therapist. 4) This step is identical to step 3, using other vocal sounds.

Similar steps were used by Salzinger, Feldman, Cowan, and Salzinger (1965) and Sulzbacher and Costello (1970) to establish vocal imitation in speech-deficient subjects.

Within the methods reviewed, vocal imitative control of subject vocalizations has been accomplished. The training techniques have been somewhat the same, those of shaping and fading (at least within a learning theory framework they are the same). But differences exist in the emphasis placed on motor imitation training. The first method carefully programs an initial repertoire of motor imitative behavior. The second neglects such a program and proceeds immediately with vocal behavior. Building a motor imitative repertoire with nonimitative children is a complex task (Baer, Peterson, and Sherman, 1967; Peterson, 1968). Whether an initial motor imitative skill facilitates the acquisition, retention, or generalization of vocal imitative behavior is an unanswered empirical question. However, such an answer seems most important for the therapist who must choose and initiate successful and economical treatment programs.

Along these lines, a recent study (Garcia, Baer, and Firestone, 1971) looked at the generalization of motor and vocal imitative behavior in severely retarded children who were initially nonimitative and nonverbal. These children were first trained to imitate a number of motor responses and then a number of short vocal responses (vowel sounds) using shaping and fading techniques. Results indicated that training motor imitative responses produced generalizations to other nontrained motor responses but not to untrained vocal responses. It was only after some vocal imitation had been established that the children began to imitate nontrained vocal responses. Although generalizations did not occur from motor to vocal imitation, it was not clear whether initial motor imitation training facilitated later vocal imitative acquisition and generalization.

Thus far we have reviewed the establishment of vocal imitative behavior. This skill has been designated as a "necessary condition" (Peterson, 1968) for the establishment of speech and has been an important component in each procedure designed to train speech to the nonverbal population. These procedures are direct applications of learning theory principles to the area of vocal behavior. Of two basic procedures shown to be successful in establishing vocal imitation, one requires the establishment of some motor imitative skills while the other neglects motor imitation completely and begins with vocal behavior. In both cases, training consists of shaping and fading procedures consistent with reinforcement theory.

From a treatment standpoint, the important issues still unanswered concern the differences in success for procedures used to establish vocal imitation. Such an answer becomes necessary for establishing economical treatment programs. Also of importance is knowledge concerning the interaction of subject variables with specific treatment programs. What effects do variables such as attentiveness, rate of vocalization and diversity of sounds have on the success of verbal imitation training, and what are the differential effects of these variables on particular training procedures? These issues are now raised owing to the abundant research which indicates that vocal imitation can be established in speech-deficient individuals, thus making refinements in these successful procedures the next logical step.

Expressive Speech. In the preceding section a number of studies were mentioned in which vocal imitation was established. In most instances these studies were also concerned with establishing expressive speech. In their detailed work with echolalic children, Risley and Wolf (1966) incorporated a number of procedures to establish a labeling vocabulary. After subjects were reliably imitating verbal demonstrations, the experimenter held up an object and asked "What is this?" When the child looked at the object, the experimenter immediately provided a verbal prompt (the object's name); reinforcement was delivered for imitating the prompt. The following steps involved lengthening the time between the question, "What is this?" and the prompt and fading out the prompt altogether. Results from these procedures indicated that the children learned to label objects when asked to do so and that labeling was dependent upon the contingent presentation of food or candy for correct labeling.

Lovaas (1968), in his work with nonverbal autistic children, described the establishment of speech after verbal imitation training. This training is similar to that described earlier (*i.e.*, a modeled vocal response plus reinforcement of imitation, followed by fading of the vocal model). Somewhat differently, the procedures call for the formation of general concepts. That is, a number of examples of each object are presented to the child so as to teach the child different classes of objects; for example, a small green *chair*, a large red *chair*, a small rocking *chair*, etc., established the general discrimination of *chair*. In an effort to make the trained language functional in the child's everyday environment, an extensive program was instituted to train receptive and expressive use of some basic prepositions (on top of, under, beside, inside) and pronouns (I-mine, you-yours, he-his). The generalization (the use of the trained vocabulary in other settings, other objects, and with other individuals) of correct usage was programmed by using various individuals as therapists and many different behaviors as objects of the verbal utterances. Results of this detailed training indicated that the children did learn to label objects verbally; but the maintenance of this behavior was dependent on the contingent delivery of food, candy, etc. for labeling. The children also used prepositions and pronouns within the context trained and to some extent in nontrained contexts.

These basic procedures were also applied to the mute population labeled as "severely retarded." Sloane, Johnston, and Harris (1968) trained nonverbal, severely retarded children in a labeling vocabulary using procedures described earlier. Following this training, children were taught a number of requests using the same basic procedures. An article of food, which independent evidence had suggested was a strong reinforcer, was shown to the subject and was paired with a vocal model which labeled the article. If the child imitated the model, he was given the article of food. The vocal model was then slowly removed (faded). This procedure was later used to establish requests for nonfood items, such as "open the door."

The research reviewed to this point has indicated that individuals who are initially mute can be trained, through imitation, to emit a number of vocal responses. An accompanying result indicates that the acquired imitative responses can come under the control of environmental stimuli which do not offer an imitative cue. Thus, verbal vocabularies including labeling, answering, and requesting have been established.

Attempts to extend speech training into the individual's everyday environment have been reported by Risley and Wolf (1967), Lovaas (1968), and Sloane, Johnston, and Harris (1968). These extensions involved the use of reinforcement-imitation-fading procedures by parents and cottage attendants. Results of such training have been reported as successful, but no meaningful data have been presented and the success has not been evaluated functionally. The recommended technique is usually described in terms of programmed generalization. The individual is reinforced for use of speech in a number of different situations (Hartung, 1970). The technique seems simple. However, the scarcity of data on this topic precludes any attempt to follow the general recommendation.

Results during acquisition of these skills indicated that many experimenter hours are required, with the initial training items requiring most of this time (Risley and Wolf, 1967; Sloane *et al.*, 1968; Lovaas, 1968). An additional finding indicated that subjects begin to use their newly acquired verbal vocabulary in settings other than those in which training took place, but usually only sparsely (Wolf, Risley, and Mees, 1964; Sloane *et al.*, 1968). Reports of this generalized use of appropriate speech have not been experimental in nature, but rather of the anecdotal type. An exception is the case of maintenance of newly acquired verbal responses such as labeling, answering questions, and requesting. Studies by Risley and Wolf (1967) and Lovaas (1968) have documented generalization and have also demonstrated the function of programmed reinforcement in maintaining these types of verbalization.

Summary. The experimental procedures used throughout these studies emphasized the *operant* analysis of language, by relying (successfully) on the programming of various stimulus consequences for the correct language responses required at each step of their programs. Many of the studies also incorporated shaping procedures, but these were well understood as a simple extension of the differential reinforcement principle (rather than as a new element in the theoretical analysis). Similarly, fading techniques had heavy use, but these too were seen as subsidiary procedures, appropriate to stimulus control of the discriminated language operant. Imitation (or modeling) was used as well, and in nearly every application outlined above. But imitation itself has undergone experimental analysis, the results of which suggest that it may be seen as a special response class of discriminated operants (Baer and Sherman, 1964; Baer, Peterson, and Sherman, 1967), rather than as a potential contradiction of the reinforcement analysis emerging from the language experiments.

Thus, it seems appropriate to conclude that an operant technology presently exists for the establishment and maintenance of imitative and expressive speech. Although these procedures are expensive in terms of therapist time, the results have been empirically evaluated as effective.

DEFICIENCIES IN THE OPERANT ANALYSIS

Despite the ongoing schedule of reinforcement-by-success outlined above, close inspection of the field nevertheless reveals several areas of neglect. Many areas should be explored systematically to maintain momentum currently evident in the field; to provide additional techniques for those persons concerned with applied treatment procedures; and to further the evaluation of the validity of this approach. These targets of future work (in increasing order of importance) should include, at least: 1) the direct comparison of the various training techniques that can be applied to the same type of language problem or deficiency; 2) the possibility that existing behaviors of the language-deficient child might serve as predictive variables for the selection of that child's best training technique; 3) note of continuing need for construction of useful training programs which are both practical in application and optimally functional for the child in his linguistic interaction with the environment; and 4) the programmed transfer, or generalization, of language behaviors from the controlled training setting in which (we know) they can be taught, to the child's "natural environment."

The need for work in these four areas exemplifies the fact that the knowledge available for improving the language of retarded children has not been optimally applied (Haviland, 1972). It is not that there has been a lack or a misdirection of effort. The great bulk of recent work has been directed at problem 3, *i.e.,* the development of procedural training sequences which bring together known effective and (where necessary) newly improvised techniques to teach a curriculum of language skills which, at the end, *ought* to result in a much improved use of language. That these programs succeed in establishing each prescribed language skill is usually self-evident to those applying the programs. However, whether these prescribed skills in fact summate to useful, functional language is still largely unexamined. Whether the skills generalize to other settings (problem 4) is rarely measured and even less often aimed for.[4]

Comparative evaluation of the various techniques available has not been pursued, and prediction of what children are best suited to these alternatives, when attempted, has been unvalidated. However, few of these lacks could have been remedied without some actual language training programs within which (or on top of which) to work. Thus, these deficiencies are inevitable to this stage in the history of the problem.

Apart from their usual (and understandable) failures to contact problem areas 1, 2, and 4, the language training programs now available or in development usually present several internal problems of their own. For example,

---

[4] But *cf.* Tawney and Hipsher (1970), who prescribed teaching some new language skills in various settings other than the one in which training usually takes place.

when these programs take the form of completely detailed step-by-step training procedures, they typically require that the child already possess basic language skills before entering the program (*e.g.,* Dunn and Smith, 1965, 1966, 1967; Dunn, Horton, and Smith, 1965; Bereiter and Engelmann, 1966; Guess, Ensminger, and Smith, 1969). However, a few very new programs are designed to accommodate the initially nonverbal, even nonimitative child. Some of these still fall short of the detailed step-by-step prescription necessary to a practical training program (one that can be applied by personnel other than the highly trained specialists of the research field), and/or they stop before a thoroughly useful level of language competence is achieved (*e.g.,* Buddenhagen, 1971; Kent, Klein, Falk, and Guenther, 1972). One (unpublished) manual assumes no vocal skills for entry to the program and offers step-by-step programming which terminates at a thoroughly useful level of language complexity, but it emphasizes receptive language, especially instruction following, rather than productive skills (Tawney and Hipsher, 1970). By contrast, the systems analysis model proposed by Bricker (1972) has specified with great thoroughness the sequential behavior steps logically involved in teaching a mute, inattentive retardate to receive and produce sentences. The model specifies 24 subprograms, each of which will require its own program of step-by-step procedures. The first program prescribes the establishment of reinforcement control. The final one cites the procedures which should establish a "pivot-open" phrase format and expand it to meaningful sentence production. The translation of the Bricker model into a complete sequence of detailed procedures presumably is still ongoing (Bricker, 1972, pp. 85–86). Paradoxically, the logic of the Bricker model is apparently so thorough that two clashing deductions present themselves immediately: 1) when finally translated into all of its implicit step-by-step training procedures, the model almost surely will succeed in producing much useful language; and 2) it will be such a lengthy program that it will not often be applied. *If so,* it will not have solved the practical problem of producing generalized functional language in deficient children.

What, then, can an operant orientation offer to the development of a remedial speech training program for nonverbal children? Initially, it can (and does) offer techniques and procedures which are effective in teaching a variety of language skills to speech-deficient children. (A major problem is to refine these techniques by directly comparing one or more procedures with the same type of speech deviation.) Second, an operant orientation provides an experimental approach to the study of language acquisition—an approach which systematically measures and manipulates those variables important to the training program and, thus, is appropriate to the empirical study of language and speech acquisition. Third, it can and has generated some language training programs which aim for comprehensive language usage as a final but programmable goal. But it has not yet shown that its programs accomplish the goal.

To alleviate these shortcomings, findings from studies by developmental psycholinguists can be helpful. These investigations provide normative data for speech development. They have indicated some fairly universal stages in language acquisition, such as the transition from single words to two-word combinations (pivot and open class words), and the use of "telegraphic" speech patterns in a child's speech. Most importantly, these studies serve to remind the language trainer of the importance of attaching meaning to the child's utterances and of the necessity for training speech and language within a context which has direct applicability and function for the child.

Miller and Yoder (1972) pointed out that *"the content for language training for retarded children should be taken from the data available on language development in normal children, and this content should be taught in the same sequence that it is acquired by the normal child"* (p. 11). Linguists have not, however, been able to determine any particular hierarchy of levels of complexity in speech and language acquisition, to determine whether it is necessary that one set of skills precedes another, or whether any number and variety of skills can be taught and learned in any order (Lenneberg, 1964). Thus, while normative data may indicate that most children use more pronouns, nouns, and verbs before they use adjectives, prepositions, and conjunctives, it is an empirical question as to whether *teaching* the former must precede the latter. It is not known whether a child must be taught to utter one- or two-word combinations before more lengthy responses are trained even though most normal children show a progression in the length of their utterances (*e.g.,* verb-object; subject-verb-object, etc.). These questions still remain problems for the development of a speech and language training program for nonverbal children.

Finally, it must be recognized that a language training program for nonverbal children may not have to follow a sequence evidenced by normal children. Almost by definition, remedial speech programs are used in those cases where normal acquisition has not occurred. And, while these programs may use training procedures which appear outwardly to be artificially contrived, it must be recognized that the procedures are used where development has already deviated from the normal pattern.

A PROPOSAL: AN EXPERIMENTAL TRAINING PROGRAM

The program described here is aimed at all of these problems. Relevant to problem 1, the program proposed here will conduct formal comparisons of the techniques available to it at various critical points in the training sequence. Relevant to problem 2, it will ask whether any of the children's preexisting vocal or verbal characteristics predict their differential responsiveness to those techniques and to the program as a whole. Relevant to problem 3, a potentially efficient program has been constructed, prescribing step-by-step procedures designed and written for application (eventually) by paraprofessionals. The program is designed for use with mute, nonimitative subjects and should produce eventual functional sentence usage, involving people, things, and their interactions, within its first sequential lesson-steps (each step a program of contingencies aimed at one further advance in language skill). Finally, relevant to problem 4, the program contains elements designed to enhance the subject's generalization to nonteaching environments. It attempts this by emphasizing the environment-controlling (hence, reinforcing) potential of the newly taught language skills. It also contains elements designed to enhance the subject's skills in expanding his language repertoire beyond that taught to him directly, and in integrating all new acquisitions and expansion with all previously taught components. These are the key characteristics which may give the program the generalized outcome essential to a truly practical program. If they succeed in creating generalized language use in the child's everyday living environments which is functional for him in those environments, then the deliberately brief character of the program (essential to its practical value) will not be disadvantageous (*cf.* Bricker's discussion of efficiency).

The model presented in this paper is the guiding framework for a training *manual,* which describes in detail specific procedures and techniques for teaching the content described below. The manual is being tested within an applied behavior analysis framework at the Kansas Neurological Institute and field tested at several other agencies and institutions. Data obtained from the experimental analysis will be used to validate, revise, or choose among specific training procedures and sequences. Thus, the manual exists primarily as a guide to the sequence of research studies, rather than as a finished recipe for producing language in mute retardates.

The experimental training program is divided into three parts. Part I provides for an initial assessment and evaluation of the child's pretraining speech and language skills. Part II describes four alternate procedures for training vocal imitation. Part III, the major section of the manual, outlines a 61-step sequence for training functional language skills.

Figure 1 presents a flow chart summarizing the order of procedures comprising the three parts.

Structure of the Training Program

Part I: Pretraining Evaluation and Assessment. The pretraining evaluation and assessment are to help the language trainer become more fully acquainted with existing behavior of the child, prior to the implementation of a language training program, as well as to conduct the more usual diagnostic assessments. During this evaluation, the trainer observes particular behavioral deficiencies and problems which could have some bearing on the child's progress. In addition, the collection and compilation of data across children who participate in this program may provide useful information for future research endeavors. These data provide baseline observations which may eventually

FLOW CHART OF EXPERIMENTAL SPEECH AND LANGUAGE
TRAINING PROGRAM

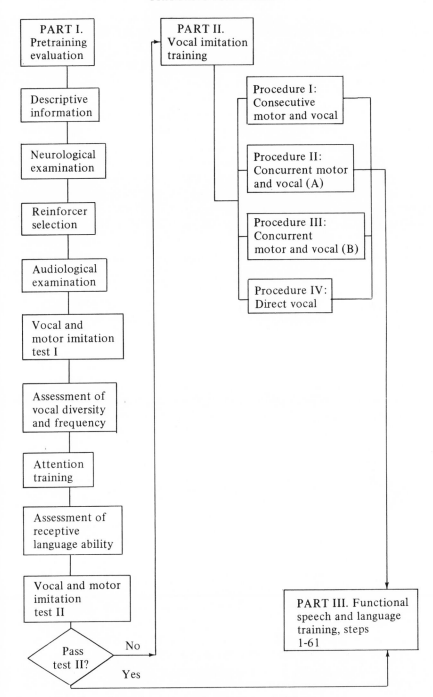

Fig. 1. Flow chart of experimental speech and language training program.

serve as predictive criteria for choice among alternative language training procedures and may also indicate the need to develop different or supplemental training procedures for certain children with divergent behavioral profiles. Possibly, this indication will be pointed enough to suggest the specific nature of the needed procedures.

Part I, as displayed in Figure 1, reveals the areas of pretraining assessments contained in the experimental manual. (Note that the pretest for vocal and motor imitation is given twice, at different positions in the sequence, to allow for possible "warm-up" effects.)

Part II: Training Vocal Imitation. The development of vocal imitation is the initial major step in a language remediation program for nonverbal children. All subsequent phases of language training are based on the premise that the child is capable of producing vocal responses which match or approximate a vocal stimulus presented by the trainer. From a treatment standpoint, the important issue concerns the criteria to evaluate differential rate of success among the various procedures now used to establish vocal imitation, which are taken to be the amount of time required for training and the accuracy with which a child can subsequently imitate new (untrained) sounds.

At least three major training procedures have been described in the literature for developing imitative speech in nonverbal children. These procedures differ essentially in their initial phase of training. In one procedure, referred to here as "consecutive motor and vocal imitation training," the teaching of nonvocal motor imitations precedes bringing the child's vocal behavior under imitative control (Baer, Peterson, and Sherman, 1967; Sloane, Johnston, and Harris, 1968). This assumes that vocal imitation is only a subclass of generalized imitation, but a very complex one, and hence is most easily established by training after establishment of generalized imitations of the less complex topography, specifically motor imitations. Motor imitations, it is assumed, are particularly useful in providing simple cases for imitation training.

In a second major procedure, referred to as "concurrent motor and vocal imitation training," motor and vocal responses are always intermixed during training. This procedure assumes that thoroughly generalized imitation will be best established only by training in widely diverse response topographies, necessarily including both motor and vocal components. Vocal imitation thus parallels motor imitation as *generalized* imitation is developed.

The third procedure, referred to as "direct vocal imitation training," assumes that motor and vocal imitations may be quite different response classes and hence that generalized imitation may be established within a vocal topography alone (or a motor topography alone). If so, the development of motor imitations need not occur in order to train vocal imitations and need not facilitate vocal imitation even when it is established first.

Four general sets of training procedures are experimentally analyzed in the present research program, derived from the three vocal imitation paradigms discussed above. (The second major procedure—concurrent motor and vocal imitation training—is subdivided into two training procedures. In one, items are trained one at a time. In the other procedure, three items are trained at a time, to criterion.) In terms of outcome, the issue is to establish vocal imitation; generalize the vocal imitation such that the child will always attempt closer and closer approximations to a modeled vocal stimulus; and finally generalize short vocal imitation to a generalized imitation of longer phoneme chains—words—which will later have functional *language* value for the child.

Experimentally, the goal is to determine the most rapid, efficient and useful technique to establish such generalized vocal imitation in a nonimitative, nonvocal child. A secondary experimental problem is the determination of the role of physical (motor) imitation training in the establishment of generalized vocal imitation as a response class.

Verbal imitation training follows as a simple extension of a generalized vocal imitation tendency, with specific shaping applied to words which will become functional for the child in part III of the training manual.

Part III: Functional Speech and Language Training. Part III of the manual describes a functional language training program, to be activated when the child has been taught to imitate vocal sounds and simple words. The training sequence presented in this section and the specific procedural options for teaching the various language skills outlined in the sequence have culminated from efforts to combine an operant orientation with numerous findings, models, and assumptions which have been described in the fields of linguistics and psycholinguistics. This training program is, of necessity, experimental in nature, and procedural options at various training points must undergo experimental analysis. Similarly, the success of the total program in generating language outside of training will require constant and detailed measurement. In the final analysis, it is the previously nonverbal child who will tell us whether the program thus developed is functional and, if so, whether it is practical, or even realistically possible.

Logic of the Training Program

Procedures for the training program have been organized across four dimensions: the *reference, control, self-extended control,* and *integration* functions of language.

Reference. The fundamental function of language is to symbolize. This requires a convenient event which can be responded *to,* and responded *with* in the same manner as some other less convenient event. When such convenient events are words, an immense gain in control is achieved for the word user. He can then respond to certain words as he would respond to the environmental events they symbolize. Response to and with words typically will be more efficient and profitable than response to and with their referents. Thus, avoidance of a sign marked "Danger! Keep away!" is more efficient than having to become acquainted through direct experience with every real-life hazard. Similarly, response with the words, "Stay back!" is more profitable in keeping children from disaster than is bodily dragging them away from every hazard which we appreciate but they do not. That a word is a substitute for something else—that it can be responded to, and responded with, as "the real world" is responded to or with—is the function of reference, put forward here as the most basic function of all in bringing a child into contact with the environment-controlling potential of language. It is assumed that the environment-controlling function of language is the ultimate reinforcer on which maintenance and expansion of language must eventually depend.

In this program, reference will be approached in its simplest but most basic two forms: as productive (spoken) labels for things and actions of importance to the child, and as receptive stimuli (spoken by another to the child) to which he can respond accurately, in both motoric and verbal modalities, by pointing to the objects labeled by another, and by answering "yes" or "no" to demonstrations accompanied by the question, "Is this (thing-label, or action-label)?" Any teaching of reference must have some environment-controlling value, but if the words (things, actions) chosen are trivial for the child, that value is correspondingly slight. For this program, an effort will be made to choose events which are of constant significance in the child's environment, whether it be in the home or an institutional setting.

Control. The lesson is only implicit, in *reference,* that labels are powerful. In this aspect of the program, that power will be made explicit, by teaching him "request" forms of language: as a productive skill, such as "I want (thing)" and "I want (action)," and later "I want (action) with (thing)" and "I want you to (action) with (thing);" and as a receptive skill which correctly acknowledges another's questions about the child's wishes, as in saying "yes" or "no" to "You want (thing)" or "You want (action)?", and later, "You want (action) with (thing)?" and "You want me to (action) with (thing)?" In effect, productive and receptive mands are being taught (in the terminology of Skinner's *Verbal Behavior*). The teaching programs of *reference* alone might eventually lead to the use of mands of the labels taught during this phase; the *control* teaching will make this progression quick and certain.

Self-extended Control. Reference and *control* trainings are meant to show the child that to the extent that he knows referents, he can manage his environment. But to a much greater extent, he is bound to find that he cannot extensively control his environment, because he does not know the necessary referents (labels) for all the things, actions, and actions-with-things he wishes. Thus, in maximizing the child's use of language to control his environment, it is important that he learn how to extend his referents, mainly by teaching him to request further instruction in the case of specific ignorances. This will be taught in the form of questions such as "What that?" in response to unknown things and "What (are) you doing?" in response to unknown actions. In effect, the child learns to request further, specific training inputs, based on his discrimination of what he does not know from what he already knows. This can be conceptualized as two simple chains controlled by two complex discriminative stimulus classes. Previously trained events produce labels, whereas events not previously trained produce questions. Although the forms of self-extended control proposed for this program are simple in themselves, the significance of their usage by the child is considered great, in that this usage can keep him in contact with the kinds of procedures he has been taught to respond to earlier. In particular, he has been taught to learn and remember what is conveyed by these teaching procedures. Thus, if the procedures do not lose that previously established function, the child becomes his own expander of his language capabilities, to that extent relieving the training program of presenting these yet untaught items. Furthermore, it makes the child the judge of what specific content he needs to learn next. From the point of view of knowing what is most functional in his current environment, he is presumably the best judge of what will maximize his contact with the environment-controlling (reinforcing) potential of language.

Integration. The power of symbolization lies largely in the capacity of individual symbols to be combined. They can be chained to accomplish an infinite variety of messages, each with its own environment-controlling potential. Together, their environment-controlling potential is so great as to stagger the descriptive abilities of even the psycholinguists. The act of combining the language skills taught in *reference, control,* and *self-extended control* is perhaps likely in children who are steadily in contact with the environment-controlling function of those skills, but it is not necessarily a certain or prompt process. Consequently, the fourth dimension of the program explicitly establishes ongoing integration of previously taught skills with currently taught skills. Furthermore, as an important part of integration, steps are programmed to be sure that the child's newly acquired techniques of self-extended control (with which he requests further instruction about what he does not yet know) are used in a functional manner (*i.e.,* are not only used to invite instruction, but are followed by storage and later use of the instruction given in answer to those requests). Thus, when the child learns to ask, "What's that?" in response to unknown things, he will also be confronted with the need to remember what he is told and to pass a receptive test of whether he remembers. If he does not remember, contingencies will be applied to promote that memory until the test is passed. A similar program is included to cover his acquisition of new action labels.

The most important research hypothesis of this program is that relatively brief instruction along these four dimensions of language usage will prove sufficient to produce the beginnings of a fundamental characteristic of "normal language"—it extends itself further without formal programming.

Content of the Training Program

The language training program is divided into six areas of emphasis. The first two categories, "persons and things" and "action with persons and things," exemplify all the essential structural components of the program. "Persons and things" begins with training to label common objects and things in the child's environment, preparatory to the acquisition of more complex speech and language skills. The concept of "yes/no" is taught and provides the basis for responding to numerous language concepts taught receptively throughout the entire training sequence. The child is also taught to ask for the names of objects he cannot identify in the "persons and things" category and to request items, using a simple sentence which includes the pronoun "I."

The "action with persons and things" category begins with training to label productively simple actions (a correlate to the object labeling taught in the "persons and things" category). Then the subject is taught to use an "I/you" discrimination; to combine pronouns, verbs, and object labels; to request that other persons engage in specific verb actions; and to ask questions about the labels of new actions. The individual training steps of this category, as well as the "persons and things" category, are repeatedly interrelated, such that the acquisition of one particular skill is expanded, refined, and rehearsed in subsequent steps. Thus, the training steps are organized within the four-dimensional structure—reference, control, self-extended control, and integration—described in the previous section.

Subsequent categories under the general heading "description of action with things" are presented as simple, similarly structured extensions of the program, to accomplish further language training in the content areas of "possession," "color," "size," and "relation." These remaining categories are not presently perceived as essential to the establishment of a basic verbal repertoire, but as additional training which adds useful (environment-controlling) precision to the child's existing repertoire. Thus, these areas could more appropriately be identified as basic educational training. The training procedures in each category are designed to 1) establish basic discriminations relevant to the stimulus dimensions for that particular concept, and 2) then teach the child to utilize this skill by engaging him in a series of statements, actions, and situations which require these discriminations for correct receptive and productive responding. The actions involved are based on the prior training of the "action with persons and things" category. These description categories are also organized sequentially in the reference, control, self-extended control, and integration dimensions of the training model, at both the productive and receptive levels, to continue and reinforce the effects those dimensions are hypothesized to accomplish.

Figure 2 presents in final outline form the 61 steps of the total program (plus an alternative training step, 4a) in the sequence of the complete manual. Each cell of the figure shows the final form of the language skill to be trained at that time. The teacher's actions and words are shown in lower case type. Each required response by the child is shown in upper case type. The sequence is self-explanatory.

Description of Training Steps

Each of the training categories contains a number of individual training steps which are sequentially arranged. The language trainer should follow the order of steps outlined, since a particular speech and language skill taught in one step usually provides the basis for extended training in subsequent steps. The "persons and things" category includes 9 training steps plus 1 alternate step. The alternate step (4a) is used to teach the yes/no discrimination if the original step 4 fails to train this important concept adequately. "Action with persons and things" includes 20 training steps (10–29). The remaining categories ("possession," "color," "size," and "relation") include 8 steps each, for a total of 61 steps, plus the alternate step, 4a.

Figure 2 presents the order of training steps as represented across the dimensions of reference, control, self-extended control, and integration. The figure describes the major stimulus provided by the trainer, plus the expected response from the child.

Training procedures for all steps in the first two categories ("persons and things," and "action with persons and things") have been written and are included in the experimental training manual. This includes 29 (plus 1 alternate) steps. The individual training steps for the remaining categories, which are subsumed under "description of action with things," must be finalized later, pending the completion of experimental training options for various steps in the first two major categories.

Outline of Training Steps. Each step follows the same outline which contains the goal, stimulus material needed for training, specific instructions for training, and a section entitled "programming for generalization."

Goal. This includes a short statement describing the exact response to be trained in the child, as well as a brief explanation as to why that particular response is being trained.

Stimulus Material. Listed for the trainer are the objects and reinforcers needed for the training step.

Instructions. The procedures to be followed in training are described in this section. For many steps, alternate training procedures are described. These alternate procedures are the subject of an experimental analysis (to be presented in a later section) to determine the most efficient training methods under specified subject parameters. Ultimately, only the most efficient training procedures will be included in the final draft of the manual. It should be stated that the training procedures described in the experimental manual

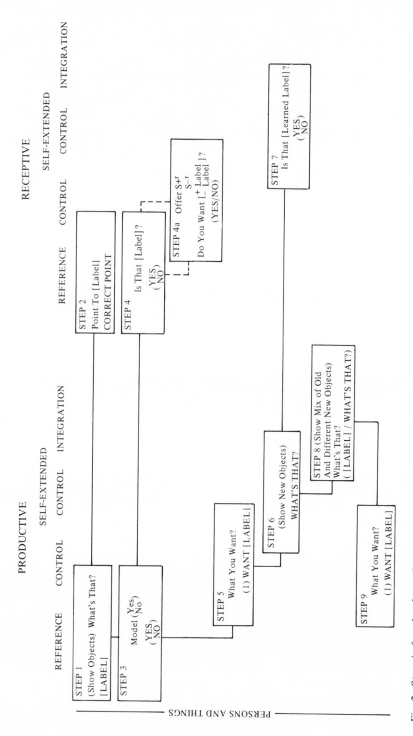

Fig. 2. Steps in functional speech and language training program.

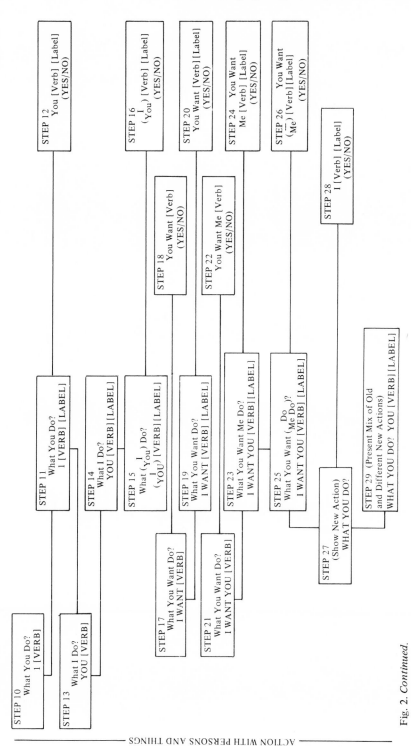

Fig. 2. Continued.

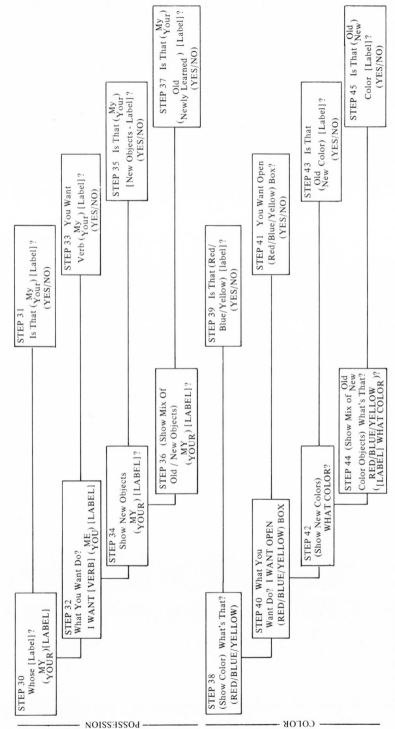

Fig. 2. *Continued.*

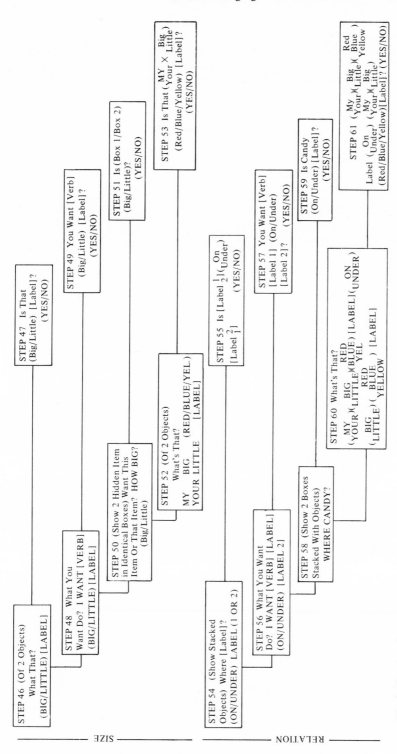

Fig. 2. Continued.

assume a certain level of sophistication with the terminology and principles of applied behavior analysis. Training instructions included in the final copy of the manual will be fully described with a minimum of technical jargon.

Programming for Generalization. All training steps include recommended procedures for extending training to the child's home or cottage setting. Experimental analyses will be made to determine the extent to which generalization occurs in natural settings, whether it be in the form of spontaneous utterances or correct responding to a more formal presentation of the particular skill trained in the laboratory.

Receptive Tests and Training Probes

Throughout the training program, the child is first taught expressively to use a certain speech skill. Training steps are then provided for teaching this same skill at the receptive level, using the yes/no response as an indication of the child's understanding of the concept. Receptive tests will be given immediately following the expressive training for a particular speech skill to determine if generalization to the receptive level does occur. If generalization occurs, the receptive level training step can be omitted altogether. If not, the child is then formally trained to respond receptively to what he has just previously learned at the expressive level. Similarly, "probes" will be used to determine the extent to which training in a skill generalizes to alternate settings and situations. These probes will assist in the over-all evaluation of the program and indicate the necessity for extended training in alternate settings and with persons other than the speech and language trainer. The receptive tests and generalization probes will be discussed more fully in the section pertaining to experimental analyses.

Generalization of the Training Program to Nonlaboratory Settings. Procedures to record and measure language acquisition during the individual steps outlined in part III of the training manual have been discussed. In each case, progress is measured as the number of sessions required to reach criterion for the response unit trained in the step. These measures, of course, provide valuable information pertaining to language acquisition under the experimental training conditions imposed in the laboratory. However, it is essential that systematic measurement be made of each child's speech usage in non-laboratory settings—settings which should contain spontaneous language usage in everyday social situations.

This evaluation will take place in a special KNI Language Training Unit. This unit, housing 16 nonverbal children, will be staffed by institutional personnel specially trained to gather data on residents' language use. Supervision of all aspects of language programming and data collection will be delegated to the Project Director. This arrangement will permit a controlled environment in which language data can be collected in a steady and systematic fashion, evaluating the generalization potential of the training program. The following measurement procedures will be utilized on the training unit to gather information on generalized and expanded language usage. They fall into two types of measures: 1) deliberate probes designed to evoke language and 2) verbatim recording of spontaneous language use.

Generalization Probes, Concurrent with Individual Training Steps, Designed to Evoke Language Use. These "probes" are designed to measure the extent to which a specific language skill trained in the controlled conditions of the laboratory generalizes to other (nontrainer) persons in different (nonlaboratory) settings. That is, does a child who is taught to label objects in step 1 of the training manual, for example, also label these same objects when presented by cottage personnel or by parents?

The generalization probes will be administered to the child before training begins for any particular step, at some point during training when the behavior is beginning to emerge, and following the successful completion of training (*i.e.*, when the child has reached criterion in the laboratory training session). Procedures for presenting the probe trials and the content (items) used in the presentations are similar to the procedures followed in the laboratory, without, however, "unnatural" programmed consequences for correct responses. But whenever presentation of a possibly reinforcing item is "naturally" appropriate to the child's response, *e.g.*, " I want milk," it certainly will be supplied whenever possible. (Indeed, the language training program is designed to make probable such "natural" contingencies on language use.) The probes will be conducted by cottage personnel under the supervision of the Project Director.

Data for the probe measures will be scored as percentages of correct responses to the items or questions presented.

Verbatim Record of Speech Usage in Small-Group Activity Sessions. These observations are especially critical to the evaluation of the language training program outlined in part III of the experimental manual. The purpose of this measurement procedure is to place the child in a social situation where his spontaneous speech can be recorded on a regularly scheduled basis, for later analysis of its content and structure. The spontaneous speech emitted by the child will be assessed for any correspondence to the speech skills taught in the current and/or recent training steps of the manual program. A major question is whether the child will spontaneously use the particular skills just taught in the laboratory and, more importantly, whether he shows expansions of either the content or structure of verbal skills trained under laboratory conditions.

Different children will come to part III of the training manual at different points in time. This will be a natural result of their differential rates of progress in the vocal imitation training in part II of the program, as well as of deliberate experimental control over their starting dates (exercised by researchers). In the long run, this will allow more careful assessment of any generalization potential of the language training sequence; since the children will be spread out over different training steps, their spontaneous language should demonstrate varying but corresponding levels of sophistication, depending on how far the child has advanced in the training sequence. This analysis will thus embody "multiple baseline" research design (Baer, Wolf, and Risley, 1968).

Procedurally, these measures will record the child's speech as expressed in an activity which is not structured for direct speech and language training. Small-group activity sessions will be the setting for such emission of spontaneous speech. These activity groups will be structured around various academically oriented skills and the development of appropriate play behavior. Each group will contain either four or five children under the immediate supervision of a Child Development Worker (institutional worker assigned to the Language Training Unit). The groups will meet daily for approximately 20-30 min. Group activities will involve playing games, working puzzles, listening to music, finger painting, coloring, sorting objects, paper and scissor exercises, etc. In one session each week, a verbatim record of each child's utterances will be recorded by an observer.

The speech *corpus* obtained during the group activity sessions will be analyzed for 1) frequency of utterances, 2) length of utterances, and 3) content and structure of utterances. Data sheets for recording speech in these activity sessions will indicate the particular step of the training sequence that the child has advanced to at that point in time.

Experimental Analyses of Training Procedures Options

Overview of Seven Experiments. In this section, seven experiments are described. Each takes place within the language training program described by the manual; and each is designed to clarify how the final manual can best be constructed, or, alternatively, how different procedures should be assigned to different subjects (on the basis of certain already existing characteristics).

Experiment 1 compares four different procedures for establishing the initial generalized vocal imitation skill necessary to begin the training program outlined in the manual. It emphasizes in particular the potentially facilitative role of *motor* imitation training as a precursor of concomitant *vocal* imitation training.

Experiment 2 compares contracted and expanded methods of vocal stimulus presentations in early training, *e.g.,* "What you want?" *vs.* "What do you want?", or "Want me open box?" *vs.* "Do you want me to open the box?", in terms of facilitating the subject's eventual use of expanded language forms.

Experiment 3 compares three different procedures for transferring vocal responses from the imitation (echoic) form resulting from the initial (premanual) training, to the object recognition form necessary for productive and receptive labeling and more advanced language behavior. The procedures will differ in the degree to which they incorporate modeling techniques in accomplishing this transition. The first procedure will model the correct response (to "What's that?", accompanied by an object) whenever an error (or no response) occurs; the second will model the correct response at first with every presentation of the object, and then gradually will model more and more intermittently on these presentations; the third will similarly accompany all initial object presentations with a model but will progressively reduce the physical aspects of the model (rather than its schedule of accompanying the object) until it is a minimal prompt (*e.g.,* "apple" reduces to "app-" and then to "a-" and finally to an open-mouth response characteristic of "a-").

Experiment 4 compares two methods of training individual recognition responses (receptive labeling behavior), either one at a time to mastery or three at a time to mastery. The question is, of three objects presented at a time, is it more economical to learn to recognize one of them, then a second, and then the third, or to learn concurrently to recognize all three?

Experiment 5 compares generalization across two developing language repertoires (expressive and receptive) during training on a range of linguistic content areas as the child progresses through the steps of the manual. The question (which has been examined experimentally using plurals as a linguistic class by Guess and Baer, 1973) is whether training on a productive (expressive) language repertoire facilitates the acquisition of a comprehensive (receptive) repertoire of the same content, or *vice versa.* Clear cut results can determine whether the manual steps are best trained in the present order of expressive first-receptive second, or the receptive repertoire should be first in the sequential training order, or perhaps that it makes little difference.

Experiment 6 compares training conducted by a single trainer who presents stimuli, models responses, reinforces desired behavior, and times-out errors, to training conducted by two trainers, one of whom plays the role of an ideal subject, answering the first trainer correctly and being reinforced for doing so. The second trainer thus could serve as a model for the real subject, potentially reducing his probability of errors (and thus maximizing his reinforcement and minimizing his time-outs). The question is whether this change results in sufficiently better learning to justify the expense of the two-trainer method. The two-trainer method may prove especially useful in the modeling necessary for training I/you discriminations.

Experiment 7 uses the two-trainer method to ask whether a stimulus-chaining procedure can be used to facilitate learning by the child at a potentially difficult transition in the program. In this experiment, the child is learning to label another's action correctly (as, *e.g.,* "you play"), after having just learned to label his own actions (*e.g.,* "I play"). "I/you" confusion is likely. In one method (not involving stimulus chaining), the label is taught directly: the first trainer presents an action, the second trainer models by correctly describing that action and being reinforced; the first trainer then asks the child to label the same action. In the stimulus-chaining method, the two trainers first go through a preliminary verbal interaction (which the subject has already learned) and chain stimuli for the now-to-be learned lesson directly to it. For example, the first and second trainers first run through a sequence of "What you want?"–"I want coke" (receives coke, starts to drink) as an entree to a "What I do?"–"You drink" training exercise involving the subject. The question is whether there is any behavioral "inertia" to be gained by preceding a difficult new response with the modeling of a familiar (already mastered) one.

REFERENCES

Baer, D. M. and Guess, D. Receptive training of adjectival inflections in mental retardates. *J. Appl. Behav. Anal.*, 1971, *4*, 129–139.
Baer, D. M. and Guess, D. Teaching productive noun suffixes to severely retarded children. *Amer. J. Ment. Defic.*, 1973, *77*, 498–505.
Baer, D. M., Peterson, R. F., and Sherman, J. A. The development of imitation by reinforcing behavioral similarity to a model. *J. Exp. Anal. Behav.*, 1967, *10*, 405–416.
Baer, D. M. and Sherman, J. A. Reinforcement control of generalized imitation in young children. *J. Exp. Child Psychol.*, 1964, *1*, 37–49.
Baer, D. M., Wolf, M. M., and Risley, T. R. Some current dimensions of applied behavior analysis. *J. Appl. Behav. Anal.*, 1968, *1*, 91–97.
Bellugi, U. The emergence of inflections and negation systems in the speech of two children. Paper presented at New England Psychological Association, 1964.
Bereiter, C. and Engelmann, S. *Teaching Disadvantaged Children in the Preschool.* Englewood Cliffs, N. J.: Prentice-Hall, 1966.
Berko, J. The child's learning of English morphology. *Word*, 1958, *14*, 150–177.
Bloom, L. Language development: Form and function in emerging grammar. *M.I.T. Press Res. Monogr.*, 1970, No. 59.
Braine, M. D. The ontogeny of English phrase structure: The first phase. *Language*, 1963, *39*, 1–13.
Bricker, W. A. A systematic approach to language training. In R. L. Schiefelbusch (Ed.), *Language of the Mentally Retarded.* Baltimore: University Park Press, 1972.
Bricker, W. A. and Bricker, D. D. A program of language training for the severely handicapped child. *Except. Child.*, 1970, *37*, 101–111.
Brown, R. Derivational complexity and the order of acquisition in child speech. Carnegie-Mellon Conference on Cognitive Processes, 1968.
Brown, R. and Fraser, C. The acquisition of syntax. *Monogr. Soc. Res. Child Develop.*, 1964, *29*, 43–79.
Buddenhagen, R. G. *Establishing Vocal Verbalizations in Mute Mongoloid Children.* Champaign, Ill.: Research Press Co., 1971.
Chomsky, N. A. *Aspects of the Theory of Syntax.* Cambridge, Mass.: MIT Press, 1965.
Chomsky, N. and Halle, M. *The Sound Pattern of English.* New York: Harper and Row, 1968.
Cook, C. and Adams, H. E. Modification of verbal behavior in speech deficient children. *Behav. Res. Ther.*, 1966, *4*, 265–271.
Dunn, L. M., Horton, K. B., and Smith, J. O. *Manual for the Peabody*

Language Development Kit (Level P). Minneapolis: American Guidance Service, 1965.

Dunn, L. M. and Smith, J. O. *Manual for the Peabody Language Development Kit* (Level 1). Minneapolis: American Guidance Service, 1965.

Dunn, L. M. and Smith, J. O. *Manual for the Peabody Language Development Kit* (Level 2). Minneapolis: American Guidance Service, 1966.

Dunn, L. M. and Smith, J. O. *Manual for the Peabody Language Development Kit* (Level 3). Minneapolis: American Guidance Service, 1967.

Fraser, C., Bellugi, U., and Brown, R. Control of grammar in imitation, comprehension, and production. *J. Verb. Learning Verb. Behav.*, 1963, *2*, 121–135.

Garcia, E. E., Baer, D. M., and Firestone, I. The development of generalized imitation within experimentally determined boundaries. *J. Appl. Behav. Anal.*, 1971, *4*, 101–112.

Garcia, E. E., Guess, D., and Byrnes, J. Development of syntax through imitation of a model. *J. Appl. Behav. Anal.*, 1973, *6*, 299–310.

Guess, D. A functional analysis of receptive language and productive speech: Acquisition of the plural morpheme. *J. Appl. Behav. Anal.*, 1969, *2*, 55–64.

Guess, D. and Baer, D. M. An analysis of individual differences in generalization between receptive and productive language in retarded children. *J. Appl. Behav. Anal.*, 1973, *6*, 311–329.

Guess, D. and Baer, D. M. Some experimental analyses of linguistic development in institutionalized retarded children. In B. B. Lahey (Ed.), *The Modification of Language Behavior*, Chap. 1. Springfield, Ill.: Charles C Thomas, 1973.

Guess, D., Ensminger, E. E., and Smith, J. O. *A Language Development Program for Mentally Retarded Children*, Vols. I and II. Project 7-0815, U.S. Office of Education, Bureau of Education for the Handicapped, 1969.

Guess, D., Rutherford, G., and Twichell, A. Speech acquisition in a mute, visually impaired adolescent. *The New Outlook for the Blind*, January, 1969.

Guess, D., Sailor, W., Rutherford, G., and Baer, D. M. An experimental analysis of linguistic development: The productive use of the plural morpheme. *J. Appl. Behav. Anal.*, 1968, *1*, 225–235.

Harrelson, A. Effects of productive speech training on receptive language. Master's thesis, University of Kansas, Lawrence, 1969.

Hartung, J. R. A review of procedures to increase verbal imitation skills and functional speech in autistic children. *J. Speech Hear. Disord.*, 1970, *35*, 204–217.

Haviland, R. T. A stimulus to language development: The institutional environment. *Ment. Retard.*, 1972, *10*, 19–21.

Hewett, P. M. Teaching speech to an autistic child through operant conditioning. *Amer. J. Orthopsychiat.*, 1965, *35*, 927–936.

Irwin, O. C. Infant speech. *Sci. Amer.*, Sept., 1949, 3–5.

Irwin, O. C. Development of speech during infancy: Curve of phonemic frequencies. *J. Exp. Psychol.*, 1942a, *37*, 187–193.

Irwin, O. C. Developmental status of speech sounds in ten feeble-minded children. *Child Develop.*, 1942b, *13*, 22–39.

Irwin, O. C. Speech development in the young child: 2. Some factors related to the speech development of the infant and young child. *J. Speech Hear. Disord.*, 1952, *17*, 269–279.

Irwin, O. C. and Chen, H. P. Development of speech during infancy: Curve of phonemic types. *J. Exp. Psychol.*, 1946, *36*, 431–436.

Isaacs W., Thomas, J., and Goldiamond, I. Application of operant conditioning to reinstate verbal behavior in mute psychotics. *J. Abnorm. Psychol.*, 1965, *70*, 155–164.

Jakobson, R., Fant, C. G., and Halle, M. *Preliminaries to Speech Analysis: The Distinctive Features and Their Correlates*, Ed. 2. Cambridge, Mass.: M.I.T. Press, 1963.

Kent, L. R., Klein, D., Falk, A., and Guenther, H. A language acquisition program for the retarded. In J. E. McLean, D. E. Yoder, and R. L. Schiefelbusch (Eds.), *Language Intervention with the Retarded*. Baltimore: University Park Press, 1972.

Kerr, N., Meyerson, L., and Michael, J. A. Procedure for shaping vocalizations in a mute child. In L. P. Ullman and L. Krasner (Eds.), *Case Studies in Behavior Modification*. New York: Holt, 1965.

Lenneberg, E. H. The capacity for language. In J. Fodor and J. Katz (Eds.), *Readings in the Philosophy of Language*. Englewood Cliffs, N. J.: Prentice-Hall, 1964.

Lenneberg, E. H. *Biological Foundations of Language*. New York: Wiley, 1967.

Lenneberg, E. H., Nichols, I. A., and Rosenberger, E. F. Primitive stages of language development in mongolism. *Res. Publ. Ass. Res. Nerv. Ment. Dis.*, 1964, *42*.

Leopold, W. F. *Speech Development of a Bilingual Child: A Linguistic Learning in the First Two Years*. Evanston, Ill.: Northwestern University Press, 1939.

Lovaas, O. I. Some studies on the treatment of childhood schizophrenia. *Res. Psychother.*, 1968, *3*, 103–121.

Lovaas, O. I., Berberich, J. P., Perloff, B. F., and Schaeffer, B. Acquisition of imitative speech by schizophrenic children. *Science*, 1966, *151*, 705–707.

Lovell, K. and Bradbury, B. The learning of English morphology in educationally subnormal school children. *Amer. J. Ment. Defic.*, 1967, *71*, 609–615.

McCarthy, D. Language development in children. In L. Carmichael (Ed.), *Manual of Child Psychology*. New York: Wiley, 1954, pp. 492–630.

McNeill, D. *The Acquisition of Language*. New York: Harper and Row, 1970.

Milisen, R. The incidence of speech disorders. In L. E. Travis (Ed.), *Handbook of Speech Pathology and Audiology*. New York: Appleton-Century-Crofts, 1972.

Miller, J. F. and Yoder, D. On developing the content for a language teaching program. *Ment. Retard.*, 1972, *10*, 9–11.

Miller, W. and Ervin, S. The development of grammar in child language. *Monogr. Soc. Res. Child Develop.*, 1964, *29*, 9–34.

Peterson, R. F. Some experiments on the organization of a class of imitative behaviors. *J. Appl. Behav. Anal.*, 1968, *1*, 225–235.

Rebelsky, F., Starr, R. H., and Luria, Z. Language development: The first four years. In Y. Brackbill (Ed.), *Infancy and Early Childhood*. New York: Free Press, 1967, pp. 289–357.

Risley, T. R. and Wolf, M. M. Experimental manipulation of autistic behaviors and generalization into the home. In R. Ulrich, T. Stachnik, and J. Mabry (Eds.), *The Control of Human Behavior*. Glenview, Ill.: Scott, Foresman, 1966, pp. 193–198.

Risley, T. R. and Wolf, M. M. Establishing functional speech in echolalic children. *Behav. Res. Ther.*, 1967, *5*, 73–88.

Sailor, W. Developing language in autistic children. Paper presented to the Ontario Speech and Hearing Association, Nov., 1970.

Sailor, W. Reinforcement and generalization of productive plural allomorphs in two retarded children. *J. Appl. Behav. Anal.*, 1971, *4*, 305–310.

Sailor, W. and Taman, T. Stimulus factors in the training of prepositional usage in three autistic children. *J. Appl. Behav. Anal.*, 1972, *5*, 183–190.

Salzinger, K. Experimental manipulation of verbal behavior: A review. *J. Gen. Psychol.*, 1959, *61*, 65–94.

Salzinger, K., Feldman, R. S., Cowan, J. E., and Salzinger, S. Operant conditioning of verbal behavior of two young speech-deficient boys. In L. Krasner and L. P. Ullman (Eds.), *Research in Behavior Modification.* New York: Holt, Rinehart and Winston, 1965.

Salzinger, S. K., Salzinger, K., Portnoy, S., Eckman, J., Bacon, P. N., Dentsch, M., and Zubin, J. Operant conditioning of continuous speech in children. *Child Develop.*, 1962, *33*, 683–695.

Schumaker, J. and Sherman, J. A. Training generative verb usage by imitation and reinforcement procedures. *J. Appl. Behav. Anal.*, 1970, *3*, 273–287.

Semmel, M. I. and Dolley, D. G. Comprehension and imitation of sentences by Down's syndrome children as a function of transformational complexity. *Amer. J. Ment. Defic.*, 1971, *75*, 739–745.

Sherman, J. A. Reinstatement of verbal behavior in a psychotic by reinforcement methods. *J. Speech Hear. Disord.*, 1963, *28*, 398–401.

Sherman, J. A. Use of reinforcement and imitation to reinstate verbal behavior in mute psychotics. Unpublished dissertation, University of Washington, Seattle, 1964.

Sherman, J. A. Use of reinforcement and imitation to reinstate verbal behavior in mute psychotics. *J. Abnorm. Psychol.*, 1965, *70*, 155–164.

Skinner, B. F. *Verbal Behavior.* New York: Appleton-Century-Crofts, 1957.

Sloane, H. N., Jr., Johnston, M. K., and Harris, F. R. Remedial procedures for teaching verbal behavior to speech deficient or defective young children. In H. N. Sloane, Jr. and B. MacAuley (Eds.), *Operant Procedures in Remedial Speech and Language Training.* Boston: Houghton-Mifflin, 1968, pp. 77–101.

Slobin, D. I. Early grammatical development in several languages, with special attention to Soviet research. In T. Bever and W. Weksel (Eds.), *The Structure and Psychology of Language.* New York: Holt, Rinehart, and Winston, 1971.

Staats, A. W. *Learning, Language, and Cognition.* New York: Holt, Rinehart, and Winston, 1968.

Sulzbacher, S. I. and Costello, J. M. A behavioral strategy for language training of a child with autistic behaviors. *J. Speech Hear. Disord.*, 1970, *35*, 256–277.

Tawney, J. W. and Hipsher, L. W. *Systematic Language Instruction.* Unpublished manual. U. S. Dept. of Health, Education, and Welfare (Grant OEG-0-8-001025 (032), Project 71205), 1970.

Wheeler, A. J. and Sulzer, B. Operant training and generalization of a verbal response form in a speech-deficient child. *J. Appl. Behav. Anal.*, 1970, *3*, 139–147.

Wolf, M. M., Risley, T. R., and Mees, H. Application of operant conditioning procedures to the behavior problems of an autistic child. *Behav. Res. Ther.*, 1964, 305–312.

Young, F. M. An analysis of certain variables in a developmental study of language. *Genet. Psychol. Monogr.*, 1941, *23*, 3–141.

CHAPTER TWENTY-TWO

ISSUES IN LANGUAGE TRAINING[1]

Kenneth F. Ruder and Michael D. Smith

Bureau of Child Research and Department of Linguistics, University of Kansas, Lawrence, Kansas 66044

Since no single language training program will meet all the needs of a group of mentally retarded children, the clinician is faced with evaluating and choosing among many and varied offerings of currently available language training programs. The following discussion is intended to serve as a guide in the selection process only in that it highlights what may be considered some of the more relevant and pragmatic issues concerned with language training of the retarded. These issues revolve around 1) the question of *what* (content) to train; 2) the selection of a suitable procedural methodology, thus determining *how* to train the necessary linguistic behaviors; and 3) assessment techniques.

Generally speaking, the language training programs proposed elsewhere in this book are based on a developmental model. Regarding the content of language training programs, Miller and Yoder (1972) advocated the use of available data on language development in normal children. Further, they stressed that such content should be taught in a sequence patterned on normal developmental trends. Gray and Ryan (1973) disputed this claim by arguing that their 40 programs need not be trained in any specific order. Guess, Sailor, and Baer (this volume) and Baer and Guess (in press) also took issue with the Miller and Yoder claim. According to these researchers, there are not sufficient empirical data on developmental progressions characteristic of normal language development from which one might determine whether or not a particular set of linguistic behaviors serves as a prerequisite to the acquisition of other linguistic behaviors. Consequently, as Guess, Sailor, and Baer indicated, whether or not a particular set of linguistic behaviors need be taught in a particular order is an empirical question which remains to be answered. Miller and Yoder's (1972) claim is difficult to evaluate but nonetheless worthy of considerable attention. Without sufficient empirical data,

[1] The preparation of this paper as well as some of the research reported herein was supported in part by Grants HD 00870 and HD 00183 from National Institute of Child Health and Development and Grant NS 10468 from National Institute of Neurological Disease and Stroke to the Bureau of Child Research, University of Kansas.

this guideline may be—at least for the present—not entirely functional as a criterion to be used in evaluating a language training program. However, in defense of Miller and Yoder, there are considerable observationally orientiated data on the content and developmental progressions characteristic of the normal acquisition process (see Bloom, 1970; Bowerman, 1973; Brown, 1973; Slobin, 1973). Hence, it might be that little is to be lost and perhaps a great deal is to be gained from structuring training programs on such data. It is possible that the results of programs modeled on the normal acquisition process will translate into strict empirical evidence in support of the implications of the observationally oriented data. (In connection with attempts to empirically motivate observationally based hypotheses, we have developed a procedure designed to measure what effects training on a particular linguistic behavior has on a nontrained behavior. This procedure will be discussed later in this chapter.)

Assuming, then, that something of value is to be gained from language training programs based on developmental models, an important criterion concerning their content is that training one behavior or set of behaviors serves as a prerequisite to the training and/or acquisition of another behavior or set of behaviors. Implicit in such models is the assumption that some terminal language behavior is specified which (for one reason or another) the language interventionist considers to be functional behavior for the particular child to be trained. Perhaps an example of such a building principle is in order. First of all, consider what might be a reasonable goal for training a language-deficient child in English; the simple active affirmative declarative sentence is the most frequently used structure and the base from which other structures are derived. A reasonable initial goal might thus be to train a child to the point where he is at least capable of using the subject-verb-object (S-V-O) string as the basic communicative structure. Selecting the S-V-O string as our initial goal does meet the requirement that the structure be of some functional utility in the child's everyday communicative needs in that it is a structure which can be used in his everyday communication.

Upon examining the semantic relations underlying the S-V-O string, one finds that those relations can be expressed as agent-action-object relations. These semantically based relations have been discussed as being pivotal to a language training program (Miller and Yoder, this volume) and have been extensively discussed as universal relations in the language acquisition process (Bloom, 1970; Brown, 1973; and Bowerman, 1973). In light of the apparent universality of the agent-action-object semantic relations, it might be well to consider the expression of these semantic relations as the pivotal aspect of a language acquisition program. Hence, inclusion of agent-action-object expressions should be considered a necessary component of any language program.

Considering the agent-action-object relations as the pivotal structure permits the form of a language training program to be two-faceted: 1) the training of behaviors leading to the expression of verbal propositions containing the agent-action-object relations and 2) the modification of the basic propositions. The first part of the program can be viewed as taking the child from expression of single word utterances which express either agent, action, or object relations to the two-word stage (expressing agent-action, action-object, and/or agent-object relations) and on to three-word expressions of these semantic relations. Expression of these semantic relations can be mapped directly onto the basic S-V-O strings of English. The second facet of such a program can be described as performing operations on the basic agent-action-object proposition. These operations can be viewed as being of two types: 1) operations on the entire proposition (*e.g.*, negation, question, tense, etc.) or 2) operations on elements within the proposition (*e.g.*, modification of nouns and verbs). An example might be helpful to illustrate the different types of operations. Given a child using one-word responses designating agent or object functions, one may modify such responses by adding a negative marker to the verbal expression such as the addition of "no," "all gone," or a simple headshake. The same operation would apply to a longer string such as a three-word S-V-O string, which could be negated in the same way or could be made into a question through the use of either rising terminal intonation or a tag such as the use of "O.K." (*e.g.*, "don't eat food, O.K."). Operations on elements within the proposition differ in that they are confined to portions of the proposition rather than the proposition as a whole. For example, one could view the use of plural inflections or adjectival modifiers with the agentive noun in the preceding example (*e.g.*, "dog eat food") as a modification only of the agentive noun, with the basic communicative intent of the proposition remaining the same.

The preceding examples are intended only to illustrate the over-all direction a language training program could take while utilizing the basic semantic relations expressed in *agent-action-object* strings. If such strings are incorporated as the pivotal structures upon which a program is based, we are provided with a workable goal, namely, the training of structures upon which can be built the more complex linguistic behaviors. Most important, it simplifies the task facing the child in that such a training program provides a cohesiveness by including explicitly related rules and structures rather than presenting the child with a series of seemingly unrelated rules.

Implicit in a model which centers around the training of agent-action-object strings are several procedural issues. The first of these issues has been discussed at some length by Miller and Yoder (this volume), namely, that new functions to be trained be built upon old forms. More specifically, this *building* principle can be stated as follows: "Old forms are used to express new functions and old functions used to express new forms." This principle simplifies the task of learning new structures and functions. In the past, such a building principle has been overlooked in the development and utilization of language training programs. Such a building principle as a primary procedural issue will be discussed later in this chapter.

Another procedural issue to be discussed in terms of language training program evaluation involves the selection of a specific training paradigm. Basically, all training paradigms can be broken down into three basic mechanical components: 1) antecedent events, including stimulus array and mode of presentation; 2) response events; and 3) subsequent events, primarily reinforcement procedures and schedules. The central question here is: given a specific linguistic structure to train, what is the most effective way to train it? The key word in the preceding statement is the word "effective." There are a number of training paradigms which are potentially capable of achieving the target behavior. The problem, then, is to determine whether one particular procedure achieves the same result in less time with less effort than another procedure. Some general issues here concern the use of imitation and comprehension procedures, the use of modeling and expansion techniques, and the question of generalization or overgeneralization of trained items to untrained items. Each of these procedural issues will be discussed in some detail in succeeding sections of this chapter.

In addition to the evaluation of the content and procedures of a language training program, there are other questions worthy of mention but which are all too often neglected by language interventionists. Among these questions are those concerned with assessment and those concerned with the utility of the structures trained. Questions regarding assessment procedures include what linguistic forms (content) should be considered in the initial evaluation. Another issue to be considered is the question of whether or not the language training program itself allows for assessment, necessarily including the assessment of individual components and procedures to determine if they are in need of revision or elimination to achieve the goal of a more efficient training program. Also ignored are issues concerned with the utility of the linguistic structures selected to be trained.

The passive structure in English, for example, would have very little functional utility for the language-impaired child or, for that matter, the normally developing child (Goldman-Eisler, 1968) and should thus be assigned a low priority rating in a language training sequence. Related to this issue, and probably more often ignored, is the seemingly external problem commonly referred to in clinical terminology as "carry-over." It is quite obvious to the everyday practitioner engaged in language training that it is important to include training on appropriate situations calling for use of a particular structure as well as direct training on that structure. That is to say, when evaluating a language training program, it is necessary to insure that there are provisions for training the child *when* and *where* it is appropriate to use the to-be-trained structures in everyday communication.

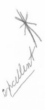

WHAT TO TRAIN–ISSUES CONCERNED WITH THE CONTENT OF A LANGUAGE TRAINING PROGRAM

The content of a language training program usually reflects the researcher's views concerning language structure and linguistic theory as they might apply to language development. Consequently, the number and types of linguistic structures selected for inclusion in a training program are representative of the researcher's theoretical persuasions. There is a need for more interaction among those involved in psycholinguistics and language training research in order to avoid inefficiency and, in turn, increase the likelihood of arriving at a reliable means of training functional language.

The content of most language training programs can be classified according to how they define the nature of linguistic structures. Linguistic structures may be defined as embodying 1) syntactically based structural relationships, 2) semantically based structural relationships, or 3) a combination of these. An example of a training program which assumes that linguistic relationships are syntactically based is one which considers two-word utterances to be realizations of *pivot + open* constructions. In contrast, a training program which assumes that linguistic relationships are semantically based is one which considers two-word utterances to be expressions of semantic relationships like *agent-action, action-object,* or *agent-object.* Language training programs of the third type view the surface forms as mapping a conceptual base (Premack, 1970). The issue here is not so much a matter of which of the above models one would subscribe to, but rather the degree to which one structures a training program based on a particular viewpoint to the exclusion of other viewpoints. Fortunately, not all training programs are as dogmatic in regard to their particular view of language structure as it might first seem. Few would deny, for instance, that, in order to be functional, language must have a conceptual base. This may be saying nothing more than that a person must have something to talk about and that, in order to be understood by members of his language community, there are certain prescribed rules which must be adhered to if the communication event is to be successful.

A central issue here concerns the amount of linguistic knowledge the researcher proposes that the subject should be exposed to and expected subsequently to absorb. As Schlesinger (this volume) and Watt (1970) pointed out, in research on the normal acquisition process, the tendency has been to work from an adult model and, hence, perhaps credit the child with too much knowledge. According to Schlesinger and Watt, it is more desirable to credit the child with as little as possible in the way of grammatically and/or semantically based knowledge. There are implications here for language training programs. For instance, a training program based essentially on surface structure would view such sentences as "The knife is cutting," "The girl is swimming," and "The baby is falling" as being identical linguistic structures. A semantically based view of language, however, would interpret these three sentences as expressing different semantic relationships. In terms of Fillmore's (1968) case grammar, for example, the sentence "The girl is swimming" expresses an *agentive* relationship (where an animate noun functions as the instigator of an activity), whereas the sentence "The knife is cutting" expresses an *instrumental* relationship (where an object is causally involved in an action). Further, in the sentence "The baby is falling," a *dative* relationship is expressed (where the animate grammatical subject is affected). The differences involved in these underlying relationships are not immediately apparent even to the normal adult speaker of English. Nonetheless, it is quite possible that a mature linguistic competence has the capacity to make these semantically based distinctions. In terms of accounting for the emerging linguistic competence of normal children, Bowerman (1973) and Brown (1973) demonstrated quite effectively that, of the available models, those based on case grammar are the most adequate. However, while a case grammar model of the type used by Bowerman and Brown may to date be the most revealing approach to the study of the acquisition process in the natural setting, it is not immediately apparent that it is, in turn, the most appropriate model for the task of language training. Perhaps a more suitable approach is one similar to that of Schlesinger (this volume) where at the outset of the acquisition process agentive expressions include those which are later treated as instrumentals and datives. Such an approach does not necessitate the inclusion of the finer distinctions entailed by instrumental and dative expressions in attempts at training structures like those mentioned above. The exclusion of the finer distinctions at the outset of training may simplify the task of a training program. That is, it may be more realistic to overlook the finer distinctions in favor of capitalizing on the surface structure similarities. Suci and Hamacher's (1972) research into the psychological dimensions of finer case distinctions in young children, as opposed to adults, supports such an approach.

   In an attempt to assess the facilitative effects of surface similarities in the presence of underlying semantic distinctions, a study was designed to train the English copula and auxiliary structures. In a preliminary study, Stremel (1973) selected several language-deficient mentally retarded (MR) children who showed no use of either the copula (to be) or use of the auxiliary (to be). Training on the copula construction was initiated for one group of subjects while the second group received initial training on the auxiliary structure. Upon reaching criterion (90% correct usage) on the copula structure, subjects in the first group were then trained on the auxiliary structure, and, likewise, for the second group of subjects, auxiliary structure training was followed by training on the copula. Procedures in either training sequence consisted of presenting the subject with a visual stimulus and a verbal model which the subject was to imitate echoically (initial production training). Gradually, the echoic response was faded until replaced by spontaneous production with the help of a visual prompt in the form of an "equal" ($/=/$) symbol to remind the subject to include "is" in the verbal response. The visual symbol was the same for both the copula and the auxiliary structures, thus treating these two linguistically distinct forms as being similar on the basis of surface topography. In all cases, the subjects learned both forms. Table 1 summarizes the data, which indicate quite clearly that, regardless of the training sequence, acquisition of the copula required less trials than acquisition of the auxiliary form, thus indicating that prior training of *to be* in the auxiliary structure did not significantly affect copula training. These data can be interpreted as demonstrating the functional independence of the copula from the auxiliary form, thus supporting the notion of linguistic and functional distinctness between two superficially similar structures. However, if one looks at the acquisition of the auxiliary, the data reflect a functional interdependence that is unidirectional, implying that copula training should precede training of the auxiliary form. While this study does not answer the question as to whether it is more efficient to train the copula and auxiliary

Table 1. Effect of Training Sequence in the Acquisition of the Copula and Auxiliary "to be"*

Subjects	Copula		Auxiliary	
	First trained (group I)	Second trained (group II)	First trained (group II)	Second trained (group I)
1	18	6	42	9
2	14	19	44	37
3	19	9	54	47
4	6	21	57	11
5	15	15	36	32
6	16	24	27	28
7	10	6	62	14
8	13	16	29	11
9		3	35	
10		0	47	
Mean	13.8	11.9	43.3	23.6
Standard deviation	4.25	8.19	11.8	14.3
	$t = 0.61$		$t = 3.19$	
	(Not significant at 0.05 level of confidence for two-tailed t-test)		(Significant beyond 0.01 level of confidence. Critical value for $t_{0.01}$ (two-tailed) $= 2.92$)	

*Group I subjects received training first in the copula and second in the auxiliary while group II subjects received training in the opposite sequence. Numerical entries are trials to 90% criterion.

forms by utilizing surface similarities as opposed to utilizing their linguistic uniqueness, it does demonstrate that language-deficient MR children are potentially capable of utilizing surface similarities.

Demonstrations like the above, indicative of how surface similarities may facilitate training, are not grounds to exclude the systematic treatment and possible facilitating effects of what might be called conceptually based semantic distinctions. Though not the intention of this particular study, it can be argued by way of analogy that the rationale underlying the laboratory research dealing with the acquisition of the mechanical principles (governing regularities of surface forms) of semantically empty languages by learning theorists has influenced operant-oriented attempts at language training, where language is viewed as a set of environmentally controlled stimulus (class)-response (class) networks. The resultant assumption has been that training programs based primarily on various imitation and differential reinforcement techniques may result in the emergence of functional language (Lynch and Bricker, 1972; Malouf and Dodd, 1972; Guess and Baer, 1973a; Salzinger, 1973). However, as Braine (1970), Malouf and Dodd (1972), and Lynch and Bricker (1972) pointed out, such an assumption leads to a misleading over-simplification of the processes underlying language development. Aware of the tendency to oversimplify, Bandura (1969, 1970), Sherman (1971), and Whitehurst (in press), agreed that much of the operant research has been too much concerned with training procedures which utilize imitation and differential reinforcement techniques to train language than with the actual processes involved. According to Bandura (1970), the consequence has been that research dealing with the role of imitation has dealt with the question of language development in a most cursory manner. Premack (1970), concurring with Bandura, pointed out that imitation-based training procedures, if successful in training selected linguistic behaviors, do not necessarily serve as plausible explanations of how subjects acquired the behaviors in question. Still, such controversy does not rule out the possibility that the development of language is in part dependent upon contingency awareness, implying that language is *in part* environmentally controlled learned behavior. Therefore, by attending to the potential of training on systematic combinations of semantically or syntactically based distinctions and, at the same time, relying on suitable procedures to induce contingency awareness (Ferster, 1972), it is possible that the goal of designing an optimal language training program is within reach.

With this goal in mind, the theoretical perspective of Premack (1970) which holds that language maps a conceptual base is worthy of much consideration. Premack views functional language as being governed by four essential principles, all of which are discussed in terms of discrimination processes. These principles are: 1) discriminations between different environmental events, 2) discrimination of symbols, 3) discriminations between different linguistic symbols, and 4) discriminations between different sequential arrangements of symbols. The first principle can be viewed as the conceptual base; the others represent the symbolic mapping of the conceptual base. Premack's (1970) analysis of functional language in terms of these four basic components or principles stems from his research with Sarah, his chimpanzee. These same principles, however, form the basis for several of the language training programs discussed in the preceding chapters as well as that recently described by Stremel and Waryas (1973). It might be noted here that Premack's interpretation of the origin and nature of functional language is not unlike that of Schlesinger (1971, this volume), who posited a conceptual base and, hence, a mapping of a conceptual base onto a surface representation.

It is becoming increasingly apparent, then, that, whereas in the past it has been possible to talk about the content of the language training program strictly in terms of the surface grammatical forms, this approach is quickly becoming inadequate. The semantically based theories of language acquisition (Bloom, 1970; Schlesinger, 1971a, b, this volume; Bowerman, 1973; Brown, 1973) have already made themselves felt with regard to specifying the content of language training programs (Stremel and Waryas, 1973; Bricker and Bricker, 1973). Some recent attempts have also been made to incorporate a Piagetian view of conceptual development into language training (Bricker and Bricker, 1973, this volume) as well as into the process of normal language acquisition. In view of this emphasis on the conceptual base for language acquisition and language training, it might do well to examine briefly some of the issues which eventually contributed to a conceptually based view of the language acquisition process and its implications for language training programs.

As much of the current developmental psycholinguistic literature (Brown, 1973; Bloom, 1973; Bowerman, 1973; Schlesinger, in press, Slobin, 1973; and Greenfield *et al.,* 1972) and a number of the preceding chapters indicate, the role of cognition in language development is receiving considerable attention. The rise of transformational theory and the advent of generative grammar (Chomsky, 1957) and their application to the formalization (*vs.* operationalization) of the acquisition process, however, predicted quite the opposite. The original claim was that cognitive abilities of the young child are much too limited to serve as a basis for the acquisition of language. In addition, it was claimed that a child's verbal environment is incapable of systematically rendering assistance to the child. In all fairness, it is necessary to mention here that the Chomskyan position was based on the state of cognitive psychology as related to linguistic theory in the late 1950's and early 1960's. During these years, too little was known about the direction of dependency between cognitive and linguistic abilities. The result was that Chomsky's attempt to develop a formal model of language and the language acquisition process was qualified with his statement that language acquisition may eventually be explained by the concept-forming abilities of the young child and the system of linguistic universals that these abilities imply (1965, p. 32). With this qualification in mind, consideration of extralinguistic factors was discouraged and the child came to be viewed as being somehow innately predisposed to acquire language (Chomsky and Miller, 1963; Chomsky, 1959, 1965, 1968; Lenneberg, 1967; McNeill, 1970, 1971). Furthermore, Chomsky's (1957) observation that, on the one hand, some sentences are meaningless but at the same time grammatical and, on the other hand, that some sentences are meaningful but at the same time ungrammatical led to the conclusion that grammar is autonomous and independent of meaning. Chomsky's generative syntax and the model of language it entails were originally designed to facilitate the mapping of syntactic structure onto semantic structure. Upon its projection into the acquisition process by nativists, it became the basis of the innateness hypothesis (Chomsky, 1965, 1968; Bever et al., 1965; Lenneberg, 1967; McNeill, 1970, 1971).

As a reaction to the assumptions and implications of Chomsky's formal model, McCawley (1968), Lakoff and Ross (1968), Fillmore (1968), and Lakoff (1971) proposed what is known as generative semantics. According to the theory of generative semantics, the grammatical structure of language is a function of semantic constraints. In contrast to Chomsky, the assumption here is that semantic representations are mapped onto syntactic structures. McCawley (1968) proposed a formation rule component designed to specify the possible semantic representations and a transformational rule component which relates the outputs of the formation rule component to surface structures. Such a semantically based theory is capable of admitting to the influence of extralinguistic factors, including cognitive-based phenomena (Olson, 1970; MacNamara, 1972) and presuppositions based, in part, on one's world view (Karttunen, 1973; Keenan, 1971, Kiparsky and Kiparsky, 1971; Lakoff, 1971; Langendoen, 1971; and Thompson, 1971).

In view of the current interest in cognition as it relates to the acquisition process, a semantically based model of language is more appealing than a syntactically based model. To distinguish better between semantically based and syntactically based models, McNeill's (1970) distinction between weak and strong linguistic universals might be referred to. Briefly, weak linguistic universals may be defined as universals that automatically appear in language because of conditions existing outside of language, namely, conditions which are a function of underlying cognitive or perceptual abilities. In contrast, strong linguistic universals are universals ". . . that appear in language because of the human communication system itself, and so are not caused by general cognitive or perceptual abilities" (p. 1064). Formalizations of the acquisition process which depend on weak universals assume that at the outset of the acquisition process language is a function of basic nonlinguistic cognitive phenomena. Such a position is neither strictly empirical nor strictly nativistic and is capable of accommodating what can be loosely called a Piagetian view of how one might begin to characterize adequately the acquisition process.

According to Sinclair (1969, 1971) and Piaget (1963, 1968, 1970), a Piagetian interpretation of the acquisition process stipulates that 1) the infant brings to the acquisition task, not a set of innate linguistic universals, but innate cognitive functions which ultimately result in universal structures of thought of which linguistic universals are a function and 2) since intelligence exists phylogenetically and ontogenetically before language, and since the acquisition of linguistic structures is a cognitive activity, cognitive structures should be used to explain at least the initial stages of language acquisition rather than *vice versa*. Slobin (1973) has expressed similar opinions regarding the role of cognition in language development. According to Slobin (1973), the child comes to the task of learning language with a set of procedures and inference rules which are the function of language independent cognitive strategies. That Slobin is not alone in considering the role of cognitive-based phenomena can be seen in a number of the preceding chapters in this volume and in the most recent work of Bloom (1973), Bowerman (1973), Brown (1973), and Schlesinger (in press).

In spite of the polemics resulting from Chomsky's (1959) criticism of Skinner (1957) and the subsequent impression that little attention has been given to what Hebb *et al.* (1971) called the "middle ground," the mainstream of developmental psycholinguistic research is sympathetic to Morton's (1970) statement that "Claims inferring that language is innate in man seem to be based on a few facts, a number of suppositions, and a great deal of faith" (p. 82). Along with the mainstream of developmental psycholinguistic research and its attempts at operationalizing the language acquisition process, a few prominent learning theorists (*e.g.,* see Braine, 1970, 1971; Palermo and Molfese, 1972) are in agreement with Verhave's (1972) claim that

> There are other alternatives in addition to the rationalist (nativist) or empiricist ones. Furthermore, these two options are not necessarily mutually exclusive or totally contradictory in all aspects. It is, for example, possible to assume that there are inherent schema (principals of organization or cognitive structures) and that these structures are crucial in determining the form of output (p. 192).

The result has been that a more or less eclectic or interactionist approach is currently being taken. Topics dominating the current research include 1) the study of cognitive prerequisites and resultant developmental progressions in relation to the question of just what is innate or specific to the acquisition of language and 2) the fundamental nature of a child's verbal environment, including questions of how it is structured and the role of motivation and/or pressure to communicate successfully.

In relation to the latter topic, it has recently been recognized that more attention must be given to the interaction of the child's verbal and nonverbal environment with his propensity to isolate and subsequently internalize (learn) the regularities embedded within the stream of speech. A notable development centers around the research of Snow (1972) and Phillips (1973), who have countered the claim that the child's verbal environment is too unstructured and, hence, incapable of exerting a significant degree of influence on the acquisition process. The research of Snow and Phillips implies that, as the child's receptive and expressive language passes through the various stages of acquisition, especially the earlier stages, it is marked by features of complexity to which parents are sensitive. The result is that parents unknowingly adjust their linguistic behavior. It ought to be mentioned here that Braine (1963a,b, 1970, 1971), though much criticized by Bever *et al.* (1965), may well have been correct in claiming that the child's verbal environment is designed to render assistance systematically to the child.

What should be of great interest to those involved in language training research is the fact that continued research into the child's interaction with his verbal environment may shed light on the status of *natural* reinforcers and their role in the development of language. The argument that reinforcement (in some form) is crucial to the development of language is difficult to reject. However, before we can isolate *natural* reinforcers, it is necessary that we first isolate what is being reinforced. As Brown and Hanlon (1970) pointed out, reinforcement in the form of social approval or disapproval is contingent not on the form of the child's statement but rather on the truth value of his statement. Contrary to various psycholinguistic interpretations, such reinforcement contingencies do not necessarily rule out the importance of reinforcement in language development. Reinforcement contingent on the truth value of a statement (and, hence, success at communicating) may very well be crucial to the development of language. Such response contingencies may later serve to motivate the child to approximate the form of adult models. That is, at the outset of the acquisition process, reinforcement may be contingent on truth value, but as time passes the reinforcement contingencies may shift to a combination of the truth value and the form of statements to a point where success at communication motivates and, at the same time, reinforces the child. Therefore, it cannot be overemphasized that in order to isolate what the *natural* reinforcers are we must first determine what is reinforced along with the accompanying contingencies. As Ferster (1972) implied, if control (noncoercive) of behavior is to be understood, an understanding of conditions which exist in the natural environment is of prime necessity. Hence, assuming that enduring control of behavior is necessary for the development and maintenance of functional language, the study of the child's interaction with his verbal environment is of the highest priority.

As for the ongoing attempts to determine the role of cognition in language development, a great deal can be said. From the standpoint of linguistic theory, they may eventually provide answers to the question of what constitutes on adequate formal model of language (Zwicky, 1972). Where practicalities are concerned, such attempts may result in adequate language training programs, where the ultimate goal is an intact *generative* language repertoire. A moment of digression is appropriate here. In the operant training literature, the term "generative" has been used in a confusing and inconsistent manner. Lahey's (1973) use of the term comes very close to that of the psycholinguist. According to Lahey, the term "generative" is used to refer to one's capacity to produce grammatical utterances and respond appropriately to utterances that one has never before experienced. Unfortunately, in contrast to Lahey, the term has been misused by the majority of those involved in language training. This is especially true in Whitehurst (1972, in press) and in various studies by Baer, Guess, and Sailor (see bibliography) where the term has been often equated with the notion of *generalization.* Consequently, linguistic repertoires that include the appropriate use of items not previously trained (modeled) but similar in topography are referred to as generative repertoires (*e.g.,* generalization of pluralization to nonmodeled items). From the psycholinguist's standpoint, claims that such repertoires are generative are misleading, especially where the claims are made that operant procedures result in generative language.

If we choose to follow a developmental model and extend the Piagetian notion that cognitive structures should be used to explain language acquisition into language training research, it can be assumed that the ideal training program must be capable of adjusting to a given subject's level of cognitive functioning. That is, the linguistic behaviors selected to be trained should not go beyond one's current level of cognitive functioning. The assumption here is that whatever is mapped onto a linguistic system is at some level a function of cognitive structure. For example, as Schlesinger (this volume) explained, "The order of acquisition of linguistic forms is dictated in part by their relative complexity and, hence, may be out of pace with the maturing concepts the child is ready to express." Obviously, a major obstacle here involves the assessment of a child's cognitive ability prior to and during training. Further, increased demands will be placed on a training program in lieu of the likelihood that language training will have to be combined with efforts to raise the child's level of cognitive functioning.

Assuming that the ideal language training program is one that not only identifies appropriate behaviors but also identifies those behaviors which are absent or in need of modification and subsequently trains all and only those structures which are necessary for a particular child's needs, in the context of a Piagetian approach it is important that the primary emphasis be placed on determining what cognitive prerequisites or conceptual behaviors are necessary to acquire and *maintain* functional use of the selected linguistic behaviors (*e.g.,* consider the implications of Mehrabian and Williams, 1971). Such considerations may lead to the establishment of specific cognitive functions or behaviors which control a range of linguistic behaviors and, as a result, cause functions underlying initially trained behaviors to shift to higher levels of functioning. In spite of the demands it places on a language training program, a Piagetian approach may facilitate the acquisition and maintenance of a structured linguistic system. Because it assigns primary emphasis to the cognitive system, and since what is mapped onto a linguistic structure is a function of the child's cognitive system, the child's ability to manipulate his environment readily (perhaps the ultimate reinforcer) is more likely to occur as a result of a Piagetian approach rather than as a result of an approach which fails to consider the role of cognition and its relationship to language.

HOW TO TRAIN—METHODOLOGICAL ISSUES IN LANGUAGE TRAINING

Most of the widely used language training programs today depend upon operant principles of behavior modification as a basic procedural model. When one examines the methodologies of these programs, there seems to be widespread agreement on at least the general principles regarding language training procedures. First, and perhaps most important, there seems to be general agreement that training sequences should be programmed. This point was mentioned earlier when it was suggested that one of the more desirable features of a training program is that it provides for the training of new functions with old forms and the training of new forms with old functions. Stremel and Waryas (1973) have patterned their program so that training progresses from simple to more complex forms and functions. Data from their program indicate that acquisition of certain aspects of language is facilitated by, if not dependent upon, a prior level of development. More specifically, their data indicate that acquisition of certain terminal structures, such as use of negative constructions (*e.g.,* don't) is facilitated by training on a set of intermediate behaviors. For example, the training of negation begins with emphasis on a nonverbal negative marker external to the basic sentence. A sentence such as "Want cookie" would then be negated by an accompanying headshake. The second step of the program involves shifting the expression of negation to a verbal marker (external to the sentence), resulting in utterances like "No want cookie" or "No boy hit girl." This procedure conforms to the principle that new forms (*e.g.,* the verbal negation marker) are taught within the scope of an already established function (*e.g.,* negating an affirmative proposition). Other sequential steps in this program involve the shifting of the negative marker to within the sentence and finally shaping the form of the negative marker to the desired terminal structure, that being *auxiliary + negative contraction.*

The utilization of intermediate steps in training programs which build upon previously acquired forms has the distinct advantage of simplifying the learning task for the child. Slobin (1971) and Brown (1973) have both noted that in the normal acquisition process children frequently acquire new forms to express the same function that a grammatically less complex form had previously expressed. The application of this principle to language training programming may be even more critical than it is to the normal acquisition process. For example, in a recent study (Ruder and Bunce, 1973), a language-delayed child was trained to use intonation differentially (declarative statements *vs.* questions) utilizing an imitation procedure. At the outset of training, the subject's verbal imitation and memory span was three words, usually spoken with a falling or declarative terminal intonation. When the constraint of differential intonation (*e.g.,* using rising or falling intonation) was added to the imitation task, training was not successful until the length of the modeled string was reduced to two words. However, once the intonation patterns were used differentially in the simpler strings, differential use was applied successfully to three-word strings, with additional training, of course. Upon reaching criterion (90% correct imitation of three-word strings), a new constraint was added—that of stress. The subject was now required to repeat all three words while, at the same time, stressing the second and utilizing the appropriate terminal intonation. As Figure 1 shows, with the additional stress constraint, imitation performance dropped from 90% correct to a low of 13%. Most of the errors made upon the introduction of the stress constraint consisted of either omitting the stress or using stress correctly at the expense of the correct use of terminal intonation. The same basic behavioral pattern was observed later in training when the length of the

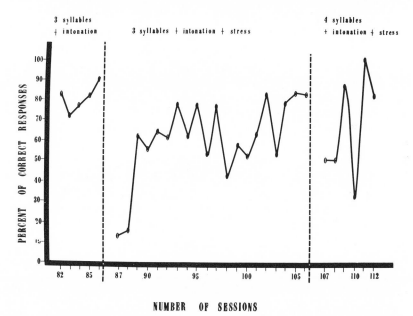

NUMBER OF SESSIONS

Fig. 1. Graphic depiction of child's performance during training on production of suprasegmental features of terminal intonation contour and stress. Initial portion of graphs shows the subject performing at a 90% criterion level in imitating three-word strings with appropriate terminal intonation contour. Performance drops drastically with the addition of a stress constraint (session 87) and again with the addition of a fourth syllable (session 107).

modeled strings was increased from three to four words. The introduction of the additional word resulted in decreased imitation accuracy, and again the inclusion of the new item resulted in a decrement primarily in the use of the structure most recently trained. Establishing the new form (the extra word) in a more elementary, previously learned structure, the unstressed model in this case, rapidly led to imitation of four-word strings with proper stress and intonation. The data from this study should not necessarily be construed as indicating a methodology for training stress and intonation patterns. The results do, however, serve to highlight the principle that new behaviors can be introduced by building upon already learned structures and functions providing that only a minimal contrast differentiates the learned forms from the forms selected to be trained. Consequently, it might be said that increased empirical verification of this principle is a challenge confronting researchers interested in language training procedures.

Additionally, procedural variables encompassed by the operant approach have been studied extensively and need not be reiterated here. It is sufficient to say that the general consensus of opinion is that the basic operant or behavior modification paradigm segmenting the clinical interaction into three classes of events (antecedent, response, and subsequent events) constitutes a powerful methodology for language intervention.

In regard to some recent claims concerning the use of operant principles in training linguistic rules, the major concern is not to question the power of the training procedure but rather to question whether or not a training program needs to go to extremes in training so as to achieve the degrees of overgeneralization that typically occur. The occurrence of overgeneralization may be desirable to emphasize the power of a particular methodology; however, it is questionable whether it is a desirable product of a language training program. As a case in point, consider the series of studies by Guess *et al.* (1968), Guess (1969), Sailor (1971), Baer *et al.* (1972), and Guess and Baer (1973a, b). The underlying theme of these studies is that the acquisition of pluralization morphology (or past tense morphology) in English is a function of stimulus control-reinforcement complexes. The result is that the three plural allomorphs ([-s], [-z], [-əz]) are considered to be arbitrarily related to the preceding noun stem, entailing the claim that phonological conditioning factors do not affect the selection of a particular plural allomorph (see Staats, 1968). Phonological theory stipulates, however, that as conditioned plural markers 1) [-əz] predictably occurs after sibilants and affricates (*e.g.,* glass + [-əz], church + [z]), 2) [-z] predictably occurs after all other voiced segments (*e.g.,* rib + [z], hill + [z], knee + [z]), and 3) [-s] predictably occurs after all other voiceless segments (*e.g.,* cat + [s]). Apparently contradicting phonological theory, the above studies demonstrated that as a result of training based on stimulus-control reinforcement procedures the phonological conditioning factors were consistently violated, principally because of the occurrence of overgeneralization. For example, the prediction would be that upon training [-əz] to appropriate stems, probe trials across stems requiring either [-s] or [-z] result in the occurrence of [-əz]. That such results are consistently obtainable through the use of stimulus-control reinforcement procedures is not denied. Witness the degree of overgeneralization found by Schumaker and Sherman (1970) in their attempt to train past tense morphology. Open to question, however, is the resultant conclusion that phonological conditioning factors are inoperative (see Cofer, 1963). It can be argued that the results obtained are strictly a function of the *immediate* effects of training. The theory of phonological conditioning predicts that data obtained from a longitudinal study would support the claim that phonological conditioning factors are operative. Unfortunately, none of the above studies report on extensive use of longitudinal data.

As previously stated, the occurrence of overgeneralization does indeed demonstrate the power of operant methodology. However, if a training program is designed to train, for example, the morphology of pluralization, it should be designed to minimize the degree of overgeneralization and take advantage of the naturally occurring phonological conditioning factors which would result in the occurrence of the remaining allomorphs with a minimum of additional training. Built into such a program would be the option to forego additional training, the expectation being that the remaining allomorphs will occur once the immediate effects of training subside. A program of this sort is in contrast to the implied approach of the preceding studies where it is assumed that all three allomorphs must be trained as separate behaviors (*e.g.*. see especially Guess, 1969; Guess and Baer, 1973a,b).

At stake in this issue is more than the efficiency of training. Again, the particular viewpoint implied in the preceding studies is that the plural allomorphs represent three different linguistic behaviors and thus can be classed as being independent of one another. Linguistically speaking, the three plural allomorphs are considered to be interdependent behaviors. That is, they are classifiable as a single linguistic behavior with three different, phonologically conditioned surface manifestations. While issues involving independent and interdependent linguistic behaviors are of interest to psycholinguistic theory, the issues have practical implications for language training as well. Basically, the major implication is that in order to approximate an optimal training procedure, linguistic behaviors which are interdependent ought to be trained concurrently rather than serially, where training in a concurrent fashion involves simultaneous training within the same modality (Schroeder and Baer, 1972). In contrast, training in a serial fashion involves the training of one behavior to criterion and then sequentially the training of another to criterion, etc. To date, the serial fashion dominates the operant literature dealing with language training, perhaps the main reason being that it allows one to demonstrate the systematic effects of the training procedure and the power of the methodology involved. The feeling here is that serial training may not serve to facilitate the development of a functional linguistic system. Training in a concurrent fashion appears to be more in line with the realities of one's linguistic environment. To speculate on what the structure of a concurrent training program might look like, it is necessary to begin with some basic assumptions concerning the form of the selected linguistic behaviors. In the case of pluralization, as mentioned above, it can be assumed that the plural allomorphs comprise a single linguistic behavior with three different physical manifestations. Such an assumption implies that training on the [-s] allomorph may in turn result in the occurrence of the appropriate, phonologically conditioned use of the [-z] and [-əz] allomorphs. Such a procedure is not meant to imply that the [-s] allomorph must be trained in order to insure the occurrence of [-z] and [-əz]. Training on [-z] or [-əz] may also result in the proper use of the plural allomorphs, that is, after the immediate effects of training and subsequent overgeneralization subside.

In reference to such a procedure one might initially assume that the choice to place emphasis on a particular plural allomorph is an arbitrary one. Yet, one ought to consider that, of the three plural allomorphs, [-s] demands least of the productive system, it is generally the first one acquired, and, because of its phonological properties, [-s] will more readily assimilate to the range of environments requiring the [-z] and [-əz] allomorphs, hence resulting in the appropriate phonologically conditioned forms of the plural affix. Consequently, placing emphasis on the [-s] allomorph could possibly minimize the degree of overgeneralization, and, perhaps in some instances, it might rule out overgeneralization (Smith et al., 1973).

When considering perceptual saliency, however, it is conceivable that placing emphasis on either the [-z] or [-əz] allomorph ([-əz] being the more perceptually salient of the two) may prove to be more efficient than placing emphasis on the [-s] allomorph. Viewing the problem of training pluralization as being representative of the many other problems encountered in attempts at training language, a question of central import is: By what method(s) can the most effective training procedure(s) be determined? Unfortunately, not enough attention has been given to the problem of determining the effectiveness of training procedures. A major reason for this lack of attention may have to do with the neglect of the content of the trained or to-be-trained linguistic behaviors. In attempting to approach a solution to the problem, a clarification of the distinction between independent and interdependent linguistic behaviors might prove helpful. The distinction can be discussed in reference to what is called componential content (CC) analysis (Smith et al., 1973). CC analysis consists of reducing linguistic behaviors to their salient features or components. For example, in the case of the morphology of pluralization and other morphologically based linguistic behaviors, the componential content includes consideration of 1) concepts mapped by particular linguistic structures, 2) grammatical principles, and 3) phonological topographies. For the purpose of an illustration, a CC analysis of the two plural allomorphs [-s] and [-z] appears as follows:

1) Linguistic concept = same (pluralization)
2) Grammatical principle = same (affixation)
3) Phonological topography = different ([s] *vs.* [z])

To assess which of the two allomorphs is more effective in terms of leading to the correct use of the other allomorph, the procedure would be first to train initially on the [-s] allomorph while systematically probing with appropriate stems for the occurrence of [-z]. If the probe accuracy of the [-z] allomorph does not meet criterion, it is subsequently trained to meet criterion. Next, as a systematic replication, the [-z] allomorph is initially trained and [-s] is systematically probed. The significant variables consist of 1) the number of trials to criterion for either [-s] or [-z] when it is initially the nontrained probe behavior and 2) the number of trials to criterion for either [-s] or [-z] when it is initially the trained behavior. The ratio of 1) over 2) serves as a probability index, referring to the probability that the nontrained behavior will or will not occur as a function of the componential content of the trained behavior. The probability index yields a sensitizing quotient which, in terms of a multiple baseline design, reflects the degree to which a trained behavior may or may not systematically effect a nontrained behavior. As Figure 2 illustrates, a sensitizing quotient of 1.0 or greater is an indication that either an equal number or more trials to criterion was required for [-z]

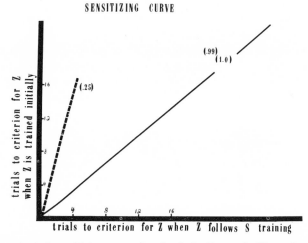

Fig. 2. Hypothetical sensitizing curve for the [-z] allomorph. The ratio of trials to criterion for acquisition of the [-z] allomorph when it is the initially trained allomorph to the trials to criterion for [-z] when it follows previous training on the [-s] allomorph is depicted as the sensitizing curve for [-z]. To determine whether it would be more efficient to train on [-z] allomorph or the [-s] allomorph, the sensitizing curve for [-z] depicted here would have to be compared to a similarly computed sensitizing curve for [-s]. The allomorph with the higher sensitizing quotient (nearest to 1 or more) should be the one selected for the initial training since the allomorph with the lower sensitizing quotient shows a greater dependence (less trials to criterion, hence a savings in training) when the other allomorph is trained first.

where [-z] was initially the nontrained probed behavior and [-s] was the initially trained behavior and, during the systematic replication, where]-z] was the initially trained behavior and [-s] was the probed behavior. From a practical standpoint either situation implies that no systematic interdependence exists among the behaviors. In contrast, a sensitizing quotient below 1.0 is indicative of a certain degree of systematic interdependence among the behaviors. The closer the sensitizing quotient is to 0.0, the greater the degree of systematic interdependence. Hence, a sensitizing quotient of 0.25 implies a greater degree of systematic interdependence than does one of 0.60.

At this point a hypothetical example may clarify matters. In the case of [-z], for instance, if 4 trials to criterion were required under the first condition (where [-s] was the trained behavior and [-z] was initially the nontrained probed behavior) and 16 trials were required under the second condition (where [-z] was initially the trained behavior), the sensitizing quotient would read 0.25, indicative of a high degree of interdependence. The resultant sensitizing curve is depicted in Figure 2. What the sensitizing quotient implies is that [-z] is sensitive to the training on [-s]. However, it is not necessarily the case that [-s] ought to be just as sensitive to the training on [-z]. For example, imagine that the number of trials to criterion for [-s] under both conditions was 12 and 16, respectively. The sensitizing quotient would then read 0.60. A comparison of the two sensitizing quotients indicates that [-s] is not as sensitive to training on [-z] as [-z] is sensitive to training on [-s]. From this hypothetical example, it can be concluded that the direction of interdependence favors training on [-s].

The value of CC analysis is that it has the potential to provide a data-based means of determining both the degree and direction of interdependence among to-be-trained linguistic behaviors. By defining linguistic behaviors in terms of a componential analysis (necessarily including consideration of linguistic concepts, grammatical principles, phonological and structural topographies) and utilization of sensitivity quotients, it may become possible to determine the effects a behavior's content has on attempts at training language. For instance, in terms of the above example, the degree and direction of interdependence among the [-s] and [-z] plural allomorphs can be considered a function of phonological topography because of the fact that [-s] and [-z] are realizations of the same linguistic concept (pluralization) and grammatical principle (affixation). Additional hypothetical examples may be cited. If one wishes to assess the effects a difference in concept might have on training, one could train the [-s] plural allomorph and probe for the [-s] possessive allomorph. In terms of CC analysis, their phonological topographies are identical (voiceless [s]) and the behaviors are governed by the same grammatical principle (affixation). Obviously, the difference has to do with the concepts underlying these behaviors. Intuitively, one would expect to find little if any systematic interdependence among these two behaviors. Nonetheless, the data from such a study could contradict one's expectations.

Consider the training of the English copula (to be) and auxiliary (to be) constructions, linguistic behaviors which differ in terms of the underlying linguistic concepts. According to Stremel's (1973) data as illustrated in Table 1, the training sequence copula-then-auxiliary (13.8 and 23.6 trials, respectively) is more facilitative than the training sequence auxiliary-then-copula (43.3 and 11.9 trials, respectively). The differences between trials to criterion of the copula form in the two training sequences is significant beyond the 0.01 level. Here then, even though the underlying linguistic concepts differ, placing emphasis on one of the behaviors (as in the copula-then-auxiliary sequence) is considerably more effective than placing emphasis on another of the behaviors (as in the auxiliary-then-copula sequence). Moving on, while holding phonological topography constant, the direction and degree of interdependence, if any, could be determined for behaviors differing in terms of the linguistic concepts and grammatical principles involved. For example, consider a case where the [-s] plural allomorph is the initially trained behavior and the [-s] subject-verb agreement marker is the probed behavior. Here the phonological topography is constant, whereas linguistic concept (semantic plural *vs.* grammatical agreement) and grammatical principle (direct affixation *vs.* discontinuous affixation) differ. Finally, we may have a situation where all three components vary, as in the case of the [-s] plural allomorph and the future tense marker "will." Intuitively, as in the case of the [-s] plural and the [-s] possessive allomorph, one would expect to find little, if any, systematic interdependence among the linguistic behaviors in the last two situations. However, in a much larger and more realistic study dealing with a multitude of to-be-trained linguistic behaviors, we might find that such behaviors are interdependent in the loose sense that one of them is typically acquired prior to the other, hence possibly serving to some limited degree as a prerequisite behavior.

It is hoped that in the future CC analysis or something similar to it will be taken into consideration when selecting to-be-trained linguistic behaviors. Determination of the degree and direction of interdependence may dictate what behaviors ought to be emphasized and what procedures might be incorporated. The long range goal of studies based on CC analysis is to demonstrate that an optimal language training program is one that incorporates concurrent training techniques with emphasis among interdependent behaviors being placed upon the behavior that is more facilitative (*i.e.,* the behavior which, according to sensitivity quotients, controls the direction and degree of interdependence).

Another prominent issue concerns the role of imitation and comprehension in the normal acquisition process and language training. As discussed earlier, imitation in particular has come under a great deal of scrutiny. In response to the previously mentioned eclectic approach and concomitant interest in the child's structured verbal environment, attempts have been made to revise the currently held definitions of imitation and subsequently assess the effects of redefinition on the hypothesis that (in the acquisition process) imitation precedes comprehension, and, in turn, comprehension precedes production (the ICP hypothesis). In the past, especially where language intervention is concerned, imitation has too often been viewed as a process involving *exact copying* of the topography and/or items of an immediately preceding model (Whitehurst, in press). Aware of the limitations of such an interpretation, Bandura (1969, 1970), Sherman (1971), and Whitehurst (in press) admitted that such an interpretation has perhaps obscured the function of imitation in the development of functional language.

If the role of imitation in the language training process has been obscured by definitional considerations, then the problem may be even more acute in the psycholinguistic literature. The research of Ervin (1964) is a primary example. Judging from the comparison of her subjects' spontaneous (*exact copy*) imitations *vs.* their free speech patterns, Ervin concluded that "There is not a shred of evidence supporting a view that progress toward adult norms of grammar arise merely from practice in overt imitation of adult sentences" (p. 172). Many were misled by Ervin's conclusion and interpreted her study to mean that imitation cannot play a significant role in the acquisition process. The most that can be said in reference to Ervin, however, is that imitation is not the sole or central means of acquiring linguistic competence. More recently, Slobin (1968), Kemp (1972), and Kemp and Dale (1973) argued that new features may enter a child's emerging linguistic behavior by way of imitating utterances more complex than his own. Agreeing that imitation may be progressive (*i.e.,* provides a means of introducing new features) leads us to the difficult task of specifying the precise role played by imitation. The issue is not clear cut, for as Kemp and Dale (1973) pointed out, there are situations where features are not imitated even though they occur in the child's free speech, and there are also situations where features are imitated even though they do not occur in free speech.

Without a doubt, future success at utilizing imitation paradigms in language training will depend on how imitation is defined. According to Whitehurst (in press), Ervin's exact copy interpretation is plainly inadequate, especially when one considers the observation that children tend to simplify adult models when imitating. A plausible alternative to the exact copy interpretation has been proposed by Whitehurst. According to Whitehurst (in press), imitation may be defined as "any behavior that matches the behavior of a previously observed model, or any characteristic or dimension of that model's behavior, such that the occurrence of the imitative behavior can be shown to be a function of the occurrence of that dimension or characteristic of the model's behavior which is matched." Such a definition, in Whitehurst's terms, ". . . allows that characteristics of the verbal model, such as complexity, length, order, or aspects of structure can be imitated without any necessity that every feature of the model be mirrored in the output." The only requirement, then, is that a specifiable subset of the total stimulus array modeled be separated out by way of abstraction and mirrored in the output. Simply stated, imitation is seen as a process whereby behavior is brought under control of a subset of a particular stimulus array.

Thus far, we have referred to imitation as being primarily an echoic process. The question as to whether or not imitation is accompanied by some degree of comprehension has been to a large part ignored. Even though Whitehurst gave no direct attention to the question of what might be called "attempts" at comprehension, underlying his interpretation is the assumption that attempts at comprehension are the heart of an imitation process that is crucial to language development. Attempts at comprehension may be defined as the tendency to attend to, to separate out, to assimilate, and, hence, to store relevant as opposed to irrelevant regularities embedded in the stream of speech. However, it is not implied here that all instances of imitation reflect attempts at comprehension. What is implied is that if imitation is to function at a maximum, especially where language intervention is concerned, attempts at comprehension are necessary.

Apparently negating the potentially facilitative role that comprehension may play, previous research has for the most part assumed that imitation precedes comprehension. This assumption has led to the proposition that intervention programs based on imitation and differential reinforcement techniques will eventually result in the emergence of functional language (Lynch and Bricker, 1972). Intuitively, it seems counterproductive to assume that, as a first goal in language training, an echoic repertoire must be established. What of the question that intervention programs based on comprehension training and differential reinforcement may facilitate subsequent imitation training and, in turn, result in the occurrence of nontrained production?

Recent research by Asher (1972) and Winitz and Reeds (1972) indicated that training based on comprehension alone (receptive language training) is more effective in eliciting verbal production than training based on imitation. Asher and Winitz and Reeds have demonstrated that training on comprehension alone resulted in verbal production in second language learning, supposedly ruling out imitation as a functional component in language training. It is quite possible, however, that the results obtained are ambiguous in that the occurrence of rehearsal or covert imitation was not effectively controlled.

Also questioning the emphasis placed on imitation-based procedures, Mann and Baer (1971) attempted to assess the effects of training on comprehension. According to Mann and Baer, comprehension training (based on antecedent events) facilitates the occurrence of productive speech, in essence supporting the claims of Asher, Winitz, and Reeds. The results and conclusions drawn stand in contradiction to the claim that receptive and productive repertoires may be functionally independent (Guess, 1969; Sailor, 1971; Guess and Baer, 1973a,b). Definitional considerations, however, obscure the comparison. In Mann and Baer (1971), for instance, production as defined is little more than elicited imitation. Witness the instructions given to their subjects for the production task: "I'm going to say some words one at a time, and I want you to say the same word after me" (p. 293). The claim, then, that comprehension training facilitates verbal production is reduced to a statement that comprehension training facilitates subsequent imitation. Thus, the results cannot be considered supportive of the claim that comprehension training alone results in verbal production in the same sense that Winitz and Reeds (1972) and Asher (1972) spoke of their comprehension training as resulting in spontaneous verbal production.

A recent study (Ruder, Smith, and Hermann, 1974) was designed to assess the functional relationship between imitation and comprehension training procedures. Initial training commenced on four Spanish lexical items (to control for previous exposure) within a verbal imitation paradigm, and four other Spanish lexical items presented within a comprehension training paradigm (in which the child was presented with a verbal stimulus and asked to select the appropriate picture from a stimulus array containing three pictures). Production probes were conducted periodically for all eight words. As expected, the echoic imitation training did not result in verbal production during the probes since the subject had no way of establishing the referential tie between the objects and the imitated models. Contrary to expectations, however, comprehension training failed to result in production. The claims of Asher, Winitz, and Reeds lead one to believe that verbal production should have been obtained as a result of comprehension training. To determine whether or not continued comprehension training might result in production, each subject continued to be trained on two of the words which were originally trained on comprehension. In addition, to assess functional interactive effects between imitation and comprehension training, for each subject the two remaining words initially trained on comprehension were trained on imitation. Likewise, two of the items trained initially on imitation were trained on comprehension. As illustrated in Figure 3, additional comprehension training did not increase production. In regard to comprehension training on words initially trained on imitation, production probes continued at zero until the 15th session. In contrast, imitation training on items initially trained on comprehension resulted in 100% performance on production probes by the 9th session, several sessions prior to the acquisition of any production in the imitation-then-comprehension training sequence. Subsequent training on imitation resulted in verbal production for all items trained on comprehension. Follow-up studies (Ruder and Hermann, 1973; and Ruder et al., 1974) supported the conclusion that it matters little whether initial training (on lexical items) is based on either imitation or comprehension. What does seem to be essential, however, is that elements of both imitation training and comprehension training are required to achieve production.

Another procedural issue in need of attention concerns the role of modeling and expansion procedures in language training. The use of modeling

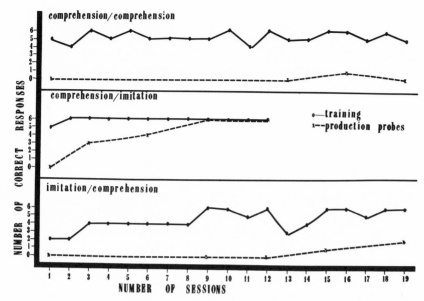

Fig. 3. Performance on verbal production probes for three subjects being trained concurrently in three different training sequences: a) comprehension training on items previously trained in comprehension, b) imitation training on items previously trained in comprehension, and c) comprehension training on items previously trained in imitation.

and expansion techniques stems initially from a study by Brown and Bellugi (1964) in which they reported that, in observing mothers and their children in the home environment, they found at least two events which they speculated play an important role in the acquisition of linguistic structures. These two events are 1) parental modeling and 2) parental expansions of the child's utterances. An example of parental modeling would be to present the child with a well formed phrase or sentence which he could then imitate or process *via* comprehension. Expansions in the Brown and Bellugi study were defined as an imitation of the child by a parent or a more knowledgeable speaker, an imitation which involved a correction or addition of some type to the child's utterance. Cazden (1965) attempted to separate the modeling and expansion events in order to assess their individual contributions to the language development process. In this particular study, modeling was found to be the more effective approach. In a later replication of this study, Feldman and Rodgon (1970) found that there was no difference between the effects of modeling and expansion on the child's acquisition of new linguistic structures.

Despite the contradictory nature of the data concerning the role of modeling and expansion in the normal language acquisition process, the initial impetus of the Brown and Bellugi (1964) study has carried over into the language training domain as well. Some form of modeling has been used as an integral part of language training studies (Fygetakas and Gray, 1968, Guess,

1969, Guess, Sailor, Rutherford, and Baer, 1968, and Schumaker and Sherman, 1970). The modeling paradigm of these experiments has consisted primarily of 1) a verbal model presented by the experimenter or the trainer, 2) an attempt at verbal imitation of the model by the subject, and 3) appropriate reinforcement. For the most part, modeling was taken to be a useful methodological approach to the training of new linguistic structures. In support of such a view, the results of the modeling studies have, in general, shown that transfer of the linguistic behavior to untrained structures does occur when several examples of the particular rule are trained within the modeling-imitation-reinforcement paradigm described above. However, as with many studies concerning language training procedures, comparison of the modeling approach to other possible approaches and attempts at determining the more efficient training approach have been largely ignored. Malouf and Dodd (1972) provided one of the few studies which compared modeling and expansion approaches to the training of linguistic structures. In essence, their training study (teaching a nonsense grammar to normal first graders) showed that expansion procedures were generally superior to simple modeling procedures. In a similar type of study, Murray (1972) found that neither modeling nor expansion, in the strict sense defined by Brown and Bellugi (1964), was effective as a training procedure for teaching morphological inflections to non-English-speaking preschoolers. The approach she found effective was one which she termed "reciprocal exchange." Reciprocal exchange was defined in the Murray study as a procedure which provides not only a model of the target linguistic structure, but also a discrimination task and a consequence which is directly related to performance on the linguistic task at hand. For example, the reinforcers in the Murray study might be viewed as examples of reinforcing the truth value of an utterance rather than reinforcing the linguistic structure *per se*. In the training of the plural morpheme, the reciprocal exchange procedure entails the modeling of both the singular and plural forms under the appropriate environmental conditions. One of the structured situations in this particular study consisted of having the experimenter and the child engage in a play activity where either could request items from a common stimulus array such as a series of pictures or toys. The procedure would begin with the experimenter saying, "I want the trucks," and selecting the multiple items corresponding to the class of trucks. If the experimenter modeled the singular form, "I want the truck," then only a single item was selected from the array of trucks. To participate, the child not only had to name the particular object he wanted but also had to mark the lexical items to indicate either singular or plural. The child was given exactly what he requested. If he intended to ask for the truck and used an inappropriate label, he was given what he asked for. By the same token, if the subject wanted all of the trucks and failed to include the proper morphological inflection (*e.g.*, the plural [-s] allomorph) he was given the single truck. Utilizing this procedure, Murray found it extremely effective in instances where a modeling procedure alone or an expansion procedure alone had failed to achieve acquisition of the intended structure by the child.

The reciprocal exchange procedure of the Murray (1972) study could be summarized as providing a structured environmental situation which has a high probability of eliciting the desired linguistic structures. The difference between this approach and many other approaches utilizing modeling, expansion, and imitation techniques lies primarily in the fact that the consequences in the reciprocal exchange procedure are directly related to the communication event rather than consisting of tangible reinforcers such as tokens or verbal praise. In this respect, the reciprocal exchange procedure might be viewed as an attempt to model a normal communication environment, one similar to the social and communicative transaction procedure utilized by Premack (1970) in training Sarah in the use of language structures.

The observation that modeling and expansion procedures were found to be inferior to the reciprocal exchange procedure in the Murray study may be partially accounted for by the fact that differential reinforcement and feedback were not utilized during the modeling or expansion conditions. Miller and Yoder (this volume) suggested that both modeling and expansion be utilized as language training procedures. In our language training programs we have likewise utilized echoic models to establish the desired verbal responses initially and have also utilized expansion procedures effectively to achieve use of particular linguistic structures without direct training or with relatively little training. In a recent study examining the use of expansions in a language training program, Stremel and Ruder (1973) found that expansions had to be defined somewhat more rigidly than the definition advanced by Brown and Bellugi (1964). In the context of the Stremel and Ruder training study, an expansion was defined as a subsequent event in response to a subject's production of a target behavior (*e.g.,* production of a *subject-verb* string). The subsequent event consisted of appropriate tangible reinforcements for production of the target behavior, as well as an *expanded* imitation of the target behavior which included the target behavior for the next level of training within the program. For example, if the target behavior being trained consisted of stringing together *subject-verb* strings and the subject correctly produced such a structure, he was reinforced (verbal praise or tokens) tangibly. This reinforcer was accompanied by the experimenter's imitation of the same *subject-verb* string, expanded to include the object (*e.g.,* the S-V-O form), which in this particular program was the target behavior for the next level of training. If the subject responded with a spontaneous production of the expanded utterance, with particular reference to inclusion of the target behavior for the next level of training, he was given a magnitude of reinforcement for such a production (two tokens instead of one). Table 2 summarizes the effect of utilizing expansion procedures for three different subjects being trained on nine different linguistic structures. As can be seen from the summary data, expansions achieved a savings of training in that six of these

592   Ruder and Smith

Table 2. Effect of Clinician's Expansions of Child's Response on Acquisition of Expanded form*

Training (target form)	Expansion (next stage in training sequence)	Number of clinician expansions	No. of trials in which subjects used expanded forms without direct training
1. Verb	Sub. + V	340	49
2. Subject + verb	Sub. + V + obj.	117	60
3. Sub. + verb + object	Sub. + V + prep. + obj.	83	11
4. Sub. + verb + prep. + obj.	Sub. + Ving + prep. + obj.	140	33
5. Adj. + noun	N + is (copula) + adj.	147	0
6. Sub. + verb + prep. + obj. (reversal)	Sub. + is (aux.) + Ving + prep. + obj.	153	0
7. Sub. + is + Ving + obj.	Sub. + is + Ving + prep. + obj.	443	87
8. Sub. + is + Ving + N + prep. + obj.	Sub. + is + Ving + N + prep. + obj. (pronoun)	403	55
9. Sub. + is + Ving + N + prep. + obj. (pronoun)	Sub. (pronoun) + is + Ving + N + prep. + obj. (pronoun)	167	0

*Entries are means for three subjects.

structures were eventually produced by the subjects before direct training on those specific structures was introduced. The remaining three structures, two of which contained some variant of either the copula (to be) or the auxiliary (to be), were not acquired *via* the expansion technique and had to be trained directly. In this sense, then, the results of this study can be interpreted as demonstrating that expansion to the next level of training can be utilized to achieve more efficient acquisition of linguistic structures in at least some instances. The fact that the expansion technique did not work with all structures cannot be explained from the present data. Suffice it to say that even if expansions can be utilized effectively for only a limited number of structures, the data seem sufficiently clear to indicate that this is probably a useful technique for language training, at least until further data contradict use of such a procedure. The procedure described here requires little extra time or effort on the part of the clinician, so that even minimal positive effects would probably warrant its inclusion. Until further data are available on the reciprocal exchange method proposed by Murray (1972), there may be reservations about its effectiveness and utility in a long range language training program, although it does show promise as a potentially powerful procedure. What is apparent from these studies utilizing modeling and expansion techniques is that considerably more research is needed before any satisfactory answer can be proposed concerning the effectiveness of these techniques and their utility for widespread use in language training.

WHAT IS THE LANGUAGE PROBLEM?—ISSUES IN LANGUAGE ASSESSMENT

One of the essential features of a language training program is its method of assessing the structures a child does not have as well as the level of the child's current language functioning. The problem of assessing the language of the nonverbal child is considerably simplified in terms of identifying specific language structures the child may or may not have (*e.g.*, being nonverbal, it is probably appropriately assumed that the child has little or no functional use of language). For the teacher faced with training the functional use of language structures to the nonverbal child, the problem is not quite so simple. One might wish to know, for example, whether or not the child has passive control of linguistic structures. That is, while the child does not use expressive speech, is he able to respond appropriately to specific linguistic stimuli on the receptive level? Going beyond the assessment for specific linguistic emphasis, one must also assess with this child, as well as with the more advanced child, the level of functioning on prerequisite behaviors (behaviors which are considered prerequisite to entering the language training program such as attending behavior, chair sitting behavior, motor imitation, etc.) Such behavior assessment should be accompanied by hearing and medical evaluations.

With regard to language assessment *per se,* one may speak of at least three types or levels of assessments: 1) informal assessment, 2) formal assessment, and 3) ongoing assessment. Informal language assessments can be broken down into two main types. The simplest level of language assessment is the parent's or teacher's reports of the child's language capacity or their impressions of the language problem. This report can be very informative and time-saving to the clinician or teacher who is assigned the task of evaluating the child's level of language functioning. If nothing else, it will at least help him narrow down the range of possible speech and language deficits and allow the clinician or teacher to develop a preliminary test battery for more formal assessments. A somewhat more structured informal assessment for a teacher consists of eliciting spontaneous speech productions from the child to be recorded for later analysis. Samples may be taken of the child's interactions with peers, parents, and teachers. Elicited speech samples, such as "Tell me the story of the three bears," or "Tell me a story about this picture," have also been found to be of considerable use in assessing or planning the language training program for individual youngsters. Lee and Cantor (1971) have provided a format for assessing a child's level of language functioning from elicited spontaneous speech samples. While the procedure allows only a gross analysis of the nature of the child's language deficit, it does provide some structure for informal language assessment. It provides a tentative identification of the functional speech and language deficits which should be considered not only for further formal language assessment but also for development of a language training program.

The second level of language assessment is one with which we are more familiar. This consists of testing for comprehension and production of specific linguistic behaviors. At the lowest levels, such assessment procedures may contain tests for verbal imitations and auditory discriminations as prerequisite behaviors for the testing of imitation, comprehension, and production of specific lexical and grammatical behaviors. The Parsons Language Sample (Spradlin, 1963) is an example of a formal assessment tool which includes evaluation of such behaviors as imitations of verbal and nonverbal models, gesture imitation, naming, comprehension of verbal and nonverbal commands, as well as including more relevant linguistic information such as the child's performance on verbal classification of objects, and verbal or gestural expression in the child's request for information. The Utah Test of Language Development (Mecham, Jex, and Jones, 1967) is another example of a formal assessment procedure for use with children with little or no verbal behavior. While such tests may provide information regarding prelinguistic behaviors or prerequisite skills, either the relationships of many of these behaviors to the language training program are not specified or their relationship to language or language training is simply not relevant to any of the language training programs in use. This is not to say that such tests have no place in the language assessment phase of the complete language training program. It simply means that many of the behaviors contained in such preverbal, prelinguistic testing are necessary, not because they have any specific relationship to language functioning, but because they represent levels of prerequisite behaviors necessary for functional interaction between clinician and child in a language training program.

The most common and frequently used formal language tests are those which test comprehension of vocabulary. Such tests as the Peabody Picture Vocabulary Test (Dunn, 1965) and the Ammons Full Range Picture Vocabulary Test (Ammons and Ammons, 1968) are representative tests. Procedures for these tests present the child with a verbal stimulus (word), and the child is asked to point to the appropriate initial stimulus (picture) which best depicts the stimulus word. Recently, Aram and Nation (1972) have adapted the comprehension form of the Peabody Picture Vocabulary Test as a vocabulary usage test (*e.g.,* a production vocabulary test). In assessing either the comprehension or production of vocabulary items, the tests just mentioned classify the test items according to age level rather than grammatical categories.

To assess the child's knowledge and use of language structure (syntax), most formal tests employ modifications of imitation-comprehension-production procedures described by Fraser *et al.* (1963). In this test, the child is asked to imitate a verbal model containing the grammatical form under test, point to a picture (from a set of three or four) which best depicts the grammatical form under test, and produce the grammatical form. The method of assessing production devised by Fraser *et al.* is one in which the child is presented with two verbal models in which all elements remain constant except the grammatical form that is being contrasted. The child is then asked to produce the appropriate grammatical forms by selecting which of two verbal models best describes a picture designed to elicit that form. Their production test might then be considered to be a form of delayed imitation. However, it is widely used as a method for controlled elicitation of specific grammatical forms under test. Lee (1969) has formalized a diagnostic test based on the approach used by Fraser *et al.* Lee's test, the Northwestern Syntax Screening Test, is a 40-item picture test which includes both comprehension and production measures. Visual stimuli consist of four pictures, the picture depicting the grammatical form under test and three foils. In the comprehension test the child is presented with a model containing the grammatical form under test and is asked to point to the picture best depicting the model sentence. Carrow (1969 and 1973) has devised a similar although somewhat more comprehensive test to measure comprehension of specific language structures. Bellugi-Klima (1968) also has developed a comprehension test for language structures based on the early Fraser *et al.* study. Her comprehension testing procedure, however, involves a set of manipulation tasks to test syntactic constructions. The Bellugi-Klima test has the advantage of providing more stimulation and motivation for the child in that he is given a more active role by being permitted to manipulate objects. Such a procedure may obviate, to some degree, the problem encountered when using visual stimuli, stimuli which may not adequately depict linguistic contrasts under test. Thus, the Bellugi-Klima test may give a more accurate picture of the child's language comprehension than do tests relying on picture stimuli.

Picture comprehension tests for assessing knowledge of grammatical structure have recently come under closer scrutiny. Goodglass *et al.* (1970) found that the results of a traditional language comprehension test can prove to be misleading especially when compared with the results of a comprehension testing procedure in which a child is presented with a single picture and given a choice of two verbal stimuli (sentences), the task being to select the sentence he prefers for the particular picture. The use of such a preference procedure and its applicability to assessing comprehension of specific linguistic structures have recently been demonstrated in a series of studies by Waryas and Stremel (1973) and Waryas and Ruder (1973a,b). In this series of studies it was found that the traditional picture comprehension test generally underestimates the child's knowledge of a particular linguistic rule (in comparison to results obtained from the preference procedure). While considerably more research remains to be done, the preliminary data indicated that the preference procedure is a simple and effective way of assessing knowledge of grammatical structure.

The preceding type of formal assessment and use of specific rules is limited in that it indicates only whether or not the child possesses a certain structure. It gives very little indication of where to begin training. Test results which show, for example, that the child does not have functional use of five particular linguistic structures do not give any indication of which of the five should be trained first or whether concurrent training should be utilized on some combination of the deficient structures. The particular language training program being used should remedy this situation somewhat if the structures to be trained are sequentially programmed. A major issue, however, concerns what to do with structures found deficient in the evaluation but which are not included in the training sequence. This is not a remote possibility. Consider, for example, that a child, being given the Illinois Test for Psycholinguistic Abilities (Kirk, *et al.*, 1968) for evaluation of language abilities, has the opportunity to make errors on a number of items which do not appear in the content of any of the language training programs discussed elsewhere in this volume. The point is simply that the assessment device, to be maximally beneficial to the clinician, should show some relevance to the particular language training program being used.

The primary method utilized by most developmentally based language training programs is built-in, ongoing assessment in the form of specifying certain prerequisite behaviors as entry requirements into a particular phase of the training program. Programs utilizing such a device can be used to test for prerequisite behaviors and, in turn, determine at which point in the program to begin training with a particular child. Once the child is *plugged into* the program, the ongoing assessment is automatic. It follows, then, that in order to progress through the stages of development, the acquisition of certain terminal behaviors at one stage of training is prerequisite to the acquisition of behaviors in succeeding stages.

Assessment, then, should be a continuous, ongoing process. A major difficulty here involves determining the content and training sequence of a language training program. As Guess, Sailor, and Baer (this volume) pointed out, there are few data presently available concerning the best training sequence for certain linguistic structures. To date, the designation of prerequisite behaviors and resultant sequencing represent probably no more than rough approximations based primarily on what we know of the normal developmental sequence.

It is obvious, then, that the problems of assessment are tied inextricably to issues concerning the content and training sequence particular to a given language training program. As such, assessment procedures, to be maximally productive, should probably be considered in a broader perspective. Not only should assessment provide for placing a child in a particular phase of a training program, but it also should provide the clinician or researcher with some feedback concerning the relevance of a particular training sequence and the prerequisite behaviors required to enter particular stages of a program. To illustrate the latter point, it is obvious that if a particular terminal behavior can be reached without going through an intervening stage, then we will want to reconsider inclusion of this intervening stage in our training sequence. Therefore, an optimal assessment procedure should be capable of providing the clinician with data concerning the training sequence which might be most effective in achieving a particular terminal goal. Utilization of data based on CC analysis (discussed previously in this chapter) may be a method of documenting quantitively the efficient direction of training.

A device utilized by Spradlin (1973) to depict a child's progress through a particular training program might also be useful for general evaluation of a program. Figure 4 is a sample of such a progress record for a child engaged in a language training program (Stremel, 1973). The progress record represented in Figure 4 includes only the major structures that have been trained. This progress record not only summarizes training sessions and the relative time required to reach a criterion performance level but also contains provisions for review of the structures once they are trained or partially trained. For instance, *question* training must progress through four stages before it is placed on review (R) in the form *WH NOUN VERBing ?* This form is reviewed until the auxiliary (is) is trained. Next, the auxiliary is incorporated into the previously trained question form. The progress record in Figure 4 does not present the various stages of training for certain structures (for reasons of simplicity) but indicates expanded training on certain structures along the time axis. For example, on *negation* training, the subject in

Figure 4 achieved the 90% criterion accuracy by the 6th week of training for negating with a headshake paired with the verbal marker (*e.g.*, "no go"). Shifting this form of negation to a more complex form (*e.g.*, "I don't want cookie") required an additional 9 weeks of training. Not only does such a report vividly and succinctly depict the child's progress, it also provides a composite view of the training procedure concerning items being trained concurrently as well as consecutively. In week 3, for example, concurrent training on verbs, negation, and limited *adjective-noun* combinations was undertaken. Training on noun-verb-noun (N-V-N) strings, however, was not initiated until criterion had been reached on V-N and N-V strings. Also evident from the above figure is that the N-N sequence which had initially been included in the training sequence as a possible prerequisite behavior to the use of N-V-N strings (on the basis of the use of such strings by normal children prior to the use of N-V-N strings) was not necessary to establishment of the N-V-N sequence. Hence, for future programming, it may not be necessary to include this structure for training consideration. The data in Figure 4 also demonstrate that only the production of the copula (is) and auxiliary (is) drops to below 50% accuracy after a period (2 weeks) of receiving no training or no review. Stremel (1973) found these data to be representative when the auxiliary and copula were trained very early. These and additional data on the copula and auxiliary suggest that these behaviors should be trained later. This example depicts the point made previously. That

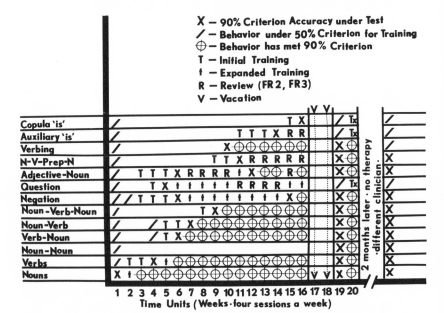

Fig. 4. Sample progress record for a child engaged in early phases of a language training program.

is, by having an assessment procedure which not only moves the child from stage to stage in the language training program but also provides an ongoing step-by-step evaluation, a more efficient training program may be developed.

SUMMARY

We have attempted to isolate some currently relevant issues pertaining to language training. These issues are concerned with 1) evaluation and selection of a language training program or battery of programs, 2) the content of a language training program, 3) language training procedures, and 4) language assessment. In the process of discussing issues in each of these areas we have probably raised as many questions as we were able to resolve. Probably the most pervasive theme is that of efficiency and utility. The ultimate goal of any language training program is to produce the desired behavior changes in the child with language problems so that he can communicate effectively. As such, the complete language training program is one that not only identifies appropriate behaviors but also identifies those behaviors which are either absent or in need of modification.

Just as an adequate grammar is capable of producing all and only the permissible strings of a particular language, an adequate language training program will identify (for training) all and only those structures which are necessary for a particular child's communicative needs. This brings us to another important generalization concerning language training programs. Aside from identifying and training relevant linguistic structures, they should also be able to identify and provide training for identification of the appropriate environmental situations which call for use of particular structures. As a final point, let us reiterate what we consider to be one of the more practical observations. That is, when one considers the diversity and scope of the language problems encountered, it is naive to assume that a single language program has been, or will be, devised which is capable of handling such a diversity of problems and individual differences in as efficient a manner as would a *battery* of language training programs which are geared and individualized to meet a particular child's language deficiencies and communicative needs.

REFERENCES

Ammons, R. B. and Ammons, H. *The Full-Range Picture Vocabulary Test,* Missoula, Mont.: Psychological Reports, 1968.

Aram, D. and Nation, J. Developmental language disorders: Patterns of language behavior. Paper presented at the American Speech and Hearing Association, San Francisco, 1972.

Asher, J. Children's first language as a model for second language training, *Mod. Lang. J.,* 1972, *56,* 133–138.

Baer, D. and Guess, D. Teaching productive noun suffixes to severely retarded children. *Amer. J. Ment. Defic.,* in press.

Baer, D., Guess, D., and Sherman, J. Adventures in simplistic grammar. In R. L. Schiefelbusch (Ed.), *Language of the Mentally Retarded.* Baltimore: University Park Press, 1972.

Bandura, A. *Principles of Behavior Modification.* New York: Holt, Rinehart and Winston, 1969.

Bandura, A. Modeling theory. In W. S. Sahakian (Ed.), *Psychology of Learning: Systems, Models, and Theories.* Chicago: Markham Publishing Co., 1970.

Bellugi-Klima, U. Evaluating the young child's language competence. Paper available through National Laboratory on Early Childhood Education, ERIC, 1968.

Bever, T. G., Fodor, J. A., and Weksel, W. On the acquisition of syntax: A critique of "contextual generalization." *Psychol. Rev.,* 1965,*72,* 467–482.

Bloom, L. *Language Development: Form and Function in Emerging Grammars,* Cambridge, Mass.: M.I.T. Press, 1970.

Bloom, L. *One Word at a Time: The Use of Single Word Utterances before Syntax.* The Hague: Mouton, 1973.

Bowerman, M. F. *Learning to Talk: A Cross-linguistic Comparison of Early Syntactic Development, with Special Reference to Finnish.* London: Cambridge University Press, 1973.

Braine, M. On learning the grammatical order of words. *Psychol. Rev.,* 1963a, *70,* 323–348.

Braine, M. The ontogeny of English phrase structure: The first phase. *Language,* 1963b, *39,* 1–13.

Braine, M. The acquisition of language in infant and child. In C. Reed (Ed.), *The Learning of Language.* New York: Appleton-Century-Crofts, 1970.

Braine, M. On two models of the internalization of grammars. In D. I. Slobin (Ed.), *The Ontogeny of Grammar.* New York: Academic Press, 1971.

Bricker, D. and Bricker, W. *Toddler Research and Intervention Project Report: Year II.* IMRID Behavioral Science Monograph 2, Institute of Mental Retardation and Intellectual Development, George Peabody College, Nashville, 1973.

Brown, R. *A First Language: The Early Stages.* Cambridge, Mass.: Harvard University Press, 1973.

Brown, R. and Bellugi, U. Three processes in the child's acquisition of syntax. *Harvard Educ. Rev.,* 1964, *34,* 133–151.

Brown, R. and Hanlon, C. Derivational complexity and the order of acquisition in child speech. In J. R. Hayes (Ed.), *Cognition and the Development of Language.* New York; Wiley, 1970.

Carrow, E. *Test for Auditory Comprehension of Language.* Austin, Tex: Urban Research Group, 1973.

Carrow, E. The development of auditory comprehension of language structure in children. *J. Speech Hear. Disord,* 1969, *32,* 99–111.

Cazden, C. Environmental assistance to the child's acquisition of grammar. Unpublished doctoral dissertation, Harvard University, Cambridge, Mass., 1965.

Chomsky, N. *Syntactic Structures.* The Hague: Mouton, 1957.

Chomsky, N. Review of Skinner's verbal behavior. *Language,* 1959, *35,* 26–58.

Chomsky, N. *Aspects of the Theory of Syntax*. Cambridge, Mass.: M.I.T. Press, 1965.

Chomsky, N. *Language and Mind*. New York: Harcourt, Brace, and World, 1968.

Chomsky, N. and Miller, G. A. Introduction to the formal analysis of natural languages. In R. D. Luce, R. R. Bush, and F. Galanter (Eds.), *Handbook of Mathematical Psychology*, Vol. 2, New York: Wiley, 1963.

Cofer, C. Comment on the paper by Brown and Fraser. In C. Cofer and B. Musgrave (Eds.), *Verbal Behavior and Learning: Problems and Processes.* New York: McGraw-Hill, 1963.

Dunn, L. M. *Peabody Picture Vocabulary Test*, Minneapolis: American Guidance Service, 1965.

Ervin, S. Imitation and structural change in children's language. In E. H. Lenneberg (Ed.), *New Directions in the Study of Language*. Cambridge, Mass.: M.I.T. Press, 1964.

Feldman, C. F. and Rodgon, M. The effects of various types of adult responses in the syntactic acquisition of two- to three-year-olds. Department of Psychology, University of Chicago, Chicago, 1970.

Ferster, J. Clinical reinforcement. *Sem. Psychiat.*, 1972, *4*, 101–111.

Fillmore, C. The case for case. In E. Bach and R. T. Harms (Eds.), *Universals in Linguistic Theory*. New York: Holt, Rinehart, & Winston, 1968.

Fraser, C., Bellugi, U., and Brown, R. Control of grammar in imitation comprehension and production. *J. Verb. Learning Verb. Behav.*, 1963, *2*, 121–135.

Fygetakas, L. and Gray, B. Programmed conditioning of linguistic competence. *Behav. Res. Ther.*, 1968, *8*, 153–163.

Goldman-Eisler, F. *Psycholinguistics: Experiments in Spontaneous Speech.* New York: Academic Press, 1968.

Goodglass, H., Gleason, J. B., and Hyde, M. Some dimensions of auditory language comprehension in aphasia. *J. Speech Hear. Res.*, 1970, *13*, 595–606.

Gray, B. and Ryan, B. A language program for the non-language child, Champaign, Ill.: Research Press, 1973.

Greenfield, P. M., Nelson, K., and Saltzman, E. The development of rule-bound strategies for manipulating seriated cups: A parallel between action and grammar. *Cognitive Psychol.*, 1972, *3*, 291–310.

Guess, D. A functional analysis of receptive language and productive speech: Acquisition of the plural morpheme. *J. Appl. Behav. Anal.*, 1969, *2*, 55–64.

Guess, D. and Baer, D. Some experimental analysis of linguistic development in institutionalized retarded children. In B. B. Lahey (Ed.), *The Modification of Language Behavior*. Springfield, Ill.: Charles C Thomas, 1973a.

Guess, D. and Baer, D. An analysis of individual differences in generalization between receptive and productive language in retarded children. *J. Appl. Behav. Anal.*, 1973b, *6*, 311–331.

Guess, D., Sailor, N., Rutherford, G., and Baer, D. An experimental analysis of linguistic development: The productive use of the plural morpheme. *J. Appl. Behav. Anal.*, 1968, *1*, 297–306.

Hebb, D. O., Lambert, W. E., and Tucker, G. R. Language, thought, and experience. *Mod. Lang. J.*, 1971, *55*, 212–222.

Karttunen, L. Remarks on presuppositions. Paper presented at the 1973 Texas Conference on Performatives, Conversational Implicature, and Presupposition, University of Texas, Austin, 1973.

602   Ruder and Smith

Keenan, E. L. Two kinds of presupposition in natural language. In C. J. Fillmore and D. T. Langendoen (Eds.), *Studies in Linguistic Semantics*, New York: Holt, Rinehart and Winston, 1971.

Kemp, J. A study of young children's spontaneous verbal imitations. Unpublished doctoral dissertation, University of Washington, Seattle, 1972.

Kemp, J. and Dale, P. Spontaneous imitations and free speech: A developmental comparison. Paper presented at the Biennial Meeting of the Society for Research in Child Development, Philadelphia, 1973.

Kiparsky, P. and Kiparsky, C. Fact. In D. D. Steinberg and L. A. Jakobovits (Eds.), *Semantics: An Interdisciplinary Reader.* New York: Cambridge University Press, 1971.

Kirk, S. A., McCarthy, J. J., and Kirk, W. D., The Illinois test of psycholinguistic ability (rev. ed.), Urbana, Ill.: University of Illinois Press, 1968.

Lahey, B. B. Introduction. In B. B. Lahey (Ed.), *The Modification of Language Behavior.* Springfield, Ill.: Charles C Thomas, 1973.

Lakoff, G. On generative semantics. In D. D. Steinberg and L. A. Jakobovits (Eds.), *Semantics: An Interdisciplinary Reader.* New York: Cambridge University Press, 1971.

Lakoff, G. and Ross, J. R. Is deep structure necessary? Indiana University Linguistics Club, 1968 (mimeographed).

Langendoen, D. T. Presupposition and assertion in the semantic analysis of nouns and verbs in English. In D. D. Steinberg and L. A. Jakobovits (Eds.), *Semantics: An Interdisciplinary Reader.* New York: Cambridge University Press, 1971.

Lee, L. L. *Northwestern Syntax Screening Test.* Evanston, Ill.: Northwestern University Press, 1969.

Lee, L. L. and Canter, S. Developmental sentence scoring: A clinical procedure for estimating syntactic development in children's spontaneous speech. *Speech Hear. Disord.,* 1971, *36,* 315–340.

Lenneberg, E. H. *Biological Foundations of Language.* New York: Wiley, 1967.

Lynch, J. and Bricker, W. Linguistic theory and operant procedures: Toward an integrated approach to language training for the mentally retarded, *Ment. Retard.,* 1972, *10,* 12-17.

MacNamara, J. Cognitive basis of language learning in infants. *Psychol. Rev.,* 1972, *79,* 1–13.

Malouf, R. and Dodd, D. Role of exposure, imitation and expansion in the acquisition of an artificial grammatical rule. *Develop. Psychol.,* 1972, *7,* 195–203.

Mann, R. and Baer, D. The effects of receptive language training on articulation, *J. Appl. Behav. Anal.,* 1971, *4,* 291–298.

McCawley, J. D. The role of semantics in grammar. In E. Bach and R. T. Harms (Eds.) *Universals in Linguistic Theory,* New York: Holt, Rinehart & Winston, 1968.

McNeill, D. The development of language. In P. Mussen (Ed.), *Carmichael's Manual of Child Psychology.* New York: Wiley, 1970.

McNeill, D. Explaining linguistic universals. In J. Morton (Ed.), *Biological and Social Factors in Psycholinguistics.* Urbana: University of Illinois Press, 1971.

Mecham, M. J., Jex, J. L., and Jones, J. D. *Utah Test of Language Development.* Box 11012, Salt Lake City, Utah: Communication Research Associates, 1967.

Mehrabian, A. and Williams, M. Piagetian measures of cognitive development for children up to age two. *J. Psycholing. Res.*, 1971, *1*, 113—126.

Miller, J. and Yoder, D. A syntax teaching program. In J. McLean, D. Yoder, and R. Schiefelbusch (eds.), *Language Intervention with the Retarded*. Baltimore: University Park Press, 1972.

Morton, J. What could possibly be innate? In J. Morton (Ed.), *Biological and Social Factors in Psycholinguistics*. Urbana: University of Illinois Press, 1970.

Murray, S. Investigation of three teaching methods for language training. Unpublished doctoral dissertation, University of Kansas, Lawrence, 1972.

Olson, D. Language and thought: Aspects of a cognitive theory of semantics. *Psychol. Rev.*, 1970, *77*, 257—273.

Palermo, D. and Molfese, D. Language acquisition from age five onwards. *Psychol. Bull.*, 1972, *78*, 409—428.

Phillips, J. Syntax and vocabulary of mothers' speech to young children: Age and sex comparisons. *Child Develop.*, 1973, *44*, 182—185.

Piaget, J. *The Origins of Intelligence in Children*. New York: Norton, 1963.

Piaget, J. Quantification, conservation and nativism. *Science*, 1968, *162*, 976—979.

Piaget, J. *Structuralism*. New York: Basic Books, 1970.

Premack, D. A functional analysis of language. *J. Exp. Anal. Behav.*, 1970, *14*, 107—125.

Ruder, K. and Bunce, B. Training suprasegmental features of speech—Effects of memory load. Unpublished manuscript, Bureau of Child Research Laboratories, Working Paper, University of Kansas, Lawrence, 1973.

Ruder, K. and Hermann, P. Imitation and comprehension procedures in establishment of a second language in first and second graders. Research Progress Report, Bureau of Child Research Laboratory, University of Kansas, Lawrence, 1973.

Ruder, K., Smith, M., and Hermann, P. Effects of verbal imitation and comprehension training on verbal production of lexical items. In L. V. McReynolds (Ed.), *Developing Systematic Procedures for Training Children's Language*, American Speech and Hearing Association Monograph, #18, Danville, Ill.: Interstate Press, 1974.

Ruder, K., Smith, M. and Murai, H. Children's responses to telegraphic and wellformed commands. Paper presented to 1973 Convention of the American Educational Research Association, New Orleans, Available from ERIC document reproduction service, 1973.

Sailor, W. Reinforcement and generalization of production of plural allomorphs in two retarded children. *J. Appl. Behav. Anal.*, 1971, *4*, 305—310.

Salzinger, K. Review of Neisser's cognitive psychology. *J. Exp. Anal. Behav.*, 1973, *19*, 369—378.

Schlesinger, I. M. Production of utterances and language acquisition. In D. Slobin (Ed.), *The Ontogenesis of Grammar*. New York: Academic Press, 1971.

Schlesinger, I. M. Acquisition of grammar—What and how should we investigate. Unpublished manuscript, 1972.

Schlesinger, I. M. Grammatical development: The first steps. In E. H. Lenneberg and E. Lenneberg (Eds.), *Foundations of Language Development*, in press.

Schroeder, G. and Baer, D. Effects of concurrent and serial training on generalized vocal imitation in retarded children. *Develop. Psychol.*, 1972, *6*, 293–301.

Schumaker, J. and Sherman, J. Training generative verb usage by imitation and reinforcement procedures. *J. Appl. Behav. Anal.*, 1970, *3*, 273–287.

Sherman, J. Imitation and language development. In H. W. Reese and L. P. Lipsitt (Eds.), *Advances in Child Development and Behavior.* New York: Academic Press, pp. 239–272, 1971.

Sinclair, H. Developmental psycholinguistics. In D. Elkind and J. H. Flavell (Eds.), *Studies in Cognitive Development: Essays in Honor of Jean Piaget.* New York: Oxford University Press, 1969.

Sinclair, H. Sensorimotor action patterns as a condition for the acquisition of syntax. In R. Huxley and E. Ingram (Eds.), *Language Acquisition: Models and Methods.* New York: Academic Press, 1971.

Skinner, B. F. *Verbal Behavior.* New York: Appleton-Century-Crofts, 1957.

Slobin, D. I. Imitation and grammatical development in children. In N. S. Endler, L. B. Boultier, and H. Osser (Eds.), *Contemporary Issues in Developmental Psychology,* New York: Holt, Rinehart & Winston, 1968.

Slobin, D. I. Universals of grammatical development of grammar. In G. B. Flores d'Acrais and W. J. LeVelt (Eds.), *Advances in Psycholinguistics.* Amsterdam: North Holland, 1971.

Slobin, D. I. Cognitive prerequisites for the development of grammar. In D. I. Slobin, and C. Ferguson (Eds.), *Studies of Child Language Development.* New York: Holt, Rinehart & Winston, 1973.

Smith, M., Ruder, K., and Stremel, K. Independent vs. interdependent linguistic behaviors: A componential analysis. Bureau of Child Research Working Paper, University of Kansas, Lawrence, 1973.

Snow, C. Mother's speech to children learning language. *Child Develop.*, 1972, *43*, 549–565.

Spradlin, J. E. The Parsons Language Sample. In Schiefelbusch, R. L. *et al.*, Language studies of mentally retarded children. *J. Speech Hear. Disord.*, Jan., Monogr. Suppl., 1963, *10*, 88.

Spradlin, J. Personal communication, 1973.

Stremel, K. Personal communication, 1973.

Stremel, K. and Ruder, K. Utilization of grammatical expansions in language training. Bureau of Child Research Working Paper, University of Kansas, Lawrence, 1973.

Stremel, K. and Waryas, C. A behavioral-psycholinguistic approach to language training. Bureau of Child Research Working Paper, University of Kansas, Lawrence, 1973.

Suci, G. and Hamacher, J. Psychological dimensions of case in sentence processing: Action role and animateness. *Linguistics,* 1972, *89*, 34–48.

Thompson, S. A. The deep structure of relative clauses. In C. J. Fillmore and D. T. Langendoen (Eds.), *Studies in Linguistic Semantics,* New York: Holt, Rinehart and Winston, 1971.

Verhave, T. A review of Chomsky's *Language and Mind. J. Psycholing. Res.*, 1972, *2*, 183–195.

Waryas, C. and Ruder, K. On the limitations of language comprehension procedures and an alternative. Unpublished manuscript, Parsons Research Center and Bureau of Child Research Laboratories, University of Kansas, Lawrence, 1973a.

Waryas, C. and Ruder, K. Children's sentence processing strategies: The double-object construction. Unpublished manuscript, Parsons Research

Center and Bureau of Child Research, University of Kansas, Lawrence, 1973b.

Waryas, C. and Stremel, K. On the preferred form of the double object construction, Unpublished manuscript, Parsons Research Center, Parsons, Kans., 1973.

Watt, W. C. On two hypotheses concerning psycholinguistics. In J. R. Hayes (Ed.), *Cognition and the Development of Language*. New York: Wiley, 1970.

Whitehurst, G. Production of novel and grammatical utterance by young children. *J. Exp. Child Psychol.*, 1972, *13*, 502–515.

Whitehurst, G. Imitation, response novelty and language acquisition. *J. Exp. Child Psychol.*, in press.

Winitz, H. and Reeds, J. The OHR method of language training. Kansas City Working Papers in Speech Science and Linguistics, No. 3, University of Missouri at Kansas City, 1972.

Zwicky, A. On the question of directionality. *J. Ling.*, 1972, *10*, 121–129.

CHAPTER TWENTY-THREE

DISCUSSION SUMMARY–LANGUAGE INTERVENTION FOR THE MENTALLY RETARDED

Barbara Bateman

Department of Special Education, University of Oregon, Eugene, Oregon 97401

Most of the discussion of language programs for mentally retarded centered on two issues: 1) the role of the normal developmental sequence of language acquisition in constructing intervention programs for developmentally deviant children and 2) the appropriateness of the goals that guide such program development. A less discussed but also important concern was how the disciplines represented in and by the conference participants can be utilized in intervention programs. A fourth recurring strand was not a topic as such, but rather a repeated acknowledgement that most of the issues dealt with are subject to empirical investigation.

RELEVANCE OF THE NORMAL LANGUAGE DEVELOPMENT SEQUENCE TO INTERVENTION PROGRAMS

The predominant discussion theme was the relevance of normal language development data and/or theory to teaching language to retardates. Miller and Yoder hold that a language program *must* be based on what is known about normal psycholinguistic development while Guess, Sailor, and Baer have based their program on an appraisal of what language forms and skills seem maximally useful to the child in controlling the environment. Ruder and Smith observed that this issue bears directly on the content and sequence of a language program but not on instructional tactics.

There was agreement that the comparative efficiency of programs based to varying degrees on knowledge of normal acquisition sequences is an empirical question, but one which will be difficult, lengthy, and expensive to answer. Two major reasons were offered in support of incorporating developmental data: 1) to increase the likelihood of the child acquiring language usage beyond that specifically programmed and 2) to facilitate teaching in those cases where the normal sequence perhaps obtains because of ease of learning (related, *e.g.,* to degree of semantic or linguistic complexity). Bowerman and Cromer concurred that it is important to ask why a given acquisition sequence normally obtains. If or when the reason is compelling, the program developer could utilize this developmental information. Miller further observed that if normal language development follows cognitive development, then developmental data would enable one to maximize the learning process by tapping into those cognitive strategies the child is using. Oller, in agreement with Miller and Yoder, observed that the current direction in psycholinguistic research is toward a semantic view, a primary focus on the determination of what the child is trying to communicate. The earlier focus was on syntactic structures. The developmentalists suggest that language teaching programs should stem from a view of language acquisition incorporating a conceptual-semantic rather than syntactic basis. The Miller-Yoder program was presented as one application of the position that data on the normal acquisition process are useful.

Baer, on the other hand, argued that developmental data are not relevant because the children being taught are not young, normal children but are older, retarded, and different. An 8-year-old retarded child with a mental age of 3 is not otherwise like a normal 3-year-old. If developmental level is critical, then the observation that a retarded child is not at the same developmental level as his normal mental age peer becomes important. A deviant population by definition demonstrates the inappropriateness of the developmental sequence for that group.

A subtle but important difference in the implications of the two positions was revealed when Chapman pointed out that developmental data would have predicted a particular problem Baer encountered in teaching yes-no and would have dictated waiting and teaching it later. Baer agreed that developmental data anticipated the difficulty, but that their decision was not therefore to wait, but rather to teach yes-no by programming the task in small units. Bricker, in an earlier discussion, suggested that given a 4-month-old does not look for a "gone" object and an 8-month-old does, one can attribute the difference either to age or to the experience of the intervening 4 months. The job of the interventionist, as viewed by Baer, is to provide or impose the appropriate intervening events.

In response to Menyuk's question as to whether all things are equally easy to teach, Baer said "No matter what the problem presented to the child, if he will not learn it on terminal contingencies, perhaps we should assume there is always a program which will lead him from where he is now to that skill. (This) assumption leads you to discover teaching techniques rather than to put problems aside and say he must not be developmentally, conceptually, (or) cognitively ready for this skill."

Considerable agreement existed that language programs can be described in terms of content, sequence, and instructional procedures. The issue of relevance of developmental data is clearly most pertinent to selection of content and to sequencing it. Comparatively few disagreements arose over instructional procedures. Those techniques such as modeling, shaping, and reinforcing, often associated with behaviorists, were widely accepted by the group, including those otherwise critical of many aspects of the behavioral focus.

GOALS FOR A LANGUAGE PROGRAM

A second major issue was whether the goals of a language program for retarded ought to be normal language usage or some lesser degree or kind of language. Many participants expressed concern that the goals or terminal behaviors of some behaviorally oriented programs were unduly limited. In response to the "limited goal" concern, Baer expressed the position that 1) some language is more useful than none and 2) we can empirically determine which program elements will facilitate the extension of language acquisition beyond the program itself. After clarification of the usage of the terms "generalization" (by behaviorists) and "generative" (by psycholinguists) there was widespread agreement that the ideal program treats whatever language it teaches in such a way that further and unlimited language acquisition may be facilitated.

Ruder and Smith urged the development of a battery of language programs rather than a program. This position was also reflected by those who felt programs should be designed for use in a variety of settings and specifically not limited to institutions. It was also stressed that parents should be fully informed about possible or likely limitations in program outcomes. In a brief but noteworthy sidelight, Bricker and Baer debated the desirability of developing programs for use in institutions, when the current trend is clearly away from institutionalization. Baer agreed that was a real and desirable trend, but countered that there are still over 200,000 institutionalized persons in need of such a program and that the wheels of de-institutionalization turn slowly. Language is clearly one of the skills most vital in the successful return of institutionalized persons to a normal community setting. The language programs being developed which are useful in improving the performance of retarded in institutions will therefore increase the numbers able to leave institutions and enhance their postinstitutional functioning.

Although no explicit discussion emerged on the topic of whether mental retardation itself might impose limits on the rate or final extent of language acquisition, casual references in other sessions suggested real differences in the participants' concepts of such limitations. It appeared that some participants routinely think in terms of normal children and their patterns of development, while others, especially those designing behaviorally oriented language programs, tend readily to envision severely retarded and deviant children. This difference may encourage the disparity in views about program goals and the relevance of developmental data to program development.

CONTRIBUTIONS OF LINGUISTICS, PSYCHOLINGUISTCS, AND COGNITIVE PSYCHOLOGY TO LANGUAGE PROGRAM DEVELOPMENT

In a sense the entire conference was addressed to the role of the contributions from linguistics, psycholinguistics, and cognitive psychology to the development of language programs. When asked what contributions were most needed, Baer (clearly speaking for most behaviorists engaged in language program development) replied that program developers needed 1) accurate and usable descriptions of language behavior and 2) data on what constitutes prerequisites for these behaviors. He added that to be useful for programming these descriptions and information on prerequisites must be stated or statable in behavioral terms. Throughout the discussion there were instances where the behavioral psychologists and other disciplines had difficulty bridging the gap between behavioral and nonbehavioral terminology. This seemed especially noticeable in discussions of the need to match language instruction to the child's cognitive level. A related difference in these two viewpoints is seen in Baer's comment that in the behavioral approach to language program development "the abstract, conceptual, cognitive or representational relationship is not the independent variable of the study, but the dependent variable; it is the outcome; it is the result of a set of specified training procedures which we applied and designed in the interests of producing not simply a one-to-one response to those procedures but a generalized response of the nature predictable by the procedures themselves and aimed at by the procedures." The developmentally oriented programmer, by contrast, sees cognitive factors as independent variables within the child which should be matched to the intended language instruction or input.

UNANSWERED QUESTIONS SUBJECT TO EMPIRICAL INVESTIGATION

Agreement prevailed throughout the discussion that unresolved issues and unanswered questions were subject to empirical investigation. For example, there was a bantering yet serious exchange on the reasons for the linguists' recent shift away from syntax and toward semantics, as the basis for acquisition, and whether programmers could therefore count on linguists to "stand still" long enough to be of help. To the relief of all, it was observed that the shift had resulted from empirical data and the reanalysis of old data, not from whimsy. Quick agreement on the feasibility and desirability of empirical resolution was reached on many matters, *e.g.,* the comparative efficacy of language programs, tactics for teaching specific language behaviors, generalizability (generative power) of various language structures, and the ease of teaching specific language forms.

Baer wisely cautioned that if any two language programs (one developmentally sequenced and one nondevelopmentally sequenced) were to run for a few years and be compared, several possible sources of interpretative confusion would exist. Perhaps one sequence might be intrinsically superior. On the other hand, the differences might, in the absence of expensive and extensive controls, be due to initial differences in populations, or superior technology in one when the curricula were comparable, or superior technology combined with an inferior curriculum (if technology outweighed curriculum), or other factors quite extraneous to the issue of the value of a developmentally based instructional sequence.

SUMMARY OF LANGUAGE PROGRAM DEVELOPMENT CONSIDERATIONS

A review of the total discussion reveals high expectations for language intervention programs. Participants recognized the need for: 1) the development and evaluation of more programs diversified by type of learner and setting; 2) comparative efficacy studies even though they are admittedly difficult and expensive; 3) programs which maximize the extension and transfer of language forms and skills specifically taught to those not taught and which ensure spontaneous use of the forms and skills in natural settings; 4) exploration of the most efficient criteria to use in content selection; 5) full consideration of program goals and empirical study of the limited language *vs.* natural language goal concepts; and 6) provision within the program for assessment of entering linguistic structures (and/or cognitive strategies) and of changes in language behavior. The challenge to program developers is truly large. The amount of assistance available from the other disciplines represented in this conference remains to be determined, but a new spirit of interdisciplinary cooperation and willingness to join together in the effort was clearly visible throughout the discussion. The "needs" side of the ledger is large indeed, but these papers and the discussion of them manifest substantial contributions. The delineation and clarification of needs are valuable in themselves but beyond that 1) issues have been pinpointed, *e.g.,* the role or nonrole of developmental data in language program development; 2) research priorities have been suggested, *e.g.,* internal and comparative studies of program efficacy; and 3) useful descriptions of two well developed language programs have been made available.

VIII EPILOGUE

BEHAVIORISM AND COGNITIVE THEORY IN THE STUDY OF LANGUAGE: A NEOPSYCHOLINGUISTICS

Arthur W. Staats

Department of Psychology, University of Hawaii, Honolulu, Hawaii 96822

One of the central goals of this author's approach has been to effect an integration of aspects of psychology that are now separate or in conflict (see Staats, 1963, 1968c, 1971a, 1972, in press; Staats, Gross, Guay, and Carlson, 1973). There has been a separatism in psychology that has had an adverse effect upon progress. One of the foremost contributors to that separatism is the antagonism between learning approaches (behaviorism, or behavior modification) and cognitive approaches (which come under many names). The conflict between the approaches has occurred in the study of language, to the detriment of this field. This chapter provides some background on the schism, illustrates some of the issues, and proposes a method of rapprochement. It will then be possible to refer to the various papers within a context relevant to all of them.

THE COGNITIVE-LEARNING SCHISM

Watson (1930) described language development as learned. The second generation behaviorists began an elaboration of this account. Within a Hullian learning theory, as examples, there were beginning theoretical statements by Cofer and Foley (1942), Osgood (1953), and Mowrer (1954). Linguistics, of course, has been a formal field of study for some time.

In 1953 there was an attempt to form an interdisciplinary approach to the study of language, at a seminar sponsored by the Social Science Research Council. The publication that ensued in 1954 was called *Psycholinguistics,* edited by Osgood and Sebeck.

The seminar first set itself the task of examining three differing approaches to the language process: (1) the linguist's conception of language as a structure of systematically interrelated units, (2) the learning theorist's conception of language as a system of habits relating signs to behavior, and (3) the information theorist's conception of language as a means of transmitting information. These various points of view were explored in order to appraise their utility for handling different problems and to discover in what respects they could be brought into a common conceptual framework (p. iv).

This characterizes one prominent spirit of the middle 1950's in the study of language. Shortly following this, the Group for the Study of Verbal Behavior was formed. It included many of the persons who were then pursuing the study of language. Those of us who were members of the group exchanged prepublication prints of our papers and met from time to time at APA meetings and so on. The group included individuals interested in verbal learning, linguistics, psycholinguistics, and learning theory. My interests in language were based on a foundation of classical conditioning (*e.g.*, Staats and Staats, 1957, 1958) and instrumental conditioning (*e.g.*, Staats, 1957; Staats, Staats, Schultz, and Wolf, 1962), as well as on the interaction between the principles of classical and operant conditioning (*e.g.*, Staats, 1961, 1968a), and included formal theory and research as well as clinical and educational applications (*e. g.*, Staats, 1957, 1964, 1970, 1972; Staats and Butterfield, 1965).

In the 1950's investigators with different orientations to the study of language were in contact, if not generally in mutually influential communication. However, this began to change. In 1957 Skinner's *Verbal Behavior* was published. In addition to its positive contributions, it presented a one-sided view of language that recognized no value in other accounts—even other learning accounts. The only guide to research given in this book was a reference to an apparatus (a "verbal summator") that could present sounds (to a subject) that seemed like language but which were not. The book, thus, did not provide impetus to the conduct of research. However, it did provide an anchoring position for one theoretical extreme.

In 1959 Chomsky wrote a scathing review of Skinner's book. This and the linguistic tradition provided an anchoring position for the other theoretical extreme in the study of language. The two positions constituted a basis for schismatic separation.

In 1959 and 1961 the general conferences on Verbal Learning and Verbal Behavior were conducted as interdisciplinary exchanges sponsored by the Office of Naval Research. However, by the 1961 conference the positions had already become partisan. I was already utilizing linguistic products in my theoretical work. In describing this behaviorist position at the 1961 conference, I indicated that it was possible to interpret language behaviors that led individuals to infer mentalistic or cognitive processes like grammatical rules (Brown and Fraser, 1961) within a straightforward S-R (learning) analysis.

In the course of the discussion Staats made methodological objections to the use of terms such as rules and strategies because they imply explanation and turn interest away from an experimental analysis of the independent variables involved. After observing that the child's verbal behavior, for example, comes to follow grammatical rules, which is itself a very important occurrence to establish by systematic observation, the task is then to make a functional analysis of the development of this behavior. The use of concepts like "rules" obscures this need (Cofer and Musgrave, 1963, p. 208).

It is interesting to note that discussion at the conference leading to this volume indicates that the concepts of rules and strategies are still current, as are behavioristic criticisms of such concepts (see Spradlin's discussion, this volume). At any rate, the responses to these methodological criticisms were strongly opposed—somewhat tempered in the published account from the 1961 conference:

> The discussion revolved around three major issues. First, there was objection to Staats' treatment of purpose in S-R terms, because of the belief that it either ignored or obscured important aspects of the problem. Second, there was discussion of his application of the conditioning paradigm to verbal responses and the nature of the processes involved in his experiments. Third, concern was expressed about the applicability of S-R principles, including reinforcement, to the processes designated by such terms as . . . [grammatical] rules, and the like (Cofer and Musgrave, 1963, p. 290).

The reference to grammatical rules concerned my response to Brown and Fraser's description of their work on the development of syntax in children. For example, they dealt with English inflections as they had been studied by Berko (1958).

> The rule in English is: a word ending in a voiceless consonant forms its plural with the voiceless sibilant . . . as in *cats, cakes,* and *lips;* a word ending in either a vowel or a voiced consonant forms its plural with the voiced sibilant . . . as in *dogs, crows,* and *ribs;* a word ending in the singular with either /s/ or /z/ forms its plural with /z/ plus an interpolated neutral vowel as in *classes* and *poses.* We all follow these rules and know at once that a new word like *bazooka* will have, as its plural bazooka/-z/, even though most speakers of English will never know the rule in explicit form (Brown and Fraser, 1961, pp. 5–7).

Berko had developed a method for studying the manner in which children evidenced correct inflections. A child was shown a small animal and told: "This is a *wug.* Now there are two of them. There are two _____." She found progressive improvement in skill in this type of grammatical speech in 1st, 2nd, and 3rd grade children and concluded that the abstract mental processes called grammatical rules develop with maturational age (Berko, 1958).

My consideration of this material, which I described in my 1963 book *Complex Human Behavior,* recognized the very significant linguistic and developmental linguistic observations of language and language development that were involved. The (Chomsky-inspired) psycholinguistic position, however, involved the inference of abstract mental processes which developed in the child with which to explain the language data. I indicated that linguistic rules or other mental processes did not have to be inferred. The grammatical language and the children's language development could be analyzed and accounted for in strict stimulus-response principles, including that of reinforcement.

The word "rules" as used here can only be thought of as a descriptive term; a person does not ordinarily say things *because* he is following a rule. Actually, in this case the S-R account is rather simple. It is suggested that the stimuli which come to control the voiceless sibilant /-s/ vocal response are, for example, the plural stimulus object [the context] and the labeling response which ends in the voiceless consonant. After the child has had many, many trials where he is reinforced for the sibilant /-s) following the voiceless consonant, this stimulus would elicit the appropriate response. After the appropriate associations have been formed between the ending of a word and the "plural" response, the appropriate ending would be expected to occur even when a novel word was introduced (Staats, 1963, pp. 177–178).

It is pertinent to note, in view of the other topics to be discussed, that this learning analysis has been fully supported in the experiments of Guess, Sailor, and Baer (Guess, Sailor, Rutherford, and Baer, 1968; Guess, 1969; Sailor, 1971). Thus, a theoretical learning theory analysis could be made of certain linguistic data to produce experimental hypotheses demonstrating learning causation—rather than mental causation that has usually been considered to be biologically determined. A major point here is the suggestion that points of combination are possible between observations and descriptions of language in linguistic study and the learning principles that suggest the conduct of manipulative, experimental research—not the inference of biologically caused mental processes. Another point, which differs from the Skinnerian methodology of nontheoretical functional analysis, is that prior theoretical analysis in stimulus-response terms can provide a basis for experimentation.

It may be noted, however, that this combination of psycholinguistic description and learning theory analysis was not influential at that time. Skinner's theory did not contain analyses leading to empirical test. And the success of Chomsky's critique of Skinner's book produced a style of vehement criticism and affirmation orthogonal to empirical research. It then became a central mission of prominent psycholinguists to disprove the credibility of learning approaches—all learning approaches—both in theoretical statements and in experiments designed to show incompatability with learning principles. For example, Fodor (1965) considered the nature of Osgood's concepts of meaning as a representational response process and rejected it as adding nothing to a straightforward one-stage stimulus-response model. He has also generally rejected learning theory approaches.

If it be said that the learning-theoretical accounts of reference psychologists have proposed have only been intended as a first step, it must be replied that they are quite certainly a first step in the wrong direction (Foder, 1966, p. 110).

In the middle 1960's, following the trend toward schism already described, a symposium was organized by Slobin to effect a crucial confrontation between psycholinguistic and learning theorists. Slobin's plan was to provide a summary of the facts of language development and have the theorists direct themselves to analysis of the language development and to the criticism of the opposing position (Slobin, 1971). Some of the issues addressed in 1967 in extending my learning theory of language to these issues and some of the responses to this analysis are relevant in the present context.

To begin, one of the important objectives of this analysis was to consider the Chomskian psycholinguistic approach within the context of a learning theory or a set of behavioral principles. The intent was to place the psycholinguistic and learning approaches in a context that indicated their relationship. I suggested that linguists such as Chomsky are concerned only with language behavior as their data. They do not make observations of the informant's learning history that may account for his language behavior, or of the biological conditions that might be involved. As a consequence, the theory of the mental processes inferred solely on the basis of observations of language is circular. Attribution of causal status over one event by a preceding event demands specification of two events. When only language behavior is observed, and grammatical rules (or deep structure), for example, are inferred as the explanatory event, then some independent specification of those allegedly causal processes must be established.

I thus suggested that Chomsky's psychological (explanatory) theory of language and language development in terms of the development of mental structures or processes (based only on observations of language behavior) did not have explanatory status. Such status could only be gained by isolation of those mental structures. In Chomsky's case, this could be by isolation of the biological mechanisms assumed to be involved. This approach had led students of language away from a concern with the environmental events (the context) and learning that had a determining effect upon language and language development. This could be seen in extreme arguments denying that context exerts any control over what the individual says (Foder, 1965). As another example that implicitly follows the paradigm, the facts of language development summarized by Slobin (1971) describe only language behavior, nothing about the nature of the learning that might have been involved, the nature of the parent-child interactions that could occur, or the context within which the language forms occur. This has been implicit in a good deal of language study (Brown and Fraser, 1963; Berko, 1958).

I made several points in referring to the lack of specification of the determing variables for language development—especially of the lack of specification of past learning conditions and present stimulus conditions.

First, the same types of detailed naturalistic observations must be made of various aspects of language that have been made of formal features such as grammar and phonology. The *functions* of various types of language must be studied as well. *In addition, the same type of detail in naturalistic observations must be made of the stimulus aspects that affect language behavior as has been made of the language behavior itself. This must include detailed observation of the language training environment of the child—which will involve both verbal and non-verbal stimulus events. In addition, detailed naturalistic observations must be made of the present stimulus situation (context) in which the language occurs.* The statement that "The golf ball hit John" is elicited by one set of stimuli, "John hit the golf ball" by another. The two statements are isomorphic with different events. It has been generally suggested (Staats, 1968b) that the nature of the physical stimulus world in which we live operates according to certain principles and we must expect that language—if it is to serve the adjustment of the speaker—must to some extent follow those principles. It should thus come as no surprise that there are language universals. After all, languages are acquired in response to events that in many respects follow the same principles everywhere (Staats, 1971a, p. 146).

It is interesting to note that a concern with the stimulus context and with the experience of the child began to develop among the more linguistically oriented researchers in the late 1960's. Bloom (1970), one of our present contributors, indicated that her research aimed to study "the development of linguistic behavior in relation to the underlying conceptual meaning of language for the child, with specific focus on the relation between children's speech and aspects of their experience related to the speech they use." Other cognitively oriented theorists have also begun to show more concern with the effects context has upon language and with the functions that language has for the user of the language (Brown, 1973a,b). These concerns—most of which fall into that long neglected area of linguistics called semantics—are reflected in some of the chapters in this volume.

Second, I also suggested that studies should be conducted in the naturalistic situation that would be of the manipulative, cause-and-effect, type—in contrast to the straight observational type of investigation.

But, in addition to the naturalistic observations, experimental-naturalistic research must be conducted. By this is meant studies where manipulations are made of learning variables and observations made of the language behavior produced—but not necessarily in the controlled conditions of the basic laboratory. . . . The manner in which grammatical forms can be produced through manipulating learning principles could be studied in the same manner, as could various other aspects of language (see Staats, 1968b). Moreover, there is also a wider opportunity to conduct more controlled laboratory experimentation on language learning. This can be done at various levels of learning beginning with the development of language in infancy—prior to the emergence of actual speech. It can also be done at points where the child is introduced to new types of language learning—for example, in learning reading (which includes various forms of language and various learning principles), in learning number language responses, writing, and so on. There are opportunities for conducting manipulative (causative) studies with normal children and with a variety of children whose language development is absent or defective. Thus, for example, retarded children, autistic children, and so on, could only benefit from research which would attempt to train them to normal behaviors—and learning principles could at the same time be tested and extended (Staats, 1971a, pp. 146–147).

Experimental-naturalistic and laboratory studies of language development have been reported (Baer and Guess, 1971, 1973; Risley and Wolf, 1967; Sailor, 1971; Sailor and Tamar, 1972; Guess, 1969; Guess, Sailor, Rutherford, and Baer, 1968; Staats, 1957, 1963, 1964, 1968a, 1971a, b; Staats and Butterfield, 1965; Staats, Staats, Schutz, and Wolf, 1962; Staats, Minke, Finley, Wolf, and Brooks, 1964; Staats, Finley, Minke, and Wolf, 1964). Moreover, in this volume, three intervention programs for training retardates in language skills have been outlined. The programs of Bricker and Bricker, Miller and Yoder, and Guess, Sailor, and Baer appear to be indicating that children with language problems can benefit from manipulative types of procedures based upon learning principles, as was suggested.

The strategy of Slobin's symposium, however, was to describe facts of language and emphasize facts that seemed most difficult for a learning theory approach to encompass. This orientation appeared in Slobin's introductory chapter where several points of this type were stressed: 1) that development of the complex phenomena of language occurs so rapidly and is completed so early in life that it does not appear to be learned, 2) that each child acquires essentially the same language even though exposed to a different language experience, 3) that the process is systematic and productive in contrast to "merely imitative or rote learned" (Slobin, 1971, p. 3).

The specific facts of language development dealt with 1) two-word utterances and pivot-open class analyses that indicate the grammatical rules of two class combinations that yield original utterances; 2) hierarchical constructions within which multiword combinations function as single units; 3) the manner in which children who have already come to use irregular verbs correctly later give those verbs regular verb endings, a progression that goes from correct usage to incorrect usage; 4) the development in the use of negatives, including incorrect double negatives that the child's parents do not use.

Each of these aspects of language development contains an incongruity, considered in terms of a nonanalytic reference to learning. It was thus my purpose to indicate acceptance of the developmental linguistic observations that had been made, and of the importance of these observations, and to show that an analytic learning treatment could deal with the observation effectively. At the same time the purpose was to indicate the learning conditions involved in a manner that would lend itself to the projection of research and treatment activities in exploration of the phenomena.

Some of these learning analyses will be referred to in exemplifying the major points of the controversy. A central aspect of the present argument, however, is to indicate the inhibitory potential of the cognitive-learning theory schism and the need for a more productive, integrative paradigm. The psycholinguist *vs.* learning schism became endowed with a vehemence that has produced out-of-hand rejection of each approach by the other, even in cases where it would have been productive to use aspects of the other. This may be illustrated by showing that, although the learning analysis was categorically rejected, its suggestions in central areas were accepted as guides for further cognitive theoretical analysis and empirical research.

Of central concern to the present discussion is the criticism of Ervin-Tripp, who reviewed the various papers of the Slobin symposium. The depth of the schism between the cognitive and learning theories apparently stood as an obstacle to showing acceptance of learning principles, concepts, and analyses that are clearly important contributions to the development of the cognitive theory of language development and its attendant research.

[1] Staats' discussion lays a good deal of emphasis on responses, rather than on input. It is common, also, in discussions of language instruction to assume that getting the learner to speak a lot, to practice, is likely to accelerate learning and the development of automatic habits. Yet surely if there is one kind of evidence we already have, it is that motoric output is not necessary to language acquisition (p. 195). [2] Reinforcement appears to play a strong role in Staats' theory of acquisition. I can't imagine what kind of interaction he has been watching, but it is rarely the case that we spend much effort correcting the formal structure of children's speech, especially two-year-olds'. . . . Brown, Cazden, and Bellugi (1969) examined mother-child interaction for two kinds of reinforcement, in relation to development: corrections, and failures to understand. They did not find that developmental rates were related to reinforcement at all. . . . If reinforcement were the dominant factor in language development, we would expect speech of children to be primarily composed of . . . requests for food and services. But on the contrary, many performances requested by children are that adults look at something. And in the end the bulk of child utterances turn out to be predicative declarations, or identifications whose social function is mysterious, and for which the reinforcement is often absent. [3] Staats assumes that secondary reinforcement gives imitation a very strong role in development, since any utterance imitative of an admired or affectionate other is likely to receive strengthening and be repeated. . . . In respect to the early stage of syntax [imitation] simply is inadequate. Even if secondary reinforcement is present when sentences are imitated, the failure to imitate successfully loses it as a mechanism for language change (pp. 196–197). [4] Staats evidently believes that the length of sentences is a simple function of training and would be easy to change (p. 198). [5] Staats, using the argument of "bread please", argues that reinforcement accounts for the order stability and the development of the sentence as a regular unit. Then we must ask several questions: Why is not "please bread" also reinforced? (Aren't the parents grateful for "please" in any location?) Why does the pattern generalize to "dolly please"? Do parents reinforce form anyway? We already know that the answer to the last question is that they do not (Ervin-Tripp, 1971, p. 199).

Ervin-Tripp is a very significant researcher and theorist in the field of psycholinguistics. However, it is suggested that the paradigm provided by the cognitive-learning schism did not establish a basis for recognizing the value of the learning analyses in the study of language. A number of points of the learning analysis were valuable suggestions for the cognitive approach. These points, however, were not accepted within the context of Slobin's symposium. As one example, the criticism that the learning theory ignored "input" conditions was of course quite reversed. The learning theory actually had criticized the unconcern with input in the Chomskian-oriented psycholinguistics. The importance of considering input (learning or experience, and so on) in specifics as well as generally, was stressed in the learning analysis. In fact, examples were used of actual experiential conditions the child faces, as the following quotation shows.

In discussing [telegraphic speech and expansion training], it is appropriate to introduce an issue that is general to various aspects of language development. The primary point is that the training conditions for the child's language are not from the speech of adults to each other—the observations that are usually the data of linguistics. The speech of adults to one another may ordinarily be considered for the young child to be "background noise." Adult speech of this type is important as it acquires conditioned reinforcing (reward) value—however, actual training of children's speech is quite different from ordinary adult communication.

When speaking to the young child, the adult's speech is ordinarily appropriate to the listener's skill development. Thus, with preverbal infants and young children, the adult will emit many more one-word utterances, or utterances that are very simple. The parent will many times say simply "Daddy . . ., Daddy" when he walks into the child's room and the child looks at him from the crib. The parent will say "Doll . . ., Doll," when the child looks at a doll. And the parent gives similar training with other objects. When the parent knows the child is hungry (that is, has not eaten) and sees the child reach for an apple on a table the parent will say "Apple . . ., Can you say apple?" In these and many other ways, the child receives a great deal of single word training.

Furthermore, even at a later stage of advancement, *much of the child's language training will consist of the parent naming an object or event as the child experiences the object or event.* Since the primary type of training involves labeling stimulus objects and events, it is to be expected that certain classes of words (for example, some nouns, adjectives, and verbs) will be acquired more quickly than others.

It is thus suggested that the child receives training which will give him a repertoire of certain words *before* other types of words and that many times these more frequent words are learned singly or in short multiple-word utterances. The parent who is a good trainer presents experience that will most effectively train the child—and this means presenting training that is not too complex for the child to respond to appropriately. For example, the parent of the child who has *just* learned to say "bread" appropriately (that is, under the control of bread and not other objects) among a very sparse repertoire of word responses, should not say to the child "If you are hungry you may have a slice of bread." The child would be unable to respond appropriately to this communication stimulus and would learn little or nothing besides. The more effective parent-trainer will simply say "Bread?" or "Want bread?" and hold up a slice for the child to see. If the child says "Bread" or "Want bread" the parent will then give the slice to the child—a very important training action that will help insure that the verbal response will be well learned, under the appropriate stimulus control.

The verbal stimuli provided the child, along with other training supports, may be gradually increased in complexity as the repertoirial skills of the child make the progression appropriate. It is a long time before the adult can converse with the child in the same manner that he would with another adult. Furthermore, adults who have more extensive language development than some other adults have to modulate their speech in accord with the person being addressed. As an example, any professor who is a good trainer will present to his students material to which they can appropriately respond—a display of inappropriate erudition has little training value (Staats, 1971a, pp. 136–137).

This line of reasoning was elaborated and tied in with an analysis of the importance of imitation in the child's language development. This elaboration was necessary since the role of imitation in language learning was apparently not generally understood:

There is a tendency in psycholinguistic statements to consider imitational behavior of children, and imitational learning, to spring from a basic characteristic of the organism involved. (Actually this error has been made by people other than cognitively oriented psycholinguists, for example, Bandura, 1962). This leads to the hypothesis—which can be readily rejected by those inclined to an antilearning orientation—that imitational *learning* is not importantly involved in language development. That is, as the psycholinguistic approach suggests, it can be seen easily that the child's speech is quite different from that of the adult's. If the child learned by imitating adult speech, then his language would be more like that of an adult.

It has already been suggested, however, that adult communication is not like the communication that occurs between adult and child. This is also true in the case of imitation. It should be noted that a child does not imitate *any* stimulus that impinges upon his sensory apparatus. A child comes to imitate through learning, not because of innate propensity. As a consequence *some* stimuli come to control imitational responses, but not others. It is not possible to go into this topic fully. However, it may be suggested that in the realm of language, as one example, the child will imitate the speech of an adult who is looking at him more than an adult looking elsewhere. The child is trained to do so (Staats, 1971a, pp. 140–141).

This was specifically indicated because a naive view of learning theory and imitation leads to incorrect expectations, as the following example indicates. "An important datum at ... [the two-word utterance] stage (and later stages) is the fact that many of the child's utterances—although consistent with *his* system—do not directly correspond to adult utterances, and do not look like reduced imitations of utterances he has heard" (Slobin, 1971, p. 5). This statement errs in its conclusion because the sample of adult's speech used is that of the adult speaking to the adult. The resemblance between adult speech and the child's speech can be seen when the sample is that of the adult speaking to the child.

To continue, however, the Chomskian position had negated the parent-child speech interaction as an influence on the child's speech development. Ervin-Tripp's rejection of the learning analysis—which included stipulation of parent-child speech interaction—was in accord with the Chomskian position. However, the specific principles of the interaction, when isolated from the learning theory involved, were accepted and used.

> Children are exposed to a great deal of speech which is not addressed to them. But they probably "tune out" a good deal that is uninteresting or too complex, just as they turn off political commentators on television. There seem to be neurological bases to attention which simply eliminate from processing and storage a good deal to which we are exposed. So we have good grounds for believing that at least at the begining the most important language in learning is the speech addressed to the child (Ervin-Tripp, 1971, p. 192).

This acceptance of the general importance of learning in the parent-child relationship had an impact upon the research activities being conducted. That is, when Slobin drafted the facts of language development for the symposium in 1967 there was no reference to the experiential environment of the child included—even though it appears that data demonstrating the learning principles involved had already been recorded. It is suggested that these data were not of interest because the Chomskian theory of language development was oriented in an antilearning direction. The learning theory of language acquisition, however, provided specific principles of parent-child speech interaction that made that data meaningful. Reports began to emerge that were in remarkable coincidence with the suggestions projected in the learning analysis that has been summarized.

Fortunately, at our Berkeley Program on Language, Society, and the Child, three of my students explored existing family tapes for evidence on the grammatical forms of speech to children as contrasted with speech to adults. . . . The syntax of speech addressed to children is simple, containing short sentences with relatively few passives, conjoined phrases, or subordinate clauses. Drach (1969) found that over two and a half times as many of these general transformations per sentence occurred in complete sentences in a women's address to adults as to her two-year-old son, and sentences were over twice as long.

Kobashigawa (1969) has shown that speech to children is highly repetitive. It contains both paraphrases and expansions of deleted material. In a sample to a two-year-old child, from a third to over half of the utterances were repeated. . . .

Most of these samples were of speech to two-year-olds. Infants may be addressed in widely varying syntax since it is not assumed they will understand. In analyzing the texts from Brown's studies, Pfuderer (1969) found that middle class mothers increased syntactic complexity with the age of the child in the two-to-three period, showing that there may be learning by the mother as well as the child. The result may be that in certain respects the input maintains a consistent relation to the child's interpretive skill (Ervin-Tripp, 1971, pp. 192–193).

Ervin-Tripp concluded her statement by saying that the "writing of childhood grammers [which had been the goal of the Chomskian psycholinguists] can only tell us that a change has occurred" not "how the changes came about" (p. 212). She said that language *acquisition* is "where the action is" (p. 212). These statements, like the others already indicated, coincide with the recommendations already made in the learning theory. Slobin (1973) has recently indicated that he considers language to be learned. He still gives a causal role to the child's cognitive development, suggesting that the child learns language in accord with his cognitive advancement. This is a change from a previous Chomskian position.

These turns in the direction of accepting the importance of learning coincide with that which was predicted. The impact of learning upon the development of the child cannot be ignored once learning is attended to. "As psycholinguists also observe the experience (learning) in the child's language development, they will be drawn into the learning theory of language along with their data—the predicted and proper denouement" (Staats, 1971b, p. 150).

Both of the psycholinguists referred to, Ervin-Tripp and Slobin, have been outstanding researchers and theorists. The fact that each of these major figures has elaborated his position to include learning principles and learning-oriented research is an important step. These and similar developments, it is suggested, represent an incipient but major turn in the study of language and in dealing with language acquisition.

NEOPSYCHOLINGUISTICS

The intent of the original psycholinguistics was to combine learning theory and linguistics and information-processing approaches in the study of language. The effort foundered on the shoals of the antagonisms between radical behaviorism and cognitive theory. Neither position provided a rationale for rapprochement, and neither did the new psycholinguistics.

Radical behaviorism has traditionally rejected the concepts and findings of cognitive theory. Skinner (1957), as a representative of radical behaviorism, did not consider cognitive theory in his book on verbal behavior. Cognitive theory, on the other hand, has had as a major goal the negation of behavioral (learning) conceptions. Chomsky (1959) represented this orientation, and Chomskian psycholinguists elaborated the orientation in both research and theory, accepting the antilearning position as a major concern.

It is suggested, thus, that there are general positions involved here that are antagonistic. The radical behavioristic approach is concerned with the manner in which the environment affects behavior. The position is deterministic; the search is for causal, elementary laws that apply across the phylogentic scale. The position rejects concepts of inferred mental processes that are not observed, that allegedly determine the individual's behavior (for example, the concept of rules). Biological variables are deemphasized, in effect at any rate, since the study is not directed toward such variables.

Cognitive theory, on the other hand, has as a main goal a description of the characteristics of the mind that determine human behavior. These are usually thought to be in large part special to man, and biologically based. Cognitive theory resists the concept that man is merely the product of his experience (learning) and insists that man is original, spontaneous, and creative.

The two basic positions have stimulated different types of research activities and different types of concepts and principles. The possibility that there could be products within each that might be important to the other has largely been ignored. The separatism provoked by the basic issues and the antagonisms have obscured this possibility.

It has been my conviction that there is a possible interdisciplinary combination. My orientation is to build a general learning theory that includes the combination of products from the approaches (Staats, 1963, 1968a,b, 1970, 1971a,b, 1972; Staats, Gross, Guay, and Carlson, 1973). It is my conclusion that this will result in the ultimate resolution of the issues. But it is quite evident that this third approach, with its basic principles anchored in a learning theory, is not acceptable to many.

A rapprochement does appear to be possible, however, on more neutral grounds. It is suggested that, for the present at any rate, the rapprochement take place only in part. That is, the deep differences in basic tenets of cognitive and learning theories must be recognized. There will continue to be controversy about these, since they are important issues that demand resolution of one kind or another. They cannot be swept under the rug and ignored. The schism between the behavioristic and cognitive approaches has occurred before, as in the nature-nurture issue in developmental psychology. After a period of strife a position, like the "interactionist" position in developmental psychology, may attempt to sweep the issue away. But this is not a real resolution. The conflict springs up again, as it has in the work of Jensen (1969) and others in the nature/nurture issue.

What must be recognized is that there are separable elements involved in both the radical behavioristic and the cognitive positions. There are in each case productive elements, even when viewed from the standpoint of the other position. These elements should not be ignored or rejected or, what is more likely because of the schism, simply overlooked or not comprehended. If some products are useful, others may also be useful. The general approach must recognize this. The theme of the neopsycholinguistics proposed is that basic differences in the approaches should be recognized and dealt with— sometimes in an adversarial way. At the same time the products of each approach should be explored by the opposition for knowledge that will be useful in developing studies of language and language development.

The militant and total separatism that we have seen has been mutually damaging. Radical behaviorism has been at fault in its rejection of the totality of the cognitive-mentalistic orientation. This was true of Watson, and it has been true of Skinner. The same criticism may be leveled at radical cognitivists, such as Chomsky, and others who accepted his out-of-hand rejection of all learning theory accounts of language.

POINTS OF RAPPROCHEMENT

It is evident that there are a number of currents among the present papers. There are those interested in applications (intervention) *vs.* those who are interested in theory of one type or another. There are those who appreciate tight experimental control *vs.* those who collect data in more naturalistic circumstances. There are those who are environmentally oriented *vs.* those who are biologically oriented. And issues centering on the behavioristic-cognitive split are evident. As a consequence of the separatism that has been discussed, the different patois in the study of language make communication difficult.

It is not possible to deal here with all the issues. Moreover, this would provide no organization. The present mission, thus, is to refer to the specific papers, primarily in the context of the possibilities of a neopsycholinguistics. Examples have already been given of the manner in which cognitive theory data can be utilized in constructing a learning theory of language (see Staats, 1963, 1968a, 1971a, b, 1972). Examples have also been given of the manner in which learning analyses can be employed by cognitively oriented psycholinguists. This volume provides additional examples that will be referred to in elaborating the theme of a neopsycholinguistics.

Morse's and Eimas' chapters are founded in what has been simply termed "cognitive theory." A goal of speech perception research is to establish the characteristics of the mind (for example, short term phonetic memory, short term auditory memory, coding rules, temporary memory buffers, control component of speech-analyzing system, and so on).

Morse's model of the development of speech perception is Chomskian in form: included are concepts of phonetic (deep) structures, speech codes (grammatical rules for speech), and utterances (surface structures). He is thus interested in the developmental investigation of a varying speech perception with age and other factors such as mental and conceptual age. Morse's approach is much like that of a developmental interactionist. His concepts are cognitive, but he does not assume biological determination, rather than learned acquisition, of advancing linguistic perceptual skills. Morse suggested valuable lines of exploration in the development of speech perception and described important areas of investigation.

Eimas presented an approach that is in the same area of study, but with a biological orientation. He cited data that infants can discriminate certain linguistically significant variations in speech sounds as indication that the child is biologically constructed to specially respond to linguistic sounds in general. He also referred to evidence that speech sounds stimulate greater cortical activity in the left hemisphere than do nonspeech sounds, which stimulate greater activity in the right hemisphere—a lateralization that one study showed to exist in 1-week-old infants. A biological theory of language development demands isolation of the biological structures involved. This line of research is thus very important.

The study of early speech perception is also very interesting. Before general conclusions can be reached, however, the various auditory stimuli that make up language sounds will have to be studied with infants. The relationships of speech perception principles to other aspects of language will require investigation. It would also be of interest to conduct similar studies with other primates to establish possible species specificities in sensory characteristics.

In terms of the neopsycholinguistic theme, it is interesting that many of the studies cited by Morse and by Eimas rely upon learning principles and procedures of experimentation. Thus, the reinforcement principle is centrally involved in testing infant speech perception. This is in line with the suggested rapprochement. Although the theoretical orientation of both Eimas and Morse is cognitive, they have not rejected the body of knowledge available to learning-oriented researchers. They in fact employ such knowledge productively.

Premack and Premack's chapter will be referred to here because it seems to have major significance at the basic level of study. The chapters by Eimas, especially, and Morse have an important bearing upon the basic biological-learning conception of language development. The evidence, for example, that infants can make linguistic discriminations presumably before they have had a chance to learn them, and that linguistic sounds stimulate different hemispheres of the brain than nonlinguistic sounds, suggests that language development is based upon biological structures. As interesting as these findings are, the confidence with which the findings can be generalized as a basis for a general conception must be tempered by the fact that the evidence is presently quite sparse.

The Premacks' work, in addition to its ingenious procedures and specific findings, lends itself to a countering interpretation. A major point of the Chomskian psycholinguistic approach is insistence on the biological foundation for language. This interpretation suggests that individuals who do not develop normal language are personally (biologically) deficient or deviant. The view holds that man has the inborn structures which (as they mature centrally) influence language development. Lesser organisms or deficient humans are thought not to have such structures. Premack and Premack's work suggests that apes are capable of learning language, or aspects of language, when a suitable response system is employed. This does not support the radical biological position. Moreover, it may be suggested that evidence we have regarding the importance of learning conditions in language development indicates that problems in language development (as in some retardates) may be due to unfortunate conditions of learning.

There are too many valuable findings in Premack and Premack's work to summarize here. But one is of special interest to me because the finding with apes parallels that which I found with young children. The Premacks found that the learning of first words is very difficult with apes. This phenomenon has been systematically studied in several different areas of language (Staats, 1968a; Staats *et al.*, 1970). For example, the first letters the child learns to write or to read require many training trials. Moreover, as the child learns additional units, the learning task requires progressively fewer trials. This learning acceleration, through experience in learning, indicates the importance of such experience in cognitive development, including language development. This suggests that the child developmentalist's prejudice against early childhood training is misplaced.

Cognitive theorists such as Ervin-Tripp have indicated new interest in the effects of experiential factors, including relationships with parents, in the child's language development. Of special interest with respect to the neopsycholinguistics described is the movement shown in some of the cognitively oriented chapters toward concern with the child's learning in his language development. Several chapters are notable in this respect, as will be indicated, without the rejection of learning theory that was so much in evidence such a brief time past.

Clark based her approach on Slobin's recent concept that the child *learns* language progressively in accordance with his cognitive development. Clark, in line with Slobin's conception of the cognitive-language relationship, proposed that the child gradually learns the adult meanings of words. She addressed herself to a number of interesting questions and made some interesting analyses. There is much agreement between these concepts and those based upon learning theory. For example, Clark suggested that an object may have a number of perceptual attributes. Similarly, a word meaning can be composed of components of meaning. As Clark indicated, a dog has shape, size, coat texture, a way of moving, and so on. She suggested that the child at the beginning picks out (responds to) one or two features as criterial for the word "dog" and gradually adds others. There is an explicit stimulus-response learning analysis of the learning of the meaning of verbal concepts (see Staats, 1961, 1968a) that has similarities and differences with Clark's model, and it would be worthwhile to relate the two theoretically and empirically. This is a recommendation that may be extended to other aspects of Clark's paper as well. Her excellent paper shows the potentiality of the new developmental linguistic liberation that enables a productive treatment of language learning conditions and effects.

Schlesinger is concerned with the relational concepts of language. The relational concepts of Chomskian psycholinguists were the "subject" and "object," according to this account. "These are specifically linguistic concepts, and the fact that they are not exhibited in the surface structure of adult speech raised the problem of how they can be learned" (Schlesinger, this volume). The Chomskian answer was that the basis of the deep structure was innate. Schlesinger made steps to recognize the importance of learning in the child's language acquisition in the Slobin symposium (Slobin, 1971). He has suggested in his chapter in this volume that "the relational concepts underlying child speech are semantic in nature and reflect the way the child perceives the world." Schlesinger recognizes the importance of the labeling training that the child receives—that the linguistic productions of adults, in interacting with the child, are paired with the situation which the adult talks about. His view is very coincident with the learning theory. As one example that "learning the grammar involves finding out how the situation connects with adult sentences referring to it" (this volume), Schlesinger suggested that the child must acquire relational concepts such as agent and action, possessor and possessed, location of object, and so on—the attainment of these being "dependent on the child's general cognitive development and not on any innate syntactic concepts" (this volume). Schlesinger's approach is very open to the learning-cognitive rapprochement of a neopsycholinguistics, and his chapter suggests important avenues of advancement.

Menyuk has written a significant paper concerned with the infant's early comprehension of the properties of language and the functions of language. The studies cited cover a range of aspects of language, including production and comprehension. Menyuk referred to methodological differences in the studies. For example, some of the studies include concern with the situational context for the language performance, and some do not. Her paper also attests to the increased emphasis upon situational (semantic) observations, and to the concern with the functions of language. Menyuk's orientation is cognitive, considering stages in the child's language development to be "a product of his biological maturation, his changing communication needs, and his ability to relate these needs to particular aspects in the language. The last is due to his perceptual development" (this volume). However, her concepts also include concern with individual and group differences in language, and with the learning context for these, as well as with possible biological bases—which makes her approach congruent with the neopsycholinguistics suggested.

Cromer's approach is also cognitive in nature and includes the biological orientation involved in such an approach. He is concerned with receptive language in the retarded. Some studies suggest that retardation, as measured by intelligence tests, means simply a delayed language development. Other studies suggest that retardation processes are abnormal and result in abnormal language development. Cromer's interests in the relationship between intelligence and language development—in a manner similar to the cognitive-language relationship evidenced in other chapters—spring from a Piagetian conception that "language is dependent on and shaped by underlying cognitive structures" (this volume). Cognitive theorists should be aware of the possibility enunciated in the context of a learning theory that cognitive abilities (such as intelligence) may be learned and in fact may be in large part the same as those designated as language abilities (Staats, 1971b). As will be indicated, the studies cited by Cromer are interpretable within this conceptual framework.

It should be noted that Cromer's chapter also demonstrated the contemporary breakdown of the cognitive-learning schism. Although committed to a traditional cognitive theory, and skillful and productive in its extension, he has shown interest in the learning theory analysis of grammatical phenomena and with the learning methodology involved in testing the learnability (by retardates) of grammatical rules.

Bloom's chapter in this volume and her other works indicate the manner in which cognitive psycholinguistics is converging (at least in certain aspects) with the learning theory of language. For example, Bloom (1970) has emphasized the child's acquisition of a labeling repertoire. The child's first sentences are seen to label relationships of objects and events in the child's environment. Moreover, although Chomskian psycholinguists originally were not interested in the child's language until it had structure (was at the two-word utterance level or beyond), a point that was also criticized by Staats (1971a), Bloom has indicated interest in the single word level of performance, and in the situational context and its effect upon language. Although immediately concerned with the development of productive language and language understanding (comprehension), and their relationship, Bloom's chapter also displays these other interests. For example, Bloom indicated concern with the demonstration that the plural morpheme is a learned verbal response. Her statement, however, "It is not clear what the subjects knew that led them to use or understand the plural morpheme" (this volume), indicates that a reference to the learning theory analysis underlying the experiments would be helpful to her in indicating what is learned, as well as the learning principles involved. Such reference would generally enhance her conceptual formulations.

It is pertinent to reiterate a suggestion to cognitive psycholinguists who are becoming interested in learning. The importance of language learning is being accepted more and more widely, but the learning conception employed is a common sense conception. A much more specified and productive learning theory of language is available that would be useful to the cognitive psycholinguists. Use of the learning theory would solve many of the problems that are now focal in their literature.

Bloom also included interest in other elements of language important in the learning theory of language, for example, imitation and images (or mental representations). She handled these within a cognitive orientation. Relating this to relevant language learning analyses would enhance their significance (see Staats, 1971b).

Ingram showed an interest in comprehension and production of language. This traditional area of study has focused upon the relationship between the two, especially in terms of the time and order of their appearance. Ingram took a rather whole-hearted cognitive approach to the questions involved. In terms of the neopsycholinguistic context described, however, it is interesting that there is no reference to the cognitive-learning schism. Although Ingram referred almost entirely to cognitively oriented studies, he did refer to the study by Guess (1969) that supported the learning hypothesis that plural morphemes can be learned, even in an incorrect (or, rather, opposite) manner. It is interesting that this result is interpreted to indicate an independence for comprehension and production. This interpretation, however, rests upon an assumption that there is some absolute "correctness" to language of this type—that plurals must properly be indicated by adding inflections. Actually, a language could be constructed in which such inflections were indicative of singular referents. Guess's results do not indicate an independence of production and comprehension—only that a child trained to respond in a manner opposite to that usual in the language will comprehend language in the manner that is in accord with his training. A case of opposite speech involving confusion of the affirmative and negative has been analyzed to suggest that learning is responsible (see Staats, 1957, 1973, pp. 197–198), in the context of suggesting the behavior modification principles to be used in correcting such "abnormal language." To continue, however, Ingram's statement of the production-comprehension issue organizes and evaluates interesting literature. Among his conclusions is that the order of emergence of comprehension and production is less central than the study of the nature of the gap between them.

Moorehead and Moorehead presented an excellent exposition of a Piagetian framework for the consideration of language development in the first several years. The general lack of interaction between Piagetian cognitive theory and learning approaches can be seen here, however. Except for several references to other chapters in this volume, Moorehead and Moorehead made no reference to learning theory and learning research in language. As with other cognitive theories, there are points where Piagetian statements are disparate from expectations from the learning theory. The radical behaviorist tradition, as exemplified by Skinner, has been to ignore cognitive theories, including Piaget's. As I indicated (Staats, 1963, 1968a, 1971a; Staats, Brewer, and Gross, 1970), it is important to deal with theories that differ from learning expectations. As with the examples already cited, where cognitive findings have been dealt with in terms of learning, dealing with such issues in learning terms can effect a resolution and advancement of knowledge relevant to both approaches.

An illustration is germane here. Piaget (1953) has said that invariance in counting, over different arrangements of the objects to be counted, does not develop in the child until the age of 6 or 7. A learning analysis has been given that suggests otherwise. Learning procedures have been employed to demonstrate that this aspect of language can be acquired by the child of 2–4 years of age (Staats, 1963, 1968a, 1971a,b; Staats *et al.*, 1970).

Such points of discrepancy are to be expected in making a cognitive-learning combination. As another example, Moorehead and Moorehead have cited Bell and Ainsworth's (1972) study of maternal responsiveness and crying. Bell and Ainsworth found that prompt and attentive physical contact and caretaking would terminate crying. A learning analysis tells us that such treatment of crying will act as a reinforcer and would be expected to result in the long run in the child *learning* to cry. Bell and Ainsworth also indicated that other modes of infant communication were negatively related to extent of crying in the sample of children—attributing this to delay in development of Piaget's means-end relations. They said that when the child's crying did not result in the desired end (contact and caretaking) he continued this type of behavior and did not advance in sensorimotor stages. The learning theory, on the contrary, suggests that crying, if reinforced (by contact and caretaking), will be learned. Furthermore, this may occur to the disadvantage of the development of other language behaviors that may be in competition with crying in its role as communication. This analysis would also account for the results of Bell and Ainsworth. The same principle, it may be added, is true of other substitutes for language, such as whining, grunting, and gesticulating in order to obtain something. The child who learns such grunting and gesticulating skills will less rapidly learn the language of requesting and labeling. The principle is that there is many times a competition in learning. Learning one skill may, by its success, preclude the learning of other language skills (Staats, 1971b, see pp. 305–306, etc.).

Different child-raising methods are implied by the differing theories. The fact of discrepancy, however, should lead to productive research and treatment activities that aim toward empirical resolution—not in antagonism, denial, or avoidance that prevents interaction of the theories. Moorehead and Moorehead's chapter helps provide a basis for such considerations.

Horton's conceptual base is that cognitive development is the basis of language development. From this basis she deduced a need for early detection of the presence or absence of cognitive structures. Horton also utilized aspects of learning. For example, a primary assumption of hers is that mothers as caretakers affect their babies' language development. This conception does not recognize the parents' roles to as great an extent as the concept that the parents constitute the primary "trainers" of the young child (Staats, 1963, pp. 411–414; 1971b), but it is an advancement over the original cognitively oriented disinterest in the role of the parents. The outcomes of Horton's research project to study how amenable to alteration is the language style of parents should prove interesting. The results of the Home Teaching Program for Parents of Very Young Deaf Children are promising. The findings that early identification, early amplification for the child, and early parent training can make deaf children's language approximate the language of normals and exceed nontreated deaf children also suggest the importance of learning in language development.

Moores has presented an absorbing chapter on a topic that is not widely considered among those concerned with language development. The fact that there appears to be prejudice (by educators in the field) against sign languages is a poignant reminder that many educational practices are based upon common sense conclusions or philosophies rather than on solid empirical or theoretical analysis.

Moores has cited a number of significant findings, for example, the superiority of deaf children with nonhearing parents over those with hearing parents on a number of intellective and language performances. These results, incidently, are what would be expected from consideration of language and intelligence as overlapping repertoires of skill. This and other results cited indicate that successful early language training is essential to later learning skills (cognitive development), as the learning acceleration phenomenon already mentioned also suggests. Moores has made an excellent and very valuable presentation of an important topic.

It is pertinent at this point to pause for a few general comments relevant to the chapters described. In treating the controversy between the Chomskian psycholinguistic and learning theories of language, a path for the complementary combining of the two was described. It was suggested that, as with the early child developmentalists in general, the investigations of developmental linguists have provided the description of behavior, albeit not the explanation of the behavior.

It should be indicated that the systematic observations made of the development of child behavior by the early developmentalists were exceedingly valuable, in their proper role. For example, the observations of child behavior development, and the various types of tests of behavior that were constructed, enable us to *place* a child with respect to his behavior development—to know if he is accelerated or retarded. This information also yields prediction of later development and enables us to take remedial steps to correct any difficulty. In addition to these important uses it should be indicated that *systematic observations and descriptions of an event are necessary before one can set about finding the determinants of the event.* Thus, detailed and systematic observations and descriptions of behavior are essential. . . .

Thus, it is well to note that linguistic information is *in principle* like the developmentalist's observations of behavior development. The linguistic observations and systematic descriptions may be extremely productive in and of themselves. This work, for example, can help specify the behavior that has to be accounted for in an explanatory psychological theory. But the *determinants* of language behavior and language development must lie either in learning circumstances or in biological events of some kind. . . . [Furthermore], Chomskian psycholinguistics does not deal with the *various* important aspects of language. His approach is restricted to only one aspect of language, the description of grammar. . . . The various repertoires that constitute a functional language for the individual are not dealt with in any way. Yet these are the bases for some of the most powerful functions of language in human learning and in human interaction. There are no principles within the Chomskian psycholinguistics theory for studying how the child learns his *various* repertoires of language or how they function in the individual's behavior and in social interaction (Staats, 1971a, pp. 115–120).

This statement suggests that both the radical cognitive position as represented by Chomsky and the radical behaviorist position as represented by Skinner are incomplete. The cognitive position in the study of language did not recognize the importance or nature of learning, of the child's experience, of his social interaction with his parents and others, of the situational context, of the various functions of language for the child, and of the various types of language, some of them (like single word utterances) having little relevance for grammatical theory. But the cognitive position has provided some very important knowledge about language and language development. Moreover, cognitively oriented investigators such as Ervin-Tripp, Slobin, and Brown have begun to fill in the deficits in the cognitive psycholinguistic approach that were dominant until very recently.

The task in this new orientation is not complete. The child's experience and learning in his language development presently are being explored. However, the question asked earlier (Staats, 1971a) still remains. Will the cognitive theorist in his new interest in learning remain content with a common sense conception of learning? There are general learning theories that have addressed themselves to the study of language (Osgood, 1953; Mowrer, 1954; Skinner, 1957; Staats, 1968a, 1971a,b). These are alternatives themselves, and alternatives to a common sense learning conception. In employing a learning conception as a basis for studying language development, it would seem reasonable to utilize the most productive learning theory of language available. In this competition a common sense conception would seem an unlikely winner.

The radical behaviorist position is also incomplete in excluding the products of the cognitive approach. The methodology of exclusion of nonbehavioral findings characteristic of radical behaviorism was as short-sighted as the radical cognitive position. Observations and concepts of language that had grown out of the cognitive approach were important to a description and

an understanding of language and language acquisition, but they were neglected. For this reason, an equally important step in the study of language
and language acquisition, as has been indicated, was to break down the
insularity of radical behaviorism. The four chapters concerning programs of
intervention for treating problems of language development indicate that this
avenue is now being accepted. Both Bricker and Bricker and Miller and
Yoder made explicit their use of the methodology of combining cognitive
psycholinguist descriptions of language as the content of the training program
with the principles and procedures of learning as the means of training. The
chapter of Guess, Sailor, and Baer and that of Ruder and Smith both include
reference to cognitive psycholinguistic observations. These efforts thus fit
very much into a neopsycholinguistics.

Bricker and Bricker have very skillfully combined the elements of learning
concepts, analyses, and procedures from different learning theories, along
with Piagetian and other psycholinguistic materials. Their learning concepts
and procedures, as well as their basic method of combination, fit very well
into a neopsycholinguistics, although they used the language of Skinner's
learning theory. In making the combination of cognitive and learning positions, Bricker and Bricker suggested that the basic controversies between the
positions are pseudo problems. Here they made some paradoxical points.
They considered the issue of whether language is learned to be a pseudo issue
because the "Skinnerian model" is not a learning theory. The argument here
is, however, semantic obfuscation concerning what constitutes a "learning
theory." In the face of the fact that Skinner's position heavily stimulated the
cognitive-learning schism in the study of language, this interpretation does
not appear to be productive. Bricker and Bricker dealt with the nativistic
position also as a pseudo issue, with the attempt to sweep it under the rug of
Piagetian interactionism. It is suggested that the issue will refuse to stay
swept, however, as illustrated by the recent declarations of Jensen and
Herrnstein and Shockley. There are substantive issues involved, not simply a
language game. A neopsycholinguistics that combines cognitive and learning
materials must accept the fact that there are basic controversies.

Bricker and Bricker were on much surer ground when they dealt with
language training methods. They have assembled an intervention program
from various learning analyses that would be expected to have positive
results. Moreover, they have developed a facility and program that involve
various types of training and include extension to home instruction and care.
They have also developed a very interesting experimental situation studying
the receptive language of young children. It should be possible to investigate
different aspects of this type of learning.

The extent to which the cognitive approach has become congruent with
aspects of a learning approach to language can be seen in the chapter by
Miller and Yoder. Unlike the Chomskian-inspired focus upon syntax and
multiple word utterances, there is interest in the child's acquisition of

semantic units. Miller and Yoder suggested that the basis of early language development is the semantic concept. This has been called the "labeling response" in learning theory terms. Within that, Miller and Yoder indicated the relational functions and substantive functions to be learned by the child at the single word, two-word, three-term, and four-term levels.

Miller and Yoder included sequencing as well as content in their analysis of a prototypical language intervention program. They suggested a functional criterion for sequencing, again in a manner congruent with the suggestions made within the learning theory. Frequency of occurrence of words in normal language was suggested as the criterion for functional importance. Another concern with function was indicated by Miller and Yoder's emphasis upon teaching the child language for communication purposes. It may be added that Miller and Yoder's suggestions for training procedures within a learning (behavior modification) paradigm are also very productive.

Guess, Sailor, and Baer have pioneered in testing the stimulus-response learning analyses of linguistic phenomena (Staats, 1963). It is not until such theoretical analyses have received empirical support that they begin to command confidence and general attention. The number of references to their experiments on pluralization, and so on, in the other chapters attests to the success of their experiments. The fact that the learning analyses by themselves were ignored and rejected from 1963 until the publication of their experimental corroboration indicates the crucial role of experimental verification. Moreover, the experimental work also gave additional impetus to the possibility of using learning principles and procedures in intervention programs. Like the Brickers, the experimental work of Guess, Sailor, and Baer referred to above and their proposed program to teach language to retarded children, by including the products of cognitive psycholinguistics, have diverged from the radical behaviorism of Skinner, in the direction that was projected (Staats, 1963, 1971a,b).

In their prototypical intervention program for work with retardates— unlike the cognitive accounts of language—Guess, Sailor, and Baer used categories of language that have emerged from the learning theories. Thus, their program deals with tacts (Skinner, 1957), or labeling training (Staats, 1971b), verbal-motor unit training (Staats, 1971b), and so on. They also introduced a new category, which they called "self-extended control," where the child is trained to ask "What that?" and is told the name of the object. Within such categories of language repertoires, various subclasses of training were outlined, as were experiments that are to be conducted. Guess, Sailor, and Baer have presented comments on methodology as well as principles and training procedures that will be valuable in the study and treatment of language problems with the mentally retarded.

Ruder and Smith discussed some of the matters relevant to language training programs, including the isolation and analysis of some of the issues involved from among the intervention programs outlined in other chapters.

They have done an excellent job, and their chapter indicates some of the important considerations involved in such intervention programs, only a few of which will be referred to here. As Ruder and Smith have indicated, the intervention programs, by including reference to language development, suggest a concern with the order of training to be conducted. As Ruder and Smith indicated—although Guess, Sailor, and Baer feel there are not enough data on developmental progressions in language development to be usable—it is important to address this issue. Cognitive theorists have frequently assumed a progression in child development that is based upon maturation. Stage theories of development include this as a heavy component. Radical behaviorism has not dealt with the possibility of a hierarchical development and in so doing has ignored an important aspect of language development and child development in general. Gagné (1965) proposed that there are different levels of learning: that there are simple principles of learning, such as those of conditioning, and more complex types of learning. Staats (1968a, 1971b), on the other hand, in proposing a hierarchical learning theory, has suggested that the basic principles of learning remain constant in development. However, this cumulative-hierarchical learning theory of the child's language-intelligence development suggests that repertoires of skills are learned by the child—according to conditioning principles—that serve as the basis for later learning. As an example, vocal imitation skills constitute such a basic behavioral repertoire. Vocal imitation must be learned, and it is thus a dependent variable to be studied. The vocal imitation repertoire, however, is a foundation repertoire for the learning of many new words. In this sense it is an independent variable that must be studied in language and dealt with in training programs. This theory suggests the way in which the considerations of cognitive theorists that required the concepts of stage theories can be treated within a learning theory which has its basis in conditioning principles. A rapprochement results that recognizes cognitive development and the explanatory effects of cognitive traits but indicates how the traits are learned. In any event, Ruder and Smith, in focusing on the issue of hierarchical progression in language, have indicated an area of study important in language intervention.

Another of the excellent points made by Ruder and Smith is the suggestion that it is unrealistic to expect that any one of the existing language intervention programs will meet all the demands of the language problems that exist. Their concept of the plural allomorphs and the training procedures they derive from the conception, however, do not agree with the learning theory analysis. Ruder and Smith consider the three plural allomorphs to "comprise a single linguistic behavior with three different physical manifestations" (this volume). Thus, training on only one allomorph will be sufficient for the child to use all these correctly. It is true that *after* the child has learned to make plural endings correctly, in *later* learning such as learning to read. training in one of the three allomorphs will generalize to the others

(Staats, 1968a, pp. 288–289). This has been indicated in an analysis suggesting that correct usage depends upon "pluralization word associations." This should not be taken, however, to indicate that the three allomorphs *originally* constitute a single linguistic behavior on some basic level. It is only that by the time the child is trained to read he has already learned all three plural allomorphs. All he has left to learn is that the letter "s" at the end of the printed word must elicit one of the plural speech forms. Originally, however, in learning to speak, each of the plural allomorphs has to be learned. There is no conceptual basis in learning theory for expecting them to be tied together as a single linguistic behavior. Nevertheless, Ruder and Smith contributed with their analysis by providing additional impetus for the type of study that should be conducted to resolve this issue.

A point may be made here, in the context of these chapters. Much contemporary behavioral work has followed Skinner's example elevating the status of empirical research and downgrading theoretical analysis. It should be recognized, however, that both activities are essential ingredients. For example, as has been suggested, the research which showed that grammatical inflections were learned was productive in the manner already indicated. However, the preceding theoretical treatment specifically analyzed grammatical inflection learning and in doing so provided a foundation for the research. Ruder and Smith, it is suggested, made a contribution in formulating a theoretical analysis of the plural allomorphs that can lead to empirical research. There are various theoretical analyses that could be employed as a basis for research on language (Staats, 1968a, 1971a, b).

INTELLIGENCE AND LANGUAGE

At various places in this book there are references to cognitive development and language development. The topic has been raised repeatedly by those of a cognitive theory orientation. The general approach sponsored by Piaget (and others), for example, holds that cognitive development depends upon processes or structures (intelligence) that are different from those involved in language development—and, moreover, that cognitive development underlies language development.

Radical behaviorism in rejecting concepts of internal mental processes has not been concerned with this issue. Radical behaviorism has not considered what constitutes intelligence, or what functions intelligence performs, or what produces individual differences in learning ability, and so on. This, actually, is one of the weaknesses of radical behaviorism.

This is not an inevitable weakness of a learning theory approach, however. A few words are appropriate here on the cognitive-language relationship because the issue has figured so prominently in the conference, and because of the inherent importance of the topic. Only a brief statement can be given here, taken from the more complete theory (Staats, 1971b). This book also described a set of procedures for *producing* language development in young children—procedures to be used with normal children as well as with remedial cases such as retardates. Because of this there is a good deal of similarity in this account and the intervention programs described here.

First, the learning theory suggests that what is referred to as cognitive development (or intelligence) is many times the same as language development. In contrast, the reigning view is that intelligence is an internal personal quality or process, and the intelligence test is looked at as the external manifestation of the internal process. When one looks at the specific items of which intelligence tests are composed, however, the cognitive-language relationship is shown. Intelligence tests are to a large degree composed of items that assess the state of the child's language development. Many items on the Stanford-Binet, for example, assess whether or not the child has acquired a repertoire of verbal labeling responses to pictures or objects (Staats, 1971b, pp. 89–90). Other items on intelligence tests measure the extent of the child's understanding of language (Staats, 1971b, pp. 67–70). For example, at the 2-year level of the Stanford-Binet the child is presented with a set of miniature objects and is told, "Show me the kitty," "Put your finger on the kitty" (Terman and Merrill, 1937, p. 75). If the child comprehends the language units by behaving appropriately, he will receive points towards his intelligence score. Many other items test the child's language imitation repertoire (Staats, 1971b, pp. 125–129). Other items measure number language skills, word association skills, and so on (Staats, 1971b).

The learning theory of language-intelligence development, thus, sees the two as closely related areas of skill which the child develops through learning. The complete account suggests that the child learns a number of repertoires of behavior in his early years. Some of the most important of these repertoires are language repertoires. The learning involves basic conditioning principles but must also include principles of a cumulative-hierarchical nature that are not stated in the basic principles. Moreover, some of these language repertoires are the same behavioral skills that are used to index intelligence. In this sense the relationship is not how cognitive processes (such as intelligence) underlie language development. The relationship is one of identity.

It should be stressed, however, in contrast to the radical behavioristic views, that the language-intelligence repertoires are considered a personality trait in the behavioral interaction learning approach being described. Many of the repertoires determine how the child (or adult) will adjust to and learn in later situations. Thus the language-intelligence repertoires are a cause, an independent variable, as well as a dependent variable. This conception, it is suggested, provides a basis for rapprochement between cognitive theory and learning theory because it recognizes the causative status of personality trait processes like intelligence and other cognitive repertoires. (This approach is now being adopted by social learning theorists such as Mischel, 1973.)

This conception also provides a basis for the interpretation of some of the results cited in previous chapters. For example, Cromer summarized a study (Graham and Graham, 1971) in which a linguistic analysis of conversational performance was correlated with mental age in retardates. The positive correlation in such studies is interpreted to indicate that the internal process of intelligence influences the rate of language development. The present suggestion is that intelligence and language are correlated because they are in good part the same thing—and this largely learned. Other studies, such as that of Lackner (1968) provide similar findings.

It is not possible here to develop this conception in detail (see Staats, 1971b). One thing that follows from the conception, however, is that the study of language development in normals and retardates is not a study of an important feature of humanness that depends for its development upon intelligence. *Language and intelligence are inextricably linked and depend upon the same types of determining events. The study of mental retardation, thus, is in good part the study of language retardation. This conception, it is suggested, helps provide a basic rationale for the concern with language of those whose primary interest is in understanding and dealing with mental retardation.*

THE NEOPSYCHOLINGUISTICS PROPOSAL

Considerable change has taken place within the cognitive-linguistic approach and the learning theory approach to language. The former has begun to recognize the importance of learning in the child's language development and of the child's interaction with his parents and others. It is beginning, also, to be concerned with the role of the context in eliciting language, as well as with the functions of language for the individual. This development should deepen, with an increasing use of a formal learning theory of language, in contrast to the present common sense notions employed.

On the other hand, investigators who were once concerned only with operant conditioning and Skinner's analysis of aspects of language in terms of operant conditioning principles are now utilizing analyses of language learning phenomena from a learning theory that includes linguistic specifications. It is thus suggested that the radical and separatistic positions of Chomskian psycholinguistics and Skinner's operant conditioning have been breached in fact. It is now time to recognize that a rapprochement, at least in part, is possible. A neopsycholinguistics that generally recognizes these possibilities can provide a productive impetus to the field. The following points summarize the suggested rapprochement.

1. Whether or not language is learned has been an issue that has been a stumbling block to rapprochement. Acceptance of the fact that language is to an important extent learned clears this obstacle. There appears now to be agreement that the context has an effect upon language and that the

nature of the interaction between the child and others is important in the child's language learning. There is also growing interest in the possibility that language has functions in the individual's adjustment.

2. Linguistics and psycholinguistics and other cognitive approaches have made important observations of language behavior and language development and have formulated important systematic (theoretical) organizations of the observations.

3. The basic learning principles have been explicitly formulated in the animal laboratory, with detail and specificity. They have been verified in the context of functional human behaviors. There are learning theories that have been elaborated in the context of language.

4. There are points where the cognitive-linguistic approach could be furthered significantly by reference to a learning theory of language. Some of the issues of concern to the cognitive approach have already been analyzed in terms of learning principles. Such analyses constitute hypotheses for experimentation.

5. There are points where learning theories of language could be (and have been) elaborated by reference to linguistic observations, concepts, and analyses. In general, the productive role of *theoretical* learning analyses of language, for behavioral research and intervention programs, should be recognized.

6. It is suggested that a neopsycholinguistics for contemporary times should utilize and expand these avenues of rapprochement. Real issues between the positions should be aired, but without continuing the separatism that has prevented productive interaction of the approaches at points of coincidence of interests and concepts.

7. It is suggested that a neopsycholinguistics of this type could result in a genuine interdisciplinary interaction in the study of language learning and language function.

REFERENCES

Baer, D. M. Behavior modification: you shouldn't. In E. A. Ramp and B. L. Hopkins (Eds.) *A New Direction for Education: Behavior Analysis,* Lawrence, University of Kansas Support and Development Center for Follow Through, 1971.

Baer, D. M. and Guess, D. Receptive training of adjectival inflections in mental retardates. *J. Appl. Behav. Anal.,* 1971, *4,* 129–139.

Baer, D. M. and Guess, D. Teaching productive noun suffixes to severely retarded children. *Amer. J. Ment. Defic.,* 1973, *77,* 498–505.

Bandura, A. Social learning through imitation. In M. R. Jones (Ed.), *Nebraska Symposium on Motivation.* Lincoln: University of Nebraska Press, 1962.

Bell, S. and Ainsworth, M. Infant crying and maternal responsiveness. *Child Develop.,* 1972, *43,* 1171–1190.

Berko, J. The child's learning of English morphology. *Word,* 1958, *14,* 150–177.

644   Staats

644   Staats

644   Staats

Bloom, L. *Language Development: Form and Function in Emerging Grammars.* Cambridge, Mass.: M.I.T. Press, 1970.

Brown, R. *A First Language: The Early Stages.* Cambridge, Mass.: Harvard University Press, 1973a.

Brown, R. Schizophrenia, language, and reality. *Amer. Psychol.,* 1973b, *28,* 395–403.

Brown, R., Cazden, C. B., and Bellugi, U. The child's grammar from 1 to 111. In J. P. Hill (Ed.) Minneapolis, Minnesota Symposium on Child Psychology: University of Minnesota Press, 1967, *2,* 28–73.

Brown, R. and Fraser, C. The acquisition of syntax. Paper delivered at the Second ONR-New York University Conference on Verbal Learning, June, 1961, Dobbs Ferry, N.Y. (Also published in C. N. Cofer and B. Musgrave (Eds.), *Verbal Behavior and Learning.* New York: McGraw-Hill, 1963.)

Chomsky, N. A review of B. F. Skinner's *Verbal Behavior. Language,* 1959, *35,* 26–58.

Cofer, C. N. and Foley, J. P. Mediated generalization and the interpretation of verbal behavior: I. Prolegomena. *Psychol. Rev.,* 1942, *49,* 513–540.

Cofer, C. N. and Musgrave, B. (Eds.) Verbal Behavior and Learning. New York: McGraw-Hill, 1963.

Drach, K. The language of the parent: A pilot study. In Working Paper 14: The structure of linguistic input to children. Language-Behavior Research Laboratory, University of California, Berkeley, 1969.

Ervin-Tripp, S. An overview of theories of grammatical development. In D. I. Slobin (Ed.), *The Ontogenesis of Grammar.* New York: Academic Press, 1971.

Fodor, J. A. How to learn to talk: Some simple ways. In F. Smith and G. A. Miller (Eds.), *The Genesis of Language: A Psycholinguistic Approach.* Cambridge, Mass.: M.I.T. Press, 1966.

Fodor, J. A. Could meaning be an r_m. *J. Verb. Learning Verb. Behav.,* 1965, *4,* 73– 1.

Gagne, R. *The Conditions of Learning.* New York: Holt, Rinehart and Winston, 1965.

Graham, J. T. and Graham, L. W. Language behavior of the mentally retarded: Syntactic characteristics. *Amer. J. Ment. Defic.,* 1971, *75,* 623–629.

Guess, D. A functional analysis of receptive language and productive speech: Acquisition of the plural morpheme. *J. Appl. Behav. Anal.,* 1969, *2,* 55–64.

Guess, D., Sailor, W., Rutherford, G., and Baer, D. M. An experimental analysis of linguistic development: The productive use of the plural morpheme. *J. Appl. Behav. Anal.,* 1968, *1,* 225–235.

Jensen, A. R. How much can we boost IQ and scholastic achievement? *Harvard Educ. Rev.,* 1969, *39,* 1–123.

Kobashigawa, B. Repetitions in a mother's speech to her child. In Working Paper 14: The structure of linguistic input to children. Language-Behavior Research Laboratory, University of California, Berkeley, 1969.

Lackner, J. R. A developmental study of language behavior in retarded children. *Neuropsychologia,* 1968, *6,* 301–320.

Maratsos, M. How to learn to talk: Some different ways. *Contemp. Psychol.,* 1972, *17,* 647–648.

McNeill, D. The capacity for the ontogenesis of grammar. In D. I. Slobin (Ed.), *The Ontogenesis of Grammar.* New York: Academic Press, 1971.

Mischel, W. Toward a cognitive social learning reconceptualization of personality. *Psychological Review,* 1973, *80,* 252–283.

Mowrer, O. H. The psychologist looks at language. *Amer. Psychol.,* 1954, *9,* 660–694.

Osgood, C. E. *Method and Theory in Experimental Psychology.* New York: Oxford University Press, 1953.

Osgood, C. E. and Sebeck, T. A. (Eds.) Psycholinguistics. *J. Abnorm. Soc. Psychol.,* Suppl., 1954, *49,* 1–203.

Pfuderer, C. Some suggestions for a syntactic characterization of baby talk style. In Working Paper 14: The structure of linguistic input to children. Language-Behavior Research Laboratory, University of California, Berkeley, 1969.

Piaget, J. How children form mathematical concepts. *Sci. Amer.,* 1953, *189,* 74–79.

Risley, T. R. and Wolf, M. M. Establishing functional speech in echolalic children. *Behav. Res. Ther.,* 1967, *5,* 73–88.

Sailor, W. Reinforcement and generalization of productive plural allomorphs in two retarded children. *J. Appl. Behav. Anal.,* 1971, *4,* 305–310.

Sailor, W. and Tamar, T. Stimulus factors in the training of prepositional usage in three autistic children. *J. Appl. Behav. Anal.,* 1972, *5,* 183–190.

Skinner, B. F. *Verbal Behavior.* New York: Appleton-Century-Crofts, 1957.

Slobin, D. I. (Ed.). *The Ontogenesis of Grammar.* New York: Academic Press, 1971.

Slobin, D. I. Cognitive prerequisites for the development of grammar. In C. A. Ferguson and S. I. Slobin (Eds.), *Studies of Child Language Development.* New York: Holt, Rinehart and Winston, 1973.

Staats, A. W. Learning theory and 'opposite speech.' *J. Abnorm. Soc. Psychol.,* 1957, *55,* 268–269.

Staats, A. W. Verbal habit-families, concepts, and the operant conditioning of word classes. *Psychol. Rev.,* 1961, *68,* 190–204.

Staats, A. W. (With contributions by Staats, C. K.) *Complex Human Behavior.* New York: Holt, Rinehart and Winston, 1963.

Staats, A. W. A case in and a strategy for the extension of learning principles to problems of human behavior. In A. W. Staats (Ed.), *Human Learning.* New York: Holt, Rinehart and Winston, 1964.

Staats, A. W. *Learning, Language, and Cognition.* New York: Holt, Rinehart and Winston, 1968a.

Staats, A. W. Social behaviorism and human motivation: Principles of the attitude-reinforcer-discriminative system. In A. G. Greenwald, T. C. Brock, and T. M. Ostrom (Eds.), *Psychological Foundations of Attitudes.* New York: Academic Press, 1968b.

Staats, A. W. A general apparatus for the investigation of complex learning in children. *Behav. Res. Ther.,* 1968c, *6,* 45–50.

Staats, A. W. Social behaviorism, human motivation, and the conditioning therapies. In B. A. Maher (Ed.), *Progress in Experimental Personality Research.* New York: Academic Press, 1970.

Staats, A. W. Linguistic-mentalistic theory versus an explanatory S-R learning theory of language development. In D. I. Slobin (Ed.), *The Ontogenesis of Grammar: A Theoretical Symposium.* New York: Academic Press, 1971a.

Staats, A. W. *Child Learning, Intelligence, and Personality.* New York: Harper and Row, 1971b.

Staats, A. W. Language behavior therapy: A derivative of social behaviorism. *Behav. Ther.*, 1972, *3*, 165–192.

Staats, A. W. Behavior analysis and token reinforcement in educational behavior modification and curriculum research. In C. E. Thoresen (Ed.), *Behavior Modification in Education.* Chicago: University of Chicago Press, 1973.

Staats, A. W. *Social Behaviorism.* Chicago: Dorsey Press, in press.

Staats, A. W. Brewer, B. A., and Gross, M. C. Learning and Cognitive Development: Representative Samples, Cumulative Hierarchial Learning, and Experimental Longitudinal Methods. Monograph of the Society for Res. in Child Dev., 1970, *8*, 35.

Staats, A. W. and Butterfield, W. H. Treatment of nonreading in a culturally deprived juvenile delinguent: An application of learning principles. *Child Develop.*, 1965, *4*, 925–942.

Staats, A. W., Finley, J. R., Minke, K. A., and Wolf, M. M. Reinforcement variables in the control of unit reading responses. *J. Exp. Anal. Behav.*, 1964, *7*, 139–149.

Staats, A. W., Gross, M. C., Guay, P. F., and Carlson, C. C. Personality and social systems and attitude-reinforcer-discriminative theory: Interest (attitude) formation, function, and measurement. *J. Personality Soc. Psychol.*, 1972, *26*, 251–261.

Staats, A. W., Minke, K. A., Finley, J. R., Wolf, M. M., and Brooks, L. O. A reinforcer system and experimental procedure for the laboratory study of reading acquisition. *Child Develop.*, 1964, *35*, 209–231.

Staats, A. W. and Staats, C. K. Attitudes established by classical conditioning. *J. Abnorm. Soc. Psychol.*, 1958, *57*, 37–40.

Staats, A. W., Staats, C. K., Schutz, R. E., and Wolf, M. M. The conditioning of textual responses using "extrinsic" reinforcers. *J. Exp. Anal. Behav.*, 1962, *5*, 33–40.

Staats, C. K. and Staats, A. W. Meaning established by classical conditioning. *J. Exp. Psychol.*, 1957, *54*, 74–80.

Terman, L. M. and Merrill, M. A. *Measuring Intelligence.* Boston: Houghton-Mifflin, 1937.

Watson, J. B. *Behaviorism.* Chicago: University of Chicago Press, 1930.

CHAPTER TWENTY-FIVE

SUMMARY

Richard L. Schiefelbusch

Bureau of Child Research, University of Kansas, Lawrence, Kansas 66045

Efforts to write a comprehensive summary of such a complex content are almost certain to be unsatisfactory unless the writer clearly states the purpose of the summary. There are many purposes for this work; therefore, several kinds of valid summaries could be written. For instance, Staats wrote an excellent analytic summary for readers interested in historical and theoretical perspectives of cognitive and behavioral approaches to language. Staats' analysis provides a basis for combining the interpreted theories of Piaget, Chomsky, and Skinner. This theoretical rapprochement may be one of the first attempts to develop a neopsycholinguistic position acceptable to both cognitive and behavioral theorists. In so doing, he also retained most tenets of learning theory.

In other parts of the book other orientations include Piagetian orientations (Morehead and Morehead), applied behavior analysis (Guess, Sailor, and Baer), developmental process (Menyuk and Miller and Yoder), generative grammar (Cromer), and cognitive functionalism (Premack and Premack, Schlesinger, Bloom). Other authors (Bricker and Bricker, Ruder and Smith) attempted to use an empiricism that combines most of the functions described by Staats. No author listed was bound by a single theory or operational strategy. Nevertheless, the views held did influence the way in which each selected and interpreted the data documenting the position developed. So it must be with this summary.

The position which guides this summary can be posed as a question: *What are the existing valid strategies which language specialists can use in developing effective intervention programs?* There are actually several other ways to pose this question. For instance, what are the strengths and weaknesses in language intervention research? What are the current successes in language intervention research? How can behavioral and cognitive systems be combined to form a viable strategy for training? These questions were all used by one or more of the authors in writing the chapters of the book.

For purposes of this summary, then, let it be said that I am interested in both the tactics and the results of important language research bearing upon training. Other issues, important as they may be, are secondary to this objective. Nevertheless, the perspectives of *language intervention* may provide excellent vantage points for examining early acquisition, receptive and productive processes, cognitive and linguistic systems, nonspeech communication, and other important areas of language. The intent is not to judge what is best to do or what any reader should eventually perceive but rather to examine important language perspectives relevant to language acquisition and intervention (of the language-retarded).

My procedure will be to summarize and interpret each section of the content and then to give an interpretative summary for the book as a whole. The intent will be to highlight these perspectives for both researchers and clinicians.

PERSPECTIVES ON INFANT SPEECH PERCEPTION

Research on infant speech perception is methodologically difficult. Butterfield and Cairns (this volume) have stated,

> The purpose of most infant researchers is to discover how infants divide and apprehend their world. This purpose recognizes that infants may perceive different dimensions than adults. Unless the infant researcher is careful, the use of adults to judge his stimuli may strangely defeat the basic purpose of his perceptual research on infants by delimiting inappropriately the stimuli he presents to children.

The same gap in adult and infant perceptions may also affect the validity of interpretations of infant responses. These and other experimental problems might be less formidable if infant researchers were to adopt individual subject designs and to see the same infant more than once. We need infant experiments designed to assess the impact of environmental interventions on infant perceptions. Such data may tell us whether speech discrimination training in infancy can be an effective part of a language intervention program for high risk infants. However, the issue of early perceptual training seems to depend upon a set of logical assumptions, each of which is largely unsubstantiated.

First is the assumption that there may be significant individual differences in speech perception among infants. Unfortunately, this assumption has not been substantiated. It is questionable whether or not these experiments were testing speech perception. Research data are needed to show the differences and the possible developmental mechanisms of speech perception. Even more critical to early intervention strategies is evidence that speech perception can be trained. Finally, there is the assumption, also unsupported, that perception (if trained) influences the acquisition of language.

The foregoing statements emphasize the research problems that still exist. Possibly, too, the statements may serve as a guide to further research. They also imply that the area of infant speech perception is potentially an important area for early intervention. The available data suggest that the infant can differentially process speech signals during early infancy. There is less evidence that nonspeech stimuli are processed in the same definitive way. What does the infant actually process? What features can be influenced by environmental stimulation? What beneficial effects can be achieved for the high risk infants through intervention? These and other questions must be answered through research before the potential of early infant stimulation can be clearly determined.

EARLY DEVELOPMENT OF CONCEPTS

In summarizing Section II, Bowerman stressed the shift from "formally defined syntactic categories and relationships" to an emphasis upon the "primacy of cognitive growth." This emphasis is indeed prominent in the Clark, Schlesinger, and Morehead and Morehead papers. Bowerman further suggested that this recent emphasis is due in large measure to the "discovery" of Piaget by developmental psycholinguists. A careful reading of Schlesinger's "Relational Concepts Underlying Language" together with Bowerman's summarization probably offers the best explanation for the recent emphasis upon cognitive and linguistic relationships.

In Schlesinger's view the relational concepts underlying child speech are semantic in nature and reflect the way the child sees the world. The child learns grammar by observing how the adult expresses these relations in speech. The child is able to perceive the direct relations between the adult forms and the semantic categories he (the child) perceives in his environment. Schlesinger and Bowerman agree that the child's language is based upon semantic concepts which he learns to express verbally. In the course of learning (using) language, he comes to acquire the abstract syntactic relational concepts. However, in Schlesinger's view the syntactic concepts (rules) do not replace the semantic concepts. The latter continue as a larger and more varied set of symbolic relations which the syntactic relations reflect, in part, and may also influence. The important point for this summary, however, is that language cannot be acquired beyond the bases of learned semantic relations. Also there may be a lag, perhaps serious in some instances, in learning and using the syntactic forms necessary for productive speech. Bowerman's summary speculation is that:

> . . . some children experience problems with language not because they
> lack the requisite underlying cognitive concepts which language encodes,
> but because they are unable to perform the feats of abstraction necessary
> to arrive at an understanding of purely formal linguistic relationships. . . .

Schlesinger offered three reasons why linguistic development may lag behind cognitive development: 1) complexity of the linguistic expression, 2) immaturity of communicative needs, and 3) saliency. These issues may serve as strategy points for language intervention procedures. It is interesting to speculate from these issues in examining the intervention strategies proposed in Sections V, VI, and VII. Apparently, the first issue bears upon the overload which the complex demands produce for some children. However, the second and third issues are amenable to environmental control.

DEVELOPMENT OF RECEPTIVE LANGUAGE

Semantic functions are also important in the early development of receptive language (Section III). However, the evidence for this assumption is largely inferential. Both Menyuk and Cromer spoke to this issue, and Spradlin confirmed this point in his summary comment. However, Bloom may have offered the clearest view of the difficulty observers have in studying receptive language. "A major problem in evaluating comprehension is that children's responses are multidetermined—what the child does depends on many things in addition to what he hears."

The concepts held by the child may be especially difficult to infer when the child is largely deficient in productive speech. The "disposition" (Premack and Premack's term), however, may be extremely important in planning a training program. Unless some knowledge about receptive language can be gained, there may be difficulty in planning for the appropriate expressive repertoires to be taught. Premack and Premack provided a rationale and a tactic for mapping the conceptual bases for language functions and forms. Bricker and Bricker and Miller and Yoder also are designing procedures for bridging the semantic and the linguistic functions.

The suggestions presented in Section III are more provocative than substantial. For instance, Menyuk speculated that children with language problems spend exceptionally long periods of time at specific stages of semantic, syntactic, and phonological development. She also speculated that the periods of arrest are due to the child's incomplete reorganization of linguistic data. Menyuk concluded that effective intervention programs require an understanding of the linguistic problems involved in reorganization and the cognitive organization and the environmental demands upon which this reorganization depends.

This last statement is indeed difficult to analyze. Nevertheless, it could be one of the first attempts to emphasize this significant issue. The first part of Menyuk's statement is similar to Bowerman's observation that the child may have difficulty mapping his semantic information onto syntactic forms. The *environmental designs* call for some delineations of environmental issues. Possibly a functional analysis of behavior design (antecedent and subsequent events) would serve the purpose. Viewed in this light, Menyuk is recommending that the "reorganization" issue requires a utilization of linguistic, conceptual, and behavioral systems. If so, Menyuk is highlighting the complexity of the problem of language delay, and, further, she is suggesting the areas that researchers should stress in designing intervention tactics. Clearly, these tactics must involve a combination of the linguistic, cognitive, and behavioral domains. Spradlin also suggested that the requirements call for collaborative research among language experts and behavioral scientists.

EXPRESSIVE AND RECEPTIVE LANGUAGE

In summarizing the developmental relationship between receptive and expressive language, Section IV, Chapman made no reference to intervention strategies or procedures. The papers by Ingram and Bloom also did not point up the intervention issues. Nevertheless, Section IV may be one of the most productive sections of the book. Ingram may have highlighted an especially important issue in suggesting that children with language disorders often have a lag in production (as compared with comprehension). He also recommended that this is a potential area for fruitful research. Bloom's chapter suggested a special issue on which meaningful research might be undertaken.

The memory load for saying a sentence is presumably greater than for understanding, inasmuch as the individual needs to recall the necessary words and their connections to say them, but these linguistic facts are immediately available to him when he hears them spoken by someone else. The child can experience a sentence as more or less independent of its parts, but saying sentences involves bringing together the elements to form a whole. In recognizing a word or a sentence, a child relates what he hears to existing perceptual schemas, but saying the word or sentence involves reconstructing an intervening representation in the form of a "symbolic image."

The two primary points to be derived from this interpretation are that speaking involves more complex processes than does the understanding of spoken forms and that the latter provides a variety of valuable language experience. He "relates what he hears to existing perceptual schemas."

It is meaningful in this context to report on an article by Winitz (1973). He posited that "in speaking, retrieval from storage is more complex than in comprehension; speech production appears to be a recall function, whereas speech comprehension implies a recognition function." Taking his strategy from observed mothers who "are [initially] happy that their children understand simple instructions and commands . . ." Winitz has devised a language teaching program based entirely upon comprehension functions. He introduced a series of graduated tasks which enable the learner to acquire knowledge of the language. He utilized strategies developed in teaching a second language (German). He then generalized the strategy to the task of teaching language forms to small children. The technique is to teach the child to comprehend grammatical structures prior to speaking grammatical forms.

The technique stimulates the child to learn the conceptual bases of language and to use the spoken forms in his own good time. Small children taught the comprehension sequences engage in "rehearsal" activities of a covert nature. They rehearse what they hear. Perhaps in this way they work through integration functions alluded to by Menyuk which enable the child to move ahead to acquire new functions.

The amount of available research bearing upon the utility of a "nonspeaking" language teaching program is extremely minimal. However, we agree with Winitz (1973) that "its application to disordered language deserves systematic exploration." The research recommended by Winitz might, in fact, be congruent with that recommended by Chapman (this volume): ". . . the relation of the child's cognitive and linguistic attainments to speaking and understanding in the natural language learning situation."

Winitz's assumption that comprehension training should precede production is supported by data currently available in research by Ruder *et al.*, 1974. Ruder (personal communication) found that children in the 1st and 2nd grades who are taught Spanish as a second language reach criterion more rapidly and more probably when they receive preliminary comprehension training than when imitation training and/or speech production training accompanies or precedes comprehension training. For some children imitation training after comprehension training was necessary for the child to reach criterion satisfactorily. Ruder also noted the tendency for rehearsal after training in perception tasks as reported by Winitz. Some children do not rehearse following comprehension training. Additional research is required for a full understanding of these phenomena.

NONSPEECH COMMUNICATION

Section V, Nonspeech Communication, evoked a number of questions about the utility of signs, plastic languages, and other modes of nonstandard speech. Two primary questions were raised about manual languages as described by Moores. First, is the symbolic content expressed in manual systems representative of a true language? The answer apparently is yes, and further, it may be a language that has value to groups of people other than the deaf. The primary issue may be that for many handicapped persons who cannot make effective use of their speech apparatus or who do not find the complex, vocal-phonological system of speech to be manageable, manual systems may be highly useful. The work of Berger (1972), Carrier (1973), and Hollis and Carrier (1973) adds emphasis to this point.

A second question relates to the communication value of nonspeech languages. For instance, do manual systems serve as satisfactory alternatives to speech and/or as supplements to it? Again, the answer seems to be yes. The rationale for this position, however, has not been universally accepted. A range of additional research is needed to delineate the utility of nonspeech communication practices. Nonspeech systems need to be studied both as language systems in their own right and in combination with speech-language systems. The apparent and predicted increase in the popularity of manual systems with the severely language-handicapped adds further urgency to the researchable issues raised by Moores and the discussion summarized by Dever.

Premack and Premack's novel language system can also be used to support the utility of a nonspeech system. However, the intervention issues raised by the Premacks are substantially different from those highlighted by Moores. The Premacks are attempting to develop a functional analysis of language. In this work they may be accomplishing several important tasks.

1. They are mapping the "concepts," or "dispositions" which chimps (and now echolalic children) have, as indicated by their behavior. The issue of translating or inferring these functional indicators from the behavior of chimps is a subtle, difficult job as they stressed at the conference. The importance of this work is that the functions can then be used to plan the operations used in instruction. Otherwise no one could determine what kind of a symbolic system to try to teach to chimps.

2. Both Moores and the Premacks demonstrated that language can be designed and taught apart from phonology and auditory processes. In other words, the basic units of language can be visual symbols or plastic words. The perceptions to be learned for symbolic functioning can be specific to the visual and tactual modalities. Then, too, the learner may have a less complex set of tasks to master on the way to developing a functional language system.

3. They are devising a language teaching system for non-language users. Beyond the level of the tangible, the plastic system could be other stages leading to a more complete, flexible system. Even then, however, certain severely limited children might desirably develop a "plastic language" as a means of developing symbolic behavior prior to acquiring a more complete language. Perhaps the important point might be that the initial overload of complex phonological receptive-motor processes can be initially set aside.

4. Perhaps most importantly, the Premacks are developing, from a behavioral base, a means for bridging to semantic or conceptual information. This makes their work relevant to the work of Bloom, Schlesinger, and others who are describing a semantic basis for the development of syntax. It is clear that Premack and Premack and Bloom are studying the same agent-action-object relations and thus are using the concrete environment in studying functional language. Language intervention programs then can be adapted from the model. For instance, Carrier is designing a program for severely retarded children using plastic strings similar to the Premacks'. The ultimate value of these interventions is not discernible at this time. However, in light of current data there is a strong possibility that plastic languages will join manual languages to form major strategies in language teaching programs for the severely retarded.

EARLY INTERVENTION

Several important issues emerge from the analysis of early intervention (Section VI). Five of the most prominent are featured in this summary: 1) Early intervention tactics should be based upon what is known about early acquisition. 2) Receptive speech training should precede early speech production training. 3) Language training, both receptive and expressive forms, should be based upon determined cognitive functions. 4) The process of language training is essentially a task of operationally mapping symbolic functions on to a formal language system (usually one with a formalized syntax and phonology). 5) Parents and other adults can be instructed to provide important extensions of language training.

Acquisition and Intervention

There seems to be a consensus that language acquisition research has a prominent place in guiding intervention strategies for small children. The strong implication is that the language processes and functions and the environmental stimuli that enable a child to acquire a language in the natural environment should be replicated in an intervention program. The "natural" conditions and the acquisition sequences must be understood, of course, before they can be replicated. The replication must include the multiple functions described by Bloom, Bricker and Bricker, Horton, Miller and Yoder, Morehead and Morehead, Schlesinger, and others.

Each tends to explain the early childhood issues in a somewhat different way. Consequently, in addition to data from which to plan, the intervention specialist must determine a strategy for interpreting the information and for turning the interrelations into useful strategies. Thus, Bricker and Bricker made use of issues explained by Morehead and Morehead (cognitive), Bloom (semantic functions), and Miller and Yoder (developmental). These interpretations were combined with their own research strategies which involve the mapping of environmental variables which alter the behavior of infants and preschoolers. In addition they have used normal preschool peers and parents as functional demonstrators and monitors for imitation training and support. The agents, actions, and objects (all important stimuli) are available features of a natural (acquisition) environment. Thus, the early intervention program utilizes extensive information about how the child learns to talk, the environmental conditions (including the behaviors of mothers and peers), and the language sequences that characterize the child's development.

Receptive and Expressive Speech Training

In the Bricker and Bricker system, receptive language functions precede expressive functions in teaching new new language forms. However, they do not use an extended receptive strategy covering many forms before introducing the expressive speech training. Also they delay the introduction of speech imitation until receptive speech training is under way. One problem in planning receptive training is the task of determining the small child's receptive speech level. In addition to the semantic features of the language *per se,* the child also has a variety of situational and contextual cues to help him determine the indicated meaning. Interestingly, however, these same dimensional cues that make accurate testing difficult also make receptive speech training rich and stimulating for the child. It is the task of the clinician-teacher to create this dimensional situation in the training setting. A flat, one-dimensional training arrangement involving stiff, unfamiliar contexts is not likely to be very stimulating for the small child. This issue, of course, applies to all forms of language instruction, including the more advanced forms of productive speech.

Language Training Based upon Cognitive Functions

The mapping of functions as described by the Premacks can also be applied to the determination of dispositions of small children. For instance, a question might be: What functions of available, familiar objects does the child understand? What conceptual actions does he perform? What communication behaviors does he display with familiar adults and familiar peers? The concepts displayed are likely to represent a basis for language acquisition, and the "training" that is most effective might be the reciprocal use of naming and labeling to give a shared symbolic reference to familiar agents, actions, and objects. The systematic extensions of semantic functions and syntactic forms enable the child and his teacher to map out further shared language features. The congruence of the physical stimuli, the semantic functions, and finally the language forms is apparent to the observers of early language acquisition and intervention.

Nevertheless, the demanding features of the intervention program may be that the natural environment, whether optimal or not, may not stimulate certain children to acquire functional language. For them, further research leading to a range of additional strategies and arrangements are likely to be required.

The Mapping of Semantic Functions to a Formal Language System

Morehead and Morehead presented a description of the sensorimotor period of early development. They explained that a significant indication that the child is ready to learn formal language is his propensity to respond to a word not just as part of the action (in play) but as an evocator of action (representation). At this point the child is able to respond to reference forms and relational syntax.

Perhaps it is possible to utilize the extensive observations that are represented by the Piagetian system of cognitive stages to map out a prelanguage and a language system. This essentially is the strategy adopted by Bricker and Bricker. The child's play behavior is used to indicate the symbolic functions that he can respond to and then the language functions that he can perform. In each case the language training is tuned to the natural and usually familiar functions performed by the child.

Perhaps Miller and Yoder have specified the key tactics: select a single frequently occurring experience; demonstrate a particular semantic relation; pair with the appropriate lexical marker; and after the child demonstrates mastery, move to multiple experiences expressing the same function. The first expansions of single word utterances should be of relational functions previously expressed. They quoted Slobin (1970), "New forms first express old functions. New functions are first expressed by old forms."

Parents as Language Trainers

Horton's program with parents of preschool deaf children is a massive demonstration of the effectiveness of parent training. Simple but direct instructions bearing upon active verbal participation by both parents and frequent reinforcement for the verbal productivity of the child apparently lead to accelerating verbal development. The program is further enhanced by parental sensitivity to the child's active behavior and to his interest in the semantic content of the experience. The parents also should use frequent redundancy in their utterances.

Turton summarized the process: ". . . the vocal and verbal productions of the child must be reinforced by the parents, corrected through feedback, and expanded in terms of lexical, semantic, and syntactic structures. The parents must . . . enhance the use of that language which has been acquired and shape those language skills which are being acquired."

LANGUAGE INTERVENTION FOR THE RETARDED

Each of the chapters in Section VII, Language Intervention for the Mentally Retarded, described complex, comprehensive strategies for language training. Each chapter made a special contribution to our general understanding of the intervention process. An important key to each contribution is included in the title. Miller and Yoder presented an *ontogenetic teaching strategy;* Guess, Sailor, and Baer undertook *to teach language;* and Ruder and Smith provided *issues* in language training. Consequently, one might summarize by pointing out that the first is a comprehensive design for accelerating language learning through a series of developmental sequences. The second is a comprehensive behavioral teaching design applied to retardates for whom normal language functioning has long since become improbable. The third is a comprehensive review of language intervention issues. Each chapter, however, accomplishes far more than covering these indicated issues and functions. A brief summary analysis should highlight the multiple contributions of each.

Miller and Yoder attempted to synthesize psycholinguistic and behavioral models. They used the psycholinguistic information to determine the content of instruction and the behavioral model to provide the strategy for teaching. The content is assumed to be semantic concepts which are related directly to the objects and events around the child. The child gradually learns to mark linguistically those objects and events he perceives conceptually. Thus the child learns increasingly how to map aspects of his experience and to use syntactic forms in functional contexts. (Ruder and Smith also discussed this point of view in great detail, crediting the Premacks, Bloom, Schlesinger, and others for the underpinnings of the approach they have developed.) Miller and Yoder have an impressive design for this mapping process and for maintaining the process through a sequence of environmentally related functions. They have made a major contribution to clinical intervention by designing the sequences and the program format. Very likely their strategies are applicable, as they claim, to all children with significant lags in language development. They do not intend for the child to conform to the program. Rather they intend that their strategies should be adapted to each child.

Guess, Sailor, and Baer pointed out that behavioral strategies for teaching language have moved from "extremely rudimentary levels" to complex and comprehensive language skills. In this relatively short but significant movement the current program designed by these authors is strategically the most comprehensive. Their program, however, does not follow the developmental format described by Miller and Yoder. Instead, they place even greater stress upon the teaching of functional language skills and extending and generalizing these skills. Thus, their greatest contribution may be in the technology of language instruction and in the functional analysis of the full range of issues involved.

Ruder and Smith also made a comprehensive attempt to overview the issues of language intervention. They seemed to agree with Premack and Premack that language maps a conceptual base. They analyzed the implications of this point for language training and have designed a comprehensive approach to research on utilization.

They also reported that a potentially significant contribution emerges from their work. They identified it as componential content (CC) analysis. Literally, they are studying the language content to clarify which linguistic behaviors are independent and which are interdependent. "The value of CC analysis is that it has the potential to provide a data-based means of determining both the degree and direction of interdependence among to-be-trained linguistic behaviors." The goal, of course, is to achieve efficiency and economy in language training data from a number of studies in which their methodological issues are researched. Several substantiated issues emerge from these data:

1. Acquisition of certain aspects of language is facilitated by, if not dependent upon, a prior level of development (this seems to support a developmental point of view).

2. The utilization of intermediate steps in training programs which build upon previously acquired forms has the distinct advantage of simplifying the learning task for the child (this seems to support the issue that training sequences should be programmed).
3. Serial training does not seem to facilitate language learning as readily as does concurrent training. This issue is illustrative of a larger problem of reducing linguistic behaviors to their salient features or components.
4. Modeling and expansion techniques (to the next level of training) seem to be useful techniques for language training.

A few features of agreement and several points of divergence may be pointed out for the three programs. Each program utilizes a behavioral management procedure with which to record and use explicit data as a method of maintaining and refining the training program. Guess, Sailor, and Baer described a comprehensive behavioral technology. All programs use a psycholinguistic approach to language structures and functions. Ruder and Smith made the most comprehensive effort to research issues of linguistic relevance. Both Miller and Yoder and Ruder and Smith used a conceptual basis for language planning and implementation. Both Guess, Sailor, and Baer and Miller and Yoder have evolved strategies for teaching language that will carry over to a range of communication contexts.

Ruder and Smith seemed to say, "Train the language events but seek the interdependency of events so that the language system can be learned with economy and functional permanence." Guess, Sailor, and Baer urged that "all essential language content cannot be taught unit by unit. The essential strategy, therefore, should be to teach the child how to acquire a functional language. The key features can be devised from a functional analysis of behavior approach to systematic language usage." The Miller and Yoder program is the most eclectic, but the range of reference points in their functional communication system includes: 1) an emphasis upon normal developmental sequence; 2) normal environmental interactions; 3) linguistic and nonlinguistic experiences; 4) a determination of a realistic set of communication exit behaviors; and 5) a unified, systematic approach to teaching. Their statement therefore is "Plan a program of sequential, developmental training steps leading to functional communication skills which are as complete and as efficient as the child's environment and his development will allow."

A FINAL SUMMARY

A series of summarizing statements about the content of this book may provide a useful afterword. Each statement has many antecedents in the content. Hopefully, each statement will predict a range of subsequent events of major proportions. Most of the statements, at this time, however, lack the conclusiveness that can only be developed by extensive research.

1. The field of language research, including research on acquisition and intervention, has bridged the cognitive and behavioral domains. The functional effect of this emerging synthesis is a more comprehensive paradigm.

2. As yet, there is no experimentally validated basis for training infant speech perceptions during the first weeks of life. However, this is assumed to be an especially promising area for research.

3. Language-delayed children may have linguistic development that lags significantly behind cognitive development. The implications of this lag for training purposes have only been preliminarily assessed.

4. Early intervention tactics should be based upon what is known about early acquisition. This recommendation covers early conceptual development, semantic precursors to formal syntax, and, finally, the emergence of receptive and productive language.

5. Receptive speech training should precede early speech production training. The receptive processes are simpler to acquire, more varied in content, and lead to productive rehearsal strategies which may be antecedent to spoken language.

6. Nonspeech systems may be used productively for deaf-retarded and for some severely retarded invididuals who have great difficulty with audible phonological systems.

7. Language training, both receptive and expressive forms, should be based upon determined cognitive functions. (Language cannot be acquired beyond the bases of learned semantic functions.)

8. The process of language training is essentially a task of operationally mapping symbolic functions onto a formal language system.

9. An important feature of language training is teaching the child how to extend his language functions and how to use language in ever widening contexts.

10. An important terminal objective in language training is efficient communication to the full extent of the acquired language.

Language acquisition, either in a normal environment or under the aegis of training, is limited to the extent of the child's conceptual development. However, through language (symbolic) experiences, conceptual attainments are probably increased. Thus, experience, language systems, and cognitive functions seem to fuse in a productive complex of observable and inferred events. A host of observers, experimenters, and managers are slowly mapping a process that may eventually help most, if not all, children to experience the joys of communicated feelings, thoughts, and impressions. Each step in this direction is indeed a step for mankind.

REFERENCES

Berger, S. L. A clinical program for developing multi model language responses in atypical children. In J. E. McLean, D. E. Yoder, and R. L. Schiefelbusch (Eds.), *Language Intervention with the Mentally Retarded.* Baltimore: University Park Press, 1972.

Carrier, J. K., Jr. Application of functional analysis and non-speech response mode to teaching language. Report 7, Kansas Center for Research in Mental Retardation and Human Development, Parsons, 1973.

Hollis, J. H. and Carrier, J. K., Jr. Prosthesis of communication deficiencies: Implications for training the retarded and deaf. Working Paper 298, Parsons Research Center, Parsons State Hospital and Training Center, Parsons, Kans., July, 1973.

Ruder, K., Smith M., and Hermann, P. Effects of verbal imitation and comprehension training on verbal production of lexical items. In L. V. McReynolds (Ed.) Developing Systematic Procedures for Training Children's Language. American Speech and Hearing Association Monograph, #18, Danville, Ill.: Interstate Press, 1974.

Slobin, D. I. Suggested universals in the ontogenesis of grammar. Working Paper 32, Language-Behavior Research Laboratory, Berkeley, April, 1970.

Winitz, H. Problem solving and the delaying of speech as strategies in the teaching of language. *ASHA* 1973, *15,* 583–586.

Index